CRC Handbook of Endocrinology

Editors

George H. Gass, Ph.D.
Chairman, Department of Basic Sciences
Oklahoma College of Osteopathic Medicine and Surgery
Tulsa, Oklahoma

and

Harold M. Kaplan, Ph.D.
Visiting Professor, Physiology Department
Acting Director, Vivarium
Southern Illinois University School of Medicine
Carbondale, Illinois

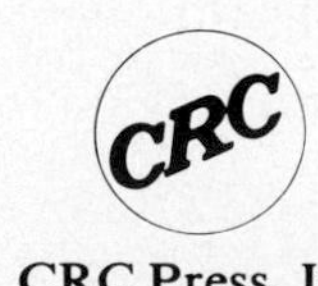

CRC Press, Inc.
Boca Raton, Florida

Library of Congress Cataloging in Publication Data

Main entry under title:

Handbook of endocrinology.

Bibliography: p.
Includes index.
1. Endocrinology—Handbooks, manuals, etc.
I. Gass, George H. II. Kaplan, Harold Morris,
1908- . [DNLM: 1. Endocrine glands—
Physiology. 2. Hormones—Physiology. WK 102
H236]
QP187.H18 612'.4 81-18079
ISBN 0-8493-3235-4 AACR2

This book represents information obtained from authentic and highly regarded sources. Reprinted material is quoted with permission, and sources are indicated. A wide variety of references are listed. Every reasonable effort has been made to give reliable data and information, but the author and the publisher cannot assume responsibility for the validity of all materials or for the consequences of their use.

Direct all inquiries to CRC Press, Inc., 2000 Corporate Blvd., N.W., Boca Raton, Florida, 33431.

International Standard Book Number 0-8493-3235-4

Library of Congress Card Number 81-18079
Printed in the United States

PREFACE

Endocrine function is reviewed in 17 topic-oriented chapters in this multi-authored handbook, emphasis being placed on the basic science approach. Each chapter includes a selected survey of the existing vast experimental literature.

The handbook was developed as a general reference source for the academic endocrinologist, teacher and researcher, and graduate and undergraduate student. It provides a source of reference for all persons interested in endocrinology and is addressed to a broad audience. The medical aspects of endocrinology, including symptoms, clinical assays, diagnosis and treatment regimens of specific diseases, are available elsewhere in many excellent texts.

Since the ultimate interest of many readers may lie in endocrine pathology, this text is directed toward developing the bases that are needed to understand endocrine action and control. The descriptions thus include anatomic and histologic data as well as physiologic and biochemical studies and interpretations. Since a unitary feature of the endocrine system is the regulation of bodily processes, the control mechanisms are emphasized. The descriptions emphasize the close alliance of the endocrine and nervous systems in homeostasis, particularly the central nature of neuroendocrine control through the hypothalamus via the pituitary to the target cells.

Overall, the reader will have access to a condensed but comprehensive survey of the chemical nature of hormones, their synthesis, secretion and transport, their actions and mechanisms of action, and their degradation and excretion, in mammals including man.

THE EDITORS

Dr. George H. Gass is presently Chairman, Department of Basic Sciences, of the Oklahoma College of Osteopathic Medicine and Surgery in Tulsa, Oklahoma. Previously he held the position of Director of the Endocrinologic Pharmacology Research Laboratory at Southern Illinois University for 18 years, during which time he was also a professor of Physiology and a professor of Medicine. He has had a very diverse career, spanning industry (Lederle Laboratories), government (Food and Drug Administration), and in university and college higher education surroundings.

Dr. Gass was awarded his doctorate at Ohio State University in 1955. His research was on the effects of androgens and their interrelationships with endocrine organs. Following graduation from Ohio State University, Dr. Gass served in the Endocrine Branch of the Food and Drug Administration in Washington, D.C. where he performed biological assay procedures, biostatistics, and endocrine research for four years before leaving to enter higher education. Dr. Gass' best known work in the Food and Drug Administration was in the co-development of the uterine weight method for estrogen assay and detection. Dr. Gass assumed his duties at Southern Illinois University, Department of Physiology, in the fall of 1959 and almost immediately upon arrival set up the Endocrinologic Pharmacology Research Laboratory. A number of students obtained their research experience under Dr. Gass in the Endocrinologic Pharmacology Research Laboratory where it was first discovered that a quantitative measure of chemical carcinogen (diethylstilbestrol)—dose response relationship of mammary tumors existed. This work has become a classic, and although published in 1964, has just recently been repeated by the National Center for Toxicological Research with Dr. Gass as a consultant.

Dr. Gass, while a member of the staff at Southern Illinois University, received a large number of honors and served on numerous occasions as a consultant for government and industry. Dr. Gass is a Fellow of the American Association for the Advancement of Science, an Alexander Van Humbolt Fellow, and a Fulbright alumnus.

He was requested to serve as a consultant for the National Center of Toxicology, Food and Drug Administration, to help determine the carcinogenicity and estrogenecity of female sex hormones, both naturally occurring and synthetic. During his 18 years at Southern Illinois University he taught physiology and pharmacology continuously. His present position as Chairman, Department of Basic Sciences, at the Oklahoma College of Osteopathic Medicine and Surgery allows him to come into intimate contact with the basic scientists in the college including those in the disciplines of human anatomy, histology, pharmacology, physiology, behavior, and biochemistry.

Dr. Harold M. Kaplan has had broad experience in many facets of biologic and medical sciences. His publications, over 200 in number, range through a diverse series of research disciplines, spanning a period of 45 years. He is an author of seven textbooks in anatomy and physiology.

Dr. Kaplan completed his doctorate at Harvard University in 1933, his research then centering on the biochemistry of lipids. After one subsequent year, on the Harvard staff, he entered teaching as a career, working successively in several universities. In his early activities he chaired the Departments of Physiology at the Middlesex Medical School, at the Middlesex Veterinary School, and then at Brandeis University. He taught at the University of Massachusetts, and then went to Southern Illinois University where he chaired the Department of Physiology for 22 years. He is currently Visiting Professor of Physiology at the Southern Illinois University School of Medicine.

Dr. Kaplan has served in a large number of capacities on a national scale, including the presidency of the American Association of Laboratory Animal Science, and also of the Illinois State Academy of Science. He was chairman of the Editorial Board of Laboratory Animal Science and is currently an associate editor of that journal. He serves on the Board of Directors of the Illinois Society for Medical Research and was on the Board of the Illinois State Academy of Science. He was for several years on the Advisory Council of the Institute of Laboratory Animal Resources. He has taught human physiology continuously since 1935.

CONTRIBUTORS

William T. Allaben, Ph.D.
Research Toxicologist
Food and Drug Administration
National Center for
Toxicological Research
Jefferson, Arkansas

Joachim Braun
Doctor of Veterinary Medicine
Universitae Muenchen
West Germany

Ulrich Braun
Doctor of Veterinary Medicine
Universitae Muenchen
West Germany

George Brenner, Ph.D.
Associate Professor of Pharmacology
Oklahoma College of Osteopathic
Medicine and Surgery
Tulsa, Oklahoma

Gerburg Buck
Doctor of Veterinary Medicine
Universitae Muenchen
West Germany

V. Chandrashekar, Ph.D.
Visiting Assistant Professor
Department of Zoology
Southern Illinois University
Carbondale, Illinois

Warren E. Finn, Ph.D.
Associate Professor of Physiology
Oklahoma College of Osteopathic
Medicine and Surgery
Tulsa, Oklahoma

Lloyd J. Forman
Assistant Professor of Medicine
University of Medicine
and Dentistry of New Jersey
School of Osteopathic Medicine
Camden, New Jersey

George H. Gass, Ph.D.
Chairman
Department of Basic Science
Oklahoma College of Osteopathic
Medicine and Surgery
Tulsa, Oklahoma

Lindsey Grandison, Ph.D.
Assistant Professor of Physiology
and Biophysics
Rutgers Medical School
University of Medicine and
Dentistry of New Jersey
Piscataway, New Jersey

Charles Hodson
Assistant Professor
Department of Obstetrics and
Gynecology
East Carolina University
School of Medicine
Greenville, North Carolina

J. G. Hurst
Associate Professor of Physiology
Department of Physiological Sciences
Oklahoma State University
Stillwater, Oklahoma

Harold M. Kaplan, Ph.D.
Visiting Professor, School of Medicine
Acting Director of the Vivarium
Southern Illinois University
Carbondale, Illinois

Werner Leidl
Professor of Veterinary Medicine
Vorstand — Gynaekologische und
Ambulatoriche Tierklinik
Universitae Muenchen
West Germany

Joseph Meites, Ph.D.
Professor of Physiology
Neuroendocrine Research Laboratory
Michigan State University
East Lansing, Michigan

Nobuhiro Miki, M.D.
Assistant Professor
Department of Internal Medicine
Division of Endocrinology
Tokyo Women's Medical College
Tokyo, Japan

Eldon L. Nelson, Jr. Ph.D.
Associate Professor of Physiology
Oklahoma College of Osteopathic Medicine and Surgery
Tulsa, Oklahoma

John J. Peluso, Ph.D.
Associate Professor of Biology
Loyola University of Chicago
Chicago, Illinois

James W. Simpkins, Ph.D.
Assistant Professor
Department of Pharmaceutical Biology
College of Pharmacy
University of Florida
Gainesville, Florida

William E. Sonntag, Ph.D.
Assistant Professor of Physiology
Neuroendocrine Research Laboratory
Department of Physiology
Michigan State University
East Lansing, Michigan

Richard W. Steger
Assistant Professor
Department of Obstetrics and Gynecology
The University of Texas
Health Science Center
San Antonio, Texas

Jimmie L. Valentine, Ph.D.
Associate Professor of Pharmacology
Department of Pharmacology
Oral Roberts University
School of Medicine
Tulsa, Oklahoma

William M. Yau, Ph.D.
Associate Professor
Department of Medical Physiology and Pharmacology
School of Medicine
Southern Illinois University
Carbondale, Illinois

ADVISORY BOARD

TABLE OF CONTENTS

HYPOTHALAMIC HORMONES AND OTHER FACTORS

Eldon L. Nelson, Jr.

HISTORICAL OVERVIEW

Only since 1955 have we formally entertained the concept that the pituitary, once recognized as the "master gland," is itself precisely controlled by regulatory agents secreted by the hypothalamus.[1,2] These hypothalamic substances controlling pituitary hormone secretion are termed "hypophysiotropic agents." For ten years there was a vigorous search for such substances, but the isolation, purification, and identification of these "hormones" ended without success. In 1965, a major effort was initiated with concurrent studies in the separate laboratories of Schally and Guillemin[3,4,5] to reinforce the then dying hypothesis of hypothalamic hormonal regulators of anterior pituitary function. They reprocessed tons of porcine and ovine brain extracts derived from previous vain attempts that had been performed to isolate corticotropin releasing factor, CRF. Their new, and quite possibly final, search was for a hormone proposed to regulate the pituitary secretion of thyroid stimulating hormone (TSH). By 1969, thyrotropin releasing hormone (TRH) was isolated, purified, and its chemical structure identified as a tripeptide (pyroGlu-His-pro-NH_2). TRH was the first hypophysiotropic hormone proven to be present in the hypothalamus. Within three years, the second hypothalamic hypophysiotropic hormone, luteinizing hormone releasing hormone (LHRH), was isolated, purified and it's decapeptide structure defined. Since then, growth hormone release-inhibitng hormone (somatostatin) has been characterized and significant progress has been made to identify other hypothalamic factors. For their creativity and perseverance, both Schally and Guillemin received the Nobel Prize in 1977. The exciting history of events of their search for the hypothalamic hypophysiotropic agents is documented in a series of articles in *Science*.[3-5]

During the subsequent years, the continuing search to understand the regulatory influence of the hypothalamus has revealed numerous other factors yet to be chemically elucidated (Table 1). It is recognized that these peptidergic agents may have important effects far beyond the regulation of pituitary endocrine secretion.[6-8] Techniques for localization and isolation of the releasing agents and other factors are described in more detail elsewhere.[7,10] Because of numerous technical difficulties, the capability of measuring hypothalamic peptides and ascertaining their location and biosynthesis is severely hindered and the studies reported are influenced by these deficiencies.[10,11] Several reviews of the state of knowledge of hypothalamic peptide biosynthesis offer excellent descriptions of the procedures and difficulties entailed.[7,12,13] It is the intent in this present chapter to present a concise, current and general description of all hypothalamic hypophysiotropic agents known to date. Literature cited here, will refer to selected recent reviews, papers of historical interest, and current papers of importance. The experimental evidence for many observations, procedures, and hypotheses are not thoroughly covered as they are presented in detail by the authors of the referenced papers. The Tables have been presented to provide concise information that would otherwise add laborious reading for those not particularly interested in the detail presented on that topic.

The discussion will first be directed to those hypothalamic hormones and factors that stimulate the release of other hormones from the pituitary, followed by a discussion of hypothalamic agents that inhibit anterior pituitary secretion. A final section will present a general description of most of the other peptide factors identified within the hypothalamus.

NOMENCLATURE

The literature contains a bewildering array of terms describing the hypothalamic regulatory agents. The present chapter employs the terminology recommended by Schally et al.[14] to delineate between factors and hormones. A hypothalamic factor is a substance shown to have regulatory effect upon the pituitary release of hormones, but which has yet to have its chemical stucture identified. A hypothalamic hormone is a chemically characterized agent shown to regulate hormonal secretion from the pituitary. Any impure extract showing "activity" is considered to contain a "factor." The abbreviations utilized for the agents will be the first abbreviations shown for each agent in Table 1.

HYPOPHYSIOTROPIC RELEASE-STIMULATING HORMONES AND FACTORS

Corticotropin Releasing Factor (CRF)

Identification

Although CRF was essentially the first hypophysiotropic substance extracted from the hypothalamus, its structure has yet to be defined. Progress has been hampered by the lack of a simple, definitive, and reliable assay for CRF activity. Some reports suggest CRF is structurally similar to either the neurohypophyseal hormone vasopressin (ADH) or the hypothalamic melanocyte stimulating hormone (MSH).[14] For some time ADH was thought to be the elusive CRF, since ADH is found in the hypothalamus and causes the secretion of adrenocorticotropic hormone (ACTH) from the anterior pituitary. Synthetic analogs of ADH have varying degrees of CRF activity.[15] A review of numerous studies comparing ADH and CRF is found elsewhere.[16] The most convincing argument that they are separate entities is the presence of substantial CRF activity in hypothalamic extracts of rats with inherited deficiency of ADH (Brattleboro strain). Most recent studies of highly purified porcine hypothalamic extracts suggest that CRF is approximately 4,000 daltons and loses its activity in the presence of trypsin or thermolysin, indicating that it is a basic polypeptide.[14]

There may be more than a single hypothalamic factor controlling ACTH release.[16]

Location and Secretion

Bioassayable CRF appears to be most concentrated in the medial basal hypothalamus,[17] though CRF activity is found not only within the hypothalamus, but throughout the brain and activity also occurs in peripheral tissues.[15,18]

The release of CRF is under the influence of central nervous system (CNS) and while there is controversy, CRF secretion usually is enhanced by serotonin (5-HT) and acetylcholine and inhibited by norepinephrine (NE) and gamma aminobutyric acid (GABA).[17] A model proposing the interaction of these agents upon CRF secretion is presented elsewhere.[16] CRF is released in an episodic fashion with a variable frequency that reflects a circadian rhythm in blood levels of ACTH and hydrocortisone. These levels are higher in the morning and lower in the evening hours.

Physiologic Role

CRF is formed within the median eminence (ME) in specific peptidergic neurons and thought to be released into the hypothalamic-hypophyseal portal system. It is then carried to the anterior pituitary where, acting upon specific cells (corticotrophs), it causes the enhanced synthesis and release of ACTH. ACTH is released into the peripheral systemic blood supply, and carried to the adrenal cortex where it acts upon specific cells, increasing the production and release of several adrenal steroids. The levels of the primary human glucocorticoid, hydrocortisone, increases in the peripheral blood

Table 1
HYPOTHALAMIC HORMONES AND FACTORS

Name	Abbreviations	Structure
Releasing Agents		
Corticotropin releasing factor	CRF	Not identified
Thyrotropin releasing hormone	TRH	pGlu-His-Pro-NH_2
Luteinizing releasing hormone	LRH, LHRH/FSHRH, GnRH, LRF	PGlu-His-Trp-Ser-Tyr-Gly-Leu-Arg-Pro-Gly-NH_2
Somatotropin releasing factor	SRF, GRF, GHRF	Not identified
Prolactin releasing factor	PRF	Not identified
Melanocyte stimulating hormone releasing factor	MRF, MSHRF	H-Cys-Tyr-Ile-Gln-Asn-OH[a]
Release-inhibiting Agents		
Somatostatin	SS, GIF, GHIF	
Prolactin release-inhibiting factor	PIF (Dopamine)[a]	3,4-dihydroxyphenylethylamine[a]
Melanocyte stimulating hormone release inhibiting factor	MIF, MSHIF	H-Pro-Leu-Gly-NH_2[a]
Other Hypothalamic Agents		
Vasopressin	ADH	Glycinamide-Arg-Pro-Cys-Tyr-Phe-Gln-Asn
Ocytocin	MLF	Glycinamide-Leu-Pro-Cys-Tyr-Ile-Gln-Asn
Substance P	SP	Arg-Pro-Lys-Pro-Gln-Gln-Phe-Gly-Leu-Met
Neurophysins		Not identified
Hypothalamic Opiates	leu- Enkephalin	Tyr-Gly-Gly-Phe-Leu-OH
	met- Enkephalin	Tyr-Gly-Gly-Phe-Met-OH
	α- Endorphin	Tyr-Gly-Gly-Phe-Met-Thr-Ser-Glu-Lys-Ser HO-Thr-Val-Leu-Pro-Thr-Gln
	β- Endorphin	Tyr-Gly-Gly-Phe-Met-Thr-Ser-Glu-Lys-Ser Asn-Lys-Phe-Leu-Thr-Val-Leu-Pro-Thr-Gln Ala-Ala-Ile-Val-Lys-Asn-Ala-His-Lys-Gly HO-Gln
	γ- Endorphin	Tyr-Gly-Gly-Phe-Met-Thr-Ser-Glu-Lys-Ser HO-Leu-Thr-Val-Leu-Pro-Thr-Gln
Neurotensin	NT	<Glu-Leu-Tyr-Glu-Asn-Lys-Pro-Arg-Arg-Pro HOOC-Leu-Ile-Tyr
Vasoactive intestinal peptide	VIP	His-Ser-Asp-Ala-Val-Phe-Thr-Asp-Asn-Tyr Lys-Val-Ala-Met-Gln-Lys-Arg-Leu-Arg-Thr Lys-Tyr-Leu-Asn-Ser-Ile-Leu-Asn-NH_2
Angiotensin II	AII	Asp-Arg-Val-Tyr-Ile-His-Pro-Phe
Cholecystokinin	CCK	Lys-Ala-Gly-Pro-Ser-Arg-Val-Ile-Met Ser-Pro-Leu-His-Gln-Asn-Asn-Lys-Ser Arg-Ile-Asp-Ser-Arg-Asp-Tyr-Met NH_2-Phe-Asp-Met-Trp-Gly

[a] Structure or substance not confirmed.

and returns to the region of the hypothalamus and pituitary where it thwarts the release of, or hampers the pituitary response to, CRF. A classic long negative-feedback regulatory mechanism is thus exemplified.

CRF and perhaps other hypothalamic hormones may possess important physiologic functions other than to act directly upon the adenohypophysis. CRF has an ubiquitous distribution within the Central Nervous System (CNS) and is found associated most often with synaptosomal fractions of brain extract. Electrical stimulation and elevated concentrations of K^+ can increase the release of CRF from isolated nerve endings of the Median Eminence (ME).[14] Both inducers of CRF release require the presence of calcium ions. CRF has been indicated in the release of other pituitary agents, β-lipotropin and β-endorphin, and it alters the level of excitability of other CNS neurons. These characteristics lead some neuroendocrinologists to speculate that CRF may be a neurotransmitter within the CNS.

Pathophysiology and Clinical Significance

Because it has not yet been specifically characterized, the clinical usefulness of CRF has not yet been elucidated. Once characterized, however, it may lead to methods to test for secondary and tertiary deficiencies of the hypothalamic-pituitary-adrenal axis. It may also catalyze the development of useful agents to prevent or diminish iatrogenic Addison's disease in those patients who receive long-term steroid therapy. Some cases of Cushing's syndome with adrenal hyperplasia are attributed to increased CRF secretion and therapeutic inhibition or antagonism of CRF secretion is a beneficial treatment.[19]

Thyrotropin Releasing Hormone (TRH)

Identification

The presence of a hypothalamic-releasing hormone for the anterior pituitary thyroid stimulating hormone (TSH) was implied in early studies that related hypothalamic function to thyroid size and activity. Hypothalamic extracts, or electrical stimulation of the hypothalamus, could increase thyroid size and function. Hypothalamic ablation or lesion results in thyroid atrophy and hypofunction.

TRH was described first as thyrotropin releasing factor (TRF), but later was characterized as a tripeptide with guarded N- and C- terminal amino acids (Table 1). TRH was the first hypothalamic hypophysiotropic hormone to be structurally identified and its sequence confirmed by chemical synthesis. Its discovery marked the beginning of our present understanding of hypothalamic regulatory hormones and gave credibility to the then budding, now burgeoning, field of neuroendocrinology.

The discovery of TRH and the procedures for its isolation and purification are presented in detail in the original studies.[20,21] Later reviews are available.[14,15] Generally, porcine or ovine hypothalamic fragments were acid-treated, and purified by gel filtration and ion-exchange chromatography. Final purification procedures involved partition chromatography, adsorption chromatography on charcoal, analytical gel filtration, and terminal purification with paper chromatography.

Biosynthesis, Localization and Degradation

TRH is synthesized *de novo* in specific brain areas by a nonribosomal TRH synthetase that requires both ATP and Mg^{++}.[12] There is some evidence TRH may be a product of proteolytic degradation of some larger moiety (prohormone), as it is distributed widely throughout the CNS where the TRH synthetase has not been found. It has been shown that in vitro biosynthesis occurs in pulsatile bursts, similar to the in vivo secretory pattern observed for TSH.[13]

Radioimmunoassay and immunohistochemical techniques, as well as microfractionation procedures, were developed to localize TRH within the CNS. These procedures and resultant studies are detailed in several excellent recent reviews.[6,9] The highest concentration of TRH is located in the medial portion of the external layer of the median eminence with moderate concentration associated with the pituitary stalk. Nerve terminals containing TRH are located not only within the hypothalamus, but are extrahypothalamic as well (Table 2).[9] Subcellular distribution of hypothalamic peptides indicate that both the hypothalamic and extrahypothalamic TRH are associated with the synaptic vesicles. Furthermore, depletion of hypothalamic TRH can be observed without concomitant change in extrahypothalamic TRH, indicating that TRH biosynthesis may occur outside the hypothalamus. This is one basis for the current premise that TRH may have a neurotransmitter function in many areas of the CNS. TRH has been discovered in all areas of the brain with the exception of the cerebellum and has been isolated in the blood, cerebrospinal fluid (CSF) and urine.

TRH degradation occurs in both the blood and tissues, but not in urine or CSF.[22] Degradation primarily involves enzymatic cleavage of the pyroGlu-His- or His-$ProNH_2$ bonds, or simple deamination of the peptide.[12] The TRH degrading peptidases are widely distributed within the CNS and peripheral tissues.

Table 2
REGIONS OF THE CNS CONTAINING THYROTROPIN RELEASING HORMONE (TRH)

Nerve Terminals Containing TRH
- Hypothalamic areas
  - Dorsomedial nucleus
  - Paraventricular nucleus
  - Perifornical region
  - Ventromedial nucleus
  - Zona incerta
  - Periventricular area
  - Suprachiasmatic nucleus
  - Ventral preoptic area
  - Medial forebrain bundle
  - Organum vasculosum lamina terminalis

  - Extrahypothalamic areas
  - Nucleus accumbens
  - Nucleus interstitialis
  - Stria terminalis
  - Lateral septal nucleus
  - Brainstem nuclei (several)
  - Ventral horn
  - Intermediolateral cell column

  - Cell Bodies Containing TRH
  - Lateral hypothalamus
  - Dorsomedial nucleus
  - Paraventricular nucleus
  - Perifornical region
  - Periventricular nucleus
  - Median eminence

Physiologic Role

TRH is a primary component of the hypothalamic-pituitary-thyroid axis. It stimulates the synthesis and secretion of the large molecular weight glycoprotein moiety, thyroid stimulating hormone (TSH), from the anterior pituitary. Plasma TSH increases within two min following the administration of TRH.[22]

The mechanism by which TRH acts is still unclear, but most likely involves stimulation of membrane-bound adenylate cyclase and the resultant elevation of intracellular cyclic adenosine monophosphate (cAMP).[23] Specific pituitary membrane receptors for TRH have been identified and their affinity appears to be directly influenced by the presence of thyroxine (T_4) and triiodothyronine (T_3).[15] A review of studies characterizing the binding phenomenon and receptor activity was published several years ago[24] and more recently updated.[23] Some recent evidence, utilizing isolated thyroid tumor cells, suggests that there is no alteration of intracellular cAMP level in the presence of TRH.[25]

The TRH stimulating effect upon pituitary secretion of TSH is modulated by the plasma levels of either T_4 or T_3. Tonic levels of TRH may establish a physiologic setpoint for TSH secretion. T_4 and T_3 determine the sensitivity of the anterior pituitary to the stimulatory action of TRH.[23] T_4 serves to inhibit the TRH effect upon the adenohypophysis, thus reducing TSH secretion, and it may also inhibit TRH secretion when administered intracranially. A short feedback regulation may also exist for TSH as it may stimulate TRH release from the hypothalamus. This positive feedback regulation is atypical of hormonal control mechanisms and is yet to be elucidated.

TRH stimulation of TSH secretion appears to be opposed by another hypothalamic hormone, somatostatin (SS). Somatostatin is discussed in more detail later in this chapter.

TRH, acting through cAMP, releases not only TSH but prolactin as well. It is uncertain, however, if TRH stimulation of prolactin release occurs within the normal physiologic environment. This stimulatory effect is unexpected, as it is recognized that the primary control of prolactin release is via an inhibitory releasing factor (discussed in more detail later in this chapter).

Normal plasma levels of TRH is approximately 60 pg/mℓ, with primary hyperthyroidism yielding values near 5 pg/mℓ. Plasma levels exceeding 100 pg/mℓ have been noted in pituitary hypothyroidism.[14]

TRH is found in the plasma of man and has a plasma half-life of 4 to 5 min, and a volume distribution of 15.7 liters.[26] TRH causes an increase in the synthesis, secretion, and release of TSH from the pituitary of several species of mammals and birds whereas it fails to affect TSH release in amphibia or fish.

A review of the CNS actions of hypothalamic hormones[8] notes that TRH may act directly upon the brain, stimulating neuronal activity and regulating various aspects of behavior. In general, TRH increases behavioral activity in animals by a mechanism that is independent of the pituitary gland. Intraventricular administration of TRH can enhance the action of several antidepressant drugs and oppose the action of depressants such as pentobarbital and chloral hydrate. TRH appears to be a CNS stimulant. Neurophysiologic studies have identified TRH sensitive neurons, some excitatory and others inhibitory. TRH, like LRH, may be a neurotransmitter. It has been found within vesicles of nerve endings and it is released from nerve terminals. It initiates CNS-dependent behavior and alters neuronal excitability of hypothalamic and extrahypothalamic neurons. These actions support the role of TRH as a neurotransmitter.

Pathophysiology and Clinical Significance

Thyroid dysfunction caused by anomalies of the pituitary gland and/or the hypothalamus may represent only 5 to 10% of the reported cases of thyroid disease. Hypothalamic dysfunction could result from either deficient or excess secretion of TRH. TRH clinically may be utilized as a tool to test for pituitary reserve of TSH, prolactin and, in certain circumstances, growth hormone.[27] Because recent studies show that TRH may be a neurotransmitter and play a role in behavior, TRH and its analogs may be candidates for drug therapy of certain psychic and behavioral diseases. Numerous synthetic analogs have been produced with varying degrees of TSH releasing activity (Table 3).

Luteinizing Hormone Releasing Hormone (LRH)

Identification

Near the turn of the 20th century, clinical observations and surgical techniques showed that the hypothalamus and pituitary are related in some undefined manner to growth of ovarian and testicular structure and development of their function.[28] Studies with crude brain and hypothalamic extracts brought to light two seemingly different factors that independently regulate the release of the pituitary gonadotropins, luteinizing hormone (LH) and follicle-stimulating hormone (FSH). These factors are found in both sexes of humans and other mammals. Originally described as "factors", but now structurally identified, these two agents are generally considered to be a single substance, luteinizing hormone releasing hormone (LRH) (Table 1).

In 1971, the structure of porcine LRH was elucidated by Schally.[29] The decapeptide hypothalamic hypophysiotropic hormone was isolated, purified, characterized, and synthesized within a remarkably short three year span. Since that time, LRH has been

Table 3
ANALOGS OF THYROTROPIN RELEASING HORMONE (TRH)[a]

Structure	TSH releasing activity (TRH = 100)
TRH = Pyr-His-Pro-NH_2	100
D-Pyr-D-His-L-Pro-NH_2	inactive
—His-Pro-NH_2	0.1
Pyr-D-His-Pro-NH_2	2-5
Pyr-His-D-Pro-NH_2	0.1
—Pro-OH	0.02
—OMe	20
—NH-NH_2	14
—NH-Me	20
—NH-Et	14
—$N(Me)_2$	0.5
—$N(Et)_2$	0.05
—NH-CH_2-CH_2-OH	16
—piperidine	0.2
—Gly-NH_2	35
—Ala-NH_2	0.5
Pyr-His-Pyrrolidine	0.2
—prolinol	1.2
—NH_2	0.003
—OMe	inactive
—Gly-NH_2	<0.02
—Ala-NH_2	0.1
—Leu-NH_2	0.04
—Val-NH_2	0.1
—Abu-NH_2	0.1
—Ile-OMe	inactive
—ILe-NH_2	inactive
—Thr-NH_2	inactive
—Met-NH_2	inactive
—Phe-NH_2	inactive
—Trp-NH_2	<0.02
Pyr-Gly-Pro-OMe	inactive
—NH_2	inactive
Pyr-Ala-Pro-NH_2	inactive
Pyr-Leu-Pro-OMe	inactive
—NH_2	0.2
Pyr-Met-Pro-NH_2	1.0
Pyr-N^π MeHis-Pro-NH_2	0.04
Pyr-N^τ MeHis-Pro-NH_2	800
Pyr-N^π MeHis-OMe	<0.0005
Pyr-N^τ MeHis-OMe	0.02
Pyr-Phe-Pro-OMe	inactive
—NH_2	10
Pyr-Tyr-Pro-NH_2	0.084
Pyr-Trp-Pro-NH_2	inactive
Pyr-Thi-Pro-NH_2	~0.2
Pyr-D-Thi-Pro-NH_2	~0.2
Pyr-Arg-Pro-NH_2	0.05
Pyr-Lys-Pro-NH_2	0.02
Pyr-Orn-Pro-NH_2	0.025
Pyr-His (Bzl)-Pro-NH_2	0.2
Pyr-β-3-pyrazolyl-Ala-Pro-NH_2	5
Acetyl-Glu-His-Pro-NH_2	inactive

Table 3 (continued)
ANALOGS OF THYROTROPIN RELEASING HORMONE (TRH)[a]

Structure	TSH releasing activity (TRH = 100)
H-Glu-His-Pro-OH	inactive
H-Glu-His-Pro-NH_2	5
N-Me-Pyr-His-Pro-NH_2	inactive
H-Pro-His-Pro-OH	inactive
—NH_2	0.01
Thiophenyl-CO-His-Pro-NH_2	0.2
Furanyl-CO-His-Pro-NH_2	0.01
Cyclopentyl-CO-His-Pro-NH_2	<0.01
Cyclobutyl-CO-His-Pro-NH_2	0.016
H-Gly-His-Pro-NH_2	inactive
H-Glu-Pro-His-OH	inactive

[a] See Reference 15.

found to be identical in structure and function in every mammal examined as well as in some birds and fishes. Though the procedures for isolation and purification are reported in detail in the original paper and others,[29,30,31] the general method involves extraction of hypothalamic fragments with either acetic acid or acidified organic solvents, followed by gel filtration with Sephadex G25, phenol extraction, ion exchange chromatography on CM-cellulose, thin layer chromatography, electrophoresis, and terminated with countercurrent distribution techniques. Although early isolation techniques revealed separate fractions for LH and FSH releasing activity, a single entity has been shown to possess both activities. Since LRH was first synthesized, many analogs have been prepared and examined (Table 4).

Biosynthesis, Localization, Degradation and Secretion

Whereas the nonribosomal *de novo* synthesis of tripeptides such as that of TRH is a possible mechanism of biosynthesis, polypeptides the size of LRH and somatostatin are less likely to be produced by this mechanism.[13] Reports of LRH biosynthesis differ and the exact mechanism is still to be proven. LRH biosynthesis occurs in both the particulate and nonparticulate fractions of hypothalamic extracts. However, the strongest evidence suggests that the synthetic mechanisms are associated with the synaptosomal fraction. Additional evidence suggests that the synthesis may result from enzymatic cleavage of a larger molecular precursor (prohormone?). Investigations regarding LRH must be tempered by the difficulty of rigorously proving the identity of the product of these experiments as LRH.

Localization of LRH within the CNS was first determined by bioassay procedures, but more recently antibodies have been prepared against LRH synthesized in the laboratory. This has resulted in the development of radioimmunoassay and histochemical procedures that have localized the distribution of LRH within the CNS and other body compartments.[7,15] LRH is primarily associated with the lateral aspects of the external layer of the median eminence, and it is found associated with the arcuate nucleus. It is also concentrated in the Organum Vasculosum Lamina Terminalis (OVLT) (Table 5). The median eminence is principally devoid of neuronal cell bodies so LRH is associated with axons and nerve terminals.[32] This association of LRH with the OVLT has generated a hypothesis of intraventricular transport of LRH to the median eminence.

Table 4
ANALOGS OF LUTEINIZING RELEASING HORMONE
(LRH)

	Structure	Biologic activity[a]
LRH	P-Glu-His-Trp-Ser-Tyr-Gly-Leu-Arg-Pro-Gly-NH_2 1 2 3 4 5 6 7 8 9 10	100
	Formyl Sar[1]	53
	NMePyr[1]	48
	3-(2-napthyl)-Ala[3]	52
	Pentamethyl Phe[3]	69
	Phe[5]	64
	D-Ala[6]	2830
	D-Leu[6]	2900
	N^{α}MeLeu[7]	102
	homoArg[8]	22
	Pro[9]ethylamide	670
	Pro[9]propylamide	380
	(D-Leu[6], des Gly[10]) LRH ethylamide	2000—5000
	(des His[2], D-Leu[6]) LRH	strong inhibitor

[a] Biologic activity is relative to either (1) stimulation of ovulation; (2) LH release in vivo; or (3) LH release in vitro. Super numerals represent the position of substitution within the LRH peptide. The term "des" refers to the omission of that amino acid in that position in the chain.

McCann[33] proposed that LRH is first secreted into the CSF, then reabsorbed by specialized cells (tanycytes) and transported to the portal vasculature. Recent immunohistochemical studies supported by lesion experiments showed that most of the LRH-containing neurons in the medial basal hypothalamus project only to the median eminence. However, some LRH neurons project from the medial preoptic area to the OVLT and suprachiasmatic nucleus. Projections also interconnect with the mammillary nuclei and terminate in the ventral tegmental area. Some LRH axons have been identified within the paraolfactory cortex, amygdala and some other extrahypothalamic regions. There is no good evidence for LRH existing within the pituitary stalk or the cerebellum.

LRH incubation with brain and serum enzymes indicates that LRH may be degraded by endopeptidases and then cleaved further by other peptidases. The endopeptidase cathepsin M is recognized as being involved in the LRH degradation process. Inactivation of LRH occurs in all areas of the CNS studied. The degrading mechanisms appear to be associated with the cytoplasm rather than with the synaptosomal mitochondria or nuclear fractions of brain extracts.

The control mechanism of LRH secretion is controversial. Some workers propose that it is regulated by dopaminergic pathways.[6] In 1979, Krulich[34] reviewed the increasing evidence that norepinephrine is the primary controlling agent for LRH secretion. Both dopamine and norepinephrine increase LRH secretion from hypothalamic fragments and synaptosomal preparations in vitro. When administered intraventricularly both increase the secretion of LH in vivo. The serotonergic system is generally thought to inhibit the secretion of LRH.

Once released from the synaptic vesicles within the median eminence, LRH diffuses into the vascular pathways of the portal system and is carried to the anterior hypophysis. LRH then binds to receptor moieties on the membrane surface of specific cells (gonadotrophs) that, in turn, secrete LH and FSH. The binding phenomenon has been studied in detail.[15,23] The mechanism by which LRH acts on the gonadotroph is presumably via activation of the membrane associated adenylatecyclase system with a

Table 5
REGIONS OF THE CNS CONTAINING LRH

Nerve terminals containing LRH
- Median eminence
- Organum vasculosum lamina terminalis

Cell bodies containing LRH
- Preoptic region
- Suprachiasmatic region
- Arcuate nucleus

resultant increase in the intracellular mediator, cyclic adenosine monophosphate (cAMP). Elevated intracellular cAMP is associated with increased intracellular Ca^{++}, and together they stimulate phosphokinase and the eventual secretion of gonadotropins LH and FSH.

Physiologic Role

Although LRH increases the pituitary secretion of both LH and FSH, the view that LRH is the releasing hormone for both LH and FHS is controversial. The LH surge that is synchronous with increased LRH can be demonstrated in the absence of FSH elevation. This dissociation of LRH influence upon LH and FSH secretion may be due to the physiologic differences in the pituitary and hypothalamic feedback actions of the end product steroids and other factors such as the putative gonadal substance, "inhibin".[23]

Numerous analogs of LRH have been developed (Table 4). The substitution of either D-alanine or D-leucine at the midglycine position increases the biologic activity of the molecule almost 30 times. A discussion of these and other analogs is detailed elsewhere.[35] McCann[33] reported a synthetic analog having as many as 5000 times the LH releasing activity as endogenous LRH. Similarly, he reported analogs with inhibitory activity as well.

The physiologic response to a single injection of LRH is characterized by an increase in LH within 15 to 30 min, with a maximal response in 30 to 45 min.[36] FSH secretion exhibits a slightly delayed onset with a relatively longer return to baseline values. The FSH response is always significantly less than the LH response except in postmenopausal, castrated, or prepubertal humans. This supports the proposal for negative feedback influence by gonadal substances upon the anterior pituitary secretion of FSH and LH.

Like TRH, LRH has been found within cell bodies and nerve terminals, identified as being involved in the neural excitability of hypothalamic and extrahypothalamic neurons and involved in the initiation of specific CNS related behavior. Because of this LRH also has been proposed as a probable CNS neurotransmitter.

Pathophysiology and Clinical Significance

There is evidence that hypogonadism can result from hypothalamic deficiency as well as from tumorous destruction of the pituitary.[36] In both of these conditions, administration of LRH appears to be beneficial in restoring gonadal function. Thus, administration of LRH can differentiate between primary and higher level gonadal deficiency. In certain disease states, such as anorexia nervosa, administration of LRH results in alteration of the relative rates of secretion of LH and FSH. FSH secretion is abnormally high in response to LRH in this disease. This response characterizes some female patients with secondary amenorrhea of presumed CNS origin. Clinical studies have demonstrated that secretion of other endocrine substances by pituitary tumors can be increased by the administration of LRH.

Table 6
AGENTS THAT CAUSE
THE RELEASE OF
GROWTH HORMONE

Glucagon
MSH
β-endorphin
Neurotension
Substance P
TRH
LRH
Beta chain of porcine hemoglobin
Vasopressin
Met-enkephalin

Acromegalic patients may have increased GH secretion and, in some cases, increased prolactin secretion in response to LRH. Such responses do not occur in the normal state.

Development of LRH analogs that are antagonists may eventually yield oral contraceptive agents having less prohibitive side effects than the current estrogen/progestin agents. In cases of female dysmenorrhea, "super LRH" analogs have been shown to possess a greater ovulatory effect without the polyovum side effects of other ovulatory agents.[33]

Somatotropin Releasing Factor (SRF)

Identification

Separation of the pituitary stalk from the hypothalamus results in a decreased secretion of growth hormone (GH, somatotropin) from the anterior pituitary.[37] Electrical or chemical stimulation of the ventromedial and arcuate nuclei within the hypothalamus increases the release of growth hormone, whereas lesions of these areas cause a reduced secretion of GH. These observations gave rise to the early speculation of the existence of a hypothalamic factor that increases GH secretion.

SRF was first isolated by Deuben and Meites[38] in 1964. Both the synthesis and secretion of somatotropin was found to be enhanced by their crude hypothalamic extracts. Further attempts to purify and characterize SRF have failed, but past efforts revealed several endogenous agents possessing growth promoting activity (Table 6). The discovery of these agents unmasked the major problem in assaying for hypothalamic hypophysiotropic agents in general.

The primary assay for SRF has been the bioassay technique of measuring the effect of the test extract on the skeletal development of mice and other animals, in vivo. With the advent of the powerful radioimmunoassay techniques, several substances were identified as SRF. Both of these assay procedures may result in error. The bioassay procedure may measure the presence of endogenous agents other than true SRF that influence growth whereas the immunoassay techniques measure substances that are immunologically similar, but which fail to possess the biologic activity of the true SRF.[14] During the last decade, several hypothalamic and CNS substances were proposed as SRF but later were discarded (Table 6).

Biosynthesis and Localization

Biosynthetic mechanisms for SRF production are as yet undefined because of the inherent difficulties with properly assaying and identifying SRF. It has been localized only within the hypothalamic ventromedial and arcuate nuclei by neurophysiologic studies.[37]

Physiologic Role

GH secretion is regulated by both a releasing factor (SRF) and a release-inhibitng hormone[37] (somatostatin, SS). The relative actions of these agents have not been fully elucidated, but there appears to be some tonic control by both agents. GH secretion is episodic and pulsatile with peak bursts occurring within hours after the initiation of sleep. This pulsatile pattern is influenced by age and increases in frequency and magnitude up to puberty and then decreases thereafter. Spontaneous bursts occur and are influenced by factors such as exercise and stress.[37] The basic controlling agent appears to be SRF since the pulsatile patterns of GH secretion disappear when the areas associated with SRF secretion are ablated. This disappearance of the normal secretory patterns of GH occurs without significant changes in the release-inhibiting hormone somatostatin. Conversely, there is little alteration of GH secretory pattern when somatostatin is chemically removed by immunologic methods.

SRF secretion is enhanced by norepinephrine, epinephrine, dopamine and serotonin. The relative importance of these agents in the control of SRF is controversial. There does not appear to be a neurotransmitter pathway that can stimulate SS release. GH, itself, may feed back upon the hypothalamus to negatively inhibit the release of SRF.

Pathophysiology and Clinical Significance

Hypersecretion or deficiency of somatotropin often results in prominent somatic alterations and pathology. Giantism, acromegaly, hyperglycemia, hyperprolactinemia, dwarfism, and amenorrhea are examples of the effects of alteration of growth hormone levels. While most of these conditions have been assumed to result from pituitary micro- or macroadenomas, it is likely that some of these diseases may result from hypothalamic dysfunction.[39] To date, there is no disease state that has been attributed exclusively to altered secretion of SRF.

Prolactin Releasing Factor (PRF)

Identification

The hypothalamus is capable of finite regulation of prolactin secretion by the anterior pituitary. It produces both a releasing agent (PRF) and a release-inhibiting agent (PIF). The inhibitory influence seems to predominate during the basal state of most mammals,reptiles, and amphibians. A stimulating influence is greatest in avian species.

A variety of agents are present within the CNS that can increase secretion of prolactin (Table 7). Biogenic amines and peptides, such as neurotensin and substance P, are potent stimulators of prolactin release in vivo.[14] Histamine, serotonin, and alpha-adrenergic agents increase prolactin secretion. Gamma aminobutyric acid (GABA) both stimulates and inhibits prolactin secretion. TRH has been investigated as the PRF because it increases prolactin secretion. Indeed, TRH stimulates the secretion of prolactin so well that it is a clinical tool for testing prolactin reserve. However, there is strong evidence to separate TRH action from that of the tonic controlling agent for prolactin secretion.[34,40] PRF activity is present in TRH-deficient extracts and there are thyroid disease states in which TRH is elevated in the absence of concomitant altered prolactin secretion. The localization and identification of PRF still remains to be elucidated.

Physiologic Role

Prolactin secretion is tonically inhibited by the inhibitory hypophysiotropic agent PIF (discussed later in this chapter) However, stimulation of prolactin secretion may involve two separate mechanisms. The elevated secretion of prolactin to acute minor stimuli such as ether-stress is rapid and of small magnitude whereas certain chronic stimuli, such as newborn suckling, cause a delayed but relatively larger release. The acute rapid release is considered to be due to an acute release of PRF overriding the tonic effects of PIF. The increased prolactin release to chronic stimuli is caused by

Table 7
CNS AGENTS THAT ALTER PROLACTIN SECRETION

Agents that stimulate prolactin secretion
- TRH
  - Neurotensin
  - Histamine
  - GABA
  - Norepinephrine
  - Serotoin
  - Substance P
  - Melatonin
  - Vasopressin
  - Prostaglandin E_1
  - Cyclic AMP

Agents that inhibit prolactin secretion
- Dopamine
  - GABA
  - Acetylcholine

diminished secretion of the inhibiting agent, PIF.[40] Some evidence has linked serotonin as a neurotransmitter for PRF release.[14] The mechanism for PRF action may involve action on the pituitary lactotroph to increase membrane permeability to Ca^{++} and a resultant increased intracellular cAMP.[40]

Melanocyte Stimulating Hormone Releasing Factor (MRF)

Identification

In a manner similar to that of prolactin and growth hormone, melanocyte stimulating hormone (MSH) secretion is thought to be regulated by two hypothalamic hypophysiotropic agents, a releasing factor (MRF) and a release-inhibiting factor (MIF). Like prolactin, the predominant influence in most animals studied is the tonic inhibition of MSH secretion, both in vivo and in vitro.[41] A primary difficulty exists in the study of hypothalamic regulation of MSH. In lower vertebrates such as amphibians, the existence and role of MSH are well documented because of its readily observable effects upon pigmentation. However, in man, the role of MSH has not been well established. Because the assays for MSH may be detecting substances other than MSH, there is controversy concerning its presence in the human body (discussed later in this chapter).

A factor within the hypothalamus of rats has been isolated that increases the pituitary release of assayable MSH. This material was purified and its structure was proposed as that of MRF.[42] The pentapeptide factor (Table 1) was thought to be the open ring fragment of oxytocin degradation, but controversy remains concerning this hypothesis. While nanogram amounts of this synthetic peptide is capable of causing the release of MSH assayable substances into the plasma of rats, a substance with this structure has not been found within the hypothalamus of any animal studied.[15]

MIF was proposed to be a tripeptide formed like the pentapeptide MRF from oxytocin, but by a different enzyme.[15] The amount of these two substances present at any time is dependent upon the relative concentrations of the prevailing enzymes in the system at that moment.

Physiologic Role

Current understanding of the role of MSH in humans remains speculative at this time and the significance of MRF (or MIF) will depend upon future developments about this hormonal system.

HYPOPHYSIOTROPIC RELEASE-INHIBITING HORMONES AND FACTORS

Somatostatin (SS)

Identification

In 1968, Krulich and co-workers[43] described two hypothalamic substances that influenced pituitary secretion of growth hormone (GH, somatotropin). One substance was inhibitory and labeled somatostatin (SS); the other stimulated GH secretion and was referred to as somatotropin releasing factor (see SRF discussed earlier in this chapter). Five years later, a more purified extract of SS was reported and shortly thereafter the chemical structure of ovine SS was elucidated.[44,45] Since then, somatostatin has been found in every mammal examined, including man, and was determined to be indistinguishable from the cyclic tetradecapeptide found earlier in sheep (Table 1). A general description of the procedures utilized in synthesis of SS is described elsewhere.[15]

Biosynthesis, Localization and Degradation

Although the biosynthetic pathways has not been determined, it appears probable that SS is derived from the catabolism of a larger, highly basic moiety, prosomatostatin.[46] Because SS has been structurally defined and synthetically prepared, highly specific radioimmunoassay and histochemical techniques have been developed to assay and localize SS. Somatostatin is distributed throughout the CNS, the peripheral nervous system and numerous other tissues of the body.[7,46] Most of the immunoreactivity within the CNS is associated with the synaptosomes of the median eminence.[6] Somatostatin has been identified within those tissues listed in Table 8, as well as the pancreas, gut and possibly the thyroid. It is the only hypophysiotropic peptide that has been found in the cerebellum.[46]

SS has been identified within the plasma of both the hepatic and pituitary portal systems, as well as within the CSF. The processes of SS degradation have not been thoroughly assessed. The relatively rapid removal from the blood (plasma half-life of 1 to 4 min) implies rapid enzymatic action. An endopeptidase similar to cathepsin M that hydrolyzes luteotropin releasing hormone and substance P discussed later in this chapter has been partially purified from hypothalamic extract and is proposed as an agent of SS degradation. Techniques for measuring SS within the peripheral plasma have not been successful until recently[47] and still await verification in humans.

Mechanism of Action

Some controversy remains concerning the mechanism by which SS exerts its effect upon the pituitary and other organs. Labrie et al.[23] proposed that SS acts to inhibit the adenylate cyclase system, thus lowering the concentration of the effective "second messenger", cyclic adenosine monophosphate (cAMP). Gerich and Patton[46] oppose that concept and propose that SS acts via alteration of membrane permeability to calcium or other ions. Perhaps both of these mechanisms exist within different tissues and species tested.

Physiologic Role

Techniques for measurement of pituitary or plasma levels of GH are not often in agreement. Outstanding differences exist between values derived by bioassay and immunoassay procedures that are not yet resolved. The descriptions presented here are generally accepted observations. Somatostatin has a strong inhibitory effect upon the secretion of growth hormone in several species including man, both in vivo and in vitro. Plasma GH increases slightly following the removal of SS by antiserum techniques. However, there is no alteration of the normal pulsatile secretory pattern of GH secretion. This suggests that SS has a tonic inhibitory effect upon GH release, but

Table 8
REGIONS OF THE CNS CONTAINING SOMATOSTATIN

- Nerve terminals containing somatostatin
  - Hypothalamic areas
    - Median eminence
    - Periventricular area
    - Ventromedial nucleus
    - Arcuate nucleus
    - Suprachiasmatic nucleus
    - Ventral premammillary nucleus
    - Organum vasculosum lamina terminalis
  - Extrahypotalamic areas
    - Stria terminalis
    - Nucleus accumbens
    - Caudate nucleus
    - Olfactory tubercle
    - Amagdaloid complex
    - Cortex (several areas)
    - Brainstem (parabrachial nucleus)
    - Spinal cord (substantia gelatinosa)
- Cell bodies containing somatostatin
  - Periventricular area
  - Zona incerta
  - Stria terminalis
  - Cortical amygdaloid nucleus
  - Dentate gyrus
  - Entorhinal area
  - Neocortex
  - Cerebellum

that higher CNS control is augmented by another pathway perhaps that of SRF. While the putative role for SRF is to control the moment to moment regulation of GH, the proposed role for SS, is that it is called into play during the onset of stress to counteract or thwart the hypersecretion of other hormones of stress, e.g., GH, TSH, insulin, glucagon, and ACTH. Numerous stressful stimuli such as surgery, acute trauma or insulin-induced hypoglycemia result in an increase of GH and other hormones that elevate blood glucose. SS is a potent inhibitor of hypophyseal TSH secretion and can inhibit ACTH and prolactin secretion during abnormal tumorous production of those agents. A role of SS is also as a physiologic regulator of glucose metabolism.

Because of the rather wide distribution of SS throughout the CNS, its association with nerve fibers, synaptosomes and secretory vesicles; its ability to diminish CNS neuronal activity, and its capacity to alter behavior of laboratory animals; SS has been proposed as a neurotransmitter. This hypothesis is supported by the unique close association of SS with the distribution of substance P (discussed later in this chapter) within the spinal cord. This implies that SS may play a neurotransmitter or regulatory role in the transmission of sensory impulses in the cord, particularly those of pain.

In addition to inhibiting the secretion of hormones such as those from the pituitary and pancreas, SS is capable of inhibiting the secretions of exocrine glands as well (Table 9).

Although there are data relating to adrenergic and serotonergic influences on GH secretion, the higher CNS control of SS secretion is not defined. As yet there are no neurotransmitters that are known to directly inhibit SS secretion.

Pathophysiology and Clinical Significance

There is currently no evidence of human pathology resulting from altered secretion of somatostatin. However, a significant increase in our understanding of such disease

Table 9
SUBSTANCES INHIBITED BY SOMATOSTATIN

Endocrine substances
- Growth hormone
- Insulin
- Glucagon
- TSH
- ACTH
- Vasoactive intestinal peptide
- Renin
- Gastrin
- Cholecystokinin
- Secretin
- Motilin
- Gastric inhibitory peptide

Nonendocrine substances
- Gastric acid
- Pancreatic fluid
- Pepsin

stated as hypothyroidism, diabetes mellitus, acromegaly, amenorrhea, Addison's disease, Cushing's disease, and Nelson's syndrome has developed from our recognition of the presence of somatostatin. Clinical use of somatostain has met with only limited success because of its wide spectrum of action and extremely short biologic half-life. Both of these characteristics have proved significantly restrictive to limit the usefulness of SS to relatively acute treatment of pituitary and pancreatic hyperfunction. Numerous analogs have been developed and tested, but the drug is still too rapidly cleared and no analog has been produced with only a single specific effect. There are several actions to any single analog synthesized. A history of the development of the analogs of SS is presented in two previous reviews.[14,15]

Prolactin Release-Inhibiting Factor (PIF)

Identification

Early investigations of prolactin revealed that its secretion was enhanced when the vascular pathways between the anterior pituitary and brain were interrupted. Additional studies showed that separate fractions of crude hypothalamic extracts could both inhibit and stimulate prolactin secretion in laboratory animals.[48] Further investigations led to the current hypothesis of the presence of two regulatory agents within the hypothalamus; PIF, a predominant inhibitory factor, and PRF a releasing factor. The latter is apparently weaker, but it has an important, influence (discussed earlier in this chapter). Although unsuccessful thus far in identifying PRF, there is increasing evidence that in most species studied PIF is identical with the neurohormone, dopamine (DA).

Elucidation of the mechanisms of prolactin secretion coincides with the demonstration that catecholamines can act directly upon the anterior pituitary to inhibit prolactin release.[40] Eventually, catecholamines and catecholamine analogs were shown to inhibit the release of prolactin both in vitro and in vivo.[14]

Later studies showed that when extracts containing PIF were treated with peptidases, there was no reduction in prolactin-inhibiting activity. PIF activity was lost, however, when catecholamines were removed from brain extracts by adsorption techniques. These studies indicated that PIF was probably not a polypeptide, but a catecholamine-like substance. Both dopamine and norepinephrine were proposed as the PIF. Dopamine has been shown to be several times more concentrated in the plasma of pituitary portal vessels than in the peripheral circulation of the rat, a concentration of DA that can physiologically inhibit prolactin secretion.[6] The immunohistologic studies of the vascular border of the median eminence show dopamine content to far exceed that of norepinephrine.[49] Major stimuli that decrease prolactin release (Table 7) appear to concomitantly diminish release of hypothalamic dopamine.[40] Estrogens have been shown to be potent stimulators of prolactin secretion, an action proposed to result from inhibition of dopamine secretion.[23] All of these observations promote the hypothesis that DA is the hypothalamic hypophysiotropic catecholamine that inhibits prolactin secretion.

Biosynthesis and Localization

If dopamine is the true PIF, then the biosynthetic mechanisms have been well defined. The enzyme system for biosynthesis of dopamine is present within the hypothalamus. Both tyrosine hydroxylase and dopa decarboxylase are found within the area mainly associated with the dense concentration of dopaminergic nerve terminals.[49] PIF is associated with the dopaminergic pathways within the hypothalamus, and the primary pathway appears to link the arcuate nucleus with the portal vasculature of the median eminence.

Physiologic Role

PIF expresses its effect on the pituitary prolactin secreting cell, the lactotroph, by preventing Ca^{++} movement through the cell membrane. Calcium ions are necessary for the activation of the cAMP-induced secretion of prolactin. By preventing Ca^{++} entry into the cell, PIF can inhibit prolactin secretion.[40] A constant secretion of PIF appears to be necessary for maintaining a tonic inhibition of prolactin release. Chronic stimuli such as suckling inhibits PIF secretion and this results in increased prolactin secretion by the lactotroph. Other acute or lesser stimuli probably increase PRF secretion; this eventually overrides the tonic effect of PIF, thus enhancing prolactin secretion. Prolactin secretion does not appear to be regulated by alteration of a single blood-borne substance. However, there is some evidence that prolactin, itself, may feedback to stimulate PIF release from the median eminence.[48]

Pathophysiology and Clinical Significance

In the past, anterior pituitary dysfunction has been attributed primarily to the presence of micro- or macro-adenomas. The current understanding of the hypothalamic influence in adenohypophyseal function has led to an awareness of the possibilities of hypothalamic dysfunction as a cause of certain types of pathology. In the most common forms of hypophyseal dysfunction, an excess secretion of GH (gigantism, acromegaly), prolactin (galactorrhea, amenorrhea), or ACTH (Cushing's disease) may involve alteration of secretion of the hypothalamic hypophysiotropic agent PIF.

Hyperprolactinemia is associated with changes in gonadal function of both men and women, resulting in oligospermia or amenorrhea. This disease has been treated primarily by surgical intervention, but morbidity and pituitary hypofunction often resulted. Because of the recognition of the hypophysiotropic influence upon prolactin secretion, there has been successful chronic treatment of these disease states by utilizing DA precursors or analogs (bromoergocryptine). New microsurgical techniques are claimed to be extremely beneficial.[50]

Melanocyte Stimulating Hormone Release-Inhibiting Factor (MIF)

Identification

Studies on lower vertebrates have brought out the influence of the pituitary melanocyte stimulating hormone (MSH) in enhancing the deposition and distribution of pigment. The role of MSH in mammalian physiology is far less apparent. This lack of understanding persists in the absence of a definitive assay procedure for MSH. Like prolactin and growth hormone, bioassays for MSH do not always agree with the immunoassay techniques that measure immunoreactive metabolites, precursors and other agents not possessing the physiologic actions of MSH. Early studies in mammals revealed the presence of hypothalamic substances that either enhanced or reduced MSH secretion, giving rise to the proposal of both an MSH releasing (MRF) and MSH release-inhibiting (MIF) factor. MRF structure still remains to be verified (discussed earlier in this chapter). In 1965, hypothalamic lesions in frogs were shown to cause increases in plasma levels of MSH and decreases in pituitary MSH content, implying the presence of tonic inhibition by a hypothalamic substance.[51] Crude hypothalmic extracts from rats were shown to block the rise in plasma MSH in vivo or prevent the depletion of pituitary MSH in vitro.[41]

In the early 1970's, a tripeptide (Pro-Leu-Gly-NH_2)[42] and a pentapeptide (Pro-His-Phe-Arg-Gly-NH_2)[52] were isolated from the stalk-median eminence. The activity of the tripeptide is at least 20 times more active in inhibiting MSH release than the pentapeptide agent and is considered the more probable MIF. However, doubt remains concerning these agents as the endogenous release-inhibiting hormones because some laboratories have not been able to show activity of these synthetic agents.[41] Endogenous aminergic agents such as catecholamines, acetylcholine, gamma aminobutyric acid, and serotonin have been proposed as possible mediators of MSH release.[53]

There is increasing evidence that MSH may not even exist in the plasma and pituitary of man, but that what is measured as MSH by immunoassay techniques is in fact the immunoreactive larger polypeptide moiety β-lipotropin, which is not physiologically active.

Physiologic Role

MIF content within the hypothalamus of experimental animals varies depending upon experimental conditions. Stress, light suckling, sound, vaginal stimulation, plasma osmolality, and adrenergic agents are reported to influence MSH secretion and therefore MIF and MRF. Because the vascular portal network is poorly developed between the hypothalamus and intermediate lobe of the pituitary, the mechanism of vascular transport of releasing factors to the pituitary has not been established. The neuronal pathway between the site of releasing factor synthesis and the intermediate lobe is well developed. In lower vertebrates MIF and MRF may be transported via axoplasmic flow. In mammals, which generally possess a poorly developed intermediate lobe, the mechanism is better defined. The MSH-producing cells are distributed within the parenchyma of the anterior pituitary which has substantial vascular pathways. It is well accepted that MSH secretion is under tonic inhibition and most likely occurs by a release-inhibiting agent associated with the median eminence. This may occur via a single MIF or by multiple agents.

A model of higher central nervous pathways for regulation of MRF and MIF secretion or for the secretion of MSH is proposed elsewhere.[41] The intriguing possibility exists that MSH may be influenced both directly and indirectly by catecholamines. Norepinephrine and other α-adrenergic agonists can inhibit MSH secretion by two pathways (1) stimulation of MIF; and (2) direct inhibition of MSH release by the pituitary. Dopamine has been shown to inhibit MSH secretion by direct action on the anterior pituitary and it has been proposed as the endogenous MIF.[53] This would enhance the role of dopamine as a hypophysiotropic agent as it is also suspected to be the inhibitory factor for prolactin release, PIF.

Pathophysiology and Clinical Significance

As yet no human disease state that is induced by altered MSH activity has been confirmed. Hyperpigmentation in patients with Addison's disease originally was attributed to increased secretion of MSH, but there is evidence to suggest that the increased MSH is in fact the physiologically inactive β-lipotropin. Additionally, MIF itself may have higher lever central nervous effects that could be involved in behavioral dysfunction or disease. Further research and data must be collected to verify an action for MIF in man. If MIF is endogenous dopamine, then the pathophysiology of altered secretion of MIF is that of the neurotransmitter, dopamine.

OTHER HYPOTHALAMIC PEPTIDES

Vasopressin (ADH)

This neurohypophyseal octapeptide hormone (Table 1) has been known since 1895, although its original discovery was with reference to its vasopressor action.[54] ADH was later shown to possess potent antidiuretic action, thus its secondary name antidiuretic hormone (ADH).

ADH is synthesized primarily in the paraventricular and supraoptic areas of the hypothalamus and neuronally transported to the posterior pituitary where it is secreted into the systemic circulation. ADH is found primarily with the hypothalamus though it has been identified within nerve terminals of the spinal cord, lateral ventricles and choroid plexes (Table 10).

Because of its important function in fluid and salt balance, its unique mechanism of transport, and the current controversial mechanisms of regulation,[55] this hypothalamic hormone is discussed more completely (see Chapter 10).

Oxytocin (MLF)

Similar in structure to vasopressin (Table 1), this octapeptide hormone possesses some of the antidiuretic actions of ADH. However, its general actions are distinct from those of ADH. Oxytocin is secreted in response to neuronal stimulation of the nipple of the mammary gland and causes the ejection of mammary milk. For this reason oxytocin is known as the milk let down factor, (MLF). It acts upon the uterine smooth muscle to promote contraction during the processes of labor. Oxytocin distribution parallels that of ADH and neurophysin (Table 10). It is discussed in detail in Chapter 10.

Substance P (SP)

This enigmatic substance is the subject of two recent brief reviews.[56,57] Substance P was first discovered in 1932 by von Euler[58] and required nearly forty years before its structure was characterizated by Chang and Leeman[59] in 1970 (Table 1). It is widely distributed throughout the CNS (Table 11), is highly concentrated in the hypothalamus, and is found within the pineal gland, pons, medulla, cortex, posterior pituitary, autonomic nerves, and spinal cord. Substance P distribution is closely associated with that of serotonin and gamma aminobutyric acid (GABA) and it is in highest concentration in the substantia nigra.[60]

The role of SP within the higher levels of the CNS is unknown. However, its role within the spinal cord and autonomic nervous system has attracted much interest and research. Substance P has been proposed as a neurotransmitter of nociceptive impulses within the afferent sensory nerves and spinal cord. It is found associated with all of the primary structures described for pain transmission. It may play a dual role in the transmission of pain impulses as it is an active neurotransmitter of nociceptive impulses in sensory nerves and spinal cord and it is also a modulating agent within the descending serotonergic fibers of the Raphe nuclei. These fibers influence the gating of pain impulses impinging upon the cord.[57]

Table 10
REGIONS OF THE CNS CONTAINING VASOPRESSIN/ OXYTOCIN/ NEUROPHYSINS

- Nerve terminals
  - Hypothalamic areas
    - Paraventricular nuclei
    - Supraoptic nuclei
    - External layer of median eminence
  - Extrahypothalamic areas
    - Lateral ventricles
    - Choroid plexus
    - Spinal cord
- Cell bodies
  - Paraventricular nuclei
  - Supraoptic nuclei
  - Suprachiasmatic nucleus
  - Triangular nucleus of the septum

Substance P release from the hypothalamus can be stimulated by electrical or chemical stimuli and appears to be dependent upon the presence of calcium and magnesium ions. Subcellular fractionation of the hypothalamus shows SP to be associated primarily with the mitochondria and synaptosome fractions. It is hydrolyzed by the peptidase cathepsin M present within the CNS.

The systemic role of SP is only conjectured. It appears to be vasoactive, hyperglycemic, and perhaps to have an influence on fluid balance.[61] There does not appear to be any direct effect of SP upon pituitary function.[9]

Neurophysins

Neurophysins are a group of cysteine-rich polypeptides found in the hypothalamus, neurohypophysis, and pineal gland.[12] They are primarily in the hypothalamus and are the binding proteins for the axonal transport of ADH and oxytocin from the hypothalamus to the posterior pituitary. The distribution of neurophysins generally parallels that of ADH and oxytocin (Table 10).

The synthesis of neurophysins is not clear, but there is evidence that two precursor molecules exist for the neurophysin and the respective neurohypophyseal hormone ADH and oxytocin.[62] These precursor moieties have yet to be identified, but the synthesis of such precursor complexes occurs in granules within the supraoptic and paraventricular nuclei. There appears to be a specific neurophysin for both ADH and oxytocin. The neurophysins are characterized thus far as having a molecular weight of 10,000 daltons and composed of 90 to 100 amino acid.[15] These hormone-neurophysin complexes are transported as granules containing hydrolases such as cathepsin D, from the hypothalamus to the posterior pituitary where they are released into the blood in response to membrane depolarization. The neurophysin complexes are degraded during the rapid transport processes, forming the free hormone and several products of degradation.

There is no known physiologic action for neurophysins other than as carrier substances for the neurohypophyseal hormones. Neurophysins, like the hormones ADH and oxytocin, are present in the pituitary of laboratory rats at birth.

Table 11
REGIONS OF THE CNS CONTAINING SUBSTANCE P

Nerve terminals
- Hypothalamic area
  - Medial preoptic nucleus
  - Periventricular area
  - Anterior hypothalamic nucleus
  - Lateral hypothalamus
  - Dorsomedial nucleus
  - Ventromedial nucleus
  - Arcuate nucleus
- Extrahypothalamic areas
  - Amygdala
  - Stria terminalis
  - Lateral septal nucleus
  - Zona reticulata
  - Interpeduncular nucleus
  - Periaqueductal central gray
  - Substantia gelatinosa
  - Parabrachial nucleus
  - Dorsal root ganglia
  - Nucleus of the solitary tract
  - Commissural nucleus
  - Habenulointerpenduncular tract
  - Striatonigral pathway
  - Marginal laminae (I and II)

Cell bodies
- Hypothalamic areas
  - Dorsomedial nucleus
  - Ventromedial nucleus
  - Premammillary nucleus
  - Lateral preoptic area
- Extrahypothalamic areas
  - Amygdala
  - Nucleus interstitialis stria terminalis
  - Medial habenular nucleus
  - Interpeduncular nucleus
  - Periaqueductal central gray
  - Dorsal tegmental nucleus
  - Commissural nucleus
  - Nucleus pallidus
  - Raphe nuclei
  - Nucleus of the solitary tract

Hypothalamic Opiates

Endogenous morphine-like substances have been identified within the hypothalamus. These substances are structurally similar (Table 1) and appear to be fragments of an even larger moiety β-lipotropin. Hypothalamic opiates are of two primary classes (1) pentapeptide enkephalins; and (2) larger polypeptide endorphins. The distribution and actions of these substances are ubiquitous. However, they do not appear to be hypophysiotropic and will not be discussed further in this chapter.

Neurotensin (NT)

This vasoactive tridecapeptide was first isolated by Carraway and Leeman[64] from bovine hypothalami in 1973. In 1975 the same laboratory unveiled the amino acid structure (Table 1).[65] Neurotensin is found distributed throughout the CNS, including

Table 12
REGIONS OF THE CNS CONTAINING NEUROTENSIN

Nerve fibers
- Stria terminalis
- Preoptic area
- Medial forebrain bundle
- Amygdaloid complex
- Ventrolateral hypothalamus
- Dorsolateral hypothalamus
- Dorsomedial hypothalamus
- Median eminence
- Pars nervosa
- Lateral hypothalamus
- Paramedial thalamus
- Lateral mammillary region
- Posterior mammillary region

Cell bodies
- Stria terminalis
- Medial preoptic area
- Lateral preoptic area
- Periventricular hypothalamus
- Anterior hypothalamic nucleus
- Lateral hypothalamic nucleus
- Paraventricular nucleus
- Arcuate nucleus
- Ventral hypothalamus
- Posterior hypothalamic nucleus
- Perifornical region
- Amygdala
- Dorsomedial nucleus

the hypothalamus, brainstem, cortex, thalamus, pituitary, and cerebellum (Table 12). Most activity is associated with synaptosomes and NT is apparently degraded by carboxypeptidases.

Neurotensin has ubiquitous systemic effects. It is hypotensive, hyperglycemic, and can increase gut motility. Neurotensin nerve fibers have been identified in the median eminence and it appears to be hypophysiotropic. Neurotensin can increase the release of LH and FSH in vitro as well as alter GH and prolactin secretion in vivo.[66] Like substance P, neurotensin is found within several neural structures associated with pain transmission.

The mechanisms of its systemic effects may be via increasing histamine release from mast cells or histaminergic pathways. Neurotensin is often described as a member of the gut-brain peptides which include the endogenous opiates, substance P, vasoactive inhibitory protein (VIP), as well as insulin, and glucagon. Neurotensin, like many other peptides, has been proposed as a neurotransmitter.[60,66]

Vasoactive Intestinal Peptide (VIP)

This 28 amino acid polypeptide (Table 1) has been identified within the small intestine, pancreatic islet cell tumors, and within the brain.[60] VIP causes vasodilation, glycogenolysis, lipolysis, insulin secretion, and water excretion by the gut.[28] It also inhibits the production of gastric acid. Although the highest concentrations within the brain are found in the cerebral cortex, VIP also is located within the nerve endings of the central amygdaloid nucleus, preoptic nucleus, and anterior hypothalamic nuclei.[60] Its physiologic role within the CNS has yet to be revealed.

Table 13
REGIONS OF THE CNS CONTAINING ANGIOTENSIN II

Nerve terminals
- Hypothalamic areas
  - External layer of median eminence
  - Dorsomedial nucleus
  - Ventral portions of hypothalamus
- Extrahypothalamic areas
  - Dorsal horn
  - Substantia gelatinosa
  - Intermediolateral cell column
  - Amygdaloid nuclei

Cell bodies
- Paraventricular nucleus
- Perifornical area

Angiotensin II (AII)

Angiotensin II is a small peptide of eight amino acids (Table 1) derived by enzymatic degradation of larger angiotensinogen produced in the liver. The physiologic role for Angiotensin II within the peripheral circulation has been generally associated with the maintenance of vascular volume and pressure. It is a potent vasoconstrictor and stimualtes the adrenal cortical secretion of the salt-retaining hormone, aldosterone. AII is a potent dipsogenic hormone that is synthesized and active within the hypothalamus, and it is widely distributed through out the CNS (Table 13). Because of the involved mechanisms of control and complex actions of AII, it is discussed at greater length in another chapter (see Chapter 11).

Cholecystokinin (CCK)

This substance was first identified as an intestinal hormone that stimulated the secretion of pancreatic enzymes. Its 33 amino acid structure (Table 1) was found to be identical with another substance that was called pancreozymin. As a result, this agent was referred to as cholecystokinin-pancreozymin for several years. The CCK identified within the brain was actually of several structural forms: a COOH terminal octapeptide (CCK-8), a less concentrated tetrapeptide (CCK-4), and a trace of the parent form, CCK-33.[60]

Like substance P and VIP, it is a gut-related peptide found within the brain. CCK is found within the hypothalamus and may be involved with the satiety center and with feeding behavior, since minute amounts of CCK-8 infused into the ventricles of rats and sheep can reduce feeding behavior.[60] Within the CNS, CCK is most concentrated within the cerebral cortex. CCK and VIP are the only gut-brain peptides found within the cells of the cerebral cortex. CCK can stimulate cortical neuronal firing and it is closely associated with dopamine in the brainstem and within sensory fibers that have cell bodies in the dorsal root ganglia. This association of CCK with sensory fibers suggests that CCK may play a role in the transmission or modulation of sensory impulses. The complete role of CCK within the brain remains to be elucidated.

REFERENCES

1. **Harris, G. W.,** *Neural Control of the Pituitary Gland,* Edward Arnold, London, 1955.
2. **Saffran, M. and Schally, A. V.,** The release of corticotropin by anterior pituitary tissue in vitro, *J. Biochem. Physiol. (Canada),* 33, 408, 1955.
3. **Wade, N., Guillemin, R. and Schally, A. V.,** The years in the wilderness, *Science,* 200, 279, 1978.
4. **Wade, N., Guillemin, R. and Schally, A. V.,** The three-lap race to Stockholm, *Science,* 200, 411, 1978.
5. **Wade, N., Guillemin, R. and Schally, A. V.,** A race spurred by rivalry, *Science,* 200, 510, 1978.
6. **Terry, L. C. and Martin, J. B.,** Hypothalamic hormones: subcellular distribution and mechanisms of release, *Ann. Rev. Pharmacol. Toxicol.,* 18, 111, 1977.
7. **Elde, R. and Hökfelt, T.,** Localization of hypophysiotropic peptides and other biologically active peptides within the brain, *Ann. Rev. Physiol.,* 41, 587, 1979.
8. **Moss, R. L.,** Actions of hypothalamic-hypophysiotropic hormones on the brain, *Ann. Rev. Physiol.,* 41, 617, 1979.
9. **Elde, R. and Hökfelt, T.,** Distribution of hypothalamic hormones and other peptides in the brain, in *Frontiers in Neuroendocrinology,* Vol. 5, Ganong, W. F. and Martini, L., Eds., Raven Press, New York, 1978, chap. 1.
10. **Jeffcoate, S. L.,** The biochemical investigation of the endocrine hypothalamus, in *The Endocrine Hypothalamus,* Jeffcoate, S. L. and Hutchinson, J. S. M., Eds., Academic Press, New York, 1978, chap. 4.
11. **Lincoln, D. W.,** Investigation of hypothalamic function: anatomical and physiological studies, in *The Endocrine Hypothalamus,* Jeffcoate, S. L. and Hutchinson, J. S. M., Eds., Academic Press, New York, 1978, chap. 2.
12. **Marks, N.,** Biotransformation and degradation of corticotropins, lipotropins and hypothalamic peptides, in *Frontiers in Neuroendocrinology,* Vol. 5, Ganong, W. G. and Martini, L., Raven Press, New York, 1978, chap. 12.
13. **McKelvy, J. F. and Epelbaum, J.,** Biosynthesis, packaging, transport, and release of brain peptides, in *The Hypothalamus,* Reichlin, S., Baldessarini, R. J., and Martin, J. B., Eds., Raven Press, New York, 1978, 195.
14. **Schally, A. V., Coy, D. H., and Meyers, C. A.,** Hypothalamic regulatory hormones, *Ann. Rev. Biochem.,* 47, 89, 1978.
15. **Sandow, J. and König, W.,** Chemistry of the hypothalamic hormones, in *The Endocrine Hypothalamus,* Jeffcoate, S. L. and Hutchinson, J. S. M., Eds., Academic Press, New York, 1978, chap. 5.
16. **Jones, M. T.,** Control of corticotropin (ACTH) secretion, in *The Endocrine Hypothalamus,* Jeffcoate, S. L. and Hutchinson, J. S. M., Eds., Academic Press, New York, 1978, chap. 11.
17. **Weiner, R. I. and Ganong, W. F.,** Role of brain monoamines and histamine in regulation of anterior pituitary secretion, *Physiol. Rev.,* 58, 905, 1978.
18. **Witorsch, R. J. and Brodish, A.,** Conditions for the reliable use of lesioned rats for the assay of CRF in tissue extracts, *Endocrinology,* 90, 552, 1972.
19. **Krieger, D. T.,** The central nervous system and Cushing's disease, *Med. Clin. North Am.,* 62, 261, 1978.
20. **Burgus, R., Dunn, T. F., Desiderio, D., Ward, D. N., Vale, W., and Guillemin, R.,** Characterization of ovine hypothalamic hypophysiotropic TSH releasing factor, *Nature (London),* 226, 321, 1970.
21. **Nair, R. M. G., Barret, J. F., Bowers, C. Y., and Schally, A. V.,** Structure of porcine thyrotropin-releasing hormone, *Biochemistry,* 9, 1103, 1970.
22. **Reichlin, S., Martin, J. B., and Jackson, I. M. D.,** Regulation of thyroid-stimulating hormone (TSH) secretion, in *The Endocrine Hypothalamus,* Jeffcoate, S. L. and Hutchinson, J. S. M., Eds., Academic Press, New York, 1978, chap. 7.
23. **Labrie, F., Borgeat, P., Drouin, J., Beaulieu, M., Lagacé, L., Ferland, L., and Raymond, V.,** Mechanism of action of hypothalamic hormones in the adenohypophysis, *Ann. Rev. Physiol.,* 41, 555, 1979.
24. **Boss, B., Vale, W., and Grant, G.,** Hypothalamic hormones, in *Biochemical Actions of Hormones,* Vol. 3, Litwack, G., Ed., Academic Press, London, 1975, chap. 4.
25. **Gershengorn, M. C., Rebecchi, M. J., Geras, E., and Arevalo, C. O.,** Thyrotropin-releasing hormone (TRH) action in mouse thyrotropic tumor cells in culture: evidence against a role for adenosine 3′, 5′-monophosphate as a mediator of TRH-stimulated thyrotropin release, *Endocrinology,* 107, 665, 1980.
26. **Leppaluoto, J., Virkkunen, P., and Lybeck, H.,** Elimination of TRH in man, *J. Clin. Endocrinol. Metab.,* 35, 447, 1972.
27. **Hershman, J. M.,** Use of thyrotropin-releasing hormone in clinical medicine, *Med. Clin. North Am.,* 62, 313, 1978.

28. **Reichlin, S.,** Introduction, in *The Hypothalamus,* Reichlin, S., Baldessarini, R. J., and Martin, J. G., Eds., Raven Press, New York, 1978, 1.
29. **Schally, A. V., Arimura, A., Baba, Y., Nair, R. M. G., Matsuo, H., Redding, T. W., Debeljuk, L., and White, W. F.,** Isolation and properties of the FSH and LH-releasing hormone, *Biochem. Biophys. Res. Commun.,* 43, 393, 1971.
30. **Matsuo, H., Baba, Y., Nair, R. M. G., Arimura, A., and Schally, A. V.,** Structure of the porcine LH- and FSH-releasing hormone. I. The proposed amino acid sequence, *Biochem. Biophys. Res. Commun.,* 43, 1334, 1971.
31. **Baba, Y., Arimura, A., and Schally, A. V.,** On the tryptophan residue in porcine LH- and FSH-releasing hormone. *Biochem. Biophys. Res. Commun.,* 45, 433, 1971.
32. **Turgeon, J. L.,** Neural control of ovulation, *Physiologist,* 223, 56, 1980.
33. **McCann, S. M.,** Actions of luteinizing hormone-releasing hormone on the pituiary and on behavior, *Med. Clin. North Am.,* 62, 269, 1978.
34. **Krulich, L.,** Central neurotransmitters and the secretion of prolactin, GH, LH, and TSH, *Ann. Rev. Physiol.,* 41, 603, 1979.
35. **Vale, W., Rivier, C., and Brown, M.,** Regulatory peptides of the hypothalamus, *Ann. Rev. Physiol.,* 39, 473, 1977.
36. **Frohman, L. A.,** Newer understanding of human hypothalamic pituitary disease obtained through the use of synthetic hypothalamic hormones, in *The Hypothalamus,* Reichlin, S., Baldessarini, R. J., and Martin, J. B., Eds., Raven Press, New York, 1978, 387.
37. **Martin, J. B., Brazeau, P., Tannenbaum, G. S., Willoughby, J. O., Epelbaum, J., Terry, L. C., and Durand, D.,** Neuroendocrine organization of growth hormone regulation, in *The Hypothalamus,* Reichlin, S., Baldessarini, R. J., and Martin, J. B., Eds., Raven Press, New York, 1978, 329.
38. **Deuben, R. and Meites, J.,** Stimulation of pituitary growth hormone release by a hypothalamic extract in vitro, *Endocrinology,* 74, 408, 1964.
39. **Pecile, A. and Olgiati, V. R.,** Control of growth hormone secretion, in *The Endocrine Hypothalamus,* Jeffcoate, S. L. and Hutchinson, J. S. M., Eds., Academic Press, New York, 1978, chap. 10.
40. **Tindal, J. S.,** Control of prolactin secretion, in *The Endocrine Hypothalamus,* Jeffcoate, S. L. and Hutchinson, J. S. M., Eds., Academic Press, New York, 1978, chap. 9.
41. **Taleisnik, S.,** Control of melanocyte-stimulating hormone (MSH) secretion, in *The Endocrine Hypothalamus,* Jeffcoate, S. L. and Hutchinson, J. S. M., Eds., Academic Press, New York, 1978, chap. 12.
42. **Celis, M. E., Taleisnik, S., and Walter, R.,** Release of pituitary melanocyte stimulating hormone by the oxytoxin fragment, H-Cys-Tyr-Ile-Gln-Asn-OH, *Biochem. Biophys. Res. Commun.,* 45, 564, 1971.
43. **Krulich, L., Dhariwal, A. P. S., and McCann, S. M.,** Stimulatory and inhibitory effects of purified hypothalamic extracts on growth hormone release from rat pituitary in vitro, *Endocrinology,* 83, 783, 1968.
44. **Brazeau, P., Vale, W., Burgus, R., Ling, N., Butcher, M., Rivier, J., and Guillein, R.,** Hypothalamic polypeptide that inhibits the secretion of immunoreactive pituitary growth hormone, *Science,* 179, 77, 1973.
45. **Burgus, R., Ling, N., Butcher, M., and Guillemin, R.,** Primary structure of somatostatin, a hypothalamic peptide that inhibits the secretion of pituitary growth hormone, *Proc. Nat. Acad. Sci. U.S.A.,* 70, 684, 1973.
46. **Gerich, J. E. and Patton, G. S.,** Somatostatin: physiology and clinical applications, *Med. Clin. North Am.,* 62, 375, 1978.
47. **Patel, Y. C., Wheatley, T., Fitz-Patrick, D., and Brock, G.,** A sensitive radioimmunoassay for immunoreactive somatostatin in extracted plasma: measurement and characterization of portal and peripheral plasma in the rat, *Endocrinology,* 107, 306, 1980.
48. **Meites, J. and Clemens, J. A.,** Hypothalamic control of prolactin secretion, *Vitam. Horm.,* 30, 165, 1972.
49. **Hökfelt, T., Elde, R., Fuxe, K., Johansson, O., Ljungdahl, A., and Goldstein, M., Luft, R., Efendic, S., Nilsson, G., Terenius, L., Ganten, D., Jeffcoate, S. L., Rehfeld, J., Said, S., Perez de la Mora, M., Possani, L., Tapia, R., Teran, L., and Palacios, R.,** Aminergic and peptidergic pathways in the nervous system with special reference to the hypothalamus, in *The Hypothalamus,* Reichlin, S., Baldessarini, R. J., and Martin, J. B., Eds., Raven Press, New York, 1978, 69.
50. **Havron, D.,** Microsurgery "the equal" of bromocriptine vs. pituitary tumors, *Med. News Int. Report,* 4, 3, 1980.
51. **Kastin, A. J. and Ross, G. T.,** MSH and ACTH activities in pituitaries of frogs with hypothalamic lesions, *Endocrinology,* 77, 45, 1965.
52. **Nair, R. M. G., Kastin, A. J., and Schally, A. V.,** Isolation and structure of another hypothalamic peptide possessing MSH-release-inhibiting activity, *Biochem. Biophys. Res. Commun.,* 47, 1420, 1972.

53. **Kastin, A. J., Schally, A. V., and Dostrzewa, R. M.,** Possible aminergic mediation of MSH release and of the CNS effects of MSH and MIF-I, *Fed. Proc.*, 39, 2931, 1980.
54. **Oliver, G. and Schafer, E. A.,** On the physiological actions of extracts of pituitary body and certain other glandular organs, *J. Physiol. (London)*, 18, 277, 1895.
55. **Bie, P.,** Osmoreceptors, vasopressin, and control of renal water excretion, *Physiol. Rev.*, 60, 961, 1980.
56. **Marx, J. L.,** Brain peptides: is substance P a transmitter of pain signals?, *Science*, 205, 886, 1979.
57. **Henry, J. L.,** Substance P and pain; an updating, *Trend Neurosci.*, 3, 95, 1980.
58. **Von Euler, U. S. and Gaddum, J. H.,** An unidentified depressor substance in certain tissue extracts, *J. Physiol. (London)*, 72, 74, 1931.
59. **Chang, M. M. and Leeman, S. E.,** Isolation of sialagogic peptide from bovine hypothalamic tissue and its characterization as substance P, *J. Biol. Chem.*, 245, 4784, 1970.
60. **Snyder, S. H.,** Brain peptides as neurotransmitters, *Science*, 209, 976, 1980.
61. **Kramer, H. J., Düsing, R., Stelkens, H., Heinrich, R., Kipnowski, J., and Glänzer, K.,** Immunoreactive substance P in human plasma: response to changes in posture and sodium balance, *Clin. Sci.*, 59, 75, 1980.
62. **Brownstein, M. J., Russell, J. T., and Gainer, H.,** Synthesis, transport, and release of posterior pituitary hormones, *Science*, 207, 373, 1980.
63. **Sinding, C., Seif, S. M., and Robinson, A. G.,** Levels of neurohypophyseal peptides in the rat during the first month of life. I. Basal levels in plasma, pituitary, and hypothalamus, *Endocrinology*, 107, 749, 1980.
64. **Carraway, R. and Leeman, S. E.,** The isolation of a new hypotensive peptide neurotensin from bovine hypothalami, *J. Biol. Chem.*, 248, 6854, 1973.
65. **Carraway, R. and Leeman, S. E.,** The amino acid sequence of a hypothalamic peptide, neurotensin, *J. Biol. Chem.*, 250, 1907, 1975.
66. **Kahn, D., Abrams, G. M., Zimmerman, E. A., Carraway, R., and Leeman, S. E.,** Neurotensin neurons in the rat hypothalamus: an immunocytochemical study, *Endocrinology*, 107, 47, 1980.

ANTERIOR PITUITARY

Richard W. Steger and John J. Peluso

INTRODUCTION

The anterior pituitary gland or the adenohypophysis is composed of the pars distalis, the pars intermedia, and the pars tuberalis. The pars distalis makes up the major portion of the anterior pituitary gland and will be the principal subject of this chapter. The existence of the pars intermedia in man is still being debated, but it is prominent in many animals living in a desert environment where its size can be correlated with a resistance to lack of water.[1] The pars intermedia is virtually absent in birds and marine mammals, but present in reptiles, amphibians, and fish. The pars tuberalis is made up of elongated cords of cells that surround the pituitary stalk and extend upward to the basal hypothalamus. The function of the pars tuberalis still has not been established due to its anatomic association with the pituitary stalk and median eminence, which makes its ablation impossible without the destruction of surrounding tissue. Midgley[2] has described luteinizing hormone-containing cells in the pars tuberalis and other histologic investigations, at the light and microscopic level, have described the presence of secretory-like granules, abundant polyribosomes, and other evidence of secretory activity.[3-5]

The anterior pituitary gland secretes six principal hormones. These include luteinizing hormone (LH) and follicle-stimulating hormone (FSH), both of which are involved in gonadal regulation; prolactin (PRL), which is involved in milk production and possibly several other metabolic processes; growth hormone (GH), involved in growth and metabolism; thyroid-stimulating hormone (TSH), which regulates thyroid activity; and adrenocorticotropic hormone (ACTH), which controls adrenal function. Melanocyte-stimulating hormone is secreted by the intermediate lobe in those species having an intermediate lobe and by the pars distalis in other species. Several other hormones or peptides, such as B-lipotropin and endorphin, are also secreted by the anterior pituitary and will be discussed elsewhere along with ACTH secretion.

HISTORICAL PERSPECTIVE

Although the function of the pituitary gland has been the subject of speculation since before the time of Aristotle, it has only been in the last century that its physiologic role has begun to be understood.[6] Aristotle believed that one of the four humors, the phlegm or pituita, passed from the brain through the pituitary and into the nasal cavity. Vesalius had a somewhat similar view of pituitary function which was not questioned until the 17th century when Schneider and Lower proposed that the nasal mucus was produced by the nasal epithelium and not by the brain.

During the mid-1800s, various clinical disorders such as delayed puberty, acromegaly, gigantism, dwarfism, and obesity began to be associated with pituitary tumors, but good endocrine studies on the pituitary gland had to await the development of a method to ablate the gland surgically. In 1910, Aschner[7] published a method to hypophysectomize dogs. A landmark series of papers were published by Smith,[8,9] who described a technique to hypophysectomize rats. From that time on literature has expanded in an explosive fashion.

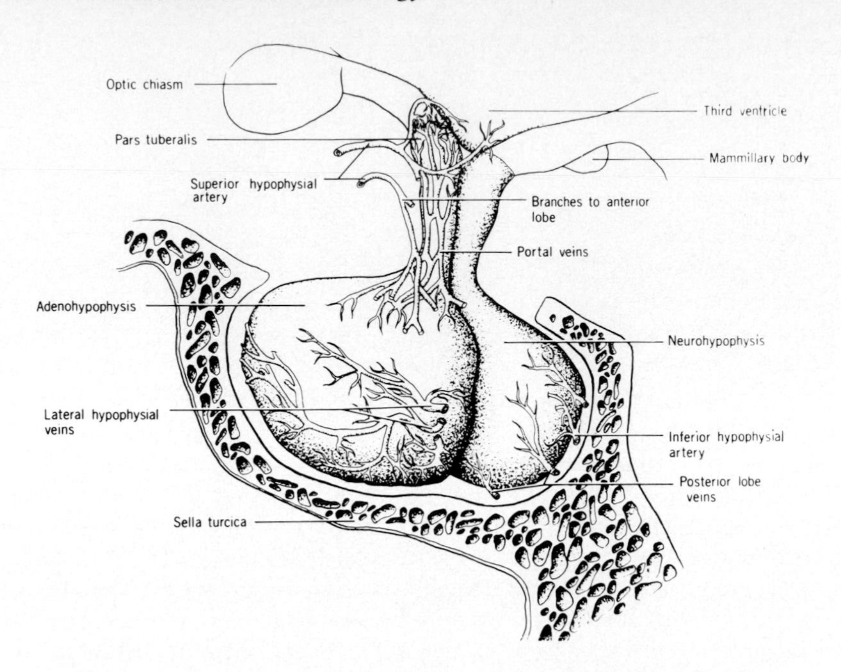

FIGURE 1. Relationship between the hypothalamus and the pituitary. Note the relationship between the blood supply and the various lobes of the pituitary gland. (Modified from a drawing by Frank Netter, CIBA Pharmaceutical Products, Division of CIBA-GEIGY Corporation, Summit, New Jersey. With permission.)

ANATOMY

Gross Anatomy

The anterior lobe of the mammalian pituitary gland, along with the intermediate and posterior lobe, is located directly below the hypothalamus in a cavity of the sphenoid bone termed the sella turcica (Figure 1). The gland is surrounded by the dura mater and is separated from the cranial cavity by the diaphragma sellae. The entire pituitary gland is approximately 10 mm × 13 mm × 6 mm and weighs about 500 mg in men and slightly more in women. The anterior lobe makes up about 75% of the gland in man. The pars intermedia is virtually absent in man and birds, but is prominent in reptiles, amphibians, fish, and some mammals.

Blood Supply

The blood supply to the anterior pituitary varies with the species, but in mammals it comes from two branches of the superior hypophysial artery (Figure 1). One branch from the superior hypophysial artery directly bathes the anterior pituitary, while the second branch enters at the level of the stalk of the median eminence, forming a capillary plexus. From this plexus, hypophysial portal vessels ultimately develop. The portal vessels collect blood from the capillary bed which is located between the hypothalamus and the median eminence and conduct the blood directly to the anterior and intermediate lobes of the pituitary. The portal vessels then develop into a second capillary plexus, bathing the cells of the anterior and the intermediate lobe of the pituitary. Venous drainage ultimately develops from this capillary plexus within the pituitary. The inferior hypophysial artery directly enters the posterior pituitary and forms a capillary network which ultimately gives rise to the venous drainage. The arterial blood which supplies the anterior and intermediate pituitary is separated from the arterial supply which perfuses the posterior pituitary.

The direction of blood flow in the vasculature of the hypothalamic-hypophysial system has been debated continually. Green and Harris[11] described flow toward the pituitary and for some time this was accepted by most investigators as the only direction of flow despite several reports of retrograde flow by Torok,[12,13] and later by Szentagothai et al.[14] Both anatomic and physiologic evidence have been presented in support of retrograde blood flow in the rat and monkey.[15,16] This backflow may be important in delivering his concentrations of pituitary hormones to the hypothalamus, making an involvement in an ultrashort feedback loop possible.

Innervation

Innervation of the anterior pituitary is limited to very fine nerve trunks which develop from the carotid plexus and accompany the arterial branches into the anterior pituitary. The nerves appear to be fine motor nerves which control the vasomotor function associated with the blood vasculature. The posterior lobe of the pituitary is very richly innervated. The latter nerves arise at the hypothalamic region and directly control the secretory rather than the vasomotor activity of the posterior pituitary gland.

Microscopic Anatomy

The pars anterior is composed of irregular cords of cells surrounded by extensive vascular channels. The channels are larger than capillaries and are lined by reticuloendothelium rather than "ordinary" endothelium. Cell types will be described in the chapters to follow on the anterior pituitary hormones, but are grouped basically into chromophobes and chromophils (Figure 2). Chromophobes are probably precursors of chromophils, the functional secretory cells of the anterior pituitary.

Cells are further classified as gonadotropes, which secrete LH and/or FSH, lactotropes which secrete PRL, somatotropes which secrete GH, thyrotropes which secrete TSH, and corticotropes which secrete ACTH.

COMPARATIVE ANATOMY (PHYLOGENY)

The pituitary gland is present in all vertebrate classes, but there are a number of unique phylogenetic changes. It does not appear that any of the protochordates have a pituitary gland.[6] A possible homologue of the adenohypophysis, Hatschek's pit, has been studied in the protochordate, Amphioxus. Hatschek's pit may have some olfactory function and it probably also secretes mucus into the oral cavity. The latter point is of interest since the glycoprotein pituitary hormones are chemically related to the mucoproteins of mucus.

It is the consensus that the adenohypophysis of vertebrates develops from exocrine tissue in the stomodeal roof.[6] The adenophypophysis was initially believed to have had an exocrine function and in phylogenetic development began to secrete directly into the blood. Several comprehensive reviews have been published which describe the evolutionary changes in the pituitary gland.[6,17]

The living cyclostomes, including lampreys (petromyzontids) and hagfish (myxinoids), have a relatively simple pituitary gland structure with distinct neural and glandular components.[6] Most of the adenohypophysial cells are chromophobic and it has not been determined whether the entire complement of hormones seen in more advanced vertebrates is present in cyclostomes.[18]

In myxinoids, two different cell types secreting an ACTH/MSH-like peptide (type 1) and a GH/PRL-like peptide (type 2) have been identified.[19] The myxinoid pituitary is poorly vascularized and hormone transport may take place in part through ependymal-like cells.[20]

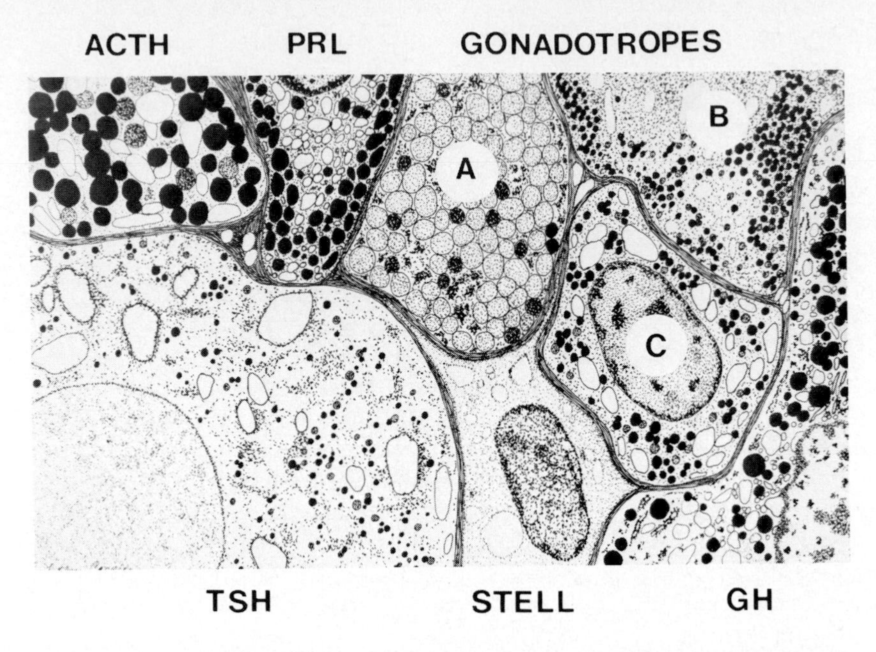

FIGURE 2. A diagram of the ultrastructure of the cells composing the anterior pituitary gland. The hormone secreted by each cell is shown in the margin. Corticotropes (ACTH-secreting cells) have granules of variable sizes and density and vesiculated endoplasmic reticulum. The lactotropes (PRL) secrete prolactin. Their granules are slightly larger and less regular than the somototropes. PRL cells are elongated with the granules often in a peripheral location. The gonadotropes show considerable variation. Gonadotrope A has large granules with variable density. The smaller granules are usually denser. Cells B and C are also gonadotropes. These cells are sparsely granulated and angular in shape. The thyrotropic cells (TSH) have small granules, 50 to 100 μm in diameter, or inconstant density. A somatotrope (GH) secretes growth hormone. These cells have large granules, active Golgi complexes and abundent endoplasmic reticulum. Stellate cells (STELL) are also interspersed among the other secretory cells of the anterior pituitary.

The adenohypophysis of petromyzontids is organized in a manner more similar to that of higher vertebrates than to that of myxinoids. Cells are arranged in cords separated by connective tissue containing capillaries.[6] Acidophils and basophils are present and several lines of evidence point to the existence of separate corticotropes, gonadotropes and somatotropes.[21-23] It has not been determined if TSH is present, but MSH is produced by the large intermediate lobe.[24-26]

The adenohypophysis of elasmobranchs (sharks, dogfish, skates, and rays) is different embryologically and anatomically from that of cyclostomes or of higher vertebrate lines.[6] The data indicate the presence of gonadotropins, TSH, ACTH, PRL, and GH in the elasmobrach adenohypophysis as well as MSH from the well developed intermediate lobe.[17,27-29] The median eminence is also well formed, as is the portal blood supply to the gland.

The teleost pituitary varies considerably among its members, but the bony fish shows in general, two distinct differences from vertebrates below them in evolution.[6] These differences include the loss of the median eminence and portal system external to the pituitary and the development of direct innervation of the pars distalis by hypothalamic neurosecretory fibers. The microscopic anatomy of the teleost pituitary has been extensively studied and the existence of lactotropes, corticotropes, somatotropes, gonadotropes, and thyrotropes has been documented.[6,18] The intermediate lobe is variable in size and secretes MSH.

The amphibian pituitary gland is similar to that of other tetrapods despite the early evolutionary diversion of this class.[6] The pituitary of frogs and toads (anurans) has a more conspicuous and developed portal system than the lungfishes have and the median eminence is more structurally specialized. In urodeles (newts and salamanders), the median eminence is less developed than in the anurans. The amphibian pituitary in both urodeles and anurans secretes prolactin, GH, TSH, ACTH, and has been reported to secrete either LH and FSH-like substances or even a single gonadotropin with LH and FSH-like properties.[30] There is an abundance of descriptions of amphibian pituitary morphologic cell types, but there is considerable controversy as to which cell type secretes a given hormone.[6]

The reptilian pituitary has similarities to both the amphibian and avian pituitary. This is compatible with the reptiles intermediate evolutionary position.[6] Crocodiles and turtles have a well developed pars intermedia and pars tuberalis and the pars distalis is divided into a cephalic and a caudal lobe. The pars tuberalis is absent in snakes and reduced or absent in lizards. Five cell-types have been described in reptiles, based on staining properties. Hormone products of the reptilian pituitary include PRH, GH, TSH, ACTH, and a single gonadotropin with LH and FSH activity.

The avian pituitary has been described in detail by Wingstrand[31] and Holmes and Ball.[6] Birds lack a pars intermedia. The cytology of the avian pars distalis has not been as extensively studied as that of the mammalian gland, but the basic structure in both seems to be similar between these classes. Two separate gonadotropins are found in the chicken[32] and are probably present in other birds. Despite the lack of an intermediate lobe, MSH is present, being located in the cephalic part of the pars distalis.[6]

EMBRYOLOGY

The pituitary gland is derived from two primordial anlagen that unite during development.[33] Thus, Rathke's pouch, an ectodermal outgrowth from the stomodeal depression, unites with the infundibular process, an outgrowth from the floor of the diencephalon. The front wall of Rathke's pouch thickens and becomes the anterior lobe, while the back wall develops into the intermediate lobe. The pars tuberalis develops from a pair of lobes which bud off from Rathke's pouch. The degree of development of these components varies markedly between species, consistent with the anatomic and functional differences of the mature gland in these species.

A small remnant of Rathke's pouch, the pharyngeal hypophysis, is left behind during development and can sometimes be found in the adult between the nasal septum and the pharyngeal tonsil. This structure is well vascularized, has some histologic resemblance to the anterior pituitary and has been reported to contain prolactin and growth hormone.

Secretory granules are found in the developing human pituitary by at least the end of the 1st trimester, but the development of secretory competence and feedback is not known.[36,37] The portal vessels are present in the 4th month, but the adult-like primary plexus develops somewhat later.[38] Anencephalic human fetuses have undeveloped adrenal cortices and, although adenohypophysial tissue is generally present, the hypothalamus is absent and therefore cannot stimulate pituitary secretion.[39]

Experimental data from laboratory animals suggest that the hypothalamo-hypophysial axis is functioning prior to the maturation of the portal system. Also, the adenohypophysis is importantly related to the fetal development of the adrenal, thyroid, gonads, and possibly other endocrine glands and tissues.[39,40]

ACKNOWLEDGMENTS

We wish to acknowledge the excellent art work of Ms. Joan Carey.

REFERENCES

1. **Legait, E. and Legait, H.,** Histophysiologie comparee de la pars intermedia de l'hypophyse, *Arch. Biol.,* 75, 497, 1964.
2. **Midgley, A. R.,** Human pituitary LH: an immunohistochemical study, *J. Histochem. Cytochem.,* 14, 159, 1966.
3. **Allanson, M., Foster, C. L., and Menzies, G.,** Some observations on the cytology of the adenohypophysis of the non-parous female rabbit, *Q. J. Microsc. Sci.,* 100, 463, 1959.
4. **Holmes, R. L.,** The pituitary gland of the female ferret, *J. Endocrinol.,* 20, 48, 1960.
5. **Cameron, E. and Foster, C. L.,** Some light- and electron-microscopical observations on the pars tuberalis of the pituitary gland of the rabbit, *J. Endocrinol.,* 54, 505, 1972.
6. **Holmes, L. and Ball, N. J.,** *The Pituitary Gland — A Comparative Account,* Cambridge University Press, London, 1974.
7. **Aschner, B.,** Über die Funktion der Hypophyse, *Pflügers Arch.,* 146, 1, 1912.
8. **Smith, P. E.,** Ablation and transplantation of the hypophysis in the rat, *Anat. Rec.,* 32, 221, 1926.
9. **Smith, P. E.,** The disabilities caused by hypophysectomy and their repair. The tuberal (hypothalamic) syndrome in the rat, *J.A.M.A.,* 88, 1958, 1927.
10. **Smith, P. E.,** Hypophysectomy and a replacement therapy in the rat, *Am. J. Anat.,* 45, 205, 1930.
11. **Green, J. D. and Harris, G. W.,** Observation of the hypophysio-portal vessels of the living rat, *J. Physiol.,* 108, 359, 1949.
12. **Rorok, B.,** Lebendbeobachtung des hypophysenkreislaufes an Hunden, *Acta Morphol. Acad. Sci. Hung.,* 4, 83, 1954.
13. **Torok, B.,** Structure of the vascular connections of the hypothalamo-hypophysial region, *Acta Anat.,* 59, 84, 1964.
14. **Szentagothai, J., Flerko, B., Mess, B., and Halasz, B.,** Hypothalamic control of the anterior pituitary, *Akademiai Kiado, (Budapest),* 81, 1962.
15. **Bergland, R. M. and Page, R. B.,** Can the pituitary secrete directly to the brain? (Affirmative anatomical evidence), *Endocrinology,* 102, 1325, 1978.
16. **Oliver, C., Mical, R. S., and Porter, J. C.,** Hypothalamic-pituitary vasculature: evidence for retrograde blood flow in the pituitary stalk, *Endocrinology,* 101, 598, 1977.
17. **Wingstrand, K. G.,** Comparative anatomy and evolution of the hypophysis, in *The Pituitary Gland,* Harris, G. W. and Donovan, B. T., Eds., University of California Press, Berkeley, 1966, 2, 59.
18. **Ball, J. N. and Baker, B. I.,** The pituitary gland: anatomy and histo-physiology, in *Fish Physiology,* Vol. 2, Hoar, W. S. and Randall, D. J., Eds., Academic Press, New York, 1969, 1.
19. **Fernholm, B.,** The ultrastructure of the adenohypophysis of Myxine glutinosa, *Z. Zellforsch. Mikrosk. Anat.,* 132, 451, 1972.
20. **Fernholm, B. and Olsson, R.,** A cytopharmacological study of the Myxine adenohypophysis, *Gen. Comp. Endocrinol.,* 13, 336, 1969.
21. **Honma, Y.,** Some evolutionary aspects of the morphology and role of the adenohypophysis in fishes, *Gunma Symp. Endocrinol.,* 6, 19, 1965.
22. **Larsen, L. O.,** Effects of hypophysectomy in the cyclostome, *lampetra fluviatilis* (L.) Gray, *Gen. Comp. Endocrinol.,* 5, 16, 1965.
23. **Molnar, B. and Szabo, Zs.,** Histological study of the hypophysis of the Transylvanian lamprey, *Acta Biol. Acad. Sci. Hung.,* 19, 373, 1968.
24. **van Oordt, P. G. W. J.,** The analysis and identification of the hormone-producing cells of the adenohypophysis, in *Perspectives in Endocrinology,* Barrington, E. J. W. and Jorgensen, C. B., Eds., Academic Press, New York, 1968, 405.
25. **Larsen, L. O. and Rothwell, B.,** Adenohypophysis, in *The Biology of Lampreys,* Vol. 2, Hardisty, M. W. and Potter, I. C., Eds., Academic Press, New York, 1972, 1.
26. **Pickering, A. D.,** Effects of hypophysectomy on the activity of the endostyle and thyroid gland in the larval and adult river lamprey, *Gen. Comp. Endocrinol.,* 18, 335, 1972.
27. **Scanes, C. G., Dobson, D., Follett, B. K., and Dodd, J. M.,** Gonadotrophic activity in the pituitary gland of the dogfish, *J. Endocrinol.,* 54, 343, 1972.
28. **Sage, M. and Bern, H. A.,** Assay of prolactin in vertebrate pituitaries by its dispersion of xanthophore pitment in the telecost, *J. Exp. Zool.,* 180, 169, 1972.
29. **deRoos, R. and deRoos, C. C.,** Presence of corticotropin activity in the pituitary gland of chondrichthyean fish, *Gen. Comp. Endocrinol.,* 9, 267, 1967.
30. **van Oordt, P. G. W. J. and DeKort, E. J. M.,** Functions of gonadotropins in adult male amphibians, *Colloq. Int. C.N.R.S., (Paris),* 177, 345, 1969.
31. **Wingstrand, K. G.,** *The Structure and Development of the Avian Pituitary,* Gleerup, London, 1951.
32. **Hartree, A. S. and Cunningham, F. J.,** Purification of chicken pituitary follicle-stimulating hormone and luteinizing hormone, *J. Endocrinol.,* 43, 609, 1969.

33. **Arey, L. B.,** The mouth and pharynx, in *Developmental Anatomy — A Textbook and Laboratory Manual of Embryology,* W. B. Saunders, Philadelphia, 1965, 213.
34. **Boyd, J. D.,** Observations on the human pharyngeal hypophysis, *J. Endocrinol.,* 14, 66, 1956.
35. **McGrath, P.,** Prolactin activity and human growth hormone in pharyngeal hypophysis from embalmed cadavers, *J. Endocrinol.,* 42, 205, 1968.
36. **Siler-Khodr, T. M., Morgenstern, L. L., and Greenwood, F. C.,** Hormone synthesis and release from human fetal adenohypophyses in vitro, *J. Clin. Endocriol. Metab.,* 39, 891, 1974.
37. **Grumbach, M. M. and Kaplan, S. L.,** Fetal pituitary hormones and the maturation of central nervous system regulation of anterior pituitary function, in *Modern Perinatal Medicine,* Gluck, L., Ed., Year Book Medical Publishing, Chicago, 1974, 247.
38. **Nieminera, K.,** Pituitary, neonate, *Acta Paediatr.,* 39, 315, 1950.
39. **Nakai, T., Kigawa, T., and Sakamoto, S.,** 3H-Leucine uptake of hypothalamic nuclei in fetal male rats and its fluctuation after castration, *Endocrinology (Japan),* 18, 353, 1971.
40. **Jost, A., DuPouy, J. P., and Gelosos-Meyer, A.,** Hypothalamo-hypophyseal relationships in the fetus, in *The Hypothalamus,* Martini, L., Motta, M., and Fraschini, F., Eds., Academic Press, New York, 605, 1970.

GROWTH HORMONE SECRETION AND NEUROENDOCRINE REGULATION

William E. Sonntag, Lloyd J. Forman, Nobuhiro Miki, and Joseph Meites

INTRODUCTION

There have been many advances in our understanding of the regulation of growth hormone (GH) secretion. Of primary importance is the knowledge that GH secretion is controlled primarily by hypophysiotropic hormones and neurotransmitters in the hypothalamus. Early experiments, using hypothalamic extracts, provided evidence for the existence of both a growth hormone releasing factor (GH-RF) and a GH release inhibiting factor (GH-RIF). The structure of GH-RIF or somatostatin has been characterized as a tetradecapeptide, but the structure of GH-RF has not yet been elucidated.

The synthesis, metabolism, and release of hypothalamic hormones are believed to be regulated by a number of neurotransmitters, including dopamine, norepinephrine, serotonin, etc. These are believed to modulate the release of hypothalamic GH-RF and somatostatin, thereby influencing pituitary GH secretion. The recent discovery of endogenous opioid peptides also in the brain suggests another level of control since the peptides can influence GH release, by acting on hypothalamic neurotransmitters or perhaps by acting directly on somatostatin or GH-RF secreting neurons.

Many other factors have been shown to influence GH release, although their mechanisms of action are not entirely clear. These include thyroid, gonadal, and adrenal hormones which may directly or indirectly influence GH synthesis or release by the pituitary or act via the hypothalmic hormones or neurotransmitters. Physiologic stimuli such as stress, exercise, sleep, and diet also can influence the secretion of GH via the hypothalamus.

For several years it has been recognized that the release of GH, as well as many other pituitary hormones, does not occur in a steady state manner. In humans, it was known that a marked surge in GH occurs during sleep. In rats, there was also evidence for large fluctuations in GH release, but the specific ultradian pattern was not recognized until serial blood samples were obtained from unanesthetized male rats. In this species, pulsatile serum GH concentrations range from less than 10 ng/mℓ to greater than 600 ng/mℓ within a period of 3.3 hr. GH is also secreted in an episodic manner in female rats, but differs from the male in that the amplitude is lower and the episodic release occurs more frequently. It is unknown if the sex related differences in the periodicity of GH secretion are influenced by gonadal steroids or are related to sexual differentiation of the brain resulting from neonatal exposure to steroid hormones. The physiologic significance of the large pulses in GH release is poorly understood.

It is generally accepted that the episodic release of GH is regulated by concomitant secretion of somatostatin and a putative GHRF, which in turn are regulated by neurotransmitters. Although there is much information on the effects of neurotransmitter agonists and antagonists on GH release, relatively little is known about the factors that regulate synthesis, metabolism, and release of hypothalamic peptides. Much of the contradictory data on the influence of neuropeptides and neurotransmitters on GH release stems from the difficulty in measuring physiologically meaningful changes in the hypothalamic peptides that regulate GH secretion.

RADIOIMMUNOASSAY OF RAT GROWTH HORMONE

Introduction

Prior to the development of a radioimmunoassay (RIA) for GH, the most sensitive bioassay measured GH activity in terms of change in width of the tibial epiphyseal growth plate in young hypophysectomized rats.[1,2] Even this sensitive bioassay was unable to detect GH concentrations less than 20 μg, which precluded analysis of blood samples from individual animals. The development of a sensitive RIA for GH that can measure hormone concentrations in blood samples as small as 200 pg provided a great advance for studies of the neuroendocrine regulation of GH.

Rat GH is usually measured by RIA using reagents provided by the National Institute of Arthritis, Metabolism and Digestive Diseases (NIAMDD). Generally, this assay is similar to RIAs for other anterior pituitary hormones, except that several precautions must be taken to insure the validity of the assay. In addition, GH is sensitive to oxidizing agents, such a chloramine T, and care must be taken to preserve immunoreactivity during iodination.

Iodination

Classically, GH has been radiolabeled using the chloramine T method and purified on Sephadex G-100.[3] However, we have found that a modification of the lactoperoxidase-glucose-oxidase method[4,5] is superior, due to the specificity of lactoperoxidase in iodinating tyrosine and the low amount of damage it causes to the hormone. After the iodination is complete, we find it preferable to stop the reaction by addition of 200 mg AG 1 × 10, 200 to 400 mesh (BioRad®, Richmond, Calif.) to absorb free isotope. The supernatant is chromatographed on Sephacryl S-200®, superfine (Pharmacia, Piscataway, N.J.), which has superior resolution, compared with Sephadex G-100. If 1.5 mℓ fractions are collected from a 1.5 × 30 cm column, the aggregate or damaged peak occurs around fractions 8 to 12 and the immunoreactive GH peak occurs around fraction 25. The free isotope peak trails around fraction 40, but does not exceed 10,000 cpm/5 μℓ due to prior absorption. The peak and the subsequent two fractions remain stable at 4°C for a minimum of 10 days and repurification of these fractions shows only a slight increase in damaged or aggregated GH.

Standard and Unknown Samples

Monkey anti-rat GH antibody (S-4) usually binds 50 to 60% of labeled GH at 1 to 6,000 dilution and GH-RP-1 produces excellent competition in a range of 0.16 ng to 5.0 ng/tube. Serum proteins may interfere with the binding of the antibody to the antigen or degrade the labeled GH. These effects must be assessed to make accurate comparisons with unknown samples. GH free plasma (obtained from hypophysectomized rats or by washing normal male serum with 20% charcoal) is added to the standard tubes in a volume comparable to that of the unknown sample to be pipetted. Since we usually run 10 and 30 μℓ aliquots of unknown plasma, three standard curves must be constructed (each with 0, 10, or 30 μℓ of GH free serum) and each unknown is analyzed with the appropriate standard curve. Failure to compare the unknowns to the appropriate standard may lead to artificially elevated GH concentrations.

Separation of Free and Bound Hormone

Free and bound GH may be separated using second antibody (goat anti-monkey γ-globulin), but we find the addition of 1 mg of Protein A bound to *Staphylococcus aureus* cells (Enzyme Center, Boston, Mass.) to be more efficien t. Using the latter technique, precipitation of bound hormone is complete within 30 min. After the addition of 2 mℓ of cold saline, all tubes are centrifuged and the supernatant aspirated. The precipitate is then counted in a γ-spectrophotometer.

Table 1
BIOLOGIC ACTIONS OF GROWTH HORMONES

1. Carbohydrate metabolism
   a. Utilization of glucose is decreased
   b. Glycogen synthesis is decreased
   c. Diabetogenic effect is increased
2. Lipid metabolism
   a. Lipogenesis is retarded
   b. Mobilization of fatty acids is stimulated without increasing fatty acid oxidation
3. Protein metabolism
   a. Transport of amino acids is stimulated
   b. Synthesis of protein is promoted
4. Electrolyte balance
   a. Nitrogen, sodium, potassium, and phosphorus are retained
   b. Excretion of calcium is increased
5. Connective tissue
   a. Collagen synthesis and turnover are increased
   b. Excretion of hydroxyproline is increased
6. Kidney
   a. Renal plasma flow and glomerular filtration rate are increased
   b. Compensatory renal hypertrophy is promoted

STRUCTURE AND FUNCTION OF GROWTH HORMONE

Introduction

GH has been investigated by numerous scientists and it has been shown that it has an important role in many metabolic functions. Major effects are listed in Table 1 and are briefly described in this section.

There is increasing evidence that at least part of the metabolic effects of GH are mediated by another group of hormones, the somatomedins, which are produced in the liver, kidney, and probably other tissues. The somatomedins are small molecular weight peptides which stimulate thymidine uptake in liver and sulfate incorporation into cartilage. Somatomedins also exhibit insulin-like effects.[6,7]

Structure of Growth Hormone

GHs in mammals are single chain polypeptides, composed solely of amino acids. The amino acid composition is very similar among the mammalian species as are the total number of amino acid residues. Canine GH has the greatest total number of amino acid residues (194 to 196), while human and sheep GH have 191 amino acid residues. Monkey GH has 192 residues and rat GH has the smallest number of residues (178).[8] It is generally accepted that these hormones are fairly uniform in molecular weight, ranging from 20,500 daltons for human GH to 26,000 for bovine GH.[9]

Function of Growth Hormone

Carbohydrate Metabolism

GH is a potent diabetogenic agent, producing hyperglycemia and an insensitivity to elevated levels of insulin. Several investigators have observed changes in carbohydrate metabolism after administration of GH or after endogenous secretion of GH. Weil[10] described the response of exogenous GH as triphasic. Initially, there is a transient hypoglycemia which may be attributed to an increase in fatty acid metabolism. In the second phase glycolysis and glycogenesis are inhibited due to feedback by the degradation products of fatty acid metabolism and therefore the concentration of glucose in the circulation begins to rise. In the third phase, the increased concentrations of glucose are magnified, resulting in a marked release of insulin.

As far as the role of endogenous GH is concerned, Rabinowitz et al.[11,12] have reported that after feeding, insulin secretion is increased whereas the level of GH is reduced. The interaction between insulin and GH promotes glucose uptake and the formation of glycogen and triglycerides. During the next phase, insulin levels decline whereas those of GH begin to rise. Protein synthesis is promoted during this period and excess storage is prevented. In the final phase, the secretion of GH increases again whereas insulin drops to basal levels. GH then provides an energy source in the form of readily available glucose and induces mobilization of fatty acids.

The diabetogenic nature of endogenously secreted GH has been shown by Schnure and Lipman.[13] These investigators reported a marked decline in glucose tolerance 90 min after the onset of sleep when GH levels are elevated. It is clear that GH plays an important role in carbohydrate metabolism, but this action cannot be viewed in isolation from its effect on lipid and protein metabolism.

Lipid Metabolism

Lipogenesis is retarded by GH. Hypophysectomized rats treated with ovine GH for four days show a reduction in the lipid content of epididymal and omental adipose tissue as compared to nontreated hypophysectomized rats.[14] Chronic administration of GH results in inhibition of glyceride synthesis and decreased body fat content.[15] Acute GH treatment of fed, intact or hypophysectomized rats decreases fatty acid synthesis in both carcass and liver. A similar effect is not observed in starved rats, since lipogenesis is already reduced in these animals.

Growth hormone facilitates mobilization of fatty acids when administered to fasted intact and hypophysectomized animals.[16] Treatment of hypophysectomized rats with GH produces a significant release of free fatty acids by epididymal adipose tissue.[17,18] Feeding reduces the magnitude of this response, but does not abolish it completely.[16]

The ability of GH to promote mobilization of free fatty acids when administered in vitro is not nearly as striking as its in vivo effect. The release of fatty acids from tissue in vitro requires high concentrations of GH, and it suggests that GH does not stimulate fatty acid mobilization by a direct action on adipose tissue.[16,19]

Early experiments suggested that GH-stimulated fatty acid oxidation, as indicated by a decrease in the respiratory quotient, increases ketogenesis and a decrease in body fat. A sensitive technique, which recognizes changes in fatty acid oxidation, is the measurement of respiratory $C^{14}O_2$ from animals intravenously injected with C^{14} palmitate.[16] Growth hormone administration fails to elicit a change in $C^{14}O_2$ production in fasted or fed hypophysectomized rats,[20] unanesthetized dogs,[21] or human diabetic subjects.[22] In vivo or in vitro administration of GH does not stimulate the oxidation of palmitate or acetate by rat liver slices or kidney homogenates.[23-25] Furthermore, neither hypophysectomy nor hypophysectomy with GH replacement produces changes in the oxidation of palmitate-C^{14} by isolated rat diaphragm.

It is possible that any changes in fat content, ketogenesis or respiratory quotient seen with GH administration are due to the inhibition of lipogenesis, and also to an increased supply of free fatty acids to tissues resulting from increased fatty acid mobilization rather than to stimulation of fatty acid oxidation per se.

Protein Metabolism

Growth hormone promotes protein synthesis, as indicated by decreased excretion of nitrogen subsequent to GH administration. More specifically, using a radioactively labeled, nonmetabolizable amino acid (α-aminoisobutyric acid-C^{14}; AIB-C^{14}), Noall et al.[26] were able to show that GH can stimulate amino acid transfer from the extracellular to the intracellular compartment. Extending this observation, Riggs and Walker[27] reported that hypophysectomy diminishes the incorporation of AIB-C^{14} into muscle, and this effect can be reversed by the administration of bovine GH.

Employing in vitro experiments, Kostyo et al.[28] found that excised diaphragm from hypophysectomized rats accumulates less AIB-C^{14} against a concentration gradient than does tissue from intact rats. Addition of either bovine or simian GH to the preparations increases the transport of AIB-C^{14} into the intracellular compartment. The transport induced by GH is equivalent to that observed in diaphragms removed from intact rats. Similarly, diaphragms from hypophysectomized rats pretreated with GH prior to sacrifice show higher intracellular levels of AIB-C^{14} after in vitro incubation in AIB-C^{14} than the diaphragms of hypophysectomized rats that are not pretreated with GH.[29]

Growth hormone can increase the intracellular transport of naturally occurring amino acids, such as glycine, alanine, serine, threonine, proline, histidine, tryptophan, glutamine, and asparagine. In addition, the diminished total amino acid content of cartilage from hypophysectomized rats is replenished in hypophysectomized rats treated with GH. Growth hormone stimulates the in vitro incorporation of labeled leucine and glycine into protein in diaphragms removed from hypophysectomzed rats. A similar response is observed in preparations of the levator ani muscle.[30]

It is clear that GH promotes the transport of naturally occurring amino acids into the cell and stimulates protein synthesis. Whether these two phenomena occur independently or are directly related remains to be established.

Other Effects of Growth Hormone

While GH administration results in the retention of minerals, such as sodium, potassium, and phosphorus, it produces an increased excretion of calcium as well as increased calcium absorption from the intestine.[16,19] This hypercalciuria may be mediated indirectly, through an effect of GH on the parathyroid gland or by the rise in plasma phosphorus also produced by GH administration.[31] The elevation of plasma phosphorus levels have been shown to be the result of an increase in kidney tubular phosphate reabsorption.[32]

Growth hormone produces an increase in urinary hydroxyproline. Jasin et al.[33] suggested that this increase represents the formation of fibrous collagen from a soluble collagen precursor. They also noted that urinary hydroxyproline levels are high in actively growing young children, supporting the growth promoting effect of GH.

The kidney is markedly affected by GH. The renal plasma flow and glomerular filtration rate are increased. Growth hormone also promotes compensatory renal hypertrophy which is absent in hypophysectomized rats.[16]

NEUROPEPTIDES THAT INFLUENCE GROWTH HORMONE

Somatostatin and Growth Hormone Releasing Factor

Introduction

Early evidence suggested the existence of a hypothalamic substance that can inhibit GH release by rat pituitary cells in vitro.[34] A tetradecapeptide which inhibits GH release was subsequently isolated by Guillemin and co-workers[35] and named growth hormone release inhibiting hormone, or somatostatin. Both synthetic and ovine somatostatin inhibit the release of GH by rat pituitary cells in vitro, and inhibit the rise in GH after the injection of sodium pentobarbital in vivo.[36]

Somatostatin inhibits the release of GH and TSH in response to several pharmacologic and physiologic stimuli.[37] In addition, chronic administration of somatostatin decreases pituitary and plasma GH.[38] Passive immunization with antisera against somatostatin demonstrates the physiologic role of this hormone in the control of GH release. Somatostatin antiserum increases basal levels of GH, reverses the inhibition of GH release by starvation or electric shock in rats, and enhances TRH mediated

TSH secretion.[39-44] Analysis of blood serial samples reveals that somatostatin antiserum increases trough GH levels, but may not affect the pulsatile nature of GH release.[45] This is convincing evidence for the existence of a GH-releasing factor (GH-RF) which may also control the release of GH.

Our laboratory proposed the existence of a GHRF in 1964 when we found that hypothalamic extracts increase the release of GH from incubated rat pituitaries in a dose-related manner.[46] GHRF is believed to be present in the ventromedial nucleus (VMN), since it has been shown that electrical stimulation of this area increases GH release whereas lesions of this area decrease GH release and result in growth retardation.[47,48] Thus, it seems likely that intermittent secretion of somatostatin may modulate the effect of a putative GHRF on GH release.

Localization

Using both RIA and bioassay, somatostatin has been localized in the median eminence, arcuate nucleus, medial preoptic area, and periventricular nucleus of the rat hypothalamus.[50] Somatostatin immunoreactivity is also found in the VMN, amygdala, mammillary bodies, and olfactory tubercle.[51-54] The inability to detect somatostatin bioactivity in the VMN is hypothesized to result from high concentrations of GHRF in this area which interfere with the somatostatin bioassay.[51]

Using immunocytochemical methods, somatostatin containing fibers have been localized in the external zone of the median eminence and VMN of guinea pigs.[55] Somatostatin nerve fibers may occur in the median eminence, forming part of the tuberoinfundibular tract.[56,57] Although perikarya were not localized in the same study, somatostatin fibers were generally localized in the arcuate, VMN, and medial basal area of the hypothalamus. Somatostatin has also been localized in the nerve endings of the organum vasculosum of the lamina terminalis (OVLT) of the rat in close proximity to the capillary network.[58] Somatostatin perikarya have been localized in the periventricular and preoptic regions of the rat hypothalamus.[59-61]

These anatomic data on the localization of somatostatin cell bodies are supported by evidence indicating that lesions of the preoptic-anterior hypothalamic area increase plasma GH whereas stimulation of this area increases somatostatin concentrations in portal blood and decreases plasma GH concentrations.[62-64]

There is increasing evidence that somatostatin is synthesized as a prohormone and is enzymatically cleaved to the mature peptide during axonal transport to the median eminence. Two higher molecular weight forms of the hormone have been reported in hypothalamic extracts[65] and there are indications that they may be released into portal blood. There is also evidence for somatostatin species in portal blood that have altered ionic charges.[66] Although hypothalamic somatostatin does not appear to be a homologous peptide, the biologic significance of the different somatostatin molecules has not been determined.

Opioid Peptides

The existence of opioid receptors in the brain has been suggested for many years by the profound analgesic and behavioral effects of plant opioid alkaloids on the mammalian central nervous system. Endocrine effects of morphine also have been suspected, based on observations of high infertility among narcotic addicts,[67-69] and evidence that morphine can initiate lactation in estrogen-primed rats.[70] Early work with morphine showed that it was a potent stimulator of GH release in many species. The recent discovery of endogenous opioid peptides and opioid receptors in the brain strongly suggest that they are involved in the neuroendocrine control of secretion of anterior pituitary hormones, including GH.

Intraventricular or systemic administration of morphine and opioid peptides, such as β-endorphin and met^5-enkephalin, can induce rapid increases in plasma GH in rats.[71-74] β-endorphin is reported to be 500 to 2000 times more potent than met^5-enkephalin.[75]

The GH stimulating activities of the opioid peptides are blocked by concomitant injection of naloxone, a specific opioid receptor antagonist.[73,74,76] The first evidence that endogenous opioid peptides have a physiologic role in the regulation of anterior pituitary hormone release was provided by the reports that naloxone alone can reduce basal serum GH and prolactin and elevate serum luteinizing hormone (LH) and follicle stimulating hormone (FSH) levels.[74,76]

The above results have been confirmed and extended by a number of investigators, although the data for GH are controversial. Both naloxone and naltrexone are reported to decrease basal serum GH levels[74,76,77] whereas neither of these drugs is known to have any effect on pulsatile GH secretion in unanesthetized, unrestrained rats.[78,79] However, we have recently found that naloxone can inhibit the GH surge induced by suckling in post partum lactating rats, suggesting that, at least under some circumstances, endogenous opioid peptides participate in the physiologic regulation of GH.[214]

In human subjects, enkephalin analogues have been found to stimulate GH release,[80] whereas naloxone can inhibit GH release induced by certain stimuli. Naloxone greatly diminishes GH release induced by arginine infusion or exercise stress, but does not influence basal GH or GH release induced by apomorphine, L-DOPA, insulin, hypoglycemia, or sleep.[78,81-84] These findings suggest that the endogenous opioid peptides have only a minor role in GH secretion in humans. However, the doses of naloxone used in human studies usually have been lower (based on the recommended dose of 0.4 mg for reversal of narcotic overdosage), than those used in animal studies (0.2 to 20.0 mg/kg), and the timing of naloxone injections has been variable. Therefore it is possible that higher doses of naloxone may have different effects on GH release than those reported.

Opioid peptides do not act directly on the anterior pituitary since they do not influence in vitro release of GH.[75,76] The opiate induced increase in GH release also does not appear to be mediated through inhibition of hypothalamic somatostatin, since opiates can stimulate GH release in rats passively immunized with antiserum to somatostatin.[72,85]

There is some evidence that opiate effects are mediated via hypothalamic neurotransmitters, which in turn can regulate the release of hypothalamic hormones into the portal vessels. Met^5-enkephalin and β-endorphin decrease dopamine and norepinephrine turnover in the median eminence[86-88] whereas serotonin turnover is increased by acute administration of morphine or β-endorphin.[89-91] Since both dopamine and norepinephrine stimulate GH release, it is unlikely that the opiate induced increase in GH is mediated through these neurotransmitters.

Although serotonin (5-HT) turnover is increased by β-endorphin, neither the 5-HT synthesis inhibitor, parachlorophenylalanine (PCPA), nor the 5-HT receptor blocker, metergoline, blocks GH release induced by morphine[92] or enkephalin analogs.[93] The GH releasing effect of an enkephalin analog is inhibited by the α-adrenergic receptor blocker, phenoxybenzamine, and by the norepinephrine synthesis inhibitor, diethyldithiocarbamate.[94] Stimulation of GH by morphine is not affected by the α-adrenergic receptor blocker, prazosin, or the catecholamine synthesis inhibitor, α-methyl-parathyrosine in rats.[77,92] Thus, the precise mechanism through which opioid peptides increase GH release remains unclear.

There is controversy about cholinergic involvement in the GH release induced by morphin or the enkephalins. In dogs, enkephalin analogs increase GH release via the cholinergic system,[93] but in rats the morphine effect on GH release is reported to be inhibited by cholinergic drugs.[77] Further study is necessary to determine the physiologic role and mechanism of brain opiates on GH secretion.

Substance P

Substance P is a decapeptide widely distributed in the brain and spinal cord. It may be important in the perception of pain and in the regulation of neuroendocrine functions.[95]

The effect of substance P on GH release is unclear since the effect appears to be dependent on the route of administration and the interaction with other peptides. Injection of substance P into the lateral ventricle of urethane-anesthetized rats decreases serum GH levels. Since this effect can be abolished by systemic injection of somatostatin antiserum, it may be concluded that substance P decreases GH by stimulating the secretion of somatostatin.[85] The same study indicates that substance P can potentiate the increase in GH resulting from intraventricular injection of β-endorphin. Administration of the opioid antagonist, naloxone, prevents the rise in GH produced by β-endorphin and substance P. It is hypothesized that substance P may modulate the opiate induced release of GH, possibly at a central level, since systemic injections of antiserum to substance P or somatostatin cannot antagonize the synergistic effect of substance P on the morphine-induced release of GH.

Contrary to the above observations, there are reports which suggest that intravenous administration of substance P to urethane-anesthetized rats increases plasma GH concentrations.[96,97] Although the opioid antagonist, naloxone, is ineffective in blocking this increase, the antihistaminergic drug, diphenhydramine, can inhibit the GH rise. This suggests that substance P may increase GH via a central histaminergic mechanism in urethane-anesthetized rats.[96]

Thyrotropin Releasing Hormone

The tripeptide, thyrotropin releasing hormone (TRH), can release GH in vitro in cows and sheep,[98,99] although in other species the action of TRH is controversial. In intact rats and man, TRH does not increase GH consistently, and it has been proposed that TRH can only increase GH under specific pathologic conditions in these species. If the pituitary is transplanted beneath the kidney capsule, intravenous administration of TRH can stimulate both the biosynthesis and release of GH.[100] This has led to the proposal that TRH has the capacity to increase GH, but the response may be tonically suppressed by hypothalamic hormones.

Bombesin

Bombesin was initially isolated from amphibian skin[101] and later reported to be present in mammalian brain.[102] Bombesin is a tetradecapeptide, and its role as a central nervous system neurotransmitter is currently under investigation.[95] Both intravenous and intracisternal administration of bombesin to steroid-primed male rats produces a considerable rise in plasma GH, although intravenous injection is more effective. The stimulatory effect of bombesin on GH secretion is blunted by the specific opioid antagonist, naloxone, as well as by somatostatin. Since bombesin is not able to increase the release of GH from rat pituitaries cultured in vitro,[102] it is hypothesized that bombesin may stimulate the release of GH via a central mechanism involving the endogenous opioid peptides.

Neurotensin

Neurotensin is a tridecapeptide found in the hypothalamus.[103] Intravenous injection of this putative neurotransmitter stimulates the release of GH in normal and estrogen-progesterone primed male rats.[96] The increase in GH is antagonized by the antihistaminergic drug, diphenhydramine. Since the addition of neurotensin to rat pituitaries cultured in vitro does not stimulate the release of GH,[96] it is suggested that the neurotensininduced release of GH may be mediated by histamine, at a central level.

Vasopressin

Vasopressin elicites the release of GH in rats[104] and humans,[105] however, the mechanism by which vasopressin promotes GH secretion varies in each of these species. In the rat, the β-adrenergic antagonist, propranolol, blocks the effect of vasopressin on GH secretion. In humans, the α-adrenergic antagonist, phentolamine, suppresses the vasopressin-induced release of GH. Vasopressin can directly stimulate GH release from the pituitary.[106] However, rats with hereditary vasopressin deficiency appear to have normal plasma GH levels. In summary, vasopressin increases circulating levels of GH via a central adrenergic mechanism which may be species dependent, and it may also stimulate the release of GH from the pituitary in vitro.

Vasoactive Intestinal Polypeptide

Vasoactive intestinal polypeptide (VIP) is present in the hypothalamus, brain, and gut in relatively high concentrations.[107] The peptide is present in hypophyseal portal blood, suggesting that it may have a role in the control of anterior pituitary function.[108] Intraventricular injection of VIP, at concentrations ranging from 4 to 500 ng, stimulates the release of GH from the pituitary.[109] This effect may be centrally mediated since VIP has no effect on GH release from the pituitary in vitro.

Summary

Many neuropeptides can influence the secretion of GH. Caution must be exercised in interpreting these data. The effects of many peptides may be dependent on the anesthetic administered, dose of the peptide, the route of administration, or nonspecific stress. Somatostatin, which inhibits the release of GH when administered intravenously, stimulates the release of GH when administered intraventricularly.[110] Although this increase may be related to ultrashort loop feedback on the release of somatostatin, it indicates some of the problems in interpreting data. Many of these peptides may participate in the regulation of GH secretion under physiologic conditions whereas others may be involved in a GH response to nonphysiologic conditions.

PUTATIVE NEUROTRANSMITTERS THAT INFLUENCE GROWTH HORMONE

Introduction

The high concentrations of biogenic amines in the hypothalamus have led to extensive studies on their role in GH secretion. Dopamine, norepinephrine and serotonin (5-hydroxytryptamine, 5-HT) have an important role in the neural regulation of GH secretion in both animals and man. These monoamines appear to act at the hypothalamic level to alter the release of somatostatin and/or GH-RF, thereby influencing GH release from the anterior pituitary gland. A number of other putative neurotransmitters influence GH secretion.

Dopamine and Norepinephrine

Dopamine and norepinephrine promote release of GH as measured by bioassay. Intraventricular administraton of either of these drugs produces a depletion of pituitary GH content in rats.[111] L-DOPA also increases basal GH levels[112] and enhances GH release induced by suckling in post partum lactating rats.[113] The effects are abolished by pretreatment with the catecholamine synthesis inhibitor, α-methyl-para-tyrosine (αmpt).[114] Since dopamine can be converted into norepinephrine, it is unclear if the major effect of dopamine is mediated by activation of dopamine receptors or because of conversion to norepinephrine.

By the use of single samples and assay of GH by RIA, it is found that dopamine and its agonists increase GH release in the rat. Two dopamine receptor agonists, apomorphine and piribedil, increase plasma GH in male rats.[115] Apomorphine also reverses the inhibition of GH induced by haloperidol, a dopamine receptor blocker. Moreoever, plasma GH release is stimulated by intraventricular injections of either dopamine or piribedil, or by systemic administration of dopamine or apomorphine in ovariectomized or ovariectomized-estrogen-progesterone-primed rats.[116] Clonidine, an α-adrenergic receptor agonist, stimulates GH release when injected intraventricularly. This increase is blocked by pretreatment with phenoxybenzamine, an α-adrenergic receptor blocker.[117] Thus, both dopamine and norepinephrine appear to stimulate GH release, as indicated by assay of single blood samples.

The recent development of serial blood sampling by cannulation of the jugular vein reveals that in the rat, plasma GH secretion occurs in a pulsatile manner with a periodicity of three to four hr.[118] Serial sampling of blood in unanesthetized unrestrained rats indicates that the GH secretory bursts are regulated by an α-adrenergic mechanism. The drugs αmpt and phenoxybenzamine abolish the spontaneous bursts of GH whereas dopamine receptor blockers have a minimal inhibitory effect. Clonidine, but not apomorphine, stimulates GH release in rats pretreated with αmpt.[119] Serial blood sampling provides a useful tool for the study of the effects of drugs on plasma GH, but the role of dopamine on the regulation of GH using different sampling procedures is unclear.

There are other reports implicating dopamine as an important neurotransmitter in the regulation of GH secretion. Pulsatile GH secretion is still evident with an increased number of secretory bursts in rats with a complete hypothalamic island produced by sectioning with a Halasz knife.[120] This technique depletes hypothalamic norepinephrine content without affecting hypothalamic dopamine content.[121] Furthermore, neonatal treatments with monosdium glutamate, which does not affect hypothalamic norepinephrine or somatostatin content, results in diminished hypothalamic dopamine content and reduced plasma GH.[122] Although these studies are not conclusive, they reinforce the importance of dopamine in the regulation of GH secretion.

Since GH secretion may be under the dual control of somatostatin and GH-RF, several studies have attempted to define the role of monoamines in the regulation of these hypothalamic hormones. Dopamine and norepinephrine are reported to stimulate the release of somatostatin from rat hypothalamic synaptosomes or fragments.[123,124] The release can be blocked by addition of pimozide or phentolamine into the incubation media.[124] These observations suggest that monoamines exert a direct action on hypothalamic somatostatin, but it does not rule out the possibility that monoamines also exert an effect on GH-RF.

Little is known about the involvement of β-adrenergic receptors in GH secretion in the rat. Propranolol, a β-adrenergic blocker, has no effect on pulsatile GH secretion,[125] but GH release induced by γ-hydroxybutyric acid (GHB), a derivative of γ-aminobutyric acid, is reported to be transiently augmented by propranolol and completely inhibited by the β-adrenergic agonist, isoproterenol.[126] Under urethane anesthesia, isoproterenol stimulates whereas propranolol inhibits GH release induced by chlorpromazine.[127] Although the specific role of β-adrenergic receptors on GH release is unclear, these results emphasize that urethane anesthesia may alter the response of GH to many drugs.

There appear to be species differences in GH responses to catecholaminergic drugs. Although data are not consistent, both dopamine and norepinephrine are involved in the release of GH in conscious dogs. L-DOPA elicits an increase in plasma GH in the dog, but this can be prevented by the α-adrenergic blocker, phentolamine[128] whereas the dopamine receptor blocker, pimozide[129] has no effect. Clonidine stimulates GH release whereas subemetic doses of apomorphine fail to increase GH.[129] Although the data suggest that norepinephrine alone is important for GH release, dopamine may play an independent role in GH release, since the GH releasing activity of L-DOPA is not influenced by treatment with fusaric acid, a potent inhibitor of dopamine-β-hydroxylase.[128]

In nonhuman primates, GH secretion may be regulated primarily by an α-adrenergic mechanism. Intravenous infusion of dopamine and norepinephrine stimuates GH release, but the GH stimulating effect of dopamine can be blocked by both phentolamine and FLA63, an inhibitor of dopamine-β-hydroxylase. Norepinephrine microinjected into the hypothalamus stimulates GH release whereas both phentolamine and dopamine suppress GH release.[130-132] In monkeys, GH release is also stimulated by clonidine and dihydroxyphenylserine (DOPS), a norepinephrine precursor, but apomorphine is effective only in emetic doses which may act as a nonspecific stress for GH release.[133] Phentolamine, but not pimozide, blocks GH release induced by amphetamine,[134] which releases both dopamine and norepinephrine from nerve terminals. These data suggest that dopamine may only increase GH through conversion to norepinephrine.

In humans, data indicate that dopaminergic and noradrenergic α-receptors are stimulatory and noradrenergic β-receptors are inhibitory to GH release. Intravenous injection of epinephrine or norepinephrine has no effect on plasma GH in man, possibly because they penetrate the blood brain barrier poorly, but oral administration of L-DOPA, the precursor of both dopamine and norepinephrine, stimulates GH release.[135]

Norepinephrine is involved in GH responses to various physiologic and pharmacologic stimuli in man. Phentolamine, an α-receptor blocker, blocks GH release induced by insulin hypoglycemia, arginine, vasopressin, L-DOPA, exercise, and stresses such as surgery and electric shock. Propranolol, a β-receptor blocker, enhances GH responses to insulin hypoglycemia, glucagon, L-DOPA and exercise. The role of noradrenergic α- and β-receptors is further supported by reports that clonidine, an α-receptor agonist, increases plasma GH and isoproterenol inhibits the vasopressin-induced increase in GH.

Dopamine also may have a distinct facilitatory role on GH secretion in man.[136-138] Subemetic doses of apomorphine stimulate GH release. Another dopaminergic drug, bromoergocryptine, produces a rise of plasma GH whereas pimozide, a dopamine receptor blocker, decreases GH response to arginine and exercise.

Serotonin

Serotonin appears to be involved in the regulation of GH secretion in the rat. When intraventricular injections of serotonin, 5-hydroxytryptamine (5-HT), are administered in the rat, plasma levels of GH increase.[139] The stimulatory effect of the serotonin precursor, 5-hydroxytryptophan (5-HTP) on GH secretion can be reversed by the structurally similar pineal hormone, melatonin, or the serotonin receptor antagonist, cyproheptadine.[140,141] Conversely, the severe depletion of brain serotonin by concomitant administration of the tyrosine hydroxylase inhibitor, p-chlorophenylalanine (PCPA), or the neurotoxin, 5,6-dihydrotryptamine, produces a marked reduction in circulating levels of GH in unanesthetized male rats.[142]

Participation of serotonin in the physiologic regulation of GH secretion in the rat is suggested by the observation that the pulsatile release of GH in unanesthetized male rats is inhibited by PCPA or the antiserotonergic drug, methysergide.[143]

Moreover, the characteristic GH pulse which occurs at the onset of the dark period is abolished by the serotonin-receptor antagonist, metergoline.[144]

The stimulatory effect of serotonin has been questioned since the report that PCPA has little effect on pulsatile GH release even though serotonin turnover is decreased.[145] When viewed together, these findings suggest that in the rat, serotonin, under some circumstances, may be an important regulator of GH secretion by the pituitary.

Findings similar to those observed in the rat have not been obtained in studies on the effects of serotonin on GH release in the dog. Müller et al.[146] reported that infusion of tryptophan, the amino acid precursor of serotonin, produces only a slight elevation in GH levels in the unanesthetized beagle. Administration of 5-HTP produces an elevated serum GH, but this effect is viewed with skepticism since 5-HTP causes dramatic side effects. PCPA has no effect on basal GH secretion, and potentiates rather than diminishes the rise in GH induced by insulin hypoglycemia. The drug 5-HTP reduces the rise in serum GH during insulin-induced hypoglycemia. Dogs maintained on a tryptophan deficient diet show no change in basal GH levels. When tryptophan is administered to these animals, it blunts rather than potentiates the insulin-induced rise in GH. Thus, in the dog, serotonin appears to be of minor importance in the regulation of GH secretion, and suppresses rather than stimulates GH release.

Generally, serotonin increases GH release in humans. Administration of 5-HTP to normal human subjects has been reported to increase[147-149] or to have no effect[150,151] on circulating levels of GH. However, cyproheptadine decreases or abolishes sleep-related GH release[152] and diminishes the rise in serum GH associated with exercise,[140] arginine infusion,[149] and insulin induced hypoglycemia.[140,147] Administration of methysergide produces a 40% decrease in peak GH values and a 35% decrease in overall mean GH concentrations.[147] Muller et al.[151] reported that L-tryptophan produces only a slight increase in plasma GH in female subjects and none in male subjects. They also found that L-tryptophan does not amplify the increase in serum GH produced by insulin-induced hypoglycemia. Thus, the physiological regulation of GH secretion by serotonin remains unclear.

Liuzzi et al.[153] cautioned that the data on the regulation of GH secretion must be viewed with reservations. Systemic administration of serotonin precursors may lead to accumulation of serotonin in cells which do not usually contain this indolamine and may also interfere with the storage or metabolism of catecholamines. There is some debate over the specificity of action of cyproheptadine, methysergide, and PCPA on the serotonergic system, and these substances may affect the catecholaminergic systems as well.

The majority of evidence leads to the conclusion that serotonin participates in the regulation of GH secretion in the rat and human. It is important to view the present data with caution.

Melatonin

Melatonin is synthesized and secreted by the pineal gland and appears to decrease the secretion of GH in the rat. Conditions which favor the secretion of melatonin correlate well with states in which growth is retarded. Sorrentini et al.[154] found that rats which are blinded or exposed to constant darkness, which increases melatonin synthesis, demonstrate a reduction in body weight, tibial length, and pituitary GH content. These effects are abolished by pinealectomy. Smythe and Lazarus[155] reported that the increase in serum GH after 5-HTP is antagonized by concomitant administration of melatonin. It is hypothesized that melatonin may antagonize the binding of serotonin to its receptor sites in the hypothalamus. Alternatively, melatonin may stimulate the metabolism of or inhibit the release of serotonin from its respective neurons.[156]

In the rat, the effect of melatonin on the pulsatile release of GH is contradictory. Ronnelkeiv and McCann[157] found that pinealectomy decreases the duration, frequency and amplitude of GH pulses as compared to sham-operated controls. The result is a reduction in mean total GH concentration. However, Willoughby[158] reported that pinealectomy has no effect on the pulsatile release of GH. It is difficult to discern the role of melatonin, if any, on the pulsatile release of GH in the rat.

In humans, the effect of melatonin on GH secretion is paradoxical. When administered to normal healthy male subjects, melatonin elevates circulating levels of GH.[159] By contrast, melatonin antagonizes the rise in GH produced by exercise or insulin hypoglycemia.[140] In humans, the effect of melatonin may be dependent on the physiologic status of the individual.

γ-Aminobutyric Acid

γ-Aminobutyric acid (GABA) is found in the hypothalamus, as well as other areas of the brain and its presence in these areas implies that GABA is a putative neurotransmitter.[160] Administration of GABA or its metabolites to rats or humans is reported to elevate circulating titers of GH.[161-163] In the urethane anesthetized male rat, injection of GABA into the lateral ventricles produces a significant rise in GH levels.[164,165] Similar results are obtained by intraventricular or intraperitoneal administration of the GABA metabolite γ-amino-β-hydroxybutyric acid (GABOB).[164,165]

Intraperitoneal injection of amino-oxyacetic acid, an agent which blocks the degradation of GABA, produces a marked rise in serum GH.[165] Intravenous administration of the potent GABA antagonist, picrotoxin, reduces plasma GH.[142,143] Our laboratory[215] found that GABA and GABA-ergic drugs, decrease serum GH levels in rats. The role of GABA or GH secretion must therefore await further study.

Little evidence is available to clarify the mechanism(s) by which GABA stimulates or inhibits the secretion of GH. Takahara et al.[165] found that GABA and amino-oxyacetic acid induce an increase in hypothalamic somatostatin content, suggesting that GABA promotes GH secretion in the rat by inhibiting the release of somatostatin by the hypothalamus. It is also possible that the effect of GABA is mediated through other neurotransmitters, a putative GHRF, or a combination of both. GABA does not have a direct effect on the pituitary, since it does not stimulate the release of GH when added to in vitro pituitary cultures.[166]

Acetylcholine

Acetylcholine (ACh) is present in high concentrations in the hypothalamus, and ACh receptors are found in the hypothalamus and pituitary gland. Several studies have been conducted to investigate the ability of acetylcholine to facilitate the release of GH by the pituitary. Casanueva et al.[167] reported that the cholinergic system stimulates the release of GH in the dog. Similarly, acetylcholine, pilocarpine (a cholinergic receptor stimulator), and the cholinesterase inhibitor, physostigmine, all promote release of GH in the rat.[168] Collu et al.[142] and Martin et al.[143] have shown that the cholinergic receptor blocker, atropine sulfate, decreases basal GH levels in the rat. Despite these findings, the participation of ACh in the physiologic release of GH is not yet clear.

Histamine

Histamine has not been established as a physiologic mediator of GH release. Rudolph et al.[169] reported that neither H_1 or H_2 agonists affects GH levels in the dog whereas the H_1 receptor antagonist, dexchlorpheniramine, significantly elevates baseline GH levels in the rat. Histamine may mediate the neurotensin and the substance P induced increase in GH.[96] However, further experimentation is necessary to establish a relationship of the histaminergic system to GH secretion.

Summary

Many putative neurotransmitters have been reported to modulate the release of GH. However, most of these experiments were performed with pharmacologic agents such as monoamine precursors, neurotransmitter agonists, and antagonists, as well as in different species of animals. Since none of these drugs are entirely specific in their actions, and there appear to be certain species differences in GH responses to these drugs, the results obtained need to be interpreted with caution. Caution also is necessary when anesthetics are used since some anesthetics alter GH responses to a number of drugs.

Much information has been obtained on the monoaminergic control of GH secretion in the rat since the development of RIA in this species. There are problems to be emphasized about this model:

1. In rats, unlike other species, even a minor stress such as handling, produces an apparent suppression of plasma GH, and daily handling (gentling) partially alleviates this effect.
2. Many anesthetics influence GH secretion. For example, pentobarbital stimulates whereas ether or urethane inhibits GH release.
3. Many of the doses of drugs used are pharmacologic and therefore have little physiologic significance. The interaction of drugs also should be carefully considered when they are administered in combination.
4. Surgical procedures, such as hypothalamic deafferentation, also must be viewed with caution, since these procedures may affect more than one hormone, as well as more than one neurotransmitter.

Nonetheless, research on all these species and the use of central acting drugs have contributed much to the elucidation of the control of GH secretion.

HORMONAL CONTROL OF GROWTH HORMONE SECRETION

Thyroid Hormones

The thyroid hormones influence the synthesis and release of GH. In the rat, thyroidectomy results in a marked reduction of both serum and pituitary GH[170-172] and abolishes the pulsatile release of GH.[173] Administration of thyroid hormone to rats increases plasma and pituitary GH within 24 hours.[172,174] In vitro incorporation of amino acids into GH is decreased by prior thyroidectomy and stimulated by thyroid hormone. It appears probable that thyroid hormones directly stimulate synthesis and release of pituitary GH.[175,176]

One characteristic of hypothyroidism in children is growth failute. The GH responses to insulin-induced hypoglycemia or arginine infusion are impaired in many hypothyroid patients.[177-179] Administration of thyroid hormone rapidly restores growth rate and normalizes the diminished GH responses to many stimuli.

Although it appears that thyroid hormones can potentiate GH release at the level of the pituitary, it has not been determined if thyroid hormones can also influence the synthesis and/or release of hypothalamic somatostatin or GH-RF, or affect the function of neurotransmitters which regulate the secretion of these hypophysiotropic hormones into the portal vessels. A recent report indicates that thyroid hormones may affect the activity of hypothalamic enzymes that metabolize somatostatin,[180] but whether this alters the concentrations of somatostatin in portal blood remains to be determined.

Estrogen and Testosterone

Estrogen and testosterone appear to have a potentiating effect on GH secretion. GH levels are increased on the day of estrus and in ovariectomized rats treated with estradiol benzoate.[181] Estrogen causes a marked increase in the pituitary sensitivity to the GH releasing activity of porcine hypothalamic extracts,[182] suggesting that estrogen acts at the level of the pituitary to sensitize the somatotroph to a putative GH-RF.

In humans, randomly sampled GH concentrations are higher in women than in men, and the increase in GH after minor activity also is greater in women.[183] The GH response to arginine infusion in women is highest at midcycle when concentrations of estrogens are elevated compared to concentrations in other phases of the menstrual cycle. Estrogen administration enhances the GH responses to arginine and exercise in children and adult men. In prepubertal children, who have low circulating gonadal steroids, the GH response to insulin hypoglycemia and arginine infusion is lower than that of adults.[185] The pulsatile release of GH becomes evident around puberty, when levels of estrogen and testosterone increase.[186]

Progesterone

Unlike estrogens, progesterone appears to have an inhibitory effect on GH secretion. Medroxyprogesterone acetate decreases the GH responses to insulin hypoglycemia or arginine infusion[187] and inhibits the sleep-related GH release in humans.[188] The elevated plasma GH levels in acromegalic patients may be reduced by medroxyprogesterone,[189] but this has not been confirmed. The mechanism by which progesterone inhibits GH secretion is unknown.

Glucocorticoids

Decreased growth in children receiving glucocorticoid therapy or suffering from chronic hypercortisolemia (Cushing's syndrome) suggests that glucocorticoids may inhibit GH secretion. The GH response to insulin hypoglycemia is impaired in patients with elevated glucocorticoids.[190-192] Little is known about the mechanism by which glucocorticoids influence GH release.

SLEEP, STRESS, AND EXERCISE EFFECTS ON GROWTH HORMONE

The major burst of GH release occurs within two hours after sleep onset in humans. About 70 to 90% of the total 24 hr secretion of GH may take place during these 2 hrs.[193-195] The nocturnal rise of GH is entrained to the onset of sleep and is not related to an intrinsic circadian rhythm, since the sleep-related secretion of GH can be reversed acutely by sleep-wake reversal.[196] The sleep-related GH release may be associated with slow-wave sleep (stage 3 and 4) defined polygraphically, but the relationship between these two phenomena does not appear to be fixed. Growth hormone secretion during sleep can occur in the absence of EEG changes of slow-wave sleep, and slow-wave sleep can occur without sleep-related GH release.

A number of attempts have been made to study the mechanism(s) of sleep-related GH secretion. Neither noradrenergic[197] nor dopaminergic blockers[193] inhibit GH release during sleep. The role of serotonin (5-HT) is controversial since three different antiserotoninergic agents are reported to increase,[198] decrease[199] or have no effect[200] on the sleep-related GH release.

A number of factors inhibit sleep-related GH secretion, including imipramine, clomiphene, medroxyprogesterone, somatostatin, obesity, fatty acids, and chronic alcoholism. An anticholinergic agent, methscopolamine, may block the GH surge during sleep without any effect on plasma prolactin or slow-wave sleep.[201] Neurotransmitters and metabolic factors thus appear to be involved in sleep-related GH secretion.

Acute physical stress or exercise stimulates GH release in many species, including man.[202,203] Physical trauma, electroshock therapy, and surgical operations result in a rise of GH in humans and GH release is also stimulated by arterial puncture and pyrogen administration. The GH response to insulin hypoglycemia may be due to stress, since GH release is associated to some degree with the severity of side effects to insulin, such as sweating, palpitation, and generalized weakness. Alpha blockers inhibit GH release induced by stress. Growth hormone secretion in nonhuman primates is also stress-responsive. A marked elevation of GH is caused by stresses such as pain, loud noise, capture, ether inhalation, hemorrhage, and aversive conditioning. Growth hormone release in rats and mice, unlike release in primates, is inhibited by stress. Somatostatin may be responsible for the stress-related inhibition of GH release in rodents.

AGE-RELATED CHANGES IN GROWTH HORMONE

Developmental Pattern of Growth Hormone

The developmental pattern of plasma GH in neonatal and prepubertal rats is difficult to assess because of the problems associated with obtaining multiple plasma samples from young animals. It is generally accepted that plasma concentrations of GH are elevated neonatally and decline steadily until days 22 to 25.[204-206] At 22 to 25 days the pulsatile release of GH appears in both male and female rats and the amplitude of the GH increases until about 45 days.[207] The increased secretion of GH in female rats immediately before the onset of puberty suggests that GH may be an important determinant of the onset of puberty in rats.[208] The early stages of puberty in humans are also characterized by enhanced pulsatile GH secretion.[186] Whether pulsatile release is a determinant of puberty, or the relection of a maturing neuroendocrine system, remains to be determined.

Although few studies are available on the ontogeny of hypothalamic somatostatin, some researchers find a high negative correlation between hypothalamic somatostatin and plasma GH.[205] Somatostatin concentration per microgram protein is claimed to increase from day 2 to day 28 and then to decline until day 50. In rats there are no sex differences. In another study,[206] somatostatin is found to increase slowly from day 10 to 36. The physiologic importance of these changes in hypothalamic somatostatin and their relation to plasma GH during development are not understood.

Aging and Growth Hormone

Early studies of age-related changes in GH are contradictory.[209] Data indicate that the pulsatile release of GH[210] and the increase in GH in response to many stimuli are diminished in old male rats.[211] Using indwelling atrial cannulae, more than 57% of young rats exhibit pulses of GH greater than 300 ng/mℓ plasma whereas only 7% of old animals have GH pulses of similar amplitude. The mean GH concentrations are significantly greater in young than in old male rats. Old male rats also have decreased hypothalamic somatostatin and pituitary GH content, compared with young animals. Although many pharmacologic stimuli are less effective in promoting GH release in old than in young rats, antiserum against somatostatin increases GH similarly in both groups. Since old male rats are capable of secreting GH if the inhibitory effect of somatostatin is removed, somatostatin may be involved in some of the age-related changes in GH.

Although trough values of GH in human males are reported not to change with age, the nocturnal surge of GH is decreased or absent.[212] The increase in GH resulting from insulin-induced hypoglycemia is diminished in aged humans.[213] Since GH participates in the growth and maintenance of many organ systems, the decline in protein synthesis, and in other processes characteristic of aging mammals may be related to a deficiency of GH secretion.

SUMMARY

There is enormous literature about the neuroendocrine regulation of growth hormone secretion. The effects of many putative neurotransmitters and neuropeptides on

GH release still remain controversial. This is partially because the action of neurotransmitter agonists and antagonists differ with the physiologic status of an organism and also because there is much difficulty in measuring the synthesis or release of hypothalamic peptides.

The demonstration of pulsatile GH secretion suggests that several neurotransmitters and neuropeptides are involved in the secretion of GH. The interaction of various systems that regulate GH secretion has only partially been studied in vertebrates and much remains to be done.

REFERENCES

1. **Greenspan, F. S., Li, C. H., Simpson, M. E., and Evans, H. M.,** Bioassay of hypophyseal growth hormone: the tibia test, *Endocrinology,* 45, 455, 1949.
2. **Wilhelmi, A. E.,** Growth hormone measurement-bioassay, in *Methods in Investigative and Diagnostic Endocrinology,* Berson, S. A. and Yalow, R. S., Eds., North Holland, Amsterdam, 1973, 296.
3. **Greenwood, R., Hunter, W., and Glover, J.,** The preparation of ^{131}I-labeled human growth hormone of high specific radioactivity, *Biochem. J.,* 89, 114, 1963.
4. **Mijachi, Y., Chrambach, A., Mecklenburg, R., and Lipsett, M. B.,** Preparation and properties of ^{125}I-LHRH, *Endocrinology,* 92, 1725, 1973.
5. **Tower, B. B., Clark, B. R., and Rubin, R. T.,** Preparation of ^{125}I polypeptide hormones for radioimmunoassay using glucose oxidase with lactoperoxidase, *Life Sci.,* 21, 959, 1977.
6. **Pecile, A. and Müller, E., Eds.,** Somatomedin: chemistry, regulation of generation, biological effects, in *Growth Hormone and Related Peptides,* Excerpta Medica, Amsterdam, 1976, 156.
7. **Pecile, A. and Müller, E. E., Eds.,** Hormone dependent growth factors: somatomedins and NILSA. Chemistry, biology, physiology, regulation of biosynthesis, in *Growth Hormone and Other Biologically Active Peptides,* Excerpta Medica, Amsterdam, 1980, 65.
8. **Frieden, E.,** Hormones of the anterior pituitary, in *Chemical Endocrinology,* Academic Press, New York, 1976, 111.
9. **Andrews, P.,** Molecular weight of prolactin and pituitary growth hormones estimated by gel filtration, *Nature,* 209, 155, 1966.
10. **Weil, R.,** Pituitary growth hormone and intermediary metabolism. I. The hormonal effect on the metabolism of fat and carbohydrate, *Acta Endocrinol. Suppl.,* 98, 1, 1965.
11. **Rabinowitz, D., Merimee, T. J., Maffezzolo, R., and Burgess, J. A.,** Patterns of hormonal release after glucose, protein and glucose plus protein, *Lancet,* 2, 434, 1966.
12. **Rabinowitz, D., Merimee, T. J., Nelson, J. K., Schultz, R. B., and Burgess, J. A.,** The influence of proteins and amino acids on growth hormone release in man, in *Growth Hormone,* Pecile, A. and Müller, E. E., Eds., Excerpta Medica, New York, 1968, 105.
13. **Schnure, J. J. and Lipman, R.,** Physiological studies of growth hormone secretion during sleep: non-suppressibility by hyperglycemia and impairment in glucose tolerance, *Proc. 52nd Meet. Endocr. Soc.,* No. 214, 1970, (Abstract).
14. **Bodel, P. T., Rubenstein, D., McGarry, E. E., and Beck, J. C.,** Utilization of free fatty acids by diaphragm *in vitro, Am. J. Physiol.,* 203, 311, 1962.
15. **Goodman, H. M.,** Effects of chronic growth hormone treatment on lipogenesis by rat adipose tissue, *Endocrinology,* 72, 95, 1963.
16. **Knobil, E. and Hotchkiss, J.,** Growth hormone, *Ann. Rev. Physiol.,* 26, 47, 1964.
17. **Knobil, E.,** Direct evidence for fatty acid mobilization in response to growth hormone administration in rat, *Proc. Soc. Exp. Bio. Med.,* 101, 288, 1959.
18. **Raben, M. S. and Hollenberg, C. H.,** Growth hormone and the mobilization of fatty acids, *Ciba Found. Colloq. Endocrinol.,* 13, 89, 1959.
19. **Root, A. W.,** Chemical and biological properties of growth hormone, in *Human Pituitary Growth Hormone,* Charles C Thomas, Springfield, Ill., 1972, 3.
20. **Franklin, M. J. and Knobil, E.,** The influence of hypophysectomy and of growth hormone administration on oxidation of palmitate-1-C^{14} by the unanesthetized rat, *Endocrinology,* 68, 867, 1961.
21. **Winkler, B., Steele, R., Altszuler, N., Dunn, A., and deBodo, R. C.,** Effects of growth hormone on free fatty acid metabolism, *Fed. Proc.,* 21, 198, 1962.

22. **Kinsell, L. W., Visintine, R. E., Michaels, G. D., and Walker, G.,** Effects of human growth hormone on lipid metabolism in diabetic subjects, *Metabolism,* 11, 136, 1962.
23. **Allen, A., Medes, G., and Weinhouse, S.,** A study of the effects of growth hormone on fatty acid metabolism in vitro, *J. Biol. Chem.* 221, 333, 1956.
24. **Bauman, J. W., Hill, R., Nejad, N. S., and Chaikoff, I. L.,** Effect of bovine pituitary growth hormone on hepatic cholesterogenesis of hypophysectomized rats, *Endocrinology,* 65, 73, 1959.
25. **Greenbaum, A. L. and Glascock, R. F.,** The synthyesis of lipids in the livers of rats treated with pituitary growth hormone, *Biochem. J.,* 67, 360, 1957.
26. **Noall, M. W., Riggs, T. R., Walker, L. M., and Christensen, H. N.,** Endocrine control of amino acid transfer. Distribution of an unmetabolizable amino acid, *Science,* 126, 1002, 1957.
27. **Riggs, T. R. and Walker, L. M.,** Growth hormone stimulation of amino acid transport into rat tissues *in vivo, J. Biol. Chem.,* 235, 3603, 1960.
28. **Kostyo, J. L., Hotchkiss, J., and Knobil, E.,** Stimulation of amino acid transport in isolated diaphragm by growth hormone added *in vitro, Science,* 130, 1653, 1959.
29. **Kipnis, D. M. and Reiss, E.,** The effect of cell structure and growth hormone on protein synthesis in striated muscle, *J. Clin. Invest.,* 39, 1002, 1960.
30. **Staehelin, M.,** *Protein Metabolism: influence of Growth Hormone Anabolic Steroids and Nutrition in Health and Disease,* Querido, A., Ed., Springer-Verlag, Basel, 1962, 521.
31. **Fraser, R. and Harrison, M.,** The effect of growth hormone on urinary calcium excretion, *Ciba Found. Colloq. Endocrinol.,* 13, 135, 1959.
32. **Corvilain, J. and Abramow, M.,** Some effects of human growth hormone on renal hemodynamics and on tubular phosphate transport in man, *J. Clin. Invest.,* 41, 1230, 1962.
33. **Jasin, H. E., Fink, C. W., Wise, W., and Ziff, M.,** Relationship between urinary hydroxyproline and growth, *J. Clin. Invest.,* 41, 1928, 1962.
34. **Krulich, L., Dhariwal, A. P. S., and McCann, S. M.,** Stimulatory and inhibitory effects of purified hypothalamic extract on growth hormone release from rat pituitary *in vitro, Endocrinology,* 83, 783, 1968.
35. **Vale, W., Brazeau, P., Grant, G., Nussey, A., Burgus, R., Rivier, J., Ling, N., and Guillemin, R.,** Premiers observations sur le mode d'action de la somatostatine un facteur hypothalamique, qui inhibe la secretion de l'hormone de croissance, *Comptes Rendus Acad. Sci.,* 275, 2913, 1972.
36. **Guillemin, R.,** Hypothalamic hormones: releasing and inhibiting factors, in *Neuroendocrinology,* Krieger, D. T. and Hughes, J. C., Eds., Sinauer, Sunderland, MA, 1980, 23.
37. **Martin, J.,** Brain regulation of growth hormone secretion, in *Frontiers of Neuroendocrinology,* Martini, L. and Ganong, W., Eds., Raven Press, New York, 12, 1976.
38. **Vale, W., Rivier, C., and Brown, M.,** Regulatory peptides of the hypothalamus, *Ann. Rev. Physiol.,* 39, 473, 1977.
39. **Arimura, A., Smith, W. D., and Schally, A. V.,** Blockade of the stress-induced decrease in blood GH by antisomatostatin serum in rats, *Endocrinology,* 98, 540, 1976.
40. **Ferland, L., Labrie, F., Jobin, M., Arimura, A., and Schally, A. V.,** Physiological role of somatostatin in the control of growth hormone and thyrotropin secretion, *Biochem. Biophys. Res. Commun.,* 68, 149, 1976.
41. **Terry, L., Willoughby, J., Brazeru, P., Martin, J., and Patel, Y.,** Antiserum to somatostatin prevents stress-induced inhibition of growth hormone secretion in the rat, *Science,* 192, 565, 1976.
42. **Tannenbaum, G. S., Epelbaum, J., Colle, E., Brazeau, P., and Martin, J. B.,** Antiserum to somatostatin reverses starvation induced inhibition of growth hormone but not insulin secretion, *Endocrinology,* 102, 1909, 1978.
43. **Hall, R., Besser, G., Schally, A., Coy, D., Evered, D., Goldie, D., Kastin, A., McNeilly, A., Mortimer, C., Phenekas, C., Tunbridge, W., and Weightman, D.,** Action of growth hormone release inhibitory hormone in healthy men and in acromegaly, *Lancet,* 2, 581, 1973.
44. **Vale, W., Rivier, C., and Guillemin, R.,** Effects of somatostatin on the secretion of thyrotropin and prolactin, *Endocrinology,* 95, 968, 1974.
45. **Martin, J. B.,** Brain mechanisms for integration of growth hormone secretion, *Physiologist,* 22, 23, 1979.
46. **Deuben, R. R. and Meites, J.,** Stimulation of pituitary growth hormone release by a hypothalamic extract, *in vitro, Endocrinology,* 74, 408, 1964.
47. **Frohman, L. A. and Bernardis, L. L.,** Growth hormone and insulin levels in weanlings, *Endocrinology,* 82, 1125, 1968.
48. **Frohman, L., Bernardis, L., and Kant, K.,** Hypothalamic stimulation of growth hormone secretion, *Science,* 162, 580, 1968.
49. **Martin, J. B., Renaud, L., and Brazeau, P.,** Pulsatile growth hormone secretion: suppression by hypothalamic ventromedial lesions and by long acting somatostatin, *Science,* 186, 538, 1974.

50. **Krulich, L., Illner, P., Fawcett, C., Quijada, M., and McCann, S. M.,** Dual hypothalamic regulation of growth hormone secretion, in *Growth and Growth Hormone,* Pecile, A. and Müller, E., Eds., Excerpta Medica, Amsterdam, 1972.
51. **Brownstein, M., Arimura, A., Sato, H., Schally, A. V., and Kizer, J.,** The regional distribution of somatostatin in the rat brain, *Endocrinology,* 96, 1456, 1975.
52. **Kizer, J., Palkovits, M., and Brownstein, M.,** Releasing factors of the circumventricular organs of the rat brain, *Endocrinology,* 98, 311, 1976.
53. **Palkovits, M., Brownstein, M., Arimura, A., Sato, H., Schally, A. V., and Kizer, J.,** Somatostatin content of the hypothalamic ventromedial and arcuate nuclei and the circumventricular organs in the brain, *Brain Res.,* 109, 430, 1976.
54. **Patel, Y., Weir, G., and Reichlin, S.,** Anatomic distribution of somatostatin in brain and pancreas islets by radioimmunoassay, *Proc. of 57th Ann. Meet. Endocr. Soc.,* No. 127, 1975, (Abstract).
55. **Hökfelt, T., Efendic, S., Johansson, O., Luft, R., and Arimura, A.,** Immunohistochemical localization of somatostatin (growth hormone release-inhibiting factor) in the guinea pig brain, *Brain Res.,* 80, 165, 1974.
56. **King, J. C., Gerall, A. A., Fishback, J., Elkind, K., and Arimura, A.,** Growth hormone-release inhibiting hormone (GH-RIH) pathway of the rat hypothalamus revealed by the unlabeled antibody peroxidase-anti-peroxidase method, *Cell Tissue Res.,* 160, 423, 1975.
57. **Sètàlò, G., Vigh, S., Schally, A. V., Arimura, A., and Flerko, B.,** GH-RIH containing neural elements in the rat hypothalamus, *Brain Res.,* 90, 352, 1975.
58. **Pelletier, G., LeClerc, R., Dube, D., Arimura, A., and Schally, A. V.,** Immunohistochemical localization of luteinizing hormone-releasing hormone (LH-RH) and somatostatin in the organum vasculosum of the lamina terminalis of the rat, *Neuroscience,* 4, 27, 1977.
59. **Alpert, L., Brawer, J., Patel, Y., and Reichlin, S.,** Somatostatin neurons in anterior hypothalamus: immunohistochemical localization, *Endocrinology,* 98, 255, 1976.
60. **Elde, R. and Parsons, J.,** Immunocytochemical localization of somatostatin in cell bodies of the rat hypothalamus, *Am. J. Anat.,* 144, 541, 1975.
61. **Hökfelt, T., Efendic, E., Hellmstrom, C., Johansson, O., Luft, R., and Arimura, A.,** Cellular localization of somatostatin in endocrine-like cells and neurons of the rat with special reference to the A cells of the pancreatic islets and to the hypothalamus, *Acta Endocrinol.,* 80, 1, 1975.
62. **Chihara, K., Arimura, A., Kubli-Garfias, C., and Schally, A. V.,** Enhancement of immunoreactive somatostatin release into hypophysial portal blood by electrical stimulation of the preoptic area in the rat, *Endocrinology,* 105, 1416, 1979.
63. **Martin, J. B.,** The role of hypothalamic and extrahypothalamic structures in the control of growth hormone secretion, in *Advances in Human Growth Hormone Research,* Raiti, S., Ed., National Institutes of Health, Washington, D.C., 1974, 223.
64. **Rice, R. W. and Critchlow, V.,** Extrahypothalamic control of stress induced inhibition of growth hormone secretion in the rat, *Endocrinology,* 99, 970, 1976.
65. **Millar, R. P., Dennis, P., Tobler, C., King, J. C., Schally, A. V., and Arimura, A.,** Presumptive prohormonal forms of hypothalamic peptide hormones, in *Cell Biology of Hypothalamic Neurosecretion,* Vincent, J. and Kordon, C., Eds., Centre National de la Recherche Scientifique, Bordeaux, France, 1977, 488.
66. **Chihara, K., Arimura, A., and Schally, A. V.,** Immunoreactive somatostatin in rat hypophysial portal blood: effects of anesthetics, *Endocrinology,* 104, 1434, 1979.
67. **Gaulden, E. C., Littlefield, D. C., Sutoff, O. E., and Seivert, A. L.,** Menstrual abnormalities associated with heroin addiction, *Am. J. Obstet. Gynecol.,* 90, 155, 1964.
68. **Hollister, L. E.,** Human pharmacology of drugs of abuse with emphasis on neuroendocrine effects, *Prog. Brain Res.,* 39, 373, 1973.
69. **Mendelson, J. H., Meyer, R. E., Ellingloe, J., Gurin, S. M., and McDougle, M.,** Effects of heroin and methadone on plasma cortisol and testosterone, *J. Pharm. Exp. Ther.,* 195, 296, 1975.
70. **Meites, J., Nicoll, S., Talwalker, P. K., and Hopkins, T. F.,** Induction and maintenance of mammary growth and lactation by neurohormones, drugs, nonspecific stresses, and hypothalamic tissue, *Proc. 1st Int. Congr. Endocrinol.,* Excerpta Medica, Copenhagen, 1960.
71. **Kokka, N., Garcia, J. F., George, R., and Elliott, H. H. W.,** Growth hormone and ACTH secretion: evidence for an inverse relationship in rats, *Endocrinology,* 90, 735, 1972.
72. **Dupont, A., Cusan, L., Garon, M., Labrie, F., and Li, C. H.,** β-Endorphine: stimulation of growth hormone release *in vivo, Proc. Natl. Acad. Sci.,* 74, 358, 1977.
73. **Rivier, C., Vale, W., Ling, N., Brown, M., and Guillemin, R.,** Stimulation *in vivo* of the secretion of prolactin and growth hormone by β-endorphine, *Endocrinology,* 100, 238, 1977.
74. **Bruni, J. F., Van Vugt, D. A., Marshall, S., and Meites, J.,** Effects of naloxone, morphine and methionine enkephalin on serum prolactin, luteinizing hormone, follicle stimulating hormone, thyroid stimulating hormone and growth hormone, *Life Sci.,* 21, 461, 1977.

75. **Cusan, L., Dupont, A., Kledzik, G. S., Labrie, F., Coy, D. H., and Schally, A. V.**, Potent prolactin and growth hormone releasing activity of more analogues of met-enkephalin, *Nature*, 268, 544, 1977.
76. **Shaar, C. J., Frederickson, R. C. A., Dininger, N. B., and Jackson, L.**, Enkephalin analogues and naloxone modulate the release of growth hormone and prolactine-evidence for regulation by an endogenous opioid peptide in brain, *Life Sci.*, 2, 853, 1977.
77. **Shaar, C. J. and Clemens, J. A.**, The effects of opiate agonists on growth hormone and prolactin release in rats, *Fed. Proc.*, 39, 2539, 1980.
78. **Martin, J. B., Tolis, G., Woods, I., and Guyda, H.**, Failure of naloxone to influence physiological growth hormone and prolactin secretion, *Brain Res.*, 168, 210, 1979.
79. **Tannenbaum, G. S., Panerai, A. E., and Friesen, H. G.**, Failure of β-endorphin antiserum, naloxone, and naltrexone to alter physiologic growth hormone and insulin secretion, *Life Sci.*, 25, 1983, 1979.
80. **Stubbs, W. A., Jones, A., Edwards, C. R. W., Delitalia, G., Jeffcoat, W. J., Rattner, S. J., and Bessner, G. M.**, Hormonal and metabolic responses to an enkephalin analogue in normal man, *Lancet*, 1, 1225, 1978.
81. **Lal, S., Nair, N. P. V., Cervantes, P., Pulman, J., and Guyda, H.**, Effects of naloxone and levallorphan on serum prolactin concentrations and apomorphine-induced growth hormone secretion, *Acta Psychiat. Scand.*, 59, 173, 1979.
82. **Morley, J. E., Baranetsky, N. G., Wingert, T. O., Carlson, H. E., Hershmman, J. M., Melmed, S., Levin, S. R., Jamison, K. R., Weitzman, R., Chang, R. J., and Varrner, A. A.**, Endocrine effects of naloxone-induced opiate receptor blockade, *J. Clin. Endocrinol. Metab.*, 50, 251, 1980.
83. **Spiler, I. J. and Molitch, M. E.**, Lack of modulation of pituitary hormone stress response by neural pathways involving opiate receptors, *J. Clin. Endocrinol. Metab.*, 50, 516, 1980.
84. **Wakabayashi, I., Demura, R., Miki, N., Ohmura, E., and Miypshi, H., and Shizume, K.**, Failure of naloxone to influence plasma growth hormone, prolactin, and cortisol secretions induced by insulin hypoglycemia, *J. Clin. Endocrinol. Metab.*, 50, 597, 1980.
85. **Chihara, K., Arimura, A., Coy, D. H., and Schally, A. V.**, Studies on the interactions of endorphins, substance P, and endogenous somatostatin in growth hormone and prolactin release in rats, *Endocrinology*, 102, 281, 1978.
86. **Ferland, L., Fuxe, K., Eneroth, P., Gustafsson, J. A., and Skett, P.**, Effects of methionine-enkephalin on prolactin release and catecholamine levels and turnover in the median eminence, *Eur. J. Pharmacol.*, 43, 89, 1977.
87. **Van Vugt, D. A., Bruni, J. F., Sylvester, P. W., Chen, H. T., Ieiri, T., and Meites, J.**, Interaction between opiates and hypothalamic dopamine on prolactin release, *Life Sci.*, 24, 2361, 1979.
88. **Van Ree, J. M., Versteeg, D. H. G., Shaapen-Kok, W. B., and DeWied, D.**, Effects of morphine on hypothalamic noradrenalin and on pituitary-adrenal activity in rats, *Neuroendocrinology*, 22, 305, 1976.
89. **Haubrich, D. R. and Blake, D. E.**, Modification of serotonin metabolism in rat brain after acute or chronic administration of morphine, *Biochem. Pharmacol.*, 22, 2753, 1973.
90. **Yarbrough, G. G., Buxbaum, D. M., and Sanders-Bush, E.**, Increased serotonin turnover in the acutely morphine treated rat, *Life Sci.*, 10, 977, 1971.
91. **Van Loon, G. R., DeSouza, E. B.**, Effects of β-endorphin on brain serotonin metabolism, *Life Sci.*, 23, 971, 1978.
92. **Martin, J. B., Audet, J., and Saunders, A.**, Effects of somatostatin and hypothalamic ventromedial lesions on GH release induced by morphine, *Endocrinology*, 96, 839, 1975.
93. **Casanueva, F., Betti, R., Frigerio, C., Cocchi, D., Mantegassa, P., and Müller, E. E.**, Growth hormone-releasing effect of an enkephalin analogue in the dog: evidence for cholinergic mediation, *Endocrinology*, 106, 1239, 1980.
94. **Kato, Y., Katakami, H., Matsushita, N., Hiroto, S., Shimatsu, A., Waseda, N., and Imura, H.**, Monoaminergic involvement in growth hormone release induced by a synthetic enkephalin analogue in the rat, *62nd Ann. Meet. Endocr. Soc.*, Abstr. 476, 1980.
95. **Snyder, S. H.**, Brain peptides as neurotransmitters, *Science*, 209, 976, 1980.
96. **Rivier, C., Brown, M., and Vale, W.**, Effects of neurotensin, substance P and morphine sulfate on the secretion of prolactin and growth hormone in the rat, *Endocrinology*, 100, 751, 1977.
97. **Kato, Y., Chihara, K., Ohgo, S., Iwasaki, Y., Abe, H., and Imura, H.**, Growth hormone and prolactin release by substance P in rats, *Life Sci.*, 19, 441, 1976.
98. **Takahara, J. A., Arimura, A., and Schally, A. V.**, Effect of catecholamines on the TRH-stimulated release of prolactin and growth hormone from sheep pituitaries *in vitro*, *Endocrinology*, 95, 1490, 1974.
99. **Convey, E. M., Tucker, H. A., Smith, V. G., and Zolman, J.**, Bovine prolactin, growth hormone, thyroxine, and corticoid response to thyrotropin-releasing hormone, *Endocrinology*, 92, 471, 1973.
100. **Giannattasio, G., Zanini, A., Panerai, A. E., Meldolesi, J., and Müller, E. E.**, Studies on rat pituitary homographs. II. Effects of thyrotropin-releasing hormone on *in vitro* biosynthesis and release of growth hormone and prolactin, *Endocrinology*, 104, 237, 1979.

101. **Anastasia, A., Erspamer, V., and Bucci, H.,** Isolation and structure of bombesin and alytesin, two analogous active peptides from the skin of the European amphibians, Bombena and Aytes, *Experientia*, 27, 166, 1971.
102. **Rivier, C., Rivier, J., and Vale, W.,** The effect of bombesin and related peptides on prolactin and growth hormone secretion in the rat, *Endocrinology*, 102, 519, 1978.
103. **Carraway, R. and Leeman, S. E.,** The isolation of a new hypotensive peptide, neurotensin, from bovine hypothalami, *J. Biol. Chem.*, 248, 6854, 1973.
104. **Kato, Y., Dupre, J., and Beck, J. C.,** Plasma growth hormone in the anesthetized rat: effects of dibutyryl cyclic AMP, prostaglandin E_1, adrenergic agents, vasopressin, chlorpromazine, amphetamine, and L-DOPA, *Endocrinology*, 93, 135, 1973.
105. **Heidingsfelder, S. A. and Blackard, W. G.,** Adrenergic control mechanism for vasopressin-induced plasma growth hormone response, *Metabolism*, 17, 1019, 1968.
106. **Wilber, J. F., Nagel, T., and White, W. F.,** Hypothalamic growth hormone-releasing activity (GRA): characterization by the *in vitro* rat pituitary and radioimmunoassay, *Endocrinology*, 89, 1419, 1971.
107. **Emson, P. C., Fahrenkrug, J., DeMuckadell, O. B. S., Jessel, T. M. and Iverson, L. L.,** Vasoactive intestinal polypeptide (VIP): vesicular localization and potassium evoked release from rat hypothalamus, *Brain Res.*, 143, 174, 1978.
108. **Said, S. I. and Porter, J. C.,** Vasoactive intestinal polypeptide (VIP): evidence for secretion in hypophyseal portal blood, *Fed. Proc.*, 37, 482, 1978, (Abstract).
109. **Vijayan, E., Samson, W. K., Said, S. I., and McCann,, S. M.,** Vaso-active intestinal peptide: evidence for a hypothalamic site of action to release growth hormone, luteinizing hormone, and prolactin in conscious ovariectomized rats, *Endocrinology*, 104, 53, 1979.
110. **Abe, H., Kato, Y., Iwasaki, Y., Chihara, K., and Imura, H.,** Central effects of somatostatin on the secretion of growth hormone in the anesthetized rat, *Proc. Soc. Exp. Biol. Med.*, 159, 346, 1978.
111. **Müller, E. E., Pra, P. D., and Pecile, A.,** Influence of brain neurohumors injected into the lateral ventricle of the rat on growth hormone release, *Endocrinology*, 83, 893, 1968.
112. **Smythe, G. A., Brandstater, J. F., and Lazarus, L.,** Serotonergic control of rat growth hormone secretion, *Neuroendocrinology*, 17, 245, 1975.
113. **Chen, H. T., Mueller, G. P., and Meites, J.,** Effects of L-DOPA and somatostatin on suckling-induced release of prolactin and GH, *Endocr. Res. Commun.*, 1, 283, 1974.
114. **Muller, E. E., Cocchi, D., Jalando, H., and Udeshini, G.,** Antagonistic role for norepinephrine and dopamine in the control of growth hormone secretion in the rat, *Endocrinology*, 92, A248, 1973.
115. **Mueller, G. P., Simpkins, J., Meites, J., and Moore, K. E.,** Differential effects of dopamine agonists and haloperidol on release of prolactin, thyroid stimulating hormone, growth hormone and lutenizing hormone in rats, *Neuroendocrinology*, 20, 121, 1976.
116. **Vijayan, E., Krulich, L., and McCann, S. M.,** Catecholaminergic regulation of TSH and growth hormone release in ovariectomized and ovariectomized, steroid-primed rats, *Neuroendocrinology*, 26, 174, 1978.
117. **Ruch, W., Jaton, A. L., Bucher, B., Marbach, P., and Doepfner, W.,** Alpha adrenergic control of growth hormone in adult male rat, *Experientia*, 32, 529, 1976.
118. **Tannenbaum, G. S. and Martin, J. B.,** Evidence for an endogenous ultradian rhythm governing growth hormone secretion in the rat, *Endocrinology*, 98, 540, 1976.
119. **Martin, J. B., Brazeau, P., Tannenbaum, G. S., Willoughby, J. O., Epelbaum, J., Terry, L. C., and Durand, D.,** Neuroendocrine organization of growth hormone regulation, in *The Hypothalamus*, Reichlin, S., Baldessarini, R. J., and Martin, J. B., Eds., Raven Press, New York, 1978, 329.
120. **Willoughby, J. O., Terry, L. C., Brazeau, P., and Martin, J. B.,** Pulsatile growth hormone, prolactin, and thyrotropin secretion in rats with hypothalamic deafferentation, *Brain Res.*, 127, 137, 1977.
121. **Weiner, R. I., Shryne, J. E., Gorski, R. A., and Sawyer, C. H.,** Changes in the catecholamine content of the rat hypothalamus following deafferentation, *Endocrinology*, 90, 867, 1972.
122. **Nemeroff, C. B., Konkol, R. J., Bissette, G., Youngblood, W., Martin, J. B., Brazeau, P., Rone, M. S., Prange, A. J. Jr., Breese, G. R., and Kizer, J. S.,** Analysis of the disruption in hypothalamic-pituitary regulation in rats treated neonatally with monosodium L-glutamate (MSG): evidence for the involvement ot tubero-infundibular cholinergic and dopaminergic systems in neuroendocrine regulation, *Endocrinology*, 101, 613, 1977.
123. **Wakabayashi, I., Miyazawa, H., Kanda, M., Miki, N., Demura, R., Demura, H., and Shizume, K.,** Stimulation of immunoreactive somatostatin release from hypothalamic synaptosomes by high (K^+) and dopamine, *Endocrinology, (Japan)*, 24, 601, 1977.
124. **Negro-Vilar, A., Ojeda, S. R., Arimura, A., and McCann, S. M.,** Dopamine and norepinephrine stimulate somatostatin release by median eminence fragments *in vitro*, *Life Sci.*, 23, 1493, 1978.
125. **Martin, J. B., Durand, D., Gurd, W., Faille, G., Audet, J., and Brazeau, P.,** Neuropharmacological regulation of episodic growth hormone and prolactin secretion in the rat, *Endocrinology*, 102, 106, 1978.

126. **Schaub, C., Bluet-Pajot, M. T., Mouonier, F., Segalen, A., and Duhault, J.,** Effects of noradrenergic agonists and antagonists on growth hormone secretion under gamma-hydroxybutyrate narcoanalgesia in the rat, *Psychoneuroendocrinology,* 5, 139, 1980.
127. **Kato, Y., Dupre, J., and Beck, J. C.,** Plasma growth hormone in the anesthetized rat: effects of dibutyryl cyclic AMP, prostaglandin E, adrenergic agents, vasopressin, chlorpromazine, amphetamine and L-DOPA, *Endocrinology,* 93, 135, 1973.
128. **Takahashi, K., Tsushima, T., and Irie, M.,** Effect of catecholamines on plasma growth hormone in dogs, *Endocrinology, (Japan),* 20, 323, 1973.
129. **Holland, F. J., Richards, G. E., Kaplan, S. L., Ganong, W. F., and Grumbach, M. M.,** The role of biogenic amines in the regulation of growth hormone and corticotropin secretion in the trained conscious dog, *Endocrinology,* 102, 1452, 1978.
130. **Steiner, R. A., Illner, P., Rolfs, A. D., Toivola, P. T. K., and Gale, C. C.,** Noradrenergic and dopaminergic regulation of GH and prolactin in baboons, *Neuroendocrinology,* 26, 15, 1978.
131. **Toivola, P. T. K. and Gale, C. C.,** Effect of temperature of biogenic amine infusion into hypothalamus of baboon, *Neuroendocrinology,* 6, 210, 1970.
132. **Toivola, P. T. K. and Gale, C. C.,** Stimulation of growth hormone release by microinjection of norepinephrine into hypothalamus of baboon, *Endocrinology,* 90, 895, 1974.
133. **Chambers, J. W. and Brown, G. M.,** Neurotransmitter regulation of growth hormone and ACTH in the rhesus monkey: effects of biogenic amines, *Endocrinology,* 98, 420, 1976.
134. **Marantz, R., Sachar, E. J., Weitzman, E., and Sassin, J.,** Cortisol and GH responses to D- and L-amphetamine in monkeys, *Endocrinology,* 99, 459, 1976.
135. **Boyd, A. E., Lebovitz, H. E., and Pfeiffer, J. B.,** Stimulation of human-growth-hormone secretion by L-DOPA, *N. Engl. J. Med.,* 283, 1425, 1970.
136. **Burrow, G. N., May, P. B., Spaulding, S. W., and Donabedian, R. K.,** TRH and dopamine interactions affecting pituitary hormone secretion, *J. Clin. Endocrinol. Metab.,* 45, 65, 1977.
137. **Leebau, W. F., Lee, L. A., and Woolf, P. D.,** Dopamine affects basal and augmented pituitary hormone secretion, *J. Clin. Endocrinol. Metab.,* 47, 480, 1978.
138. **Kaptein, E. M., Kletzky, O. A., Spencer, C. A., and Nicoloff, J. T.,** Effects of prolonged dopamine infusion on anterior pituitary function in normal males, *J. Clin. Endocrinol. Metab.,* 51, 488, 1980.
139. **Collu, R., Fraschini, F., Visconti, P., and Martini, L.,** Adrenergic and serotonergic control of growth hormone secretion in adult male rats, *Endocrinology,* 90, 1231, 1972.
140. **Smythe, G. A. and Lazarus, L.,** Suppression of human growth hormone secretion by melatonin and cyproheptadine, *J. Clin. Invest.,* 54, 116, 1974.
141. **Smythe, G. A., Brandstater, J. F., and Lazarus, L.,** Serotonergic control of rat growth hormone secretion, *Neuroendocrinology,* 17, 245, 1975.
142. **Collu, R., Du Ruisseau, P., and Tachè, Y.,** Role of putative neurotransmitters in prolactin, GH and LH response to acute immobilization stress in male rats, *Neuroendocrinology,* 28, 178, 1979.
143. **Martin, J. B., Durand, D., Gurd, W., Faille, G., Audet, J., and Brazeau, P.,** Neuropharmacological regulation of episodic growth hormone and prolactin secretion in the rat, *Endocrinology,* 102, 106, 1978.
144. **Arnold, M. A. and Fernstrom, J. D.,** Serotonin receptor antagonists block a natural, short-term surge in serum growth hormone levels, *Endocrinology,* 103, 1159, 1978.
145. **Eden, S., Bolle, P., and Modegh, K.,** Monoaminergic control of episodic growth hormone secretion in the rat: effects of reserpine, alpha-methyl-p-tyrosine, p-chlorophenylalanine, and haloperidol, *Endocrinology,* 105, 523, 1979.
146. **Müller, E. E., Udeschini, G., Secchi, C., Zambotti, F., Panerai, A. E., Vicentini, L., Cocola, F., and Mantegazza, P.,** Inhibitory role of the serotonergic system in hypoglycemia-induced growth hormone release in the dog, *Acta Endocrinol.,* 82, 71, 1976.
147. **Bivens, C. H., Lebovitz, H. E., and Feldman, J. M.,** Inhibition of hypoglycemia induced growth hormone secretion by the serotonin antagonists cyproheptadine and methysergide, *N. Engl. J. Med.,* 289, 236, 1973.
148. **Imura, H., Nakai, Y., and Yoshimi, T.,** Effect of 5-hydroxytryptophan (5-HTP) on growth hormone and ACTH release in man, *J. Clin. Endocrinol. Med.,* 36, 204, 1973.
149. **Nakai, Y., Imura, H., Sakurai, H., Kurahachi, H., and Yoshimi, T.,** Effect of cyproheptadine on human growth hormone secretion, *J. Clin. Endocrinol. Metab.,* 38, 446, 1974.
150. **Benkert, O., Laakman, G., Souvatzoglou, A., and Von Werder, K.,** Missing indicator function of growth hormone and luteinizing hormone blood levels for dopamine and serotonin concentration in the human brain. *J. Neural Trans.,* 34, 291, 1973.
151. **Müller, E. E., Brambilla, F., Cavagnini, F., Peracchi, M., and Panerai, A.,** Slight effect of L-tryptophan on growth hormone release in normal human subjects, *J. Clin. Endocrinol. Metab.,* 39, 1, 1974.

152. **Chihara, K., Kato, Y., Maeda, K., Matsukura, S., and Imura, H.**, Suppression by cyproheptidine of human growth hormone and cortisol secretion during sleep, *J. Clin. Invest.*, 57, 1392, 1976.
153. **Liuzzi, A., Panerai, A. E., Chiodini, P. G., Secchi, C., Cocchi, D., Botalla, L., Silvestrini, F., and Müller, E. E.**, Neuroendocrine control of growth hormone secretion: experimental and clinical studies, in *Growth Hormone and Related Peptides*, Pecile, A. and Müller, E. E., Eds., Excerpta Medica, Amsterdam, 236, 1976.
154. **Sorrentino, S., Schalch, D. S., and Reiter, R. J.**, Environmental control of growth and growth hormone, in *Growth and Growth Hormone*, Pecile, A. and Müller, E. E., Eds., Excerpta Medica, Princeton, New Jersey, 1972, 330.
155. **Smythe, G. A. and Lazarus, L.**, Growth hormone regulation by melatonin and serotonin, *Nature*, 244, 230, 1973.
156. **Anton-Tay, F., Chow, C., Anton, S., and Wurtman, R. J.**, Brain serotonin concentration: elevation following intraperitoneal administration of melatonin, *Science*, 162, 277, 1968.
157. **Rønnelkeiv, O. K. and McCann, S. M.**, Growth hormone release in conscious pinealectomized and sham-operated male rats, *Endocrinology*, 102, 1694, 1978.
158. **Willoughby, J. O.**, Pinealectomy mildly disturbs the secretory patterns of prolactin and growth hormone in the unstressed rat, *J. Endocrinol.*, 86, 101, 1980.
159. **Smythe, G. A. and Lazarus, L.**, Growth hormone response to melatonin in man, *Science*, 184, 1373, 1974.
160. **Baldessarrini, R. J. and Karobath, M.**, Biochemical physiology of central synapses, *Ann. Rev. Physiol.*, 35, 273, 1973.
161. **Fioretti, P., Melis, G. B., Paoletti, M., Parodo, G., Caminiti, F., Corsini, G. U., and Martini, L.**, Gamma-amino-β-hydroxybutyric acid stimulates prolactin and growth hormone release in normal women, *J. Clin. Endocrinol. Metab.*, 47, 1336, 1978.
162. **Takahara, J., Yunoki, S., Yakushiji, W., Yamauchi, J., Yamane, Y., and Ofuji, T.**, Stimulatory effects of gamma-hydroxybutyric acid on growth hormone and prolactin release in humans, *J. Clin. Endocrinol. Metab.*, 44, 1014, 1977.
163. **Cavagnini, F., Invitti, C., Pinto, M., Maraschini, C., Di Landro, A., Dubini, A., and Marelli, A.**, Effect of acute and repeated administration of gamma aminobutyric acid (GABA) on growth hormone and prolactin secretion in man, *Acta Endocrinol.*, 93, 149, 1980.
164. **Abe, H., Kato, Y., Chihara, K., Ohgo, S., Iwasaki, Y., and Imura, H.**, Growth hormone release by gamma-aminobutyric acid (GABA) and gamma-amino-β-hydroxybutyric acid (GABOB) in the rat, *Endocrinology (Japan)*, 24, 229, 1977.
165. **Takahara, J., Yunoki, S., Hosogi, H., Yakushiji, W., Kageyama, J., and Ofuji, T.**, Concomitant increases in serum growth hormone and hypothalamic somatostatin in rats after injection of gamma-amino-butyric acid, aminooxyacetic acid, or gamma-hydroxybutyric acid, *Endocrinology*, 106, 343, 1980.
166. **Vijayan, E. and McCann, S. M.**, Effects of intraventricular injection of gamma-aminobutyric acid (GABA) on plasma growth hormone and thyrotropin in conscious ovariectomized rats, *Endocrinology*, 103, 1888, 1978.
167. **Casanueva, F., Betti, R., Frigerio, C., Cocchi, D., Mantegazza, P., and Müller, E. E.**, Growth hormone-releasing effect of an enkephalin analog in the dog: evidence for cholinergic mediation, *Endocrinology*, 106, 1239, 1980.
168. **Bruni, J. F. and Meites, J.**, Effects of cholinergic drugs on growth hormone release, *Life Sci.*, 23, 1351, 1978.
169. **Rudolph, C., Richards, G. E., Kaplan, S., and Ganong, W. F.**, Effect of intraventricular histamine on growth hormone secretion in dogs, *Neuroendocrinology*, 29, 169, 1979.
170. **Reichlin, S.**, Regulation of somatotrophic hormone secretion, in *The Pituitary Gland*, Harris, G. W. and Donovan, B. T., Eds., Butterworths, London, 1966, 270.
171. **Peake, G. T., Birge, C. A., and Daughaday, W. H.**, Alterations of radioimmunoassayable growth hormone and prolatin during hypothyroidism, *Endocrinology*, 92, 487, 1973.
172. **Hervas, F., Morreale de Escobar, G., and Escobar del Rey, F.**, Rapid effects of single small doses of L-thyroxine and triido-L-thyronine on growth hormone, as studied in the rat by radioimmunoassay, *Endocrinology*, 97, 91, 1975.
173. **Takuchi, A., Suzuki, M., and Tsuchiya, S.**, Effects of thyroidectomy on the secretory profiles of growth hormone, thyrotropin and corticosterone in the rat, *Endocrinology, (Japan)*, 25, 381, 1978.
174. **Coiro, V., Braverman, L. E., Christianson, D., Fang, S., and Goodman, H. M.**, Effect of hypothyroidism and thyroxine replacement on growth hormone in the rat, *Endocrinology*, 105, 641, 1979.
175. **Samuels, H. H., Tsai, J. S., and Clinton, R.**, Thyroid hormone action: a cell-culture system responsive to physiological concentrations of thyroid hormones, *Science*, 181, 1253, 1973.
176. **Tsai, J. S. and Samuels, H. H.**, Thyroid hormone action: stimulation of growth hormone and inhibition on prolactin secretion in cultured GH^1 cells, *Biochem. Biophys. Res. Commun.*, 59, 420, 1974.

177. **Iwatsubo, H., Omori, K., Okada, Y., Fukuchi, M., Miyai, K., Abe, H., and Kumahara, Y.,** Human growth hormone secretion in primary hypothyroidism before and after treatment, *J. Clin. Endocrinol. Metab.*, 27, 1751, 1967.
178. **Kato, H. P., Youlton, R., Kaplan, S. L., and Grumbach, M. M.,** Growth and growth hormone. III. Growth hormone release in children with primary hypothyroidism and thyrotoxicosis, *J. Clin. Endocrinol. Metab.*, 29, 346, 1969.
179. **MacGillivray, M. H., Aceto, T. Jr., and Frohman, L. A.,** Plasma growth hormone responses and growth retardation in hypothyroidism, *Am. J. Dis. Child.*, 115, 273, 1968.
180. **Dupont, A., Merand, Y., and Barden, N.,** Effect of propylthiouracil and thyroxine on the inactivation of somatostatin by rat hypothalamus, *Life Sci.*, 23, 2007, 1978.
181. **Dickerman, E., Dickerman, S., and Meites, J.,** Influence of age, sex, and estrous cycle on pituitary and plasma GH levels in rats, in *Growth and Growth Hormone*, Excerpta Medica, Milan, 1971, 252.
182. **Malacara, J. M., Valverde, R., and Reichlin, S.,** Elevation of plasma radioimmunoassayable growth hormone in the rat induced by porcine hypothalamic extract, *Endocrinology*, 91, 1189, 1972.
183. **Frantz, A. G. and Rabkin, M. T.,** Effects of estrogen and sex difference on secretion of human growth hormone, *J. Clin. Endocrinol. Metab.*, 25, 1470, 1965.
184. **Merimee, T. J., Fineberg, S. E., and Tyson, J. E.,** Fluctuation of human growth hormone secretion during menstrual cycle: response to arginine, *Metabolism*, 18, 606, 1969.
185. **Illig, R. and Prader, A.,** Effect of testosterone on growth hormone secretion in patients with anorxia and delayed puberty, *J. Clin. Endocrinol. Metab.*, 30, 615, 1970.
186. **Finkelstein, J. W., Roffwarg, H. P., Boyar, R. M., Kream, J., and Hellman, L.,** Age-related changes in the twenty-four hour spontaneous secretion of growth hormone, *J. Clin. Endocrinol. Metab.*, 35, 655, 1972.
187. **Simon, S. M., Schiffer, M., Glick, S. M., and Schwartz, E.,** Effect of medroxyprogesterone acetate upon stimulated release of growth hormone in men, *J. Clin. Endocrinol. Metab.*, 27, 1633, 1967.
188. **Lucke, C. and Glick, S. M.,** Effect of medroxyprogesterone acetate on the sleep-induced peak of growth hormone secretion, *J. Clin. Endocrinol. Metab.*, 33, 851, 1971.
189. **Lawrence, A. M. and Kirsteins, L.,** Progestins in the medical management of active acromegaly, *J. Clin. Endocrinol. Metab.*, 30, 646, 1970.
190. **Frantz, A. G. and Rabkin, M. T.,** Human growth hormone: clinical measurement response to hypoglycemia and suppression by corticosteroids, *N. Engl. J. Med.*, 271, 1375, 1964.
191. **Hartog, M., Graafar, M. A., and Fraser, R.,** Effect of corticosteroids on serum growth hormone, *Lancet*, 2, 376, 1964.
192. **Krieger, D. T. and Glick, S. M.,** Growth hormone and cortisone responsiveness in Cushing's syndrome: relation to a possible central nervous system etiology, *Am. J. Med.*, 52, 25, 1972.
193. **Takahashi, K., Kipnis, D. M., and Daughaday, W. H.,** Growth hormone secretion during sleep, *J. Clin. Invest.*, 47, 2079, 1968.
194. **Honday, Y., Takahashi, K., Takahashi, S., Azimi, K., Irie, M., Sakuma, M., Tsushima, T., and Shizume, K.,** Growth hormone secretion during nocturnal sleep in normal subjects, *J. Clin. Endocrinol. Metab.*, 29, 20, 1969.
195. **Parker, D. C., Sassin, J. F., Mace, J. W., Gotlin, R. W., and Rossman, L. G.,** Human growth hormone release during sleep: electroencephalographic correlation, *J. Clin. Endocrinol. Metab.*, 29, 871, 1969.
196. **Sassin, J. F., Parker, D. C., Mace, J. W., Gotlin, R. W., Johnson, L. C., and Rossman, L. G.,** Human growth hormone release: relation to slow-wave sleep and sleep-waking cycles, *Science*, 165, 513, 1969.
197. **Lucke, C. and Glick, S. M.,** Experimental modification of the sleep-induced peak of growth hormone secretion, *J. Clin. Endocrinol. Metab.*, 32, 729, 1971.
198. **Mendelson, W. B., Jacobs, L. S., Reichman, J. D., Othmer, E., Cryer, P. E., Trivedi, B., and Daughaday, W. H.,** Methysergide: suppression of sleep-related prolactin secretion and enhancement of sleep-related growth hormone secretion. *J. Clin. Invest.*, 56, 690, 1975.
199. **Chihara, K., Kato, Y., Maeda, K., Matsukura, S., and Imura, H.,** Suppression by cyproheptadine of human growth hormone and cortisol secretion during sleep, *J. Clin. Invest.*, 57, 1393, 1976.
200. **Malarkey, W. B. and Mendell, J. R.,** Failure of a serotonin inhibitor to effect nocturnal GH and prolactin secretion in patients with Duchenne muscular dystrophy, *J. Clin. Endocrinol. Metab.*, 43, 889, 1976.
201. **Mendelson, W. B., Sitaram, N., Wyatt, R. J., Gillin, J. C., and Jacobs, L. S.,** Methscopolamine inhibition of sleep-related growth hormone secretion, *J. Clin. Invest.*, 61, 1683, 1978.
202. **Reichlin, S.,** Regulation of somatotropic hormone secretion, in *Handbook of Physiology*, Section 7, Endocrinology, Vol. 4, Part 2, Greep, P. O. and Astwood, E. B., Eds., American Physiological Society, Williams & Wilkins, Baltimore, 1975, 405.

203. **Martin, J. B., Reichlin, S., and Brown, G. M., Eds.,** Regulation of growth hormone secretion and its disorders in *Clinical Neuroendocrinology,* Chap. 7, E. A. Davis Co., Philadelphia, 1977, chap. 7, p. 147.
204. **Ojeda, S. and Jameson, H.,** Developmental patterns of plasma and pituitary growth hormone (GH) in the female rat, *Endocrinology,* 100, 881, 1977.
205. **Walker, P., Dussault, J., Alvardo-Urbina, G., and Dupont, A.,** The development of the hypothalamopituitary axis in the neonatal rat: hypothalamic somatostatin and pituitary and serum growth hormone concentrations, *Endocrinology,* 101, 782, 1977.
206. **Sonntag, W. E.,** Luteinizing hormone releasing hormone and somatostatin in the anterior and posterior hypothalamus during development of the male and female rat, *Doctoral Dissertation,* Tulane University, New Orleans, 1979.
207. **Eden, S.,** Age- and sex-related differences in episodic growth hormone secretion in the rat, *Endocrinology,* 105, 555, 1979.
208. **Ramalay, J. A. and Phares, C. K.,** Delay of puberty onset in females due to suppression of growth hormone, *Endocrinology,* 106, 1989, 1980.
209. **Finch, C. E.,** The regulation of physiological changes during mammalian aging, *Q. Rev. Biol.,* 51, 49, 1976.
210. **Sonntag, W. E., Steger, R. W., Forman, L. J., and Meites, J.,** Decreased pulsatile release of growth hormone in old male rats, *Endocrinology,* 107, 1875, 1980.
211. **Sonntag, W. E., Forman, L. J., Miki, N., Steger, R. W., Ramos, T., Arimura, A., and Meites, J.,** Effects of CNS active drugs and somatostatin antiserum on GH release in young and old rats, *Neuroendocrinology,* 33, 73, 1981.
212. **Carlson, H. E., Gillin, J. C., Gorden, P., and Snyder, F.,** Absence of sleep-related growth hormone peaks in aged normal subjects and in acromegaly, *J. Clin. Endo. Metab.,* 34, 1102, 1972.
213. **Laron, Z., Doron, M., and Amikan, B.,** Plasma growth hormone in men and women over 70 years of age, in *Medicine and Sport, Vol. 4, Physical Activity and Aging,* Karger, New York, 1970, 126.
214. **Meiki, N. and Meites, J.** Unpublished data, 1981.
215. **Bruni, J. and Meites, J.,** Unpublished data, 1981

REGULATION OF THYROID STIMULATING HORMONE SECRETION

James W. Simpkins

INTRODUCTION

The central nervous system (CNS) exerts a profound influence on homeostatic processes in the body, in part through its regulation of the secretion of trophic hormones from the anterior pituitary gland (AP, adenohypophysis). In response to both enteroceptive and exteroceptive stimuli, specialized peptidergic neurons in the brain synthesize and release neurohormones (small peptides) which reach the anterior pituitary gland and modify the rate of trophic hormone secretion. These peptidergic neurons act as neuroendocrine transducers, receiving input from the autonomic nervous system and providing output through the release of the peptide hormones.

A physiologic relationship between the CNS and the AP has long been suggested for the regulation of thyroid stimulating hormone (TSH) secretion. Electrolytic lesions of the hypothalamus produce profound thyroid atrophy[1] whereas electrical stimulation of the hypothalamus increases thyroid activity.[2] Since these effects are not observed following electrical stimulation of the AP,[2,3] it is considered that the hypothalamic region of the brain exerts a regulatory influence on AP activity.

Additional evidence to test the influence of the hypothalamus on TSH secretion is obtained by transection of the hypothalamo-hypophyseal connections. This separates the hypothalamus from the AP. As early as 1923, Dott[4] observed that this procedure results in atrophy of the thyroid gland. This observation was later confirmed both by pituitary stalk transection[5] and by transplantation of the AP from its *in situ* location to the anterior chamber of the eye or under the renal capsule.[6]

In the past 30 years, intensive research has been conducted to elucidate the mechanisms by which the CNS regulates secretion of TSH from the AP. The present review attempts to describe the current status of understanding (i) the brain areas involved in TSH regulation; (ii) the neuronal pathways and the neurotransmitters involved in TSH regulation; (iii) the mechanisms by which CNS information is transferred to the AP; and (iv) the site of feedback action of thyroid hormones on TSH secretion. Factors (chemical, surgical, environmental, and pathologic) which modify the secretion of TSH are simply listed, with references, in Tables 1 and 2.

ANATOMIC CORRELATES OF TSH SECRETORY MECHANISM

Hypothalamus

A variety of experimental approaches has been employed to define the regions of the brain which influence the secretion of TSH. Surgical removal of the neocortex[7] and of the forebrain[8] does not dramatically alter thyroid function. Massive removal of brain tissue, leaving only the hypothalamus and its attachment to the AP, has little effect on basal thyroid function or response to goitrogens.[9] These results indicate that the basal secretory rate of TSH and its response to removal of thyroid hormones are mediated by the hypothalamus-pituitary complex. Small electrolytic lesions within the hypothalamus indicate that destruction of areas in the medial basal hypothalamus, extending from the anterior hypothalamus to the median eminence, interferes with normal thyroid function.[10-14] Studies utilizing electrical stimulation have demonstrated that these same areas respond to electrical stimulation by increasing AP-TSH secretion.[15]

Although the primary TSH releasing factor, thyrotropin-releasing hormone (TRH),

Table 1
FACTORS WHICH ENHANCE TSH SECRETION

Chemical	Ref.
Thyrotropin releasing hormone (TRH)	19, 40, 45—48
Noradrenergic stimulants	53—58
Antithyroid drugs	33, 36—38, 40, 41
Histamine	75, 76
Surgical	
Thyroidectomy	19, 32, 33, 36—38, 40
Electrical stimulation of preoptic area and medial basal hypothalamus	15, 23, 39
Local cooling of the preoptic area	21,22
Environmental	
Decreased ambient temperature	19, 23, 24, 39
Pathologic	
Primary hypothyroidism	40

Table 2
FACTORS WHICH DECREASE TSH SECRETION

Chemical	Ref.
Increased serum thyroid hormones	33, 37, 38, 41, 47, 48
Somatostatin	82
Anti-TRH antibodies	81
Dopaminergic stimulants	63—69
Drugs which interfere with CNS noradrenergic neurotransmission	53—58
Morphine and methionine-enkephalin	77, 78
Glucocorticoids	40, 79
Growth hormone	40
Surgical	
Destruction of the medial basal hypothalamus	10—14
Transection of the hypothalamopituitary stalk	5
Environmental	
Stress	40, 70
Increased ambient temperature	19, 23, 24, 39, 40
Pathologic	
Hypohtalamic (tertiary) hypothyroidism	40, 80
Pituitary (secondary) hypothyroidism	40, 80

is located throughout the CNS in extrahypothalamic tissue, highest concentrations are found in the hypophysiotrophic area of the hypothalamus. Areas of the hypothalamus which respond to electrical stimulation with increased TSH release have high TRH concentrations.[17] Nerve terminals in the median eminence of the hypothalamus contain extremely high concentrations of TRH, indicating the primary importance of this hypothalamic hormone is the regulation of TSH secretion.[18]

The preoptic area of the ventral diencephalon appears to plan an important role in the response of the TSH secretory mechanism to changes in ambient temperature.[19] Electrolytic lesions of this area have no effect on basal TSH secretion, but have been reported to block the TSH increase induced by acute cold exposure.[20] Local cooling of the preoptic area results in an enhanced thyroid activity, presumably mediated by enhanced TSH secretion.[21,22] It is recognized that some preoptic-anterior hypothalamic neurons are thermosensitive, responding to alteration in body core temperature.[19] Acute exposure to low ambient temperature results in a prompt hypersecretion of TSH,[19,23,24] presumably mediated through the preoptic area-anterior hypothalamus.[20]

The Hypophyseal Portal System

Popa and Fielding[25] observed that the blood vessels supplying the anterior pituitary gland are part of a portal system connecting the sinusoids of the AP with a capillary plexus in the median eminence of the hypothalamus. They speculated that blood flows from the AP to the hypothalamus. Soon, thereafter, Houssay et al.[26] and Wislocki and King[27] observed movement of the blood from the hypothalamus to the AP. In mammals, except the rabbit, 100% of the blood supply to the AP appears to flow through the portal vessels. However, Bergland and Page[28] suggesed that under certain conditions blood can flow back from the AP to the hypothalamus, Porter et al.[29] observed extremely high levels of anterior pituitary hormones (including TSH) in hypophyseal portal blood. The observations suggest that AP hormones may travel back to the hypothalamus via portal vessels and reach the CNS in high concentrations, perhaps thereby regulating their own secretion through a short loop feedback mechanism.

For TRH, as well as for the other hypothalamic hormones which have been conclusively identified, i.e., luteinizing hormone-releasing hormone (LHRH) and somatostatin, the highest concentrations in the brain are found in the median eminence.[30] Dense clusters of TRH nerve terminals are located in the median eminence adjacent to the capillary plexus of hypophyseal portal vessels.[18] TRH has been identified in hypophyseal portal blood[31] and is the most potent known stimulus to TSH release from the AP.[19] It is now widely held that TRH, when released from nerve terminals in the median eminence, is delivered to the AP by intricate portal vessels and thereby stimulates the secretion of TSH. Thus, this median eminence-hypophyseal portal system appears to by a final common pathway by which CNS information is integrated into an appropriate TSH secretory response.

Anterior Pituitary Thyrotrophs

The anterior pituitary gland is a heterologous structure containing parenchymal cells which synthesize and secrete numerous polypeptide and glycoproteins.[32] The polypeptides include prolactin, growth hormone (GH), corticotropin (ATCH), and melanotropin (MSH). The glycoproteins are thyroid stimulating hormone (TSH), luteinizing hor mone (LH), and follicle-stimulating hormone (FSH).

The initial separation of cell types in the anterior pituitary gland utilized dye staining techniques and subsequent characterization of cellular microanatomy. Pituitary cells containing glycoproteins (TSH, LH, or FSH) stain most intensely with basic dyes and are thus classified as basophils. The polypeptide-containing cell either stains well with acidic dyes (acidophils) or does not stain well by conventional methods (chromophobes). These classical histologic techniques have been replaced by immunofluorescence techniques which allow specific staining of anterior pituitary cell for the hormone which they produce. This procedure has provided convincing evidence that the known anterior pituitary trophic hormones are all produced in separate cells.

Thyrotrophs normally make up 2 to 4% of the parenchymal cells of the anterior pituitary gland[33] and are located primarily in the ventromedial area of the lateral lobes of the anterior pituitary gland. These cells often occur in clusters and are frequently associated with capillaries of the hypophseal portal system.[34,35] Primary hypothyroidism in human patients[36] and thyroidectomy in the rat[33] results in an increase in the number of thyrotrophs and a dramatic alteration in their staining characteristics, indicative of a depletion of TSH from the thyrotrophs. High circulating concentrations of thyroid hormone cause regression of pituitary throtrophs. In contrast, TRH appears to have little effect on the number or the cytology of pituitary thyrotrophs. The latter observation suggests that TRH does little more to the thyrotroph than enhance the exocytosis of TSH-containing granules.[32]

NEGATIVE FEEDBACK OF THYROID HORMONES ON TSH SECRETION

The hypothalamus-pituitary-thyroid axis is an excellent example in neuroendocrinology of a self-regulatory, neuroendocrine system. Following the administration of extremely small doses of thyroxine (T_4), serum TSH in both human subjects[37] and in rats[38] decreases in proportion to the levels of serum T_4 present. The normal "setpoint" for the feedback regulation of TSH secretion is extremely sensitive, since only small deviations in serum T_4 or triiodothyronine (T_3) result in appropriate adjustments in serum TSH concentrations. Serum TSH concentrations can remain remarkably constant for long periods of time.

The setpoint for TSH regulation can be overridden by increased secretion of TRH from the hypothalamus. Thus, in response to low ambient temperature, a rapid surge in TSH secretion occurs.[39] Similarly, intravenous administration of TRH results in an extremely rapid hypersecretion of TSH.[40] Both of these pituitary responses to TRH can be blocked by elevating serum T_4.[41] Likewise, progressively increasing the dosage of TRH can partially overcome the inhibitory effects of T_4. Apparently, a competition exists in the pituitary between the TSH releasing effects of TRH and the TSH inhibiting effects of thyroid hormone. A primary site for the inhibitory action of T_4 on TSH secretion appears to be the pituitary gland.

An alternative site of the negative feedback of thyroid hormone on TSH secretion is the hypothalamus. Implantation of crystalline T_4 results in reduced TSH secretion, presumably through the reduced secretion of hypothalamic TRH.[42,43] These conclusions have become suspect by virtue of the observation that following hypothalamic implantation many substance are quickly distributed to the anterior pituitary gland.[44] The inhibition of TSH secretion following hypothalamic implantation of T_4 may be due simply to its diffusion to the pituitary. It is very likely that the primary site of action of thyroid hormones is in the anterior pituitary gland.

TRH appears to stimulate the release of TSH following its interaction with plasma membrane receptors on thyrotrophs.[43-46] Following the interaction with its receptor, TRH stimulates adenylate cyclase, resulting in the accumulation of cyclic nucleotides and, through a yet undefined mechanism, the exocytosis of secretory granules and the release of TSH. In contrast, the thyroid hormone inhibition of TSH secretion appears to require the *de novo* synthesis of protein.[47,48] This observation has led to the speculation that thyroid hormones stimulate the synthesis of a protein which blocks the TSH releasing effects of TRH.

INFLUENCE OF CENTRAL NEURONAL SYSTEMS ON TSH SECRETION

Inasmuch as thyroid hormones appear to exert their negative feedback effects on TSH secretion by an action on the anterior pituitary gland, the role of the hypothalamus appears to be to provide the primary stimulation for TSH secretion. In this regard,

TRH secretion may be regulated by a variety of autonomic input to the medial basal hypothalamus. Those neuronal systems which impinge upon the TRH neurons and thereby modify its secretion will now be considered.

Noradrenergic Neurons

The central noradrenergic system originates from cell bodies located in the locus coeruleus and midbrain reticular areas.[49] From these regions, axons travel via the medial forebrain bundle to provide the noradrenergic innervation of the hypothalamus as well as the remainder of the brain.[49,50] Disruption of the noradrenergic tract innervating the hypothalamus leads to profound depletion of hypothalamic norepinephrine (NE) and the enzymes which lead to its biosynthesis.[49,51,52] These observations plus the absence of hypothalamic noradrenergic cell bodies indicate that the entire hypothalamic NE supply originates from extrahypothalamic areas.

Noradrenergic neurons exert a stimulatory influence on TSH secretion, apparently by enhancing the synthesis and release of TRH from the hypothalamus. Using an in vitro preparation, Reichlin and collaborators[53] observed that NE stimulates TRH synthesis whereas depletion of NE decreases the rate of TRH production. Consistent with these observations are reports that pharmacologic disruption of NE biosynthesis blocks TSH release. Thus, α-methylparatyrosine, which blocks the synthesis of all catecholamines and diethyldithiocarbonate and disulfiram (which block the conversion of dopamine to NE) prevents the cold-induced stimulation of TSH release.[54-57] Depletion of catecholamines with reserpine or blockade of the α-adrenergic receptor with phentolamine suppresses the TSH response to cold.[55] The cold-induced increase in TSH can be restored in α-methylparatyrosine treated animals by treatment with the α-adrenergic receptor agonist, clonidine.[56] Further, the hypersecretion of TSH in hypothyroid patients can be attenuated through the blockade of NE synthesis.[58]

These data provide pharmacologic support to the concept of a stimulatory NE input into the secretion of TSH. However, it has not been conclusively demonstrated that NE turnover is accelerated in conditions of enhanced TSH secretion (i.e., decreased ambient or core body temperature, and primary hypothyroidism). In view of the observation that about 95% of hypothalamic afferents do not form true synapses,[59] it is possible that NE acts as a neuromodulator rather than as a true neurotransmitter, in regulating TSH secretion. In this role, NE can modify the action of other substances on TRH neurons, but not itself alter activity in the TRH neurons. The mechanisms by which NE stimulates TRH-TSH secretion remain to be elucidated.

Dopaminergic Neurons

Hypothalamic Dopamine (DA) innervation probably originates from DA systems which are confined to the hypothalamus. The primary hypothalamic DA system involved in hormone secretion is the tuberoinfundibular system. This arises from a tightly-packed band of cell bodies located in the arcuate nucleus and the lateral periventricular nucleus.[60,61] Axons from the cell bodies pass ventrally, to terminate in the external layer of the median eminence. Kizer et al.[62] claims that there is a DA input to the median eminence from the substantia nigra.

Pharmacologic evidence indicates that DA exerts an inhibitory influence on TSH secretion. The specific DA receptor agonists, apomorphine and piribedil, are reported to inhibit basal TSH levels,[63] to block the cold-induced rise in serum TSH,[64,65] and to attenuate the increase in TSH induced by thyroidectomy.[63] Bromergocryptine, another DA receptor agonist, is also said to block the cold-induced rise in serum TSH.[64] Intravenous administration of DA decreases serum TSH,[66] which is apparently a direct effect of DA on the AP, since DA inhibits the TRH-induced release of TSH.[67-69] Thus, DA can exert an inhibitory influence on TSH secretion by inhibiting hypothalamic TRH release or by blocking the TSH releasing effect of TRH at the level of the AP.

Serotonergic Neurons

In contrast to the evidence implicating NE and DA in the regulation of TSH secretion, there is no consistent evidence as to the role of serotonergic neurons in this regulation. Mueller et al.[70] demonstrated that both restraint stress and L-tryptophan administration increase serotonin turnover and decrease TSH secretion. However, parachlorophenylalanine, which depletes brain serotonin, decreases[71] or does not alter[72] TSH secretion. More studies on the role of serotonin in TSH secretion are needed. Since serotonin is implicated in the generation of rhythmic alterations in brain function and hormone secretion,[73] this neurotransmitter may be involved in production of the daily rhythm in TSH secretion.[74] This has not yet been experimentally evaluated.

Other Putative Neurotransmitter Systems

The central nervous system contains numerous substances which are neurotransmitters or neuromodulators. However, their significance in the control of TSH secretion has not been adequately studied. Histamine and opioid peptides have been studies with respect to TSH regulation, although these studies are preliminary in nature.

Histamine

Blockade of histamine biosynthesis attenuates the TSH release induced by cold-ambient temperatures.[75] Also, histamine releses TSH from anterior pituitaries, in vitro.[76]

Opioid Peptides

Acute morphine administration results in decreased TSH secretion[77] and decreased thyroid function.[78] A similar observation has been made using methionine enkephalin, a penta-peptide found in high concentrations in the hypothalamus.[77]

The TSH decreasing effect of morphine is diminished with chronic administration, indicating that tolerance develops. This has been long known for the antinociceptive effects of morphine. The inability of naloxone, a morphine receptor antagonist, to increase TSH secretion, even at high doses, suggests that endogenous opioid peptides may not play a physiologic role in suppressing TSH secretion. Additional study is needed to document the role of opioid peptides in the regulation of TSH secretion.

SUMMARY

Circulating levels of TSH are determined by the rate of its secretion by pituitary thyrotrophs. The rate of TSH secretion is in turn determined by the stimulatory influence of hypothalamic TRH and the inhibitory influence of serum thyroid hormones. Both TRH and thyroid hormones appear to compete at the thyrotroph to determine TSH secretion. The central noradrenergic system exerts a stimulatory effect on TRH-TSH secretion whereas dopaminergic and opioid neurons have an inhibitory effect. The interaction between aminergic and TRH containing neurons appear to occur primarily in the medial basal hypothalamus, where autonomic information is transduced into an appropriate signal for TSH secretion.

REFERENCES

1. **Cahane, M. and Cahane, T.,** Sur certaines modifications des glandes endocrines apres endocrines apres une lesion dienciphalizue, *Rev. Franc. Endocrinol. Nutrit. Metab.*, 14, 472, 1936.
2. **Harris, G. W. and Wood, J. W.,** The effect of electrical stimulation of the hypothalamus or pituitary gland on thyroid activity, *J. Physiol. (London)*, 143, 246, 1958.

3. **Markee, J. E., Sawyer, C. H., and Hollinshed, W. H.**, Activation of the anterior hypophysis by electrical stimulation in the rabbits, *Endocrinology*, 38, 345, 1946.
4. **Dott, N. M.**, An investigation into the function of the pituitary and thyroid glands. Part I. Technique of their experimental surgery and summary of results, *Q. J. Exp. Physiol.*, 13, 241, 1923.
5. **Mahoney, W. and Sheehan, D.**, The pituitary-hypothalamic mechanism: experimental occlusion of the pituitary stalk, *Brain*, 59, 61, 1936.
6. **Harris, G. W.**, Neural control of the pituitary gland, *Physiol. Rev.*, 28, 139, 1948.
7. **Greer, M. A. and Shull, H. F.**, Effect of ablation of neocortex on ability of pituitary to secrete thyrotropin in the rat, *Proc. Soc. Exp. Biol. Med.*, 94, 565, 1957.
8. **Beugen, L. Van and Van der Werff Ten Bosch, J. J.**, Rat thyroid activity and cold response after removal of frontal parts of the brain, *Acta Endocrinol.*, 37, 470, 1961.
9. **Matsuda, K., Greet, M. A., and Duyck, C.**, Neural control of thyrotropin secretion: effect of forebrain removal on thyroid function, *Endocrinology*, 73, 462, 1963.
10. **Greer, M. A.**, Evidence of hypothalamic control of the pituitary release of thyrotrophin, *Proc. Soc. Exp. Biol. Med.*, 77, 603, 1951.
11. **Greer, M. A.**, Demonstration of thyroidal response to exogenous thyrotropin in rats with anterior hypothalamic lesions, *Endocrinology*, 77, 755, 1955.
12. **Bogdanove, E. M. and Halmi, N. S.**, Effects of hypothalamic lesions and subsequent propylthiouracil treatment on pituitary structure and function in the rat, *Endocrinology*, 53, 274, 1953.
13. **D'Angelo, S. A. and Traum, K.**, An experimental analysis of the hypothalamic-hypophysial-thyroid relationship in the rat, *Ann. New York Acad. Sci.*, 72, 239, 1958.
14. **Florsheim, W. H.**, The effect of anterior hypothalamic lesions on thyroid function and goiter development in the rat, *Endocrinology*, 62, 783, 1958.
15. **Martin, J. B. and Reichlin, S.**, Plasma thyrotropin (TSH) response to hypothalamic electrical stimulation and to injection of synthetic thyrotropin-releasing hormone, *Endocrinology*, 90, 1079, 1972.
16. **Quijada, M., Krulich, L., Fawcett, C., Sundberg, D., and McCann, S.**, Localization of TSH-releasing factor (TRF). LH-RF, and FSH-RF in the rat hypothalamus, *Fed. Proc.*, 30, 197-199, 1971.
17. **Brownstein, M., Palkovits, M., Saavedra, J. M., Bassiri, R. M., and Utiger, R. D.**, Tyrotropin-releasing hormone in specific nuclei of the brain, *Science*, 185, 267, 1974.
18. **Hokfelt, T.**, Distribution of thyrotropin-releasing hormone (TRH) in the central nervous system as revealed with immunocytochemistry, *Eur. J. Pharmacol.*, 34, 389, 1975.
19. **Reichlin, S., Martin, J. B., Mitnick, M., Boshans, R. L., Grimm, Y., Bollinger, J., Gordon, J., and Malacara, J.**, The hypothalamus in pituitary-thyroid regulation, *Rec. Prog. Horm. Res.*, 28, 229, 1972.
20. **D'Angelo, S. A.**, Hypothalamus and endocrine function in persistent estrous rats at low environmental temperature, *Amer. J. Physiol.*, 199, 701, 1960.
21. **Andersson, B., Ekman, L., Gale, C. C., and Sundsten, J. W.**, Activation of the thyroid gland by cooling of the pre-optic area in the goat, *Acta Physiol. Scand.*, 54, 191, 1962.
22. **Andersson, B., Ekman, L., Gale, C. C., and Sundsten, J. W.**, Control of thyrotrophic hormone (TSH) secretion by the "heat loss center," *Acta Physiol. Scand.*, 59, 12, 1963.
23. **Golsteine-Golaire, J., Vanhaelst, L., Bruno, O. D., Leclercq. R., and Copinschi, G.**, Acute effects of cold on blood levels of growth hormone, cortisol and thyrotropin in man, *J. Appl. Physiol.*, 29, 622, 1970.
24. **Fisher, D. A. and Odell, W. D.**, Acute release of thyrotropin in the newborn, *J. Clin. Invest.*, 48, 1670, 1969.
25. **Popa, G. T. and Fielding, U.**, A portal circulation from the pituitary to the hypothalamic region, *J. Anat. (London)*, 54, 88, 1930.
26. **Houssay, B. A., Biasotti, A., and Sammertino, R.**, Modifications fonctionelles de l'hypophyse apres les lesions infundibulotuberiennes chez le crapoud, *C. R. Lebd. Seanc. Soc. Bio. (Paris)*, 120, 725, 1935.
27. **Wislocki, G. B. and King, L. S.**, The permeability of the hypophysis and hypothalamus to vital dyes, with a study of the hypophyseal vascular supply, *Am. J. Anat.*, 58, 421, 1926.
28. **Page, R. B., Munger, B. L., and Bergland, R. M.**, Scanning microscopy of pituitary vascular casts, *Am. J. Anat.*, 146, 273, 1976.
29. **Oliver, C., Mical, R. S., and Porter, J. C.**, Hypothalamic-pituitary vasculature: evidence for retrograde blood flow in the pituitary stalk, *Endocrinology*, 101, 598, 1977.
30. **Brownstein, M. J., Palkovits, M., Saavedra, J. M., and Kizer, J. S.**, Distribution of hypothalamic hormones and neurotransmitters within the diencephalon, in *Frontiers in Neuroendocrinology*, Vol. 4, Martini, L. and Ganong, W. F., Eds., Raven Press, New York, 1976, 1.
31. **Wilber, J. F. and Porter, J. C.**, Thyrotropin and growth hormone releasing activity in hypophyseal portal blood, *Endocrinology*, 87, 807, 1970.

32. **Baker, B. L.**, Functional cytology of the hypophyseal pars distalis and pars intermedia, in *Handbook of Physiology, Section 7*, Vol. 4, Knobil, E. and Sawyer, W. H., Eds., American Physiological Society, Washington, D.C., 1974, 45.
33. **Bogdanove, E. M.**, Local actions of target gland hormones on the rat adenohypophysis, in *Cytologie de l'Adenohypophyse*, Benoit, J. and Da Lage, C., Eds., Centre National de la Recherche Scientifique, Paris, 1963, 163.
34. **Baker, B. L. and Yu, Y. Y.**, The thyrotropic cell of the rat hypophysis as studied with peroxidase-labeled antibody, *Am. J. Anat.*, 131, 55, 1971.
35. **Purves, H. D. and Griesbach, W. E.**, The site of thyrotrophin and gonadotrophin production in the rat pituitary studied by McManus-Hotchkiss staining for glycoproteins, *Endocrinology*, 49, 244, 1951.
36. **Ezrin, C. and Murray, S.**, The cells of the human adenohypophysis in pregnancy, thyroid disease and adrenal cortical disorders, in *Cytologie de l'Adenohypophyse*, Benoit, J. and Da Lage, C., Eds., Centre National de la Recherche Scientifique, Paris, 1963, 183.
37. **Reichlin, S. and Utiger, R. D.**, Regulation of the pituitary-thyroid axis in man: the relationship of TSH concentration to free and total thyroid thyroxine level in plasma, *J. Clin. Endocrinol.*, 27, 251, 1967.
38. **Reichlin, S.**, Measurement of TSH in plasma and pituitary of the rat by a radioimmunoassay utilizing bovine TSH: effect of thyroidectomy on thyroxine replacement, *Endocrinology*, 87, 1022, 1970.
39. **Martin, J. B. and Reichlin, S.**, Neural regulation of the pituitary-thyroid axis, in *Proceedings of the Sixth Midwest Conference on the Thyroid*, Kenny, A. D. and Anderson, R. R., Eds., University of Columbia Press, Missouri, 1970, 1.
40. **Martin, J. B., Reichlin, S., and Brown, G. M.**, Regulation of TSH secretion and its disorders, in *Clinical Neuroendocrinology*, F. A. Davis, Philadelphia, 1977, Chap. 9.
41. **Snyder, P. J. and Utiger, R. D.**, Inhibition of thyrotropin response to thyrotropin-releasing hormone by small quantities of thyroid hormones, *J. Clin. Invest.*, 51, 2077, 1972.
42. **Chambers, W. F. and Sobel, R. J.**, Effect of thyroxineagartube application to the rat hypothalamus, *Neuroendocrinology*, 7, 37, 1971.
43. **Kajihara, A. and Kendall, J. W.**, Studies on the hypothalamic control of TSH secretion, *Neuroendocrinology*, 5, 53, 1969.
44. **Florsheim, W. H.**, Control of thyrotrophin secretion, in *Handbook of Physiology, Section 7*, Vol. 4, Knobil, E. and Sawyer, W. H., Eds., American Physiological Society, Washington D.C., 1974, 449.
45. **Grant, G.**, Interaction of thyrotropin-releasing factor with membrane receptors of pituitary cells, *Biochem. Biophys. Res. Commun.*, 46, 23, 1972.
46. **Labrie, F., Barden, N., Poirier, G., and De Lean, A.**, Binding of thyrotropin-releasing hormone to plasma membranes of bovine anterior pituitary gland, *Proc. Nat. Acad. Sci. U.S.A.*, 69, 283, 1972.
47. **Bowers, C. Y., Lee, K. L., and Schally, A. V.**, A study on the interaction of the thyrotropin-releasing factor and L-triiodothyronine: effects of puromycin and cycloheximide, *Endocrinology*, 82, 75, 1968.
48. **Vale, W., Burgus, R., and Guillemin, R.**, On the mechanism of action of TRF: effects of cycloheximide and actinomycin on the release of TSH stimulated *in vitro* by TRF and its inhibition by thyroxine, *Neuroendocrinology*, 3, 34, 1968.
49. **Loizou, L. A.**, Projections of the nucleus locus coeruleus in the albino rat, *Brain Res.*, 15, 563, 1969.
50. **Ungerstedt, U.**, Stereotaxic mapping of the monoamine pathways in the rat brain, *Acta Physiol. Scand. Suppl.*, 367, 1, 1971.
51. **Anden, N. E., Dahlstrom, A., Fuxe, K., Larsson, K., Olson, L., and Ungerstedt, U.**, Ascending noradrenaline neurons from the pons and the medulla oblongata, *Experientia*, 22, 44, 1966.
52. **Brownstein, M. J., Palkovits, M., Saavedra, J. M., and Kizer, J. S.**, Distribution of hypothalamic hormones and neurotransmitters within the diencephalon, in *Frontiers in Neuroendocrinology*, Vol. 4, Martini, L. and Ganong, W. F., Eds., Raven Press, New York, 1976, 1.
53. **Reichlin, S. and Mitnick, M.**, Biosynthesis of hypothalamic hypophysiotropic factors, in *Frontiers in Neuroendocrinology*, Ganong, W. F. and Martini, L., Eds., Oxford University Press, London, 1973, 61.
54. **Kotani, M., Onaya, T., and Yamada, T.**, Acute increase of thyroid hormone secretion in response to cold and its inhibition by drugs which act on the autonomic or central nervous system, *Endocrinology*, 92, 288, 1973.
55. **Tuomisto, J., Ranta, T., Mannisto, P., Saarinen, A., and Leppaluoto, J.**, Neurotransmitter control of thyrotropin secretion in the rat, *Eur. J. Pharmacol.*, 30, 221, 1975.
56. **Annunziato, L., DiRenzo, G., Lombardi, G., Scopacasa, F., Schettini, G., Preziosi, P., and Scapagnini, U.**, The role of central noradrenergic neurons in the control of thyrotropin secretion in the rat, *Endocrinology*, 100, 738, 1977.

57. **Krulich, L., Giachetti, A., Marchlewska-Koj, A., Hefco, E., and Jameson, H. E.,** On the role of the central noradrenergic and dopaminergic systems in the regulation of TSH secretion in the rat, *Endocrinology,* 100, 496, 1977.
58. **Yoshimura, M., Hachiya, T., Ochi, Y., Nagasaka, A., Takeda, A., Hidaka, H., Refetoff, S., and Fang, V. S.,** Suppression of elevated serum TSH levels in hypothyroidism by fusaric acid, *J. Clin. Endocrinol. Metab.,* 45, 95, 1977.
59. **Descarries, L., Watkins, K. C., and Lapierre, V.,** Noradrenergic axon terminals in the cerebral cortex of the rat. III. Topometric ultrastructural analyses, *Brain Res.,* 133, 197, 1977.
60. **Fuxe, K.,** Cellular localization of monoamines in the median eminence and in the infundibular stem of some mammals, *Acta Physiol. Scand.,* 58, 383, 1963.
61. **Fuxe, K. and Hokfelt, T.,** Further evidence for the existence of tuberoinfundibular dopamine neurons, *Acta Physiol. Scan.,* 66, 245, 1966.
62. **Kizer, J. S., Palkovits, M., and Brownstein, M. J.,** The projections of the A8, A9 and A10 dopaminergic cell bodies: evidence for a neuro-hypothalamic-median eminence dopaminergic pathway, *Brain Res.,* 108, 363, 1976.
63. **Mueller, G. P., Simpkins, J. W., Meites, J., and Moore, K. E.,** Differential effects of dopamine agonists and haloperidol on release of prolactin, thyroid stimulating hormone, growth hormone and luteinizing hormone in ras, *Neuroendocrinology,* 20, 121, 1976.
64. **Ranta, T., Mannisto, P., and Tuomisto, J.,** Evidence for dopaminergic control of thyrotropin secretion in the rat, *J. Endocrinol.,* 72, 329, 1977.
65. **Chen, H. J., Simpkins, J. W., Mueller, G. P., and Meites, J.** Effects of pargyline on hypothalamic biogenic amines and serum prolactin, LH and TSH in male rats, *Life Sci.,* 21, 533, 1977.
66. **Vijayan, E., Krulich, L., and McCann, S. M.,** Catecholaminergic regulation of TSH and growth hormone release in ovariectomized, steroid-primed rats, *Neuroendocrinology,* 26, 174, 1978.
67. **Besses, G., Burrow, G., Spaulding, S., and Donabedian, R.,** Dopamine infusion acutely inhibits the TSH and prolactin response to TRH, *J. Clin. Endocrinol. Metab.,* 41, 985, 1975.
68. **Burrow, G. N., May, P. N., Spaulding, S. W., and Donabedian, R.,** TRH and dopamine interactions affecting pituitary hormone secretion, *J. Clin. Endocrinol. Metab.,* 45, 65, 1977.
69. **Nilsson, K. O., Wide, L., and Hokfelt, B.,** The effect of apomorphine on basal and TRH stimulated release of thyrotrophin and prolactin in man, *Acta Endocrinol.,* 80, 220, 1975.
70. **Mueller, G. P., Twohy, C. P., Chen, H. T., Advis, J. P., and Meites, J.,** Effects of L-tryptophan and restraint stress on hypothalamic and brain serotonin turnover, and pituitary TSH and prolactin release in rats, *Life Sci.,* 18, 715, 1976.
71. **Shopsin, B., Shenkman, L., Sanghui, I., and Hollander, C. S.,** Toward a relationship between the hypothalamic pituitary-thyroid axis and the synthesis of serotonin, *Adv. Biochem. Psychopharmacol.,* 10, 279, 1974.
72. **Kardon, F., Marcus, R. J., Winokur, A., and Utiger, R. D.,** Thyrotropin-releasing hormone content of rat brain and hypothalamus: results of endocrine and pharmacologic treatments, *Endocrinology,* 100, 1604, 1977.
73. **Moore, R. Y.,** Central neural control of circadian rhythms, in *Frontiers in Neuroendocrinology,* Vol. 5, Ganong, W. F. and Martini, L., Eds., Raven Press, New York, 1978, 185.
74. **Vanhaekt, L., Van Cauter, E., Degaute, J. P., and Goldstein, J.,** Circadian variations of serum thyrotropin levels in man, *J. Clin. Endocrinol. Metab.,* 35, 479, 1972.
75. **Onaya, T. and Hashizume, K.,** Effects of drugs that modify brain biogenic amine concentrations on thyroid activation induced by exposure to cold, *Neuroendocrinology,* 20, 47, 1976.
76. **Bowers, C. Y., Wu, B., and Folkers, K.,** Mechanisms involved in release of thyroid stimulating hormone (TSH) and other pituitary hormones, in *Anatomical Neuroendocrinology,* Stumpf, W. E. and Grant L. D., Eds., Karger, Basel, 1975, 333.
77. **Meites, J., Bruni, J. F., Van Vugt, D. A., and Smith, A. F.,** Relation of endogenous opioid peptides and morphine to neuroendocrine functions, *Life Sci.,* 24, 1325, 1979.
78. **Lomax, P., Kokka, N., and George, R.,** Thyroid activity following intracerebral injection of morphine in the rat, *Neuroendocrinology,* 6, 146, 1970.
79. **Hershman, J. M. and Pittman, J. A. Jr.,** Control of thyrotropin secretion in man, *N. Engl. J. Med.,* 285, 997, 1971.
80. **Fleisher, N., Lorente, M., Kirkland, J., Kirkland, R., Clayton, G., and Calderon, M.,** Synthetic thyrotropin-releasing factor - a test of pituitary thyrotropin reserve, *J. Clin. Endocrinol. Metab.,* 34, 617, 1972.
81. **Kock, Y., Goldhaber, G., Fireman, I., Zor, U., Shani, J., and Tai, E.,** Suppression of prolactin and thyrotropin secretion in the rat by antiserum to thyrotropin-releasing hormone, *Endocrinology,* 100, 1476, 1977.
82. **Vale, W., Rivier, C., Brazeau, P., and Guillemin, R.,** Effect of somatostatin on the secretion of thyrotropin and prolactin, *Endocrinology,* 95, 668, 1974.

ACTH OF THE ANTERIOR PITUITARY

Lindsey Grandison

INTRODUCTION

Recent developments in the biosynthesis of adrenocorticotropin (ACTH) during the past three years have radically broadened the significance of ACTH. No longer can ACTH be considered as only an anterior pituitary hormone acting on the adrenal cortex. ACTH must now be interpreted as one of a family of polypeptides cleaved from a common precursor. It is clear that several cell types synthesize this precursor and can even produce different sets of end products. The responses to these products are diverse and in many cases incompletely identified. The following discussion will focus on the anterior pituitary adrenal aspects of ACTH, but will indicate that this is only one part of a general and diverse system of intercellular communication.

BIOSYNTHESIS OF ACTH AND RELATED POLYPEPTIDES

Corticotrophs

The corticotrophs are cells located in the anterior pituitary gland that synthesize and secrete ACTH. This cell type comprises approximately 16% of the total cell number in male rats.[1] These cells are stellate-shaped in rats with 200 nm secretory granules located around the periphery of the gland.[2] These morphologic characteristics are species dependent and, for instance, in the human a round shaped cell is observed. Corticotrophs undergo hypertrophy and hyperplasia following adrenalectomy.[3] The controversy concerning the cell type giving rise to corticotrophs apparently has been resolved by immunocytochemical straining to indicate that the histochemically characterized cell type, the basophile, give rise to ACTH producing cells.[4]

ACTH Biosynthesis in Corticotrophs

Characterization of the relationship among ACTH and related peptides as well as the secretion of these polypeptides is best achieved through a description of ACTH biosynthesis. ACTH is a polypeptide of 39 amino acids (Figure 1) found in blood, the pituitary, the hypothalamus, and the placenta. It has recently been demonstrated that cells secreting ACTH synthesize a large precursor molecule. ACTH and other hormones derive from the degradation of this precursor into smaller polypeptide fragments.[5] This precursor molecule is referred to as 31K (its apparent molecular weight of 31,000), pro-opiocorticotrophin or pro-ACTH/β-endorphin. No single designation at present is in usage. The complete amino acid sequence for the precursor has been revealed by cloned DNA.[6] As the nascent polypeptide chain is being synthesized, complex oliosaccharides may be added, resulting in two different forms of the precursor, a protein or a glycosylated protein. The absence or addition of the carbohydrate moiety is characteristic of the species and cell type producing the precursor. Both forms can be produced by one cell. Subsequent cleavage of the precursor into intermediate and end products apparently is the same for both the protein and glycosylated protein. These cleavages occur where there are pairs of basic amino acids and at different rate (Figure 2). Thus, the 31K precursor after processing is found to first yield fragments of 22,000 apparent mol wt (22K or pro-ACTH/β-endorphin intermediate) and 11,700 (11.7K or β-lipotrophin). Each of these fragments then undergoes further breakdown. The 22K yields ACTH of 4,500 apparent mol wt for the protein or 13,400 for the glycosylated protein. β-Lipoprotein can be degraded to an alpha lipotropin and a beta endorphin. The precursor, intermediate products, and end products are contained within the corticotroph secretory granule.

Amino Acid Sequence of Human ACTH

1	2	3	4	5	6	7	8	9	10
ser –	tyr –	ser –	met –	glu –	his –	phe –	arg –	trp –	gly
lys –	pro –	val –	gly –	lys –	lys –	arg –	arg –	pro –	val
lys –	val –	tyr –	pro –	asn –	gly –	ala –	glu –	asp –	glu
ser –	ala –	glu –	ala –	phe –	pro –	leu –	glu –	phe –	

FIGURE 1. Amino acid sequence of human ACTH.

Biosynthetic Pathway of ACTH in the Corticotrophs of the Anterior Pituitary

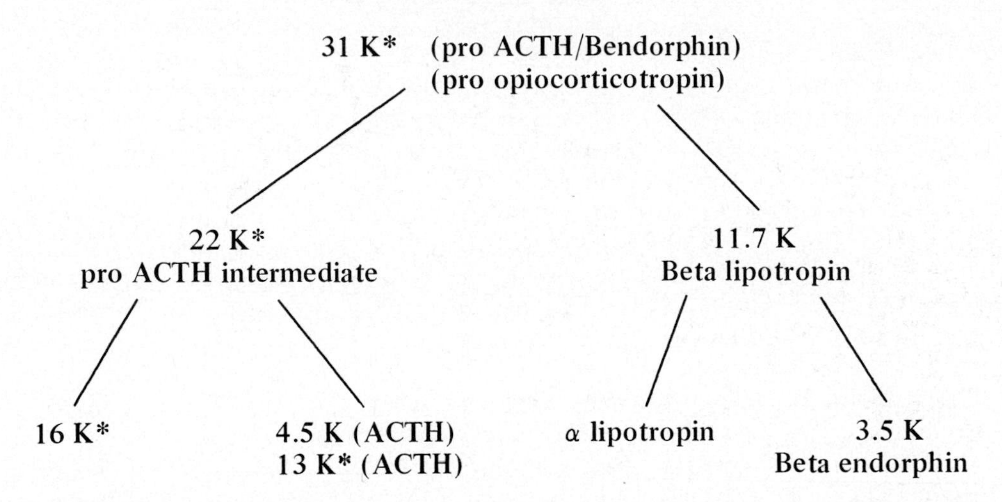

*** Indicates that the molecule can exist in two forms glycosylated or unglycosylated, e.g., 13 K (ACTH) is a glycosylated form of ACTH while the 4.5 K is the unglycosylated form.**

FIGURE 2. Biosynthetic pathway of ACTH in the corticotrophs of the anterior pituitary.

When the corticotrophs are stimulated to release, ACTH along with the other molecules are released into the blood. Parallel release of ACTH and β-endorphin/β-lipotropin following stress has been observed.[7] The biologic significance of ACTH release from the corticotrophs into the blood is well appreciated; however, the physiologic significance of the other polypeptides secreted along with ACTH into the peripheral circulation is currently an area of active interest.

The above description appears to be the process occurring in the corticotrophs. There are other cells in which the same or a similar gene for the precursor molecule is expressed. These include the cells of the intermediate lobe of the pituitary,[5] certain neuronal cell groups located in the basomedial hypothalamus,[8] and the placenta.[9] Within the hypothalamus, ACTH and β-endorphin are likewise produced. In the intermediate lobe, a further processing of the end products occurs (Figure 3). ACTH is degraded to α-MSH (ACTH-1-18) and CLIP (corticotropin-like intermediate peptide,

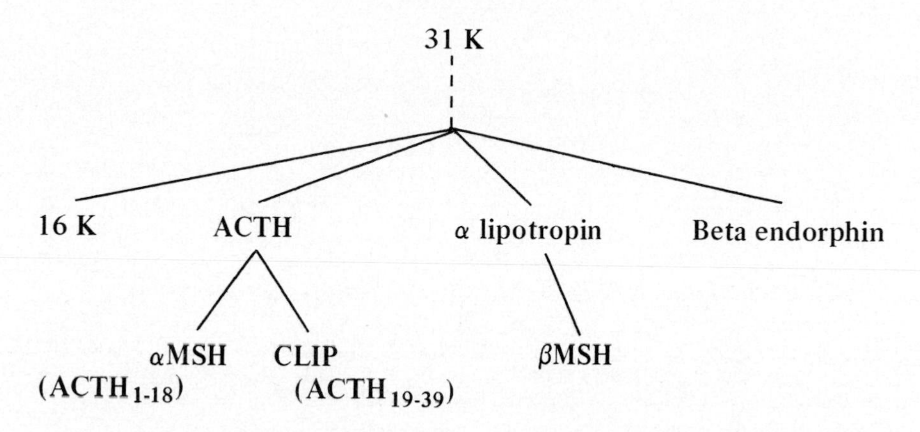

FIGURE 3. Biosynthetic pathway of aMSH in the cells of the intermediate lobe of the pituitary.

ACTH 19-39) while a α-lipotropin may be processed to β-MSH. Table 1 indicates the cell types produces pro-ACTH/endorphin and the major secretory products. The secretion of hormones from these independent cell types is regulated differently according to the characteristic of the particular cell type.

REGULATION OF ANTERIOR PITUITARY ACTH SECRETION

Regulation of ACTH secretion involves the interaction of several control mechanisms. These include as major components the trophic stimulation produced by the hypothalamus and negative feedback inhibition resulting from the adrenal glucocorticoids.

Corticotrophin Releasing Factor (CRF)

The hypothalamus has been shown to be essential for continued ACTH secretion and for ACTH release in response to stress.[10] The hypothalamus exerts a trophic effect on anterior pituitary ACTH secretion. Extracts of the hypothalamus or the stalk medium eminence (SME), site of releasing factor secretion into the hypophyseal portal blood, pare capable of releasing ACTH when injected into rats or when incubated with pituitary cells in vitro.[2,11,12] Observations such as these have led to the proposal of a hypothalamic releasing factor which stimulates ACTH release, corticotrophin releasing factor (CRF). Although, CRF was one of the first described, its isolation and structuralidentification are still proceeding. Progress in this area has been hampered by the loss of CRF activity during purification. It is clear that extracts of the hypothalamus, the SME or the posterior pituitary when purified yield separate fractions which are active in releasing ACTH.[13-15] At least two active fractions have been partially purified from each of these sources. Further purification has established that one fraction is identical to vasopressin, the posterior pituitary hormone, whereas other fractions are distinct from it. Controversy exists over the significance of vasopressin as a physiologic regulator of ACTH release.

In Table 2 the observations considered in the evaluation of vasopressin as a CRF are summarized. The role of vasopressin in the regulation of ACTH release has been suggested to include not only that of a CRF, but also as a releaser of CRF, or as a

Table 1
SITES OF PRO ADRENOCORTICOTROPHIN/ ENDORPHIN SYNTHESIS

Corticotrophs of the anterior pituitary	ACTH βLPH-some βBLPH
Cells of the intermediate lobe of pituitary	MSH βendorphin βMSH
Neurons of the hypothalamus	ACTH βendorphin
Placenta	ACTH βLPH αMSH βendorphin

Table 2
OBSERVATION ON VASOPRESSIN STIMULATION OF ACTH RELEASE

Supporting a physiologic role	Against a physiologic role
Vasopressin stimulated ACTH release *in vitro* and *in vivo.*[12] Vasopressin is found in hypophyseal portal blood at a concentration of 13.5μg/mℓ approximately 300 to 1000 times concentration in peripheral blood.[17]	Dose of vasopressin required for stimulation of release is 1000 times physiologic dose producing antidiuresis[22] nonparallel response curves of vasopressin and crude CRF activity extracted from stalk median eminence.[23]
The median eminence is directly innervated by vasopressin containing neurons.[18,19]	Only 20 to 50% of CRF activity can be accounted for by vasopressin content of stalk median eminence extracts.[24]
Electrical stimulation of paraventricular neurons (site of vasopressin containing cell bodies) stimulates ACTH release in the rat.[20]	Different distribution of CRF and vasopressin in hypothalamus.[25] Nonparallel secretion of vasopressin and ACTH.[26]
Adrenalectomy increases ACTH release and increases vasopressin in the median eminence.[20]	
Reduced ACTH response to submaximal stress in Brattleboro rat.[21]	

modulatory which potentiates the action of a separate CRF. Although vasopressin releases ACTH, its participation in the regulation of ACTH release during physiologic events has not been established at present.

In addition to vasopressin, other fractions of hypothalamic extract are active in stimulating ACTH release. The pioneering work of Saffran and Schally, and Schally and Guillemin provided clear evidence of a CRF distinct from vasopressin.[11-13] Others have subsequently confirmed CRF activity and in one case indicated that CRF activity resulted from the mixture of two separate fractions.[16] (See Addendum)

The distribution of CRF activity within the hypothalamus has been mapped.[25-27] The median eminence and medial basal hypothalamus contain the highest content, with lower activity observed elsewhere in the hypothalamus.

Attempts to determine the origin of CRF-containing cell bodies has produced divergent conclusions. Isolation of the medial basal hypothalamus when accompanied by histologic determination for the completeness of the cut has been observed to reduce SME-CRF activity to undetectable levels.[28] Severance of the anterolateral but not caudal connections of the hypothalamus reduces SME-CRF activity, suggesting that CRF-containing cell bodies are located outside the medial basal hypothalamus and project to it through the anterior-lateral hypothalamus. However, other investigations have not concurred in these conclusions.[25,29] Nor does agreement exist concerning the effectiveness of medial basal hypothalamic deafferentation on stress induced ACTH release.[30]

In addition to a hypothalamic - posterior pituitary CRF, Brodish has described ACTH releasing activity in the blood.[31] This tissue CRF produces a different time course for response; peak ACTH stimulation occurs 1 hr after injection, unlike hypothalamic CRF which produces maximal ACTH release by twenty minutes. However, the source and physiologic significance of tissue CRF activity remains to be determined.

Neurotransmitter Regulation of CRF Release

The activity of CRF-containing neurons is undoubtedly modulated by neurons impinging on them. Attempts have been made to characterize the neurotransmitter of neuronal groups affecting CRF-containing neurons and consequently ACTH secretion. The approach most extensively utilized is to mimic or inhibit the action of one neurotransmitter and observe the effect on ACTH release. The extensive investigation of neurotransmitter involvement has produced an appreciation for the complexities associated with this regulatory process and the differences among species. An inhibitory role for norepinephrine and GABA, and presumably noradrenergic and GABAergic neurons, has been indicated by several experimental approaches. A stimulatory role has been suggested for acetylcholine and cholinergic neurons. Less clear is the effect of serotonin, since both stimulatory and inhibitory actions have been observed. Such data may reflect the different roles of this neurotransmitter in the regulation of ACTH release during different physiologic conditions; i.e., basal release, circadian rhythms, stress, and feedback inhibition. Similar difficulties are also associated with the interpretation of the involvement of other neurotransmitters in the regulation of ACTH release. Histamine has recently been observed to be stimulatory to ACTH release, but its participation has not been as extensively examined. Table 3 lists, in an incomplete manner, some of the approaches used and the major findings.

Negative Feedback

Another mechanism controlling ACTH release is the negative feedback action of the glucocorticoids. Following release of ACTH, synthesis of glucocorticoids in the adrenal is stimulated, resulting in a rise in plasma glucocorticoid concentration. High plasma concentrations of glucocorticoids can reduce subsequent ACTH secretion.

The negative feedback control of ACTH release is based primarily on observations made in adrenalectomized and stressed animals. Adrenalectomy reduces endogenous glucocorticoids and is associated with an elevation in ACTH release. Stress also induces ACTH release and stimulates it to even higher levels in adrenalectomized rats. Replacement of glucocorticoids blocks the stress associated release of ACTH in both intact and adrenalectomized rats. The glucocorticoids have been observed to have a feedback action at the hypothalamus, the anterior pituitary, and at extrahypothalamic CNS sites. The relative importance of feedback at each of these sites and the mechanisms operating during physiologic events to produce feedback inhibition have not been established. However, various characteristics of feedback and several actions by which glucocorticoids can diminish ACTH secretion have been described.

Characteristics

The rise in ACTH secretion following stress has been extensively used to investigate glucocorticoid feedback of ACTH release. Glucocorticoids when given before stress block the expected rise in ACTH.[53] However, the type of stimuli used as a stressor is

glucocorticoid dexamethasone is especially effective. Blockade of ACTH secretion is due to an action of the glucocorticoids on the release of ACTH and also on synthesis. Stimulation of ACTH release by CRF is blocked by concurrent glucocorticoid treatment. Both fast and delayed feedback inhibition have been reported for release of ACTH in vitro.[64]

Of concern is the participation of feedback at the pituitary during physiologic processes. The occupancy of pituitary glucocorticoid receptors is increased following stress or administration of glucocorticoids.[65] However, other observations suggest that the effect of feedback at the pituitary is of lesser significance than negative feedback at other sites. Glucocorticoid treatment which blocks stress induced ACTH release, does not reduce pituitary responsiveness to a partially purified CRF.[66-68]

The hypothalamus is another site at which glucocorticoids can act to reduce ACTH secretion. However, the number of cells within the hypothalamus that glucocorticoids act on is relatively small.[69] Nuclear accumulation of tritiated glucocorticoids in the hypothalamus is low in comparison to that in the hippocampus, septum, or amygdala. As with other brain areas little transcortin-like material is present in the hypothalamus and consequently no differential binding of dexamethasone versus corticosterone occurs.

Implantation of glucocorticoids into the hypothalamus reduces pituitary and plasma ACTH as well as hypothalamic CRF activity.[70] Implants of glucocorticoids into the hypothalamus, but not the anterior pituitary of rabbits, is effective in blocking stress induced ACTH release. Much of the additional evidence for a hypothalamic site of glucocorticoid negative feedback comes from investigations in which CRF activity is measured after experimental treatment. Table 4 provides a summary of the observations on experimentally induced changes in CRF activity.

In addition to the hypothalamus, other brain regions have been reported to participate in glucocorticoid negative feedback, although their role and relative importance under physiologic conditions are undetermined.[71]

It is clear from the above that glucocorticoids can feed back to reduce ACTH secretion. Plasma concentrations of ACTH are prevented from rising to the high post adrenalectomy levels by basal levels of glucocorticoids. Administration of glucocorticoids, especially the potent synthetic corticoid dexamethasone, is associated with reduced ACTH release. However, under physiologic conditions, increases in plasma glucocorticoid concentration are not always associated with inhibition of ACTH. The increase in glucocorticoid release following stress was observed to have no effect on the ACTH response to subsequent stress.[72] This contrasts with the observation that infusion of glucocorticoid over a duration matching release after stress was effective in preventing stress induced ACTH release. Apparently, under these circumstances, additional factors which have been incompletely illucidated have a greater effect on regulation of ACTH release than glucocorticoid negative feedback.

ASSAY OF ACTH

For accurate measurement of ACTH, both the physiochemical properties and secretory patterns of ACTH must be taken into account. The manner of sample collection influences the observed blood concentration of ACTH, independent of assay method. Stress is a potent stimulus for ACTH release and subsequently should be minimized. Furthermore, release of ACTH shows a diurnal rhythm and occurs episodically. These factors must be considered before comparison among sample populations can be validly made. Precautions following sample collection are also necessary since ACTH is rapidly degraded by blood proteases and has a high affinity for binding to glass.

Several methods are currently used to quantify ACTH. These include radioimmu-

Table 4
EVIDENCE SUPPORTING A HYPOTHALAMIC SITE FOR GLUCOCORTICOID NEGATIVE FEEDBACK

Measurement of hypothalamic content of CRF activity after treatment *in vivo.*
- Glucocorticoids block stress induced increase in hypothalamic CRF activity.[73]
- Glucocorticoids lower pituitary and plasma ACTH content and hypothalamic CRF.[74]
- Dexamethasone reduced stress induced CRF activity in parallel with its inhibition of stress induced release of glucocorticoids.[75]

Measurement of hypothalamic CRF activity released *in vitro.*
- Treatment with glucocrticoids *in vivo* reduces release of CRF activity from hypothalamic fragments *in vitro.*[76]
- Release of CRF activity from hypothalamic fragments *in vitro* is reduced by addition of glucocorticoids to the incubation media.[77]
- Stimulation by neurotransmitters of CRF release from hypothalamic fragments *in vitro* is reduced by addition of glucocorticoids to the incubation media or by admin istration of glucocorticoids to the rats donating the hypothalami.[78]
- Release of CRF activity from hypothalamic synaptasomes is reduced by addition of glucocorticoids to the media.[79]

Table 5
ASSAY OF ACTH

General consideration regardless of assay procedure
- ACTH release is episodic
- Stress stimulates ACTH release
- ACTH is rapidly degraded in blood
- ACTH absorbs to glass

Considerations associated with assay

Assay types	Comments
Radioimmunoassay	Antiserum specificity, instability of iodinated tracer Applicable for large sample numbers
Isolated adrenal cell/glucocorticoid	Inhibitors of ACTH stimulated glucocorticoid synthesis present in sera
Cytochemical	Extremely sensitive

noassay (RIA),[80] bioassay[81] (stimulation of glucocorticoid synthesis), and cytochemistry.[82] Table 5 lists these procedures and the advantages and considerations for each.

Chief among the assay methods is RIA, a procedure lending itself to analysis of a large number of samples. There are several considerations for the RIA of ACTH which are specific to this hormone. Since ACTH derives from a precursors, antibodies to ACTH have the potential to react with ACTH and its precursors. Blood concentration of ACTH precursors is low. In tissue samples ACTH precursors may react with ACTH antibodies, indicating the presence of ACTH even though processing may normally proceed to α-MSH. As with all RIA procedures, thorough characterization of antibody specificity is required. The iodinated ACTH molecule used as a trace in ACTH-RIA has been observed to be less stable than many other iodinated polypeptides. When the above considerations are appropriately accounted for, ACTH-RIA has proven invaluable in assaying large numbers of samples.

Bioassay has also been extensively used for determination of ACTH. In one well characterized method, isolated adrenal cells are exposed to sample and the resultant stimulation of glucocortocoid synthesis is measured.[81] Some sample pretreatment of blood is recommended since inhibitors of ACTH-stimulated glucocorticoid synthesis have been observed in rat and human plasma.

The most sensitive procedure presently available for ACTH quantification is cytochemical.[82] In this procedure adrenal slices are exposed to sample and the depletion of ascorbic acid is measured. The ascorbic acid is allowed to react with a reducing reagent and the density of the product is measured by microdensitometry. The great increase in sensitivity of this procedure requires extensive labor, equipment, and skill. Consequently, the number of samples that can be processed is limited.

PATTERNS OF ACTH SECRETION

Circadian Rhythm

Secretion of ACTH is not uniform but rather it displays certain patterns. The most obvious is a circadian variation in plasma ACTH and glucocorticoid concentration. In the rat a nocturnal animal, peak ACTH and glucocorticoid secretion occurs between 1600 and 2000 hr.[83] This pattern is normally entrained to the lighting schedule and is partially regulated by the activity of the suprachiasmatic nucleus. However, other brain sites may participate or take over this function in suprachiasmatic nucleus-lesioned rats.[84] A restricted feeding schedule has been observed to set ACTH rhythms in suprachiasmatic lesioned rats. In man peak ACTH secretion occurs between 0600 and 0800 hr. Approximately 50% of total cortisol production in humans takes place during the 6 hr period immediately before and after waking.[85] Over the remaining time, ACTH secretion and cortisol production is low. In addition to the circadian rhythm there is an epsiodic pattern of secretion. ACTH is released in bursts which occur throughout the day. Total ACTH secretion is dependent on the magnitude and duration of each episode.

Although ACTH release and glucocorticoid production display similar patterns, a direct timed relationship does not necessarily exist between these two events. All increases in ACTH have not been followed by a rise in glucocorticoid production. Furthermore, adrenal sensitivity to ACTH changes. In the rat there is an estimated 12-fold greater response to ACTH during peak glucocorticoid secretion than during its nadir.[86]

Stress

Under physiologic conditions one of the most potent environmental stimuli inducing ACTH release is stress. Some of the stimuli which have experimentally been observed to induce ACTH release, and by convention are regarded as stress, include ether exposure, hemorrhage, leg-break, injection of drugs, and restraint.

CLINICAL ASPECTS OF ACTH SECRETION

Profound endocrine and metabolic abnormalaties develop from excess ACTH/glucocorticoid secretion. Cushing's syndrome refers to the clinical manifestations resulting from chronically elevated glucocorticoids. In severe forms the physical appearance is changed. Redistribution of fat deposits occur so that fat accumulates in the trunk, head, and neck region. A moon-face appearance, a buffalo hump, and fat deposits at the nape of the neck develop. In contrast, muscle tissue in the arms and legs is reduced. Skin is easily bruised and purple striations are observed on the abdomen and upper arms. Wound healing is prolonged. Such changes reflect the perturbation of metabolism resulting from excess glucocorticoids. Protein catabolism is increased while fat synthesis is favored. In the liver, increased glucose production occurs and there is a decreased peripheral utilization. Both conditions lead to the development of diabetes mellitus in these individuals. Edema can result from mineralocorticoid activity of a high concentration of glucocorticoids. Bone metabolism is also affected and results in osteoporosis.

The excess production of glucocorticoids in Cushing's syndrome results from one of three causes (1) pituitary-dependent adrenal hyperplasia (excess ACTH, Cushing's disease); (2) ACTH producing ectopic tumors; and (3) adrenal carcinoma. Measurement of nonstressed ACTH and corticoid plasma concentration and the response to dexamethasone allows a differentiation among these three causes. In individuals with Cushing's disease or an ectopic ACTH-producing tumor, plasma levels of ACTH show no diurnal rhythm. Morning and evening plasma concentrations of ACTH are similar and elevated in comparison to the evening concentrations of ACTH secretion in normal patients. Depending upon the severity of the condition, morning ACTH plasma concentration of patients with Cushing's disease or ectopic ACTH-producing tumors may not be different from the ACTH concentration found in normal individuals during the morning peak in secretion. Patients with adrenal carcinoma have low ACTH plasma concentrations due to negative feedback effect of elevated glucocorticoids. Differentiation between Cushing's disease and ectopic ACTH-producing tumors is based on negative feedback sensitivity. Individuals with Cushing's disease are less sensitive to glucocorticoid negative feedback than normal, but at high doses of exogenous glucocorticoids, ACTH secretion is reduced. In contrast, ectopic ACTH-producing tumors are not responsive to glucocorticoid negative feedback.

The cause of excess ACTH production in Cushing's disease in many cases has been established to result from a microadenoma. The possibility of increased ACTH secretion resulting from hypersecretion of CRF has been suggested, but at present this condition has not been well established.

In the above description, the clinical conditions result from excess glucocorticoids. In some instances following bilateral adrenalectomy, a rapidly growing microadenoma producing ACTH develops. The rapidly increasing concentrations of ACTH produce a condition referred to as Nelson's syndrome. It is associated with increased skin pigmentation. Additional clinical manifestations may result from the growth of the adenoma, producing a physical compression and consequential disruption of function in surrounding structures.

ADDENDUM

Two peptides have been identified recently to have CRF activity and may thus be CRF's.[87]

REFERENCES

1. **Nakane, P. K., Setalo, G., and Mazurkiewicz, J. E.,** The origin of ACTH cells in the rat, in *ACTH and Related Peptides: Structure Regulation and Action,* Kreiger, D. T. and Ganong, W. F., Eds., New York Academy of Science, New York, 1977, 201.
2. **Siperstein, E. R. and Miller, K. J. S.,** Further cytophysiologic evidence for the cells that produce adrenocorticotrophic hormone, *Endocrinology,* 86, 451, 1970.
3. **Siperstein, E. R. and Miller, K. J.,** Hypertrophy of the ACTH-producing cell following adrenalectomy: a quantitative electron microscope study, *Endocrinology,* 93, 1357, 1973.

4. **Baker, B. L. and Drummond, J.,** The cellular origins of corticotropin and melanotropin as revealed by immunochemical staining, *Am. J. Anat.,* 134, 395, 1972.
5. **Eipper, B. A. and Mains, R. E.,** Structure and biosynthesis of pro ACTH-endorphin and related peptides, *Endocrinol. Rev.,* 1, 1, 1980.
6. **Nakanishi, S., Inoue, A., Kita, T., Nakamura, M., Chang, A. C. Y., Cohen, S. N., and Numa, S.,** Nucleotide sequence of cloned c DNA for bovine corticoptropin-β-lipotropin precursor, *Nature,* 278, 423, 1979.
7. **Guillemin, R., Vargo, T., Rossier, J., Minick, S., Ling, N., Rivier, C., Vale, W., and Bloom, F. E.,** Beta endorphin and adrenocorticotropin are secreted concomitantly by the pituitary gland, *Science,* 197, 1367, 1977.
8. **Bloom, F. E., Rossier, J., Battenberg, E. L. P., Bayin, A., French, E., Henriksen, S. J., Siggins, C. R., Segal, D., Brown, R., Ling, N., and Guillemin, R.,** β Endorphin: cellular localization, electrophysiological and behavorial effects, *Adv. Biochem. Psychopharmacol.,* 18, 89, 1978.
9. **Liotta, A. S. and Kreiger, D. T.,** *In vitro* biosynthesis and comparative postranslational processing of immuno-reactive precursor corticotropin/endorphin by human placental and pituitary cells, *Endocrinology,* 106, 1504, 1980.
10. **Dunn, J. and Critchlow, V.,** Pituitary-adrenal function following ablation of medial basal hypothalamus, *Proc. Soc. Exp. Biol. Med.,* 142, 749, 1973.
11. **Saffran, M., Schally, A. V., and Benfey, B. G.,** Stimulation of the release of corticotropin from the adrenohypophysis of a neuro-hypophysial factor, *Endocrinology,* 57, 439, 1955.
12. **Guillemin, R. and Rosenberg, B.,** Humoral hypothalamic control of anterior pituitary: a study with combined tissue cultures, *Endocrinology,* 57, 599, 1955.
13. **Saffran, M. and Schally, A. V.,** Corticotropin-releasing factor isolation and chemical properties, in *ACTH and Related Peptides, Structure, Regulation and Action,* Kreiger, D. T. and Ganong, W. F., Eds., New York Academy Science, New York, 1977, 395.
14. **Gillham, B., Insall, R. L., and Jones, M. T.,** Perspectives on corticotrophin-releasing hormone (CRH), in *Interaction within the Brain Pituitary-Adrenocortical Systems,* Jones, M. T., Gillhan, B., Dallman, M. F, and Chattopadhyay, S., Eds., Academic Press, New York, 1979, 41.
15. **Gilles, G. and Lowry, P. J.,** The relationship between vasopressin and corticotropin releasing factor, in *Interaction within the Brain Pituitary Adrenocortical Systems,* Jones, M. T., Gillham, B., Dallman, M. F., and Chattopadhyay, S., Eds., Academic Press, New York, 1979, 51.
16. **Pearlmutter, A. F., Rapino, R., and Saffran, M.,** The ACTH-releasing hormone of the hypothalamus requires a cofactor, *Endocrinology,* 97, 1336, 1975.
17. **Zimmerman, E. A., Carmel, P. W., Husain, M. K., Ferin, M., Tannenbaum, M., Frantz, A. G., and Robinson, A. G.,** Vasopressin and neurophysin: high concentration in monkey hypophysial portal blood, *Science,* 182, 925, 1973.
18. **Silverman, A. J. and Zimmerman, E. A.,** Ultrastructural immunocytochemical localization of neurophysin and vasopressin in the median eminence and posterior pituitary of the guinea pig, *Cell Tissue Res.,* 159, 291, 1975.
19. **Dierickx, K., Vandesande, F., and Demay, J.,** Identification in the external region of the rat median eminence of separate neurophysin-vasopressin and neurophysin oxytocin containing nerve fibers, *Cell Tissue Res.,* 168, 141, 1976.
20. **Zimmerman, E. A., Stillman, M. A., Recht, L. D., Antuwes, J. L., and Carmel, P. W.,** Vasopressin and corticotropinreleasing factor: an axonal pathway to portal capillaries in the zona externa of the median eminence containing vasopressin and its interaction with adrenal corticoids, in *ACTH and Related Peptides Structive Regulation and Action,* Krieger, D. T. and Ganong, W. F., Eds., New York Academy Science, New York, 1977, 405.
21. **Yates, F. E., Russell, S. M., Dallman, M. F., Hedge, G. A., McCann, S. M., and Dhariwal, A. P. S.,** Potential by vasopressin of corticotropin release induced by corticotropin-releasing factor, *Endocrinology,* 88, 3, 1971.
22. **Nichols, B. and Guillemin, R.,** Endogenous and exogenous vasopressin in ACTH release, *Endocrinology,* 60, 664, 1957.
23. **Portanova, R. and Sayers, G.,** Isolated pituitary cells: CRF like activity of neurohypophysial and related polypeptides, *Proc. Soc. Exp. Biol. Med.,* 143, 661, 1973.
24. **Gillies, G. and Lowry, P. J.,** The relationship between vasopressin and corticotropin-releasing function, in *Interaction within the Brain-Pituitary Adrenocortical Systems,* Jones, M. T., Gillham, B., Dallman, M. F., and Chattopadhyay, Eds., Academic Press, New York, 1979, 51.
25. **Kreiger, D. T., Liotta, A., and Brownstein, M. J.,** Corticotropin-releasing factor distribution in normal and Brattleboro rat brain and effects of defferentation, hypophysectomy and steroid treatment in normal rats, *Endocrinology,* 100, 227, 1977.
26. **Nagareda, C. G. and Gaunt, R.,** Functional relationship between the adrenal cortex and posterior pituitary, *Endocrinology,* 48, 560, 1951.

27. **Lang, R. E., Heinzvoist, K., Fehn, H. L., and Pfeiffer, E. F.,** Localization of corticotropin-releasing activity in the rat hypothalamus, *Neurosci. Lett.,* 2, 19, 1976.
28. **Makara, G. B.,** The site of origin of corticoliberin (CRF), in *Interaction within the Brain-Pituitary Adrenocortical System,* Jones, M. T., Gillham, B., Dallman, M. F., and Chattopadhyay, S., Eds., Academic Press, New York, 1979, 97.
29. **Yasuda, N. and Greer, M. A.,** Rat hypothalamic corticotropin-releasing factor (CRF) content remains constant despite marked acute or chronic changes in ACTH secretion, *Neuroendocrinology,* 22, 48, 1976.
30. **Feldman, Conforti, S. N., Chowers, I., and Davidson, J. M.,** Pituitary-adrenal activation in rats with medial basal hypothalamic islands, *Acta Endocrinologica,* 63, 405, 1970.
31. **Brodish, A.,** Extra-CNS corticotropin-releasing factors, in *ACTH and Related Peptides, Structure Regulation and Action,* Kreiger, D. T. and Ganong, W. F., Eds., New York Academy Science, New York, 1977, 420.
32. **Van Loon, A. R., Hilger, L., King, A. B., Boryczka, A. T., and Ganong, W. F.,** Inhibitory effect of L-dihydroxyphenyl-alanine on the adrenal venous 17 hydroxy corticosteroid response to surgical stress, *Endocrinology,* 88, 1401, 1971.
33. **Van Loon, G. R., Scapagmini, U., Cohen, R., and Ganong, W. F.,** Effect of the intraventricular administration of adrenergic drugs on the venous 17 hydroxysteroid response to surgical stress in the dogs, *Neuroendocrinology,* 8, 257, 1971.
34. **Ganong, W. F., Kramer, N., Salmon, J., Reid, I. A., Lovinger, R., Scapagnini, U., Boryczka, A. T., and Shackelford, R.,** Pharmacological evidence for inhibition of ACTH secretion by a central noradrenergic system in the dog, *Neuroscience,* 1, 167, 1976.
35. **Rose, J. C., Goldsmith, P. C., Hellan, F. J., Kaplan, S. L., and Ganong, W. F.,** Effect of electrical stimulation of the canine brain stem on the secretion of ACTH and growth hormone (GH), *Neuroendocrinology,* 22, 352, 1976.
36. **Hillhouse, E. W., Burden, J. L., and Jones, M. T.,** The effect of various putative neurotransmitters on the release of corticotropin-releasing hormone from the hypothalamus of the rat *in vitro.* I. the effect of acetycholine and noradrenalin, *Neuroendocrinology,* 17, 1, 1974.
37. **Buckingham, J. C. and Hodges, J. R.,** The secretion of corticotropin-releasing hormones. *In vitro* effects of neurotransmitter substances, drugs and cortisosteroids, in *Interactions within the Brain-Pituitary Adreno Cortical System,* Jones, M. T., Gillham, B., Dallman, M. F., and Chattopadhyay, S., Eds., Academic Press, New York, 1979, 115.
38. **Makara, G. B. and Stark, E.,** Effect of gamma-aminobutyric acid (GABA) and GABA antagonist drugs in ACTH release, *Neuroendocrinology,* 16, 178, 1974.
39. **Markara, G. B. and Starke, E.,** *Interaction between Putative Neuro-Transmitters in the Brain,* Garahini, S., Pujsland, J. F., and Samanin, R., Raven Press, New York, 1978.
40. **Burden, J. L., Hillhouse, E. W., and Jones, M. T.,** The inhibitary action of GABA and melatonin on the release of corticotropin-releasing hormone from rat hypothalamus *in vitro, J. Physiol.,* 239, 116, 1974.
41. **Kreiger, H. P. and Kreiger, D. T.,** Chemical stimulation of the brain: effect on adrenal corticoid release, *Am. J. Physiol.,* 218, 1632, 1970.
42. **Edwardson, J. A. and Bennett, G. W.,** Modulation of corticotropin-releasing factor release from hypothalamic synaptosomes, *Nature,* 251, 425, 1974.
43. **Naumenko, E. V.,** Effect of local injection of 5 hydroxytryptamine into rhinencephalic and mesencephalic structures on pituitary adrenal function in guinea pigs, *Neuroendocrinology,* 5, 81, 1969.
44. **Abe, K. and Hiroshige, T.,** Changes in plasma corticosterone and hypothalamic CRF levels following intraventricular injection or drug induced changes in brain biogenic amines in the rat, *Neuroendocrinology,* 14, 195, 1974.
45. **Fuller, R. W., Snoddy, H. D., and Molloy, B. B.,** Pharmacologic evidence for a serotonin neural pathway involved in hypothalamic pituitary adrenal function in rats, *Life Sci.,* 19, 337, 1976.
46. **Jones, M. T., Hillhouse, E. W., and Burden, J. L.,** The effect of various putative neurotransmitters on the secretion of corticotropin-releasing hormone from the rat hypothalamus *in vitro*; a model of the neurotransmitters involved, *J. Endocrinol.,* 69, 1, 1976.
47. **Kreiger, D. T. and Luria, M.,** Effectiveness of cyproheptadine in decreasing plasma ACTH concentrations in Nelson's syndrome, *J. Clin. Endocrinol. Meth.,* 43, 1879, 1976.
48. **Telegdy, G. and Dermes, I.,** The role of serotonin in the regulation of the hypophysis-adrenal system, in *Brain-Pituitary Adrenal Interrelationships,* Brodish, A. and Redgate, E. S., Eds., Karger, Basel, 1973, 332.
49. **Van Loon, G. R.,** Brain catecholamines and ACTH secretion, in *Frontiers in Neuroendocrinology,* Ganong, W. F. and Martini, L., Eds., Oxford Press, New York, 1973, 209.
50. **Vernikos-Danellis, J., Berge, P. A., and Barchas, J. D.,** Brain serotonin and pituitary adrenal function, *Prog. Brain Res.,* 39, 301, 1973.

51. **Scapagnini, U., Moberg, C. P., Van Loon, G. R., de Groot, J., and Ganong, W. F.**, Relation of brain 5 hydroxytryptamine content to the diurnal variation in plasma corticosterone in the rat, *Neuroendocrinology*, 7, 90, 1971.
52. **Rudolph, C., Richards, G. E., Kaplan, S., and Ganong, W. F.**, Effect of intraventricular histamine on hormone secretion in dogs, *Neuroendocrinology*, 26, 169, 1979.
53. **Sayers, G. and Sayers, M.**, Regulation of pituitary adrenocorticotrophic activity during the response of the rat to acute stress, *Endocrinology*, 40, 265, 1947.
54. **Dallman, M. F. and Yates, F. E.**, Anatomical and functional mapping of central neural input and feedback pathways of the adreno-cortical system, *Mem. Soc. Endocrinol. (London)*, 17, 39, 1968.
55. **Gann, D. S. and Cryer, G. S.**, Feedback control of ACTH secretion by corticol, in *Brain-Pituitary-Adrenal Interrelationship*, Brodish, A. and Redgate, E. S., Eds., Karger, Basel, 1973, 197.
56. **Sirett, N. E. and Gibbs, F. P.**, Dexamethasone suppression of ACTH release: effect of the interval between steroid administration and the application of stimuli known to release ACTH, *Endocrinology*, 85, 355, 1969.
57. **Yates, F. E. and Brennen, D.**, *Hormonal Control System*, Stear, E. B. and Kadish, A. H., Eds., American Elsevier, New York, 1973.
58. **Watanabe, H., Orth, D. N., and Toft, D. O.**, Glucocorticoid receptors in pituitary tumor cells I cytosol receptors, *J. Biol. Chem.*, 248, 7625, 1973.
59. **Smelik, P. G.**, Some aspects of corticosteroid feedback actions, in *ACTH and Related Peptides: Structure Regulation and Action*, Kreiger, D. T. and Ganong, W. F., Eds., New York Academy of Science, New York, 1977, 580.
60. **Jones, M. T., Tiptaft, M., Brush, F. R., Fergusson, D. A. N., and Neane, R. L. B.**, Evidence for dual corticosteroid-receptor mechanisms in the feedback control of adrenocorticotrophin secretion, *J. Endocrinol.*, 60, 223, 1974.
61. **DeKloet, E. R. and McEwen, B. S.**, A putative glucocorticoid receptor and a transcortin like macromolecule in pituitary cytosol, *Biochem. Biophys. Acta*, 421, 115, 1976.
62. **McEwen, B. S., DeKloet, R., and Wallach, G.**, Interactions *in vivo* and *in vitro* of corticoids and progesterone with cell nuclei and soluble macromolecules from rat brain regions and pituitary, *Brain Res.*, 105, 129, 1976.
63. **Olpe, H. R. and McEwen, B. S.**, Glucocorticoid binding to receptor-like proteins in rat brain and pituitary: ontogenic and experimentally induced changes, *Brain Res.*, 105, 121, 1976.
64. **Smelik, P. G.**, Some aspects of corticosterone feedback actions, in *ACTH and Related Peptides: Structure Regulation and Action*, Kreiger, D. T. and Ganong, W. F., Eds., New York Academy Science, New York, 1977, 580.
65. **McEwen, B. S., Wallach, G., and Magnus, C.**, Corticosterone binding to hippocampus: immediate and delayed influences of the absence of adrenal secretion, *Brain Res.*, 70, 321, 1974.
66. **Takebe, K., Kunita, H., Sakakura, M., Horiuchi, Y., and Mashimo, K.**, Suppressive effect of dexamethasone on the rise of CRF activity in the median eminence induced by stress, *Endocrinology*, 89, 1014, 1971.
67. **Vernikos-Danelles, J.**, Effect of stress adrenalectomy, hypophysectomy and hydrocortisone on the corticotropin releasing activity of rat median eminence, *Endocrinology*, 76, 122, 1965.
68. **Russell, S. M., Dhariwal, A. P. S., McCann, S. M., and Yates, F. E.**, Inhibition by dexamethasone of the *in vivo* pituitary response to corticotropin-releasing factor (CRF), *Endocrinology*, 85, 512, 1969.
69. **Stumpf, W. E. and Sar, M.**, Glucocorticoid and mineral corticosteroid hormone target sites in the brain: autoradiographic studies with corticosterone, aldosterone and dexamethasone, in *Interaction with the Brain-Pituitary Adrenocortical System*, Jones, M. T., Gillhan, B., Dallman, M. F., and Chattopadhyay, S., Eds., Academic Press, 1979, 137.
70. **Chowers, I., Conforti, N., and Feldman, S.**, Effects of corticosteroids on hypothalamic corticotropin releasing factor and pituitary ACTH content, *Neuroendocrinology*, 2, 193, 1967.
71. **McEwen, B. S.**, Adrenal steroid feedback in neuroedocrine tissues, in *ACTH and Related Peptides: Structure, Regulation and Action*, Kreiger, D. T. and Ganong, W. F., Eds., New York Academy of Science, New York, 1977, 658.
72. **Dallman, M. F. and Jones, M. T.**, Corticosteroid feedback control of ACTH secretion: effect of stress induced corticosterone secretion on subsequent stress responses in the rat, *Endocrinology*, 92, 1367, 1973.
73. **Sato, J., Sato, M., Shinsako, J., and Dallman, M. F.**, Corticosterone induced changes in hypothalamic corticotropin releasing factor (CRF) content after stress, *Endocrinology*, 97, 265, 1975.
74. **Vernikos-Danellis, J.**, Effect of acute stress on the pituitary gland: changes in blood and pituitary ACTH concentrations, *Endocrinology*, 72, 574, 1963.
75. **Takebe, K., Konita, H., Sakakura, M., Horiuchi, Y., and Mashimo, K.**, Suppressive effect of dexamethasone on the rise of CRF activity in the median eminence induced by stress, *Endocrinology*, 89, 1014, 1971.

76. **Jones, M. T., Hillhouse, E., and Burden, J.,** Secretion of corticotropin releasing hormone *in vitro,* in *Frontiers in Neuroendocrinology,* Martins, L. and Ganong, W. F., Eds., Raven Press, New York, 1976, 195.
77. **Jones, M. T., Gillhan, B., Mahmoud, S., and Holmes, M. C.,** The characteristics and mechanism of action of corticosteroid negative feedback at the hypothalamus and anterior pituitary, in *Interaction within the Brain Pituitary Adrenocortical System,* Jones, M. T., Gillhan, D., Dallman, M. F., and Chattopadhyay, S., Eds., Academic Press, New York, 1979, 1963.
78. **Jones, M. T. and Hillhouse, E. W.,** Structure activity relationship and the mode of action of corticosteroid feedback on the secretion of corticotrophin releasing factor (corticoliberin), *J. Steroid Biochem.,* 7, 1189, 1976.
79. **Edwardson, J. A. and Bennett, G. W.,** Modulation of corticotrophin releasing factor from hypothalamic synaptosomes, *Nature,* 251, 425, 1974.
80. **Yalow, R. S., Glick, S. M., Roth, J., and Berson, S. A.,** Radioimmunoassay of human plasma ACTH, *J. Clin. Endornol. Metab.,* 24, 1218, 1964.
81. **Sayers, G.,** Bioassay of ACTH using isolated cortex cells, in *ACTH and Related Peptides: Structure, Regulation and Action,* Kreiger, D. T. and Ganong, W. F., Eds., New York Academy Science, New York, 1977, 220.
82. **Chayen, J., Daly, J. R., Loveridge, N., and Bitensky, L.,** The cytochemical processing of hormones, *Rec. Prog. Horm. Res.,* 32, 33, 1976.
83. **Retiene, K., Zimmerman, E., Schindler, W. J., Neuenschwander, E., and Lipscomb, H. S.,** A correlative study of endocrine rhythms in rats, *Acta Endocrinol.,* 57, 615, 1968.
84. **Kreiger, D. T.,** Circadian periodicity of plasma ACTH levels, in *ACTH and Related Peptides: Structure Regulation and Action,* Kreiger, D. T. and Ganong, W. F., Eds., New York Academy Science, New York, 1977, 561.
85. **Weitzman, E. D., Fukushma, D., Nogeire, C., Roffwarg, H., Gallagher, T. F., and Hellman, L.,** Twenty-four hour pattern of the episodic secretion of cortisol in normal subjects, *J. Clin. Endocrinol. Metab.,* 33, 14, 1971.
86. **Dallman, M. F., Engeland, W. C., Rose, J. C., Wilkinson, C. W., Shinsako, J., and Siedenburg, F.,** Nycthemeral rhythm in adrenal responsiveness to ACTH, *Am. J. Physiol.,* 235, 210R, 1978.
87. **Vale, W.,** Characterization of the 41-residue ovine hypothalamic peptide that stimulates secretion of the corticotropin and beta endorphine, *Science,* 213, 1397, 1981.

THE GONADOTROPES

Richard W. Steger and John J. Peluso

INTRODUCTION

The gonadotropes are responsible for the synthesis and release of hormones that control both the gametogenic and steroidogenic function of the male or female gonad. In the lower vertebrates only one gonadotropin may exist, but in mammals a separate follicle stimulating hormone (FSH) and luteinizing hormone (LH) are found. Luteinizing hormone is also known as interstitial cell stimulating hormone (ICSH) in the male.

The following section will review the anatomy of the gonadotropes as well as the chemistry of LH and FSH and the factors regulating LH and FSH release. The major emphasis will be on data from primates, principally man, and from the laboratory rat where the most extensive body of research exists.

CYTOLOGY OF THE GONADOTROPES

Many investigators have attempted to differentiate LH and FSH secreting cells from other cell types of the anterior pituitary gland. Although the gonadotropes can usually be identified by morphologic means, it is still not entirely clear whether one cell type secretes both LH and FSH or whether there are two distinct cell types.

A number of histologic techniques have been used to differentiate the gonadotrope from other cell types. These techniques have been reviewed by Romeis[1] and by Holmes and Ball.[2] In man, gonadotropes fit into the delta cell classification of Romeis.[1] They are either ovoid or polyhedral in shape and contain a fine, PAS-positive granulation. In the rat, gonadotrophic cells are also ovoid in shape and PAS-positive.[3,4] Under the electron microscope, many dense 150 to 200 mμ granules are observed.[3,5] Ribosomes are generally less numerous than in lactotropes and the Golgi apparatus is often arranged in a spherical configuration in the perinuclear area.

Numerous workers have attempted to differentiate LH and FSH secretory gonadotropes from each other, using a variety of techniques. A differential granulation of gonadotrophic cells was described by Purves and Griesback,[6] who assocaited these differences with LH vs FSH secreting cells. Using the PAS-methyl blue technique to monitor pituitary changes after castration, Hildebrand et al.[7] came up with contradictory results. Several ultrastructural studies have described differences in gonadotropes based on nuclear shape, distribution of secretory glanules, rough endoplasmic reticulum appearance, and changes following castration and/or FSH injections, but conclusive differences in LH and FSH cells have not been agreed upon.[4,5,8] There is even disagreement on cell types when using the potentially more powerful immunohistologic techniques. Rennels,[4] using an immunofluorescent procedure, showed distinct LH and FSH cells, whereas Nakane,[9,10] using the peroxidase technique, found gonadotropes containing both LH and FSH. Moriarty,[11] using electron microscopic-immunocytochemical techniques, described two distinctive LH cell types in female rats, but only one type in male rats. She also showed that the "FSH cell" contains LH. An attempt to isolate secretory granules from pituitary cells showed that both LH and FSH were associated with granules of the same size and density.[12]

CHEMISTRY

Luteinizing hormone (LH) is a glycoprotein hormone with a molecular weight ranging from 26,000 in man to 44,500 in the horse.[13] The active LH molecule consists of a unique β subunit coupled to an α subunit which is similar, if not identical, to the α subunit of FSH, thyroid stimulating hormone (TSH) and human chorionic gonadotropin (hCG). In most cases, these subunits have little or no intrinsic biologic activity, but can be recombined with restoration of full biologic potency. In fact, hybrids of α and β subunits from different hormones can be produced that retain activity of the parent molecule from which the β subunit has been isolated.[14] The α subunit appears to contain most of the recognition sites for the receptor. Both subunits may be synthesized in the same cell type of the anterior pituitary.

The amino acid composition of LH from various species is similar, suggesting that the primary structures are similar.[13,15] Luteinizing hormone has a very high content of proline and cystine, but probably only human LH contains any tryptophan.[13] The amino acid composition of the α and β subunits is different, accounting for the ability to separate the units by countercurrent distribution, ion-exchange chromatography and/or gel-filtration.

Carbohydrate moieties make up about 12 to 20% of LHs molecular weight, with a number of quantitative and qualitative differences among species.[13,15] Mannose, galactose, fucose, glucosamine, and galactosamine have been found in all preparations examined. Sialic acid residues occur in several species, including man, where they may contribute up to 2% of the molecular weight.[15] The carbohydrate composition of the α and β subunits is dissimilar.

Follicle stimulating hormone (FSH) is a glycoprotein made up of an α and β subunit, but has not been as extensively studies as LH due to its lower pituitary concentration and its high lability.[13] It is also difficult to remove all traces of LH activity from FSH preparations and this has caused great difficulties in the physiologic and chemical characterization of FSH.

Despite the similarity of their α subunits, the amino acid composition of LH and FSH are markedly different. The carbohydrate content of FSH is stated differently depending on the laboratory, but basically FSH contains the same components as LH does. Sialic acid appears to be necessary to maintain the hormone in the circulation, although desialylated FSH is found to be active in vitro.[16]

There is increasing amounts of evidence for changes in gonadotropin structure and/or potency in various physiologic states. Thus, gonadectomy and/or steroid administration change the ratio of immunoassayable to bioassayable LH and FSH.[18,20] One factor that may affect this ratio is the degree of hormone sialylation.[22]

BIOLOGIC ACTIONS

FSH stimulates follicular development in the ovary and plays an important role in spermatogenesis in the male. Luteinizing hormone stimulates ovulation and steroidogenesis within the ovary and stimulates steroidogenesis by the Leydig cells of the testis. Besides a possible ultrashort feedback action on the hypothalamus or pituitary, it appears that all LH and FSH actions are exerted at the level of the gonads.

ASSAYS OF GONADOTROPINS

In several species, LH and FSH are routinely measured in blood, tissue, and incubation media by radioimmunoassay (RIA.) The National Institute of Arthritis and Metabolic Digestive Diseases (NIAMDD) routinely supplies kits for the measurement of rat and human LH and FSH. Numerous other assay procedures are described in the literature (see review by Moudgal et al.[23]). Despite the relative ease, precision, and sensitivity of RIA procedures, it is now being realized that there are many instances where the biologic and immunologic potency of a hormone changes.[18-21] Thus, RIA can sometimes underestimate or overestimate the biologic activity of the actual circulating hormone. Human LH-RIAs often employ an antibody against the β subunit of LH to increase specificity and also to overcome the problems with cross-reactivity to human chrionic gonadotropin which are found in the plasma of pregnant women.

Numerous biologic endpoints of LH and FSH action have been utilized as bioassays. The classical LH bioassay, developed by Parlow,[24] measures ovarian ascorbic acid depletion (OAAD) after LH administration, but assays measuring ventral prostate growth in hypophysectionized rats[25] or ovarian interstitial cell repair[26] have also been utilized. The Steelman and Pohley assay, based on FSH induced ovarian weight gain in immature rats, has probably been the most utilized FSH bioassay.[27] These assays are expensive, time consuming and lack the sensitivity to measure basal hormone levels in intact animals which is often in the range of nanograms per milliliter (approximately 10^{-11} *M*).

Recently, a sensitive and precise bioassay based on the ability of LH to stimulate testosterone production by rat interstitial cells (RICT assay) has been developed.[19] Radioreceptor assays utilizing LH receptors isolated from corpus luteum or Leydig cells are also being used.

SYNTHESIS OF GONDOTROPINS

Gonadotropin biosynthesis appears to occur similarly to protein synthesis in all cell types. The peptide chain is assembled on the ribosomes with some of the carbohydrate moieties being added in the rough endoplasmic reticulum and the terminal sugars being added in the Golgi apparatus.[28] The regulation of α and β subunit synthesis is not clear, but the amount of α subunit production appears to be greater than that of β subunit.[29] Free α subunits can be found in plasma whereas free β subunits are rarely seen.

Luteinizing hormone and FSH are stored in granules which are released by exocytosis upon stimulation with gonadotropin releasing hormone (GnRH) (see previous section). There are two storage pools of LH. One is rapidly released by GnRH and the second is a reserve pool.[30] The first pool appears to consist of granules in close proximity to the cell membrane. The lack of an immediate FSH response to GnRH could reflect the absence of a "ready-releasable" pool of FSH.[31]

METABOLISM AND EXCRETION OF GONADOTROPINS

Luteinizing hormone and FSH are metabolized principally by the liver and kidney, although a small fraction is probably metabolized by the gonads.[31] The plasma half-life of human LH and human FSH is approximately 30 min and 3 hr, respectively. The differences in half-life correlate well with differences in sialic acid content. This is supported by the finding that enzymatically desialylated hormones have very short half lives due to rapid hepatic uptake.[32,33]

CONTROL OF GONADOTROPIN SYNTHESIS AND RELEASE

Introduction

The release of pituitary LH and FSH is ultimately controlled by the central nervous system upon activation of the hypothalamic peptide, gonadotropin releasing hormone

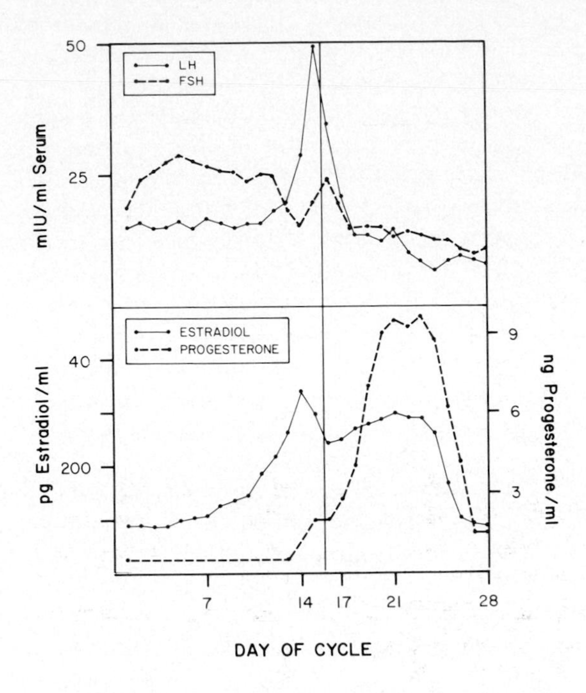

FIGURE 1. Changes in serum hormone levels and ovarian follicular development in the human menstrual cycle. (Hormonal data from Taymor, M. L., Berger, M. J., Thompson, I. S., and Karam, K., *Amer. J. Gynecol.*, 114, 445, 1972; Morphologic data from Block, E., *Acta Endocrinol.*, 8, 33, 1951. With permission.)

(GnRH). The release of GnRH and the sensitivity of the pituitary to GnRH stimulation is under a complex control system responsive to gonadal feedback and a number of environmental cues. The following sections will describe these factors as well as the areas in the central nervous system and the neurotransmitters involved in the regulation of LH and FSH release.

Gonadotropin Releasing Hormone (GnRH)

GnRH Induced LH and FSH Release

The release of both LH and FSH is controlled by the hypothalamic peptide, gonadotropin releasing hormone (GnRH). There is presently no solid evidence for the existence of a separate FSH releasing factor.[34-36]

Gonadotropin releasing hormone is a decapeptide (Figure 1) tht has been isolated from several species and it has also been synthesized. The GnRH molecule appears identical in mammalian species, but there are contradictory reports of the heterogeneity of GnRH across the major vertebrate classes.[37-40] Although GnRH is generally assumed to release only LH and FSH, it has also been shown to release GH in acromegliacs[41] and prolactin in women.[42]

The ability of GnRH to release LH and FSH has been clearly demonstrated in numerous species and appears to be essential for regulation of LH and FSH in a variety of physiologic states. Immunization against GnRH blocks ovulation in both sheep and rats and has also been shown to block the post ovariectomy rise in LH and FSH.[43-45] Increased GnRH levels have been described in the portal blood during the LH surge in rats and monkeys.[46]

GnRH appears to release LH and FSH in a manner similar to the mechanisms of action of other protein or peptide hormones. Thus, GnRH binds to a high affinity receptor and, in turn, stimulates the synthesis or release of one or several intracellular second messengers. Cyclic AMP levels in the pituitary are increased specifically by hopothalamic extracts or synthetic GnRH.[47] Cyclic AMP or inhibitors of cAMP breakdown have been shown to stimulate LH release. Calcium may also be involved as a second messenger in gonadotropin release.[48,49]

The release of LH and FSH in response to exogenous GnRH varies markedly according to dose, method and route of administration, as well as the physiologic state and steroid milieu. Thus, a divergence of LH and FSH release can be produced by several experimental means and this fact has been used as an argument for the existence of only one releasing factor for both LH and FSH.

In general, a single bolus injection of GnRH is more effective in releasing LH than FSH whereas GnRH infusions release LH and FSH equally.[50-52] Gonadotropin releasing hormone also appears to have a "self-priming" effect in that an appropriately timed second dose of GnRH is more effective in releasing LH and FSH than the initial one in releasing LH.[55] The priming effect has also been demonstrated in vitro, confirming the suggestion that the effect is mediated directly in the pituitary gland.[56,57] The timing of the two GnRH doses is of importance since the pituitary gland is actually desensitized after a prolonged period of time or after multiple GnRH injections.[58] These phenomena appear to relate to the existence of a "ready-releasable" and a "nonreleasable" or storage pool of gonadotropins in the pituitary.[30] The priming effect could also be due to changes in LHRH receptors on the gonadotropes,[59,60] but this hypothesis has been argued against by Pickering and Fink,[6] who showed a priming effect when increased potassium was used as the second stimulus. Several reports show that GnRH priming has a differential effect on LH and FSH release, but the reports are contradictory.[53,54,62]

In the rhesus monkey, both the timing and dose of GnRH are important in controlling pituitary response. Thus, in monkeys with hypothalamic lesions blocking endogenous GnRH secretion or constant GnRH infusions had little effect on LH and FSH release whereas pulsatile infusion of GnRH released both FSH and LH.[63,64] Changes in the amplitude of the GnRH pulses changed the ratio of LH to FSH secretion.

Several lines of evidence point to the importance of gonadal steroids in regulating pituitary responsiveness to GnRH and such studies ave been reviewed by Fink.[65] There exists a marked variation in the response to GnRH during the human menstrual cycle, with increased reponsiveness seen during the late follicular phase and possibly the luteal phase.[66,67] The increased sensitivity appears to be related to elevated estrogen levels. There is, likewise, considerable evidence suggesting that the rat pituitary is more sensitive to GnRH during the times of the ovarian cycle associated with increased estrogen secretion.[54,55] In ovariectomized rats, estrogen replacement has been shown to increase GnRH responses.[68,69] The timing of the estrogen treatment is important since investigators have demonstrated both stimulatory and inhibitory effects.[70] A direct effect of estrogen on GnRH response in women has also been demonstrated.[71,72]

The direct stimulatory effect of E_2 on pituitary LH and FSH responses can also be demonstrated in vitro and the data suggest that the effect is due to an increased sensitivity of the release mechanism rather than to an increase in gonadotropin synthesis.[73] A differential estrogen effect on LH vs. FSH release has been observed which could relate to a divergent release of these hormones.[74]

Progesterone alone has no apparent effect on GnRH response in vitro[73] although, in vivo, progesterone can be stimulatory or inhibitory depending on the time of administration in relation to GnRH administration.[75,76] Progesterone in vitro, however, increases the ratio of FSH to LH in the pituitary and stimulates basal and maximal FSH release.[73] The progesterone effect on FSH is potentiated by estrogen. Progesterone also seems to inhibit the sensitizing effect of E_2 on response to GnRH.[73,77]

Androgens appear to inhibit basal LH release as well as LH release in response to GnRH both in vivo and in vitro.[73,78] Androgens have the opposite effects on FSH release and thus markedly affect the ratio of basal or stimulated LH/FSH release.[73,78-81]

The physiologic importance of ovarian steroids on GNRH response is perhaps most clearly demonstrated in a recent publication by Knobile and co-workers,[64] who demonstrated that the primate menstrual cycle can be maintained in hypothalamic lesioned monkeys (no endogenous GnRH) by a long term unvarying replacement regimen of one intravenous GnRH pulse/hr. Thus, in the monkey, the ovary appears to be the major factor controlling the cyclic release of pituitary LH and FSH whereas a bolus of endogenous or exogenous GnRH seems to be necessary for the gonadotropin surge and ovulation in the rat.

Two recent papers have described a significant increase in the number of GnRH receptors in the rat pituitary between metestrus and early proestrus.[59,60] The receptor number decreases rapidly after the LH surge, suggesting a physiologic basis for changes in pituitary sensitivity throughout the rat estrous cycle. In both studies, the number of receptors were positively correlated with serum estradiol concentrations, but it could not be determined if the effect of estrogen was exerted directly on the pituitary or indirectly through a selfpriming effect mediated by increased hypothalamic GnRH release. Gonadotropin releasing hormone receptor affinity remained constant throughout the cycle. Clayton et al.[60] demonstrated that GnRH receptors were decreased in lactating rats which showed decreaed GnRH responses when compared to cycling controls.

GnRH Localization

Many procedures have been used to determine the localization of GnRH in the central nervous system of several laboratory species. Several investigators have sectioned the rat brain and assayed GnRH content in the various tissue blocks.[82] Gonadotropin releasing hormone was found in a band extending from the medial preoptic area (MPOA) caudally to the median-eminence arcuate region (ME-arcuate). Similar studies were carried out using microdissection procedures to dissect out specific nuclei for GnRH assay.[83] Gonadotropin releasing hormone has also been studied by numerous investigators using immunohistochemical techniques at both the light and electron microscopic levels.[84,89] In these studies, it was observed that the greatest concentration of GnRH is in the median eminence with lesser amounts in both the arcuate nucleus and the preoptic area of the hypothalamus. Gonadotropin releasing hormone is also found in the premammilliary area. This is unexpected, since this region does not appear to be involved in the regulation of any of the hypothalamic releasing hormones. By using the drug, colchicine, which prevents the axonal transport of the releasing factors, it appeared that the cell bodies of the neurons which compose the preoptic nucleus, arcuate nucleus and septal hypothalamic areas are the sites for the synthesis of GnRH.[90] However, these observations have not been confirmed and there are still contentions about the sites of GnRH synthesis. In humans, the greatest concentration of GnRH occurs in the pituitary stalk.[91]

Using immunohistocheimical techniques, GnRH has been found in several extrahypothalamic sites. GnRH has been found in the pineal glands of rats, sheep, and monkeys.[95] Cells rostral to the anterior commissure within the paraolfactory area and in the organum vasculosum of the laminal terminalis in rats also contain GnRH.[89,90] These anterior locations may have particular significance since (1) GnRH excites sexual activity in both male and female rats under conditions in which gonadal activity is maintained at a constant level;[93] and (2) GnRH can control the firing rates of individual hypothalamic neurons.[94] Thus, these observations suggest that GnRH can act within the brain as a neurotransmitter agent and modify sex drive.

Synthesis and Degradation of GnRH

Relatively little work has been done on the biosynthesis of GnRH. Preliminary studies indicate that particulate-free hypothalamic extracts incubated in the presence of 21 essential amino acids, ATP, and magnesium, form GnRH as determined by bioassay.[96] Hypothalamic tissue slices can incorporate radioactive amino acids into a peptide which shows the physiologic and chemical characteristics of GnRH.[97] Fractions of hypothalamic tissue enriched in mitochondria have been shown to be capable of synthesizing GnRH, suggesting that the mitochondria are the site of GnRH synthesis.[98] However, to date the mechanism by which GnRH is synthesized cannot be established with certainly.

Hypothalamic extracts have been shown to contain factors which actively degrade the decapeptide GnRH.[99-100] These factors appear to be endopeptidases. It has been proposed that GnRH degrading enzymes may serve a functional or physiologic role in decreasing GnRH secretion and subsequent LH and FSH secretion. The rate of breakdown of GnRH either at its site of synthesis and/or at the interaction with its receptors may be an important regulator of GnRH secretory rate and has been proposed as a mechanism of general control of LH and FSH. However, the degrading enzyme systems appear to be relatively nonspecific in regard to their substrate requirements.

Negative Feedback Control of Gonadotropin Release

Negative Feedback

Gonadal steroids have a potent inhibitory or negative feedback effect on LH and FSH release. The inhibitory effect of steroids on gonadotropin secretion in humans and laboratory species is clearly demonstrated by the marked rise in both LH and FSH seen after ovariectomy.[101-103] A similar phenomenon is observed at the menopause when ovarian steroid production is severely attenuated and also in several abnormal conditions associated with abnormally low gonadal activity.[103,104] The rise of FSH after castration is generally more rapid than that of LH and the increases generally occur more rapidly in the male than in the female.[105-108] The release of LH in intact and gonadectomized animals is pulsatile in nature; however, the amplitude of the pulses is much greater after castration.[109,110] The pulsatile release of LH appears to be due in turn to a pulsatile release of GnRH, although a pulsatile release of LH in response to a constant infusion of GnRH has been demonstrated in an in vitro perfusion system.[65,109,111]

The data from various feedback experiments must be carefully evaluated since the dose, timing, pattern, and method of steroid replacement as well as steroid clearance rates will affect the results.[106] Single injections, infusions, or implants of estrogen decrease gonadotropin levels in ovariectomized females.[101,106,112-114] The sensitivity of castrate males to estrogen is somewhat less, especially in regard to FSH suppression.[115-117] Testosterone is effective in lowering LH in the castrate male, but FSH levels are more difficult to suppress unless the animal is also given estrogen.[115-118] Immediate androgen replacement after castration is more effective than delayed replacement in lowering both LH and FSH levels.

The negative feedback effect of progesterone on LH and FSH secretion is equivocal, but several studies have shown a synergism between estrogen and progesterone to inhibit gonadotropin in ovariectomized but not intact monkeys.[118] Estrogen and progesterone may also be synergistic in the ovariectomized rat, where it appears that lowering of estrogen and progesterone to "physiologic levels" suppresses LH, but not FSH, to normal tonic levels.[106,120-122] Progesterone may serve as the most important negative feedback hormone in the sheep, thus illustrating the difference of hormonal effects, among species.[123]

The principal site of steroid negative feedback action in the rat appears to be in the medial basal hypothalamus,[124] although activity at the pituitary level may initially be of some importance.[125,126] Estrogen receptors have been isolated from both of these areas and this supports the view of a direct estrogen effect.[127,128] Castration has been shown to deplete hypothalamic GnRH content presumably by increasing release whereas steroid replacement increases GnRH content.[129] Data from castrate or postmenopausal women indicate increased levels of GnRH in the peripheral blood. The levels are reduced by estrogen replacement.[130,131]

Ultrashort Loop Feedback

Luteinizing hormone and FSH may alter their own level of secretion by acting directly on the brain or pituitary. The physiologic significance of this "short-loop" feedback is questionable, but probably of minor importance, since very high FSH and LH levels are maintained in castrated male and females of many, if not all, species. Nevertheless, it has been demonstrated that hCG inhibits LH but not FSH secretion in oophorectomized women or castrated rabbits.[132-135] This effect was seen shortly after castration, but was lost by 6 months in women and by 6 weeks in rabbits. It has also been shown that hCG blocks the estrogen-induced release of LH in long-term castrated rhesus monkeys.[136] Experiments by Patritti-Laborde et al.[137] have demonstrated that human LH inhibits the response of the rabbit pituitary to GnRH both in vivo and in vitro, indicating a direct inhibitory effect of LH on the pituitary.

Nonsteroidal Negative Feedback (Inhibin)

Several workers have been seeking a factor that can selectively suppress FSH but not LH since, following castration, FSH rises at a faster rate than does LH and since steroid replacement fails to suppress serum FSH levels to the same relative degree as LH levels.[106] A nonsteroidal factor found in ovarian follicular fluid and testicular extracts has been shown to selectively suppress FSH release in both in vivo and in vitro tests.[138-141] This substance, termed inhibin or folliculostatin, appears to be a peptide of greater than 20,000 mol wt.[142,143] The presence of inhibin in follicular fluid during the follicular phase of the cycle, but not the luteal phase, suggests this substance may play a role in regulating FSH secretion during a specific stage of the cycle.[144] Inhibin has also been found in rat ovarian venous blood during the estrous cycle where it appears that the LH surge may reduce inhibin levels allowing for the rise of FSH seen during late proestrus and early estrus.[145,146]

Positive Feedback

Besides the negative feedback role of ovarian streoids, ovarian estrogens under appropriate conditions exert a stimulating or positive feedback action on LH and FSH release. This action is seen in both estrogen primed ovariectomized and intact females during the estrous or menstrual cycle. Several investigators have shown that there is no positive feedback release of LH in the intact or castrated male rat,[118,147,148] but a positive feedback effect of estradiol has been reported in the male marmoset monkey.[149] Data concerning positive feedback release of LH in men are inconclusive.[150,151] The lack of positive feedback in male rats is apparently due to the exposure of the hypothalamus to androgens shortly after birth, since female rats exposed to androgens before day 5 of life show the masculine response to steroids.[151] Androgen exposure may not have the same importance in the monkey.[152]

The stimulatory effects of steroids were first demonstrated by Holweg[153] who used estrogen to induce ovulation and corpora lutea formation in prepubertal rats. Everett[154] showed that estrogen could advance the time of ovulation in rats and since that time several investigators have shown that antiestrogens block the spontaneous surge of LH and ovulation in intact cycling animals. Progesterone either advances or delays ovulation depending on whether it is given in late diestrus (or early proestrus) or early in diestrus.[155,157,158] Progesterone has a synergistic effect with estrogen on LH release and ovulation in the intact rat.[6]

In the ovariectomized rat or ewe, estrogen causes three to four daily LH surges.[123,124,160] Progesterone alone has no effect on LH release, but it does potentiate the action of estrogen.[161,162] Although progesterone potentiates the LH surge induced by estrogen, it blocks the release of LH seen on subsequent days in rats given estrogen alone.[163] Thus, in the intact rat, estrogen from developing follicles may serve to initiate a daily signal for LH release which is extinguished by the proestrus surge of progesterone. Estrogen probably stimulates LH release in the rat both by stimulating pituitary response to LHRH and by increasing hypothalamic LHRH release. Hypothalamic deafferentation or anterior hypothalamic lesions disrupt positive feedback in the female rat, suggesting that the anterior hypothalamic preoptic area is the locus for the generation of the positive feedback response.[164,165] It appears that although progesterone mediated positive feedback may involve the preoptic area, estrogen induced LH may involve limbic circuits.[166] Likewise, there may be separate areas for the positive feedback control of FSH release.[167] The neural control of LH release will be discussed more fully in the next section.

Estrogen or estrogen plus progesterone also stimulate LH release in women and nonhuman primates.[168-170] However, these effects may involve an action principally at the pituitary since, unlike in the rat, hypothalamic deafferentation of the monkey does not disrupt LH release.[171]

Neural Control of Gonadotropin Secretion

A neural control of gonadotropin secretion was postulated even before experimental measurements because of the observable effects of a variety of environmental factors on reproductive function.[172,173] The anatomic relationship between the brain and pituitary also led investigators to study neural control of pituitary function.

An association between certain brain lesions and gonadal dysfunction in both man and various animals provided some of the earliest insights into the neural control of gonadotropin secretion. In 1912, Aschner[174] induced gonadal atrophy in dogs by producing lesions in the hypothalamus, and similar experiments with similar results in a variety of species soon followed.[162] In 1937, Harris demonstrated that electrical stimulation of the hypothalamus can induce rabbits to ovulate.[173]

Norepinephrine was first demonstrated in the brain by Holtz[175] and, in the late 40s and early 50s, Sawyer and co-workers[176,177] showed that adrenergic or cholinergic drugs can induce ovulation in rats and rabbits and anticholinergic and antiadrenergic drugs can block ovulation. Since that time there has been a continually increasing body of data concerning the role of neurotransmitters in controlling gonadotropin release, presumably by controlling the release of hypothalamic GnRH.

Most investigators agree that norepinephrine (NE) is the principal neurotransmitter, stimulating both tonic and phasic LH and FSH release in the male and female rat. Much less is known about LH release in humans or other species. Administration of α-methyl-paratyrosine, which lowers hypothalamic NE and dopamine (DA) levels, blocks the LH surge in intact proestrus rats as well as the positive feedback release of LH in the ovariectomized steroid treated rat.[178,179] These effects can be reversed by administration of dihydroxy-phenylserine (DOPS) which selectively increases NE, but not by L-DOPA which principally increases dopamine levels. The neurotoxin, 6 hydroxydopamine, which depletes hypothalamic NE, also blocks the LH surge induced by progesterone injection.[180,181] Similarly, dopamine-β-hydroxylase inhibitors selectively lower NE levels and inhibit LH release.[178]

Additional evidence for the positive effects of NE on LH release come from deafferentation and turnover studies. Hypothalamic deafferentation, which causes a 60% depletion of hypothalamic NE, but little change in DA levels, effectively blocks the proestrus LH surge in the rat.[112,182] Castration increases hypothalamic NE synthesis and content in male and female rats whereas steroid replacement reverses this effect.[183-185] Norepinephrine turnover has also been shown to increase prior to the proestrus or the steroid (positive feedback) induced LH surge.[186-188] Peripheral NE levels are elevated in periovulatory women, but the relationship to hypothalamic NE changes is not known.[189-190] It appears that NE may be acting through the LHRH neuron to control LH release.[191]

Despite the large body of evidence for a stimulatory role of NE in LH release, several reports of an inhibitory effect have been published. These reports suggest that the steroid milieu may be of importance in predicting the effect of NE. Thus, the intraventricular injection of NE inhibits LH release in untreated ovariectomied rats, but increases LH release in ovariectomized steroid primed rats.[109,192]

The role of DA in controlling LH and FSH release is not clear and is the subject of considerable debate. Evidence for a stimulatory effect of DA has been published by several laboratories using a variety of techniques. Schneider and McCann,[193,194] using relatively large doses of DA, demonstrate that DA stimulates both LH and FSH release in an in vitro hypothalamic-pituitary coincubation system as well as in the ovariectomized rat primed with estrogen and progesterone. Intraventricular DA injections are shown to increase GnRH levels in portal and peripheral blood.[195] Dopamine has also been reported to release GnRH from synaptosomes prepared from sheep hypothalamus and median eminence and from rat hypothalamus.[196-198] The latter effects are steroid dependent and can be blocked by the DA receptor blocker, pimozide. Finally, pimozide can depress the LH surge in rats and women.[199,200]

An inhibitory role of DA has also been supported by numerous studies. Dopamine could not induce ovulation in proestrus, in ovariectomized steroid primed rats, or in rats made constantly estrous by exposure to constant illumination.[177,201,202] In contrast to in vitro studies discussed in the previous paragraph, Miyachi and co-workers[203] found that DA inhibits GnRH release from rat hypothalami. A variety of DA agonists inhibit basal LH release in castrated rats.[204,205] In women, DA infusion induces a significant decline in LH which is most pronounced during the preovulatory phase of the menstrual cycle.[206] The DA agonists, L-DOPA, and bromocryptine, have similar effects.[207]

Further evidence for an inhibitory role of DA comes from studies correlating LH release with hypothalamic DA turnover. Thus, a decrease in DA turnover precedes the proestrus LH surge or the steroid induced LH surge in ovariectomied rats.[186-188,208] Various hyperprolactinemic states are often associated with decreased LH release and increased DA turnover, giving still another line of evidence for the inhibitory effect of DA on LH release.[209-211]

In an attempt to reconcile the confusion about DA effects on LH and FSH release, Vijayan and McCann[212] demonstrated that low doses of DA stimulate LH release in steroid primed rats, whereas high doses of DA suppress LH in castrated rats. It has also been suggested that in some cases DA may be taken up in NE neurons and converted to NE which, in turn, induces LH release.[213] In summary, it appears that both the relative degree of dopaminergic stimulation and the steroid background are important in determining LH and FSH release rates. The physiologic significance of the dopaminergic control of LH release, however, has still not been elucidated.

The serotonergic system also has major effects on gonadotropin release. Serotonin (5-hydroxytryptamine; 5-HT) has direct inhibitory action on the gonads and this action was not taken into account in many early studies.[214] However, intraventricular injections of 5-HT or stimulation of the raphe nucleus, which releases endogenous 5-HT, have been shown to inhibit LH and FSH release in castrated rats.[194,215] The precursor of 5-HT, 5-hydroxytryptophane (5-HTP), blocks both the LH surge and ovula tion,[216-217] while turnover of 5-HT appears to decrease prior to the LH surge in sheep.[218] The negative feedback effect of estrogen in the rat appears to be associated with increases in midbrain 5-HT levels and 5-HT turnover.[219-220]

Although 5-HT seems inhibitory to basal LH release in the rat, evidence is accumulating to show that it may, in some instances, be stimulatory to cyclic or phasic LH release. Parachlorophenylalanine (PCPA), which depletes 5-HT, can block ovulation if given at an appropriate time and this blockade can be reversed by the 5-HT precursor, 5-HTP.[216,221] This effect of 5-HT appears to amplify rather than trigger the LH surge.

Although the majority of studies are concerned with hypothalamic NE, DA, and 5-HT, other brain areas and their neurotransmitters have been reported to affect gonadotropin release. Atropine, an anticholinergic agent, blocks ovulation, while acetylcholine has been shown to release LH and FSH in both in vivo and in vitro systems.[222,223] Other investigators have not been successful in evaluating the influence of the cholinergic system on LH release and much work needs to be done.[224]

Histamine is found in large concentrations in the hypothalamus and reportedly releases LH and FSH.[225,226] γ-aminobutyric acid (GABA) also releases LH after intraventricular injection.[212,227] The pineal hormone, melatonin, has an inhibitory effect on gonadotropin release and may mediate the effects of light on gonadal function.[228] Some investigators claim that pineal secretions other than melatonin are of more importance in this regard. The recent discovery of endogenous opiate peptides and their inhibitory effects on LH and FSH release has opened up a new area of investigation. Opiate peptides may be involved both in prepubertal and old age changes in LH release in the rat, as well as in normal cyclic changes, possibly by influencing the turnover of hypothalamic NE, DA, and/or 5-HT.[229-231] Endogenous opiates have been implicated in the control of LH secretion during the human menstrual cycle.[232]

An increasing body of literature is strongly supportive of prostaglandins as important mediators of LH and FSH release, possibly through hypothalamic mechanisms or by direct action on the pituitary gland. Prostaglandins of the E series stimulate LH and FSH release in the rat, perhaps through a direct action on the GnRH neuron.[233] Inhibitors of prostaglandin synthesis inhibit ovulation[234] and brain prostaglandin production appears to be under estrogen regulation.[235]

Although this section has been principally concerned with hypothalamic or anterior-hypothalamic preoptic area neurotransmitter relationships to gonadotropin secretion, extrahypothalamic structures such as the amygdala, hippocampus, and midbrain are undoubtedly involved in gonadotropin regulation, although their role is unclear. It appears that, in the rat, limbic structures are not essential for ovulation, but they may modulate gonadotropin release. In freely moving rats, the hippocampus is inhibitory to LH release and the amygdala seems to modulate the timing and amplitude of the LH surge.[236] Studies with other rat models have given contradictory results and have been described in an excellent review by Ellendorff.[237]

PATTERNS OF MALE GONADOTROPIN RELEASE

Fetal and Neonatal

Serum LH and FSH in the human male become detectable as early as the 9th or 10th fetal week, although pituitaries from the 5th to 7th week are capable of secreting LH and FSH in culture.[238,239] The fetal pituitary is fairly resistant to GnRH stimulation, possibly due to high levels of exogenous GnRH, since cultured fetal pituitaries are responsive to GnRH.[240,241] Gonadotropin levels peak at midgestation and then decline toward term.[238] Mean FSH levels are lower in the male than in the female fetus, possibly due to high testosterone levels in the former.[242] The decrease in gonadotropins toward term is most likely due to increasing sensitivity of negative feedback mechanisms.[238,242]

Prepubertal and Pubertal

Serum LH and FSH levels fluctuate somewhat during the first few months and thereafter remain low until puberty.[243,244] In males, LH levels gradually increase through puberty, whereas serum FSH increases earlier and levels out near the end of puberty.[238,242] Luteinizing hormone and, to a lesser extent, FSH, fluctuate throughout the day in pubertal boys with noticeable rises of LH associated with periods of sleep.[245] Testosterone levels parallel LH secretion, although increasing FSH secretion may be important in potentiating the testosterone response to LH. The increases in LH secretion during puberty are probably secondary to increased GnRH release, but it has also been demonstrated that pituitary response to GnRH increases at puberty.[246,249] With the exception of high LH levels seen at day 10 to 12, gonadotropin levels remain low until puberty, when they rise to adult levels.

Adult

Gonadotropins in adult men are released in a pulsatile fashion which is characterized by a rapid secretion over a 10 to 15 min period followed by a decrease over a 50 to 60 min period. The LH pulses are of a greater magnitude than the FSH pulses and they are usually, but not always, in synchrony.[31] Mean gonadotropin levels generally remain constant from puberty until about 50 years of age, when levels of LH and FSH gradually increase, possibly due to altered testicular function.[105] In the old male rat, gonadotropin levels are slightly attenuated.[105]

PATTERNS OF FEMALE GONADOTROPIN RELEASE

Fetal and Neonatal

The human female fetal gonadotropin profile is similar to that of the male, although FSH levels are somewhat higher. For up to 2 years after birth, FSH levels fluctuate between relatively low values to near normal adult levels, but then remain low until puberty.[242,243] Luteinizing hormone levels fall by four months and remain low.

Puberty

With the approach of puberty, gonadotropin levels rise, with FSH rising earlier than LH.[242,243] Follicle stimulating hormone secretion shows fluctuations at the beginning of puberty, while LH pulsations are not clearly evident until just before menarche. The cyclic adult pattern of LH and FSH release is usually established shortly after the menarche, although cycles are generally irregular at first.

In the female rat, neonatal levels of LH and FSH are relatively high, but drop to low levels by day 4.[248,249] Follicle stimulating hormone is elevated between days 10 and 20, while LH levels are variable, being high in some rats, but low in others. From days 10 to 20, gonadotropin levels drop and remain low until regular cycles are established at puberty (approximately day 37 to 40).

Adult

The Menstrual Cycle

The median length of the menstrual cycle is 28 days, but this varies considerably among women. The cycle is also usually irregular at the beginning and end of the reproduction years, as well as during postpartum and lactation.[31,105,250] The menstrual cycle is usually divided into follicular, ovulatory, and luteal phases, each associated with a specific hormonal profile (See Figure 1).

The early follicular phase overlaps with the previous late luteal phase and is characterized by a rise in FSH and possibly in LH. Ovarian steroid secretion is fairly constant during this phase. In the week prior to the LH surge and ovulation, ovarian estrogen secretion increases, FSH levels decrease slightly and LH either increases slightly or remains constant. During the ovulatory phase there is a precipitous drop in estrogen levels followed by a surge of LH and FSH. Ovulation follows some 18 to 24 hr later.

After ovulation, the granulosa cells of the ovulating follicle luteinize and begin to secrete relatively large amounts of progesterone. Luteinizing hormone and FSH levels decrease slowly until menstruation and the beginning of the next cycle.

The Estrous Cycle

The rat estrous cycle is 4 days in length, but has many similarities to the menstrual cycle.[101,106] During the preovulatory period, diestrus 1 and 2, LH and FSH levels are relatively low, but estrogen levels are gradually increasing.[251,252] Estrogen levels peak on the morning of proestrus, and that afternoon a surge of LH, FSH, prolactin, and progesterone is seen. Ovulation occurs 8 to 10 hr later in estrus. Follicle stimulating hormone levels are still elevated on the morning of estrus, but LH, estradiol and progesterone remain low unless pregnancy or pseudopregnancy ensue.

Several other patterns of reproductive cycles are seen in other species. Most species, including the human female and rats, ovulate spontaneously, but animals such as cats and rabbits ovulate only in response to mating or experimental procedures such as LH (or hCG) injection.[253] In these reflex ovulators, the ovary contains mature follicles which ovulate in response to an LH surge induced by coitus. There are also many animals such as sheep that are classified as seasonal breeders, since they show extrous cycles only during certain periods of the year.[254] The cycles in these animals are strongly influenced by environmental cues, daylight length being one of the more important.

Pregnancy and Lactation

Maternal LH and FSH are virtually undetectable during human pregnancies, although the placenta produces a chorionic gonadotropin (hCG) that is very similar to LH in its biologic action.[255] Luteinizing hormone and FSH remain at low to normal levels during lactation, but the cyclic release and ovulation are usually suppressed at least during the immediate postpartum period.[257]

REFERENCES

1. **Romeis, B.,** Innersekretorische Drusen, II. Hypophyse in *Handbuch der Mikroskopischen Anatomie des Menschen,* Vol. 6, von Mollendorff, W., Ed., Springer-Verlag, Basel, 1940, Part 3.
2. **Holmes, R. L. and Ball, N. J.,** *The Pituitary Gland-A Comparative Account,* Cambridge University Press, London, 1974.

3. **Baker, B. L.,** Functional cytology of the hypophysial pars distalis and pars intermedia, in *Handbook of Physiology, Section 7,* Vol. 4, Knobil, E. and Sawyer, W. H., Eds., American Physiological Society, Washington, D.C., 1974, 45.
4. **Rennels, E. G.,** Gonadotrophic cells of rat hypophysis, in *Cytologie de l'Adenohypophyse,* Benoit, J. and DeLage, C., Eds., Centre National de la Recherche Scientifique, Paris, 1963, 201.
5. **Farquhar, M. G. and Rinehart, J. F.,** Electron microscopic studies of the anterior pituitary gland of castrate rats, *Endocrinology,* 54, 516, 1954.
6. **Purves, H. D. and Griesbach, W. F.,** Changes in gonadotrophs of the rat pituitary after gonadectomy, *Endocrinology,* 56, 374, 1955.
7. **Hildebrand, J. E., Rennels, E. G., and Finerty, J. C.,** Gonadotrophic cells of the rat hypophysis and their relation to hormone production, *Zschr. Zellforsch.,* 46, 400, 1957.
8. **Kurosumi, K.,** Functional classification of cell types of the anterior pituitary gland accomplished by electron microscopy, *Saibokaku Byorigaku Zasshi,* 29, 329, 1968.
9. **Nakane, P. K.,** Simultaneous localization of multiple tissue antigens using the peroxidase-labeled antibody method: a study on pituitary glands of the rat, *J. Histochem. Cytochem.,* 16, 557, 1968.
10. **Nakane, P. K.,** Classifications of anterior pituitary cell types with immunoenzyme histochemistry, *J. Histochem. Cytochem.,* 18, 9, 1970.
11. **Moriarty, G. C.,** Electron microscopic-immunocytochemical studies of rat pituitary gonadotrophs: a sex difference in morphology and cytochemistry of LH cells, *Endocrinology,* 97, 1215, 1975.
12. **Costoff, A. and McShan, W. H.,** Isolation and biological properties of secretory granules from rat anterior pituitary glands, *J. Cell Biol.,* 43, 564, 1969.
13. **Sairam, M. R. and Papkoff, H.,** Chemistry of pituitary gonadotrophins, in *Handbook of Physiology, Section 7,* Vol. 4, Part 2, Knobil, E. and Sawyer, W. H., Eds., American Physiological Society, Washington, D. C., 1974, 111.
14. **Saxena, B. B. and Rathnam, P.,** Chemical and immunological characteristics of the subunits of human pituitary FSH and LH, in *Structure-Activity Relationships of Protein and Polypeptide Hormones — Part 1,* Margoulies, M. and Greenwood, F. C., Eds., *Excerpta Med. Int. Congr. Ser.,* 241, 122, 1971.
15. **Kathan, R. H., Reichert, L. E., Jr., and Ryan, R. J.,** Comparison of the carbohydrate and amino acid composition of bovine, ovine and human luteinizing hormone, *Endocrinology,* 81, 45, 1967.
16. **Ryan, R. J., Jiang, N. S., and Hanolon, S.,** Some physical and hydrodynamic properties of human FSH and LH, *Rec. Prog. Horm. Res.,* 26, 105, 1970.
17. **Morell, A. G., Gregoriadis, G., Scheinberg, I. H., Hickmann, J., and Ashwell, J.,** The role of sialic acid in determining the survival of glycoproteins in the circulation, *J. Biol. Chem.,* 146, 1461, 1971.
18. **Bogdanove, E. M., Campbell, G. T., Blair, E. D., Mula, M. E., Miller, A. E., and Grossman, G. H.,** Gonadal-pituitary feedback involves qualitative change: androgens alter the type of FSH secreted by the rat pituitary, *Endocrinology,* 95, 219, 1974.
19. **Dufau, M. L., Hodgen, G. D., Goodman, A. L., and Catt, K. J.,** Bioassay of circulating LH in the Rhesus monkey comparison with radioimmunoassay during physiological changes, *Endocrinology,* 100, 1557, 1977.
20. **Weick, R. F.,** A comparison of the disappearance rates of LH from intact and ovx rats, *Endocrinology,* 101, 157, 1977.
21. **Lucky, A. W., Rebar, R. W., Rosenfield, R. L., Roche-Bender, N., and Helke, J.,** Reduction of the potency of LH by estrogen, *N. Engl. J. Med.,* 300, 1034, 1979.
22. **Peckham, W. D., Kamaji, T., Dierschke, D. L., and Knobil, E.,** Gonadal function and the biological and physiochemical properties of follicle stimulating hormone, *Endocrinology,* 92, 1600, 1973.
23. **Moudgal, N. R., Muralidhar, K., and Madhwa Raj, H. J.,** Pituitary gonadotropins, in *Methods of Hormone Radioimmunoassay,* 2nd ed., Jaffe, B. M. and Behrman, H. R., Eds., Academic Press, New York, 1979, 173.
24. **Parlow, A. F.,** Bioassay of pituitary luteinizing hormone by depletion of ovarian ascorbic acid, in *Human Pituitary Gonadotropins,* Albert, A., Ed., Charles C Thomas, Springfield, Mass., 1961, 300.
25. **Greep, R. O., VanDyke, H. B., and Chew, B. F.,** Use of anterior lobe of prostate gland in the assay of metakentrin, *Proc. Soc. Exp. Biol. Med.,* 46, 644, 1941.
26. **Evans, H. M., Simpson, M. E., Tolksdorf, S., and Jensen, H.,** Biological studies of the gonadotropic principles in sheep pituitary substance, *Endocrinology,* 25, 529, 1939.
27. **Catt, K. J., Ketelslegers, J. M., and Dufau, M. L.,** Receptors for gonadotropic hormones, in *Methods Recep. Res.,* Blecher, M., Ed., Marcel Dekker, New York, 1976, (Part 1), 175.
28. **Farguhar, M. G., Skutelsky, E. H., and Hopkins, C. R.,** Structure and function of the anterior-pituitary and dispersed pituitary cells, in *Ultrastructure in Biological Systems, Vol. 7, The Anterior Pituitary,* Tixier-Vidal, A. and Farguhar, M. G., Eds., Academic Press, New York, 1975, 83.
29. **Edmonds, M., Moliton, M., Pierce, J. G., and Odell, W. D.,** Secretion of a subunit of LH by the anterior pituitary gland, *J. Clin. Endocrinol. Metab.,* 41, 551, 1975.

30. **Bremmer, W. J. and Paulsen, C. A.,** Two pools of LH in the human pituitary: evidence from constant administration of LH-releasing hormone, *J. Clin. Endocrinol. Metab.*, 39, 811, 1974.
31. **Catt, K. J. and Pierce, J. G.,** Gonadotropic hormones of the adenohypophysis, in *Reproductive Endocrinology*, Yen, S. S. C. and Jaffe, R. B., W.B. Saunders, Philadelphia, 1978, 34.
32. **Ashwell, G. and Morell, A. G.,** The role of surface carbohydrates in the hepatic recognition and transport of circulating glycoproteins, *Adv. Enzymol.*, 41, 99, 1974.
33. **VanHall, E. V., Vaitukaitis, J. L., Ross, G. T., Hickman, J. W., and Ashwell, G.,** Effects of progressive desialylation on the rate of disappearance of immunoreactive hCH from plasma in rats, *Endocrinology*, 89, 11, 1971.
34. **Arimura, A. and Schally, A. V.,** Hypothalamic LH- and FSH-releasing hormone: re-evaluation of the concept that one hypothalamic hormone controls the release of LH and FSH, in *Biological Rhythms in Neuroendocrine Activity*, Kawakami, M., Ed., Igaku Shoin, Tokyo, 1974, 73.
35. **Schally, A. V.,** Aspects of hypothalamic regulation of the pituitary gland, *Science*, 202, 13, 1978.
36. **Guillemin, R.,** Peptides in the brain: the new endocrinology of the neuron, *Science*, 202, 390, 1978.
37. **Alpert, L. C., Brawer, J. R., Jackson, I. M. D., and Reichlin, S.,** Localization of LHRH in neurons in frog brain (Rana pipiens and Rana catesbeiana), *Endocrinology*, 98, 910, 1976.
38. **Deery, D. J.,** Determination by radioimmunoassay of the luteinising hormone-releasing hormone (LHRH) content of the hypothalamus of the rat and some lower vertebrates, *Gen. Comp. Endocrinol.*, 24, 280, 1974.
39. **Jeffcoate, S. L., Sharp, P. J., Fraser, H. M., Holland, D. T., and Gunn, A.,** Immunochemical and chromatographic similiarity of rat, rabbit, chicken and synthetic luteinizing hormone releasing hormones, *J. Endocrinol.*, 62, 85, 1974.
40. **King, J. A. and Millar, R. P.,** Heterogeneity of vertebrate luteinizing hormone-releasing hormone, *Science*, 206, 67, 1979.
41. **Faglia, B.,** Elevations in plasma growth hormone concentrations after LRH in patients with active acromegaly, *J. Clin. Endocrinol. Metab.*, 37, 338, 1973.
42. **Yen, S. S. C.,** Induction of PRL release by LRF and LRF-agonist, *Life Sci.*, 26, 1963, 1980.
43. **Arimura, A., Debeljuk, L., and Shally, A. V.,** Blockade of the preovulatory surge of LH and FSH and of ovulation by anti-LH-RH in rats, *Endocrinology*, 95, 323, 1974.
44. **Koch, Y., Chobsieng, P., Zor, U., Fridkin, J., and Lindner, H. R.,** Suppression of gonadotropin secretion and prevention of ovulation in the rat by antiserum to synthetic gonadotropin-releasing hormone, *Biochem. Biophys. Res. Commun.*, 55, 623, 1973.
45. **Clarke, I. J., Fraser, H. M., and McNeilly, A. S.,** Active immunization of ewes against luteinizing hormone releasing hormone, and its effects on ovulation and gonadotropin, prolactin and ovarian steroid secretion, *J. Endocrinol.*, 78, 39, 1978.
46. **Eskay, R. L., Oliver, C., Ben-Jonathan, N., and Porter, J. C.,** Hypothalamic hormones in portal and systemic blood, in *Hypothalamic Hormones*, Motta, M., Crosignani, P., and Martini, L., Eds., Academic Press, New York, 1975, 125.
47. **Makino, T.,** Study on the intracellular mechanism of LH release in the anterior pituitary, *Am. J. Obstet. Gynecol.*, 115, 606, 1973.
48. **Samli, M. H. and Geschwind, I.,** Some effects of energy-transfer inhibitors and of Ca^{++}-free or K^{+}-enhanced media on the release of luteinizing hormone (LH) from the rat pituitary gland in vitro, *Endocrinology*, 82, 225, 1968.
49. **Wakabayashi, K., Kumberi, I. A., and McCann, S. M.,** In vitro response of the rat pituitary to gonadotrophin-releasing factors and to ions, *Endocrinology*, 85, 1046, 1969.
50. **Arimura, A., Debeljuk, L., and Schally, A. V.,** Stimulation of FSH release *in vivo* by prolonged infusion of synthetic LHRH, *Endocrinology*, 91, 529, 1972.
51. **Greeley, G. H., Jr., Allen, M. B., and Mahesh, V. B.,** FSH and LH response in the rat after intravenous, intracarotid or subcutaneous administration of LHRH, *Proc. Soc. Exp. Biol. Med.*, 147, 859, 1974.
52. **Blake, C. A.,** Simulation of the early phase of the proestrous follicle-stimulating hormone rise after infusion of luteinizing hormone-releasing hormone in phenobarbital-blocked rats, *Endocrinology*, 98, 461, 1976.
53. **Aiyer, M. S., Chiappa, S. A., and Fink, G.,** A priming effect of luteinizing hormone releasing factor on the anterior pituitary gland in the female rat, *J. Endocrinol.*, 62, 573, 1974.
54. **Castro-Vasquez, A. and McCann, S. M.,** Cyclic variations in the increased responsiveness of the pituitary to luteinizing hormone-releasing hormone (LHRH) induced by LHRH, *Endocrinology*, 97, 13, 1975.
55. **Fink, G., Chiappo, S. A., and Aiyers, M. S.,** Priming effect of LHRH elicited by preoptic stimulation and by intravenous infusion and multiple injections of the synthetic decapeptide, *J. Endocrinol.*, 69, 359, 1976.

56. **Edwardson, J. A. and Gilbert, D.**, Application of an in-vitro perfusion technique to studies of luteinizing hormone release by rat anterior hemi-pituitaries: self-potentiation by luteinizing hormone releasing hormone, *J. Endocrinol.*, 68, 197, 1976.
57. **Pickering, A. J. M. C. and Fink, G.**, Priming effect of luteinizing hormone releasing factor: *in-vitro* and *in-vivo* evidence consistent with its dependence upon protein and RNA synthesis, *J. Endocrinol.*, 69, 373, 1976.
58. **Foster, J. P.**, The response of the pituitary gland to hypothalamic stimulation, in *Control of Ovulation*, Crighton, D. B., Haynes, N. B., Foxcroft, G. R., and Lamming, G. E., Eds., Butterworths, London, 1978, 101.
59. **Savoy-Moore, R. T., Schwartz, N. B., Duncan, J. A., and Marshall, J. C.**, Pituitary gonadotropin-releasing hormone receptors during the rat estrous cycle, *Science*, 209, 942, 1980.
60. **Clayton, R. N., Solano, A. R., Garcin-Vela, A., Dufaud, M., and Catt, K. J.**, Regulation of pituitay receptors for GnRH during the rat estrous cycle, *Endocrinology*, 107, 699, 1980.
61. **Pickering, A. and Fink, G.**, Priming effect of luteinizing hormone releasing factor: *in-vitro* studies with raised potassium ion concentrations, *J. Endocrinol.*, 69, 453, 1976.
62. **Wise, P. M., Rance, N., Barr, G. D., and Barraclough, C. A.**, Further evidence that LHRH also is FSH-RH, *Endocrinology*, 104, 940, 1979.
63. **Belchetz, P. E., Plant, T. M., Nakai, Y., Keogh, E. J., and Knobil, E.**, Hypophysial responses to continuous and intermittent delivery of hypothalamic GnRH, *Science*, 202, 631, 1978.
64. **Knobil, E., Plant, T. M., Wildt, L., Balchetz, P. E., and Marshall, G.**, Control of the rhesus monkey menstrual cycle: permissive role of hypothalamic gonadotropin-releasing hormone, *Science*, 207, 1371, 1980.
65. **Kao, L. W. L., Gunsalus, G. L., Williams, G. H., and Weisz, J.**, Response of the perifused anterior pituitaries of rats to synthetic gonadotropin releasing hormone: a comparison with hypothalamic extract and demonstration of a role for potassium in the release of luteinizing hormone and follicle-stimulating hormone, *Endocrinology*, 101, 1444, 1977.
66. **Nillius, S. J. and Wide, L.**, Variation in LH and FSH response to LH-releasing hormone during the menstrual cycle, *J. Obstet. Gynaecol. Br. Commonw.*, 79, 865, 1972.
67. **Yen, S. S. C., Vandenberg, G., Rebar, R., and Ehara, Y.**, Variation of pituitary responsiveness to synthetic LRF during different phases of the menstrual cycle, *J. Clin. Endocrinol. Metab.*, 35, 931, 1972.
68. **Libertun, C., Cooper, K. J., Fawcett, C. P., and McCann, S. M.**, Effects of ovariectomy and steroid treatment on hypophyseal sensitivity to purified LH-releasing factor (LRF), *Endocrinology*, 94, 518, 1974.
69. **Aiyer, M. S., Soad, M. C., and Brown-Grant, K.**, The pituitary response to exogenous luteinizing hormone releasing factor in steroid-treated gonadectomized rats, *J. Endocrinol.*, 69, 255, 1976.
70. **Libertun, C., Orias, R., and McCann, S. M.**, Biphasic effect of estrogen on the sensitivity of the pituitary to luteinizing hormone-releasing factor (LRF), *Endocrinology*, 94, 1094, 1974.
71. **Yen, S. S. C., Vandenberg, G., and Siler-Khodr, T. M.**, Modulation of pituitary responsiveness to LRF by estrogen, *J. Clin. Endocrinol. Metab.*, 39, 170, 1974.
72. **Jaffe, R. B. and Keyes, W. R., Jr.**, Estradiol augmentation of pituitary responsiveness to GnRH in women, *J. Clin. Endocrinol. Metab.*, 39, 850, 1974.
73. **Labire, F., Drouin, J., Ferland, L., Lagace, L., Beaulieu, M., DeLean, A., Kelly, P. A., Caron, M. G., and Raymond, V.**, Mechanism of action of hypothalamic hormones in the anterior pituitary gland and specific modulation of their activity by sex steroids and thyroid hormones, *Rec. Prog. Horm. Res.*, 34, 25, 1978.
74. **Drouin, J., Lavoie, M., and Labrie, F.**, Effect of gonadal steroids on the luteinizing hormone and follicle-stimulating hormone response to 8-bromo-adenosine 3′,5′-monophosphate in anterior pituitary cells in culture, *Endocrinology*, 102, 358, 1978.
75. **Martin, J. E., Tyrey, L., Everett, J. W., and Fellows, R. E.**, Estrogen and progesterone modulation of the pituitary response to LRF in the cyclic rat, *Endocrinology*, 95, 1664, 1974.
76. **Debeljuk, L., Arimura, A., and Schally, A. V.**, Effect of estradiol and progesterone on the LH release induced by LH-releasing hormone (LHRH) in intact diestrous rats and anestrous ewes, *Proc. Soc. Exp. Biol. Med.*, 139, 774, 1972.
77. **Greeley, G. H., Allen, M. B., and Mahesh, V. B.**, Potentiation of luteinizing hormone release by estradiol at the level of the pituitary, *Neuroendocrinology*, 18, 233, 1975.
78. **Drouin, J. and Labrie, F.**, Selective effect of androgens on LH and FSH release in anterior pituitary cells in culture, *Endocrinology*, 98, 1528, 1976.
79. **Swerdloff, R. S. and Odell, W. D.**, Feedback control of male gonadotrophin secretion, *Lancet*, 2, 683, 1968.
80. **Swerdloff, R. S., Walsh, P. C., and Odell, W. D.**, Control of LH and FSH secretion in the male: evidence that aromatization of androgens to estradiol is not required for inhibition of gonadotrophin secretion, *Steroids*, 20, 13, 1972.

81. **Denef, C., Hautekeete, E., Dewals, R., and DeWolf, A.,** Differential control of LH and FSH secretion by androgens in rat pituitary cells in culture: Functional diversity of subpopulations separated by unit gravity sedimentation, *Endocrinology,* 106, 724, 1980.
82. **Ramirez, V. D. and Kordan, C.,** Localization and subcellular distribution of hypothalamic hormones: studies on luteinizing hormone-releasing hormone (LH-RH), in *Hypothalamic Hormones — Proceedings of the Serona Symposia,* Motta, M., Crosignani, P. G. and Martini, L., Eds., Academic Press, New York, 6, 57, 1975.
83. **Palkovits, M., Arimura, A., Brownstein, M., Schally, A. V., and Saavedra, J. M.,** Luteinizing hormone-releasing hormone (LHRH) content of the hypothalamic nuclei in rat, *Endocrinology,* 95, 554, 1974.
84. **Barry, J., DuBois, M. P., Poulain, P., and Leonardelli, J.,** Caracterisation et topographie des neurones hypothalamiques immunoreactifs avec des anticorps anti-LRF de syntheses, *C. R. Acad. Sci. [D] (Paris),* 276, 3191, 1973.
85. **Pelletier, G., Labrie, F., Puviani, R., Arimura, A., and Schally, A. V.,** Immunohistochemical localization of luteinizing hormone-releasing hormone in the rat median eminence, *Endocrinology,* 95, 314, 1974.
86. **Zimmerman, E. A., Hsu, K., Ferin, M., and Kozlowski, G.,** Localization of gonadotropin-releasing hormone (Gn-RH) in the hypothalamus of the mouse by immunoperoxidase technique, *Endocrinology,* 95, 1, 1974.
87. **Naik, D. V.,** Immunoreactive LH-RH neurons in the hypothalamus identified by light and fluorescent microscopy, *Cell Tissue Res.,* 157, 423, 1975.
88. **Naik, D. V.,** Immuno-electron microscopic localization of luteinizing hormone-releasing hormone in the arcuate nuclei and median eminence of the rat, *Cell Tissue Res.,* 157, 437, 1975.
89. **Samson, W. K.,** LHRH distribution in the rat with special reference to mesencephalic sites which contain both LHRH and single neurones responsive to LHRH, *Neuroendocrinology,* 31, 66, 1980.
90. **Hartter, D. E. and Ramirez, V. D.,** The effect of ions, metabolic inhibitors and colchicine on luteinizing hormone-releasing hormone release from superfused rat hypothalami, *Endocrinology,* 107, 375, 1980.
91. **Okon, E. and Koch, Y.,** Localization of GnRH and TRH in human brain by radioimmunoassays, *Nature,* 263, 345, 1976.
92. **Kizer, J. S., Palkovits, M., and Brownstein, M. J.,** Releasing factors in the circumventricular organs of the rat brain, *Endocrinology,* 98, 311, 1976.
93. **Moss, R. L., Dudley, C. A., Foreman, M. M., and McCann, S. M.,** Synthetic LRF: a potentiator of sexual behavior in the rat, in *Hypothalamic Hormones,* Motta, M., Crosignani, P. G., and Martini, L., Eds., Academic Press, New York, 1975, 269.
94. **Muller, E. E., Nistico, G., and Scapagnini, U., Eds.,** *Neurotransmitters and Anterior Pituitary Function,* Academic Press, New York, 1977, 212.
95. **White, W. F., Hedlung, M. T., Weber, G. F., Rippel, R. H., Johnson, E. S., and Wilbes, J. F.,** The pineal gland: a supplemental source of hypothalamic-releasing hormones, *Endocrinology,* 94, 1422, 1974.
96. **Hall, R. W. and Steinberger, E.,** Synthesis of LH-RH by rat hypothalamic tissue *in vitro, Neuroendocrinology,* 21, 111, 1976.
97. **Kordic, D. and Kniewald, Z.,** Incorporation of 14C-amino acids into rat hypothalamus *in vitro, Endocrinol. Exp.,* 11, 3, 1977.
98. **Johansson, K. N. G., Currie, B. L., and Tolkers, K.,** Biosynthesis of the LH-releasing hormone in mitochondrial preparations and by a possible pantetheine-template mechanism, *Biochem. Biophys. Res. Commun.,* 49, 656, 1972.
99. **Griffiths, E. C.,** Peptidase inactivation of hypothalamic releasing hormones, *Horm. Res.,* 7, 179, 1976.
100. **Kuhl, H., Rosniatowski, C., and Tauberl, H. D.,** The regulatory function of a pituitary LH-RH degrading enzyme in the feedback control of gonadotropins, *Acta Endocrinol.,* 86, 60, 1977.
101. **Schwartz, N. B., Dierschke, D. J., McCormack, C. E., and Waltz, P. W.,** Feedback regulation of reproductive cycles in rats, sheep, monkeys and humans, with particular attention to computer modelling, in *Frontiers in Reproduction and Fertility Control,* Greep, R. O. and Koblinsky, M. A., Eds., Massachusetts Institute of Technology Press, Cambridge, 1977, 55.
102. **McCann, S. M.,** Regulation of secretion of follicle-stimulating hormone and luteinizing hormone, in *Handbook of Physiology, Section 7,* Vol. 4, Part 2, Greep, R. O. and Astwood, E. B., Eds., American Physiological Society, Washington, D.C., 1974, 489.
103. **Yen, S. S. C. and Tsai, C. C.,** The effect of ovariectomy on gonadotropin release, *J. Clin. Invest.,* 50, 1149, 1971.
104. **Yen, S. S. C., Tsai, C. C., Vandenberg, G., and Rebar, R.,** Gonadotropin dynamics in patients with gonadal dysgenesis: a model for the study of gonadotropin regulation, *J. Clin. Endocrinol. Metab.,* 35, 897, 1972.

105. **Steger, R. W., Huang, H. H., and Meites, J.,** The effects of old age on the male and female reproductive system, in *CRC Handbook Physiology in Aging,* Masoro, E. J., Ed., CRC Press, Boca Raton, 1981, 331.
106. **Savoy-Moore, R. T. and Schwartz, N. B.,** Differential control of FSH and LH secretion, in *Int. Rev. Physiol.,* Greep, R. O., Ed., University Park Press, Baltimore, 22, 203, 1980.
107. **Brown-Grant, K. and Grieg, F.,** A comparison of changes in the peripheral plasma concentrations of luteinizing hormone and follicle-stimulating hormone in the rat, *J. Endocrinol.,* 65, 389, 1975.
108. **Gay, F. L. and Midgley, A. R., Jr.,** Response of the adult rat to orchidectomy and ovariectomy as determined by LH radioimmunoassay, *Endocrinology,* 84, 1359, 1969.
109. **Galo, R. V.,** Neuroendocrine regulation of pulsatile LH release in the rat, *Neuroendocrinology,* 30, 122, 1980.
110. **Soper, B. D. and Weick, R. F.,** Hypothalamic and extrahypothalamic mediation of pulsatile discharges of LH in the ovariectomized rat, *Endocrinology,* 106, 348, 1980.
111. **Carmel, P. C., Araki, S., and Ferin, M.,** Pituitary stalk portal blood collection in rhesus monkeys: evidence for pulsatile release of gonadotropin-releasing hormone, *Endocrinology,* 99, 243, 1976.
112. **Blake, C. A.,** Effects of estrogen and progesterone on luteinizing hormone release in ovariectomized rats, *Endocrinology,* 101, 1122, 1977b.
113. **Goodman, R. L.,** A quantitative analysis of the physiological role of ovarian steroids in the control of LH secretion in the rat, *Fed. Proc., Fed. Am. Soc. Exp.,* 36, 152, 1977.
114. **Bogdanove, E. M., Nolin, J. M., and Campbell, G. T.,** Qualitative and quantitative gonad-pituitary feedback, *Rec. Prog. Horm. Res.,* 31, 567, 1975.
115. **Kalra, S. P., Ajika, K., Krulich, L., Fawcett, C. P., Quijada, M., and McCann, S. M.,** Effects of hypothalamic and preoptic electrochemical stimulation on gonadotropin and prolactin release in proestrous rats, *Endocrinology,* 88, 1150, 1971.
116. **Gay, V. L. and Dever, N. W.,** Effects of testosterone propionate and estradiol benzoate — alone or in combination — on serum LH and FSH in orchidectomized rats, *Endocrinology,* 89, 161, 1971.
117. **Damassa, D. A., Kobashigawa, D., Smith, E. R., and Davidson, J. M.,** Negative feedback control of LH by testosterone: a quantitative study in male rats, *Endocrinology,* 99, 736, 1976.
118. **Karsch, F. J., Dierschke, D. J., and Knobil, E.,** Sexual differentiation of pituitary function: apparent difference between primates and rodents, *Science,* 179, 484, 1973.
119. **Dierschke, D. J., Yamaji, T., Karsch, F. J., Weick, R. F., Weiss, G., and Knobile, E.,** Blockade by progesterone of estrogen-induced LH and FSH release in the rhesus monkey, *Endocrinology,* 92, 1496, 1973.
120. **McPherson, J. C., III, Costoff, A., and Mahesh, V. B.,** Influence of estrogen-progsterone combinations on gonadotropin secretion in castrate female rats, *Endocrinology,* 97, 771, 1975.
121. **Steger, R. W. and Peluso, J. J.,** Hypothalamic-pituitary function in the old irregularly cycling rat, *Exp. Aging Res.,* 5, 303, 1979.
122. **DePaolo, L. V. and Barraclough, C. A.,** Interactions of estradiol and progesterone on pituitary gonadotropin secretion: Possible sites and mechanisms of actions, *Biol. Reprod.,* 20, 1173, 1979.
123. **Karsch, F. J., Legan, S. J., Ryan, K. D., and Foster, D. L.,** The feedback effects of ovarian steroids on gonadotropin secretion, in *Control of Ovulation,* Crighton, D. B., Haynes, N. B., Foxcroft, G. R., and Lamming, G. E., Eds., Butterworths, London, 1978, 29.
124. **Blake, C. A.,** A medial basal hypothalamic site of synergistic action of estrogen and progesterone on the inhibition of pituitary luteinizing hormone release, *Endocrinology,* 101, 1130, 1977.
125. **Blake, C. A., Norman, R. L., and Sawyer, C. H.,** Localization of the inhibitory actions of estrogen and nicotine on release of luteinizing hormone in rats, *Neuroendocrinology,* 16, 22, 1974.
126. **Negro-Vilar, A., Orias, R., and McCann, S. M.,** Evidence for a pituitary site of action for the acute inhibition of LH release by estrogen in the rat, *Endocrinology,* 92, 1680, 1973.
127. **Stumpf, W. E.,** Estrogen-neurons and estrogen-neuron systems in the periventricular brain, *Am. J. Anat.,* 129, 207, 1970.
128. **Pfaff, D. and Keiner, M.,** Atlas of estradiol-concentrating cells in the central nervous system of the female rat, *J. Comp. Neurol.,* 151, 121, 1973.
129. **Chen, H. T., Geneau, J., and Meites, J.,** Effects of castration, steroid replacement and hypophysectomy on hypothalamic LHRH and serum LH, *Proc. Soc. Exp. Biol. Med.,* 156, 127, 1977.
130. **Seyler, L. E., Jr. and Reichlin, S.,** Luteinizing hormone-releasing factor (LRF) in plasma of postmenopausal women, *J. Clin. Endocrinol. Metab.,* 37, 197, 1973.
131. **Rosenblum, N. B. and Schloaff, S.,** Gonadotropin-releasing hormone radioimmunoassay and its measurement in normal human plasma, secondary amenorrhea and postmenopausal syndrome, *Am. J. Obstet. Gynecol.,* 124, 340, 1976.
132. **Miyake, A., Tanizawa, O., Aono, T., Yasuda, M., and Kurachi, K.,** Suppression of luteinizing hormone in castrated women by the administration of human chorionic gonadotropin, *J. Clin. Endocrinol. Metab.,* 43, 928, 1976.

133. **Miyake, A., Aono, T., Kinugasa, T., Tanizawa, O., and Kurachi, K.**, The time course change after castration in short-loop negative feedback control of LH by hCG in women, *Acta Endocrinol.*, 88, 1, 1978.
134. **Molitch, M., Edmonds, M., Jones, E. E., and Odell, W. D.**, Short-loop feedback control of luteinizing hormone in the rabbit, *Am. J. Physiol.*, 230, 907, 1976.
135. **Patritti-Laborde, N. and Odell, W. D.**, Short-loop feedback of luteinizing hormone: dose-response relationships and specificity, *Fertil. Steril.*, 30, 456, 1978.
136. **Silverman, A. Y., Smith, C. G., Siler-Khodr, T. M., and Asch, R. H.**, hCG blocks the estrogen-induced LH release in long-term castrated rhesus monkeys: evidence for an ultrashort-loop negative feedback, *Fertil. Steril.*, 35, 74, 1981.
137. **Patritti-Laborde, N., Wolfsen, A. R., Heber, D., and Odell, W. D.**, Site of short-loop feedback for luteinizing hormone in the rabbit, *J. Clin. Invest.*, 64, 1066, 1979.
138. **Davies, R. V., Main, S. J., and Setchell, B. P.**, Inhibin: evidence for its existence — Methods of bioassay and nature of the active material, *Int. J. Androl.*, (Suppl. 2), 102, 1978.
139. **Franchimont, P.**, Inhibin: a new gonadal hormone, *Ann. Endocrinol.*, 41, 3, 1980.
140. **LaGace, L., Labrie, F., Lorenzen, J., Schwartz, N. B., and Channing, C. P.**, Selective inhibitory effect of porcine follicular fluid on follicle stimulating hormone secretion in anterior pituitary cells in culture, *Clin. Endocrinol.*, 10, 401, 1979.
141. **Schwartz, N. B. and Channing, C. P.**, Evidence for ovarian "inhibin": suppression of the secondary rise in serum FSH levels in proestrus rats by injection of porcine follicular fluid, *Proc. Natl. Acad. Sci. U.S.A.*, 74, 5721, 1977.
142. **Chari, S.**, Chemistry and physiology of inhibin, *Endokrinologie*, 70, 99, 1977.
143. **Lorenzen, J. R., Channing, C. P., and Schwartz, N. B.**, Partial characterization of FSH suppressing activity (folliculostatin) in porcine follicular fluid using the metestrous rat as an *in vivo* bioassay model, *Biol. Reprod.*, 19, 635, 1978.
144. **Chappel, S. C., Holt, J. A., and Spies, H. G.**, Inhibin differences in bioactivity within human follicular fluid in the follicular and luteal stages of the menstrual cycle, *Proc. Soc. Exp. Biol. Med.*, 163, 310, 1980.
145. **DePaolo, L. V., Shander, D., Wise, P. M., Barraclough, C. A., and Channing, C. P.**, Identification of inhibin-like activity on ovarian venous plasma of rats during the estrous cycle, *Endocrinology*, 105, 647, 1979.
146. **Shander, D., Anderson, L. D., and Barraclough, C. A.**, Follicle-stimulating hormone and luteinizing hormone affect the endogenous release of pituitary follicle-stimulating hormone and the ovarian secretion of inhibin in rats, *Endocrinology*, 106, 1047, 1980.
147. **Karsch, F. J. and Foster, D. L.**, Sexual differentiation of the mechanism controlling the pre-ovulatory discharge of luteinizing hormone in the sheep, *Endocrinology*, 97, 373, 1975.
148. **Taleisnik, S., Caligaris, L., and Astrada, J. J.**, Sex difference in hypothalamic-hypophysial function, in *Steroid Hormones and Brain Function*, Sawyer, C. H. and Gorski, R. A., Eds., University of California Press, Los Angeles, 1971, 171.
149. **Hodges, J. K. and Heran, J. P.**, A positive feedback effect of oestradiol on LH release in the male marmoset monkey, *Callithrix jacchus*, *J. Reprod. Fertil.*, 52, 83, 1978.
150. **Kulin, H. E. and Reiter, E. O.**, Gonadotrophin and testosterone measurements after oestrogen administration to adult men, pre-pubertal boys, and men with hypogonadotrophism: evidence for maturation of positive feedback in the male, *Pediatr. Res.*, 10, 46, 1976.
151. **Harlan, R. E. and Gorski, R. A.**, Steroid regulation of LH secretion in normal and androgenized rats at different ages, *Endocrinology*, 101, 741, 1977.
152. **Plant, T. M.**, The effects of neonatal orchidectomy on the developmental pattern of gonadotropin secretion in the male Rhesus monkey (*Macaca mulatta*), *Endocrinology*, 106, 1451, 1980.
153. **Hohlweg, W.**, Veränderungen des Hypophsen-vorderlappens und des Ovariums nach behandlung mit grossen Dosen von Follikelhormon, *Klin. Wochenschr.*, 13, 92, 1934.
154. **Everett, J. W.**, Progesterone and estrogen in the experimental control of ovulation time and other features of the estrous cycle in the rat, *Endocrinology*, 43, 389, 1948.
155. **Labhsetwar, A. P.**, Role of estrogens in spontaneous ovulation: Evidence for positive feedback in hamsters, *Endocrinology*, 90, 941, 1972.
156. **Spies, H. G. and Niswender, G. D.**, Effect of progesterone and estradiol on LH release and ovulation in Rhesus monkeys, *Endocrinology*, 90, 257, 1972.
157. **Schwartz, N. B.**, A model for the estrous cycle regulation in the rat, *Rec. Prog. Horm. Res.*, 25, 1, 1969.
158. **Zeilmaker, G. H.**, The biphasic effect of progesterone on ovulation in the rat, *Acta Endocrinol. (Kbh)*, 51, 461, 1966.
159. **Docke, F. and Dorner, G.**, A possible mechanism by which progesterone facilitates ovulation in the rat, *Neuroendocrinology*, 4, 139, 1969.

160. **Caligaris, L., Astrada, J. J., and Taleisnik, S.,** Release of LH induced by estrogen injection into ovariectomized rats, *Endocrinology,* 88, 810, 1971.
161. **Caligaris, L., Astrada, J. J., and Taleisnik, S.,** Biphasic effect of progesterone on the release of gonadotropin in rats, *Endocrinology,* 89, 331, 1971.
162. **DePaolo, L. V. and Barraclough, C. A.,** Interactions of estradiol and progesterone on pituitary gonadotropin secretion: possible sites and mechanisms of action, *Biol. Reprod.,* 20, 1173, 1979.
163. **Freeman, M. C., Dupke, K. C., and Croteau, C. M.,** Extinction of the estrogen-induced daily signal for LH release in the rat: a role for the proestrous surge of progesterone, *Endocrinology,* 99, 223, 1976.
164. **Halasz, B.,** The endocrine effects of isolation of the hypothalamus from the rest of the brain, in *Frontiers in Neuroendocrinology,* Ganong, W. F. and Martini, L., Eds., Oxford University Press, New York, 1969, 307.
165. **Blake, C. A., Weiner, R. I., Gorski, R. A., and Sawyer, C. H.,** Secretion of pituitary luteinizing hormone and follicle stimulating hormone in female rats made persistently estrous or diestrous by hypothalamic deafferentation, *Endocrinology,* 90, 855, 1972.
166. **Kawakami, M., Yoshioka, E., Konda, N., Arita, J., and Visessuvan, S.,** Data on the sites of stimulatory feedback action of gonadal steroids indispensable for luteinizing hormone release in the rat, *Endocrinology,* 102, 791, 1978.
167. **Kawakami, M., Artia, J., Yoshioka, E., Visessovan, S., and Akema, T.,** Data on the sites of the stimulatory feedback action of gonadal steroids indispensable for follicle-stimulating hormone release in the rat, *Endocrinology,* 103, 752, 1978.
168. **Krey, L. C., Butler, W. R., and Knobil, E.,** Surgical disconnection of the medial basal hypothalamus and pituitary function in the rhesus monkey. I. Gonadotropin secretion, *Endocrinology,* 96, 1073, 1975.
169. **Helmond, F. A., Simons, P. A., and Hein, P. R.,** The effects of progesterone on estrogen-induced luteinizing hormone and follicle-stimulating hormone release in the female rhesus monkey, *Endocrinology,* 107, 478, 1980.
170. **Odell, W. D. and Swerdloff, R. S.,** Progesterone-induced luteinizing and follicle stimulating hormone surge in post-menopausal women: a simulated ovulatory peak, *Proc. Nat. Acad. Sci. U.S.A.,* 61, 529, 1968.
171. **Attard, B.,** Monkey pituitary E receptors and the biphasic action of E on gonadotropin secretion, *Nature,* 185, 252, 1980.
172. **Marshall, F. H. A.,** Exteroceptive factors in sexual periodicity, *Biol. Rev.,* 17, 68, 1942.
173. **Harris, G. W.,** *Neural Control of the Pituitary Gland,* E. Arnold London, 1955.
174. **Aschner, B.,** Über die Funktion der Hypophyse, *Pflügers Arch.,* 146, 1, 1912.
175. **Holtz, P.,** Dopa decarboxylase, *Naturwissenschaften,* 27, 724, 1939.
176. **Sawyer, C. H., Markee, J. E., and Townsend, B. F.,** Cholingeric and adrenergic components of the neurohumoral control of LH release in the rabbit, *Endocrinology,* 44, 18, 1949.
177. **Sawyer, C. H.,** Some recent developments in brain-pituitary-ovarian physiology: first Geoffrey Harris memorial lecture, *Neuroendocrinology,* 17, 97, 1975.
178. **Kalra, S. P. and McCann, S. M.,** Effects of drugs modifying catecholamine synthesis on plasma LH and ovulation in the rat, *Neuroendocrinology,* 15, 79, 1974.
179. **Kalra, P. S., Kalra, S. P., Krulich, L., Fawcett, C. P., and McCann, S. M.,** Involvement of norepinephrine in transmission of the stimulatory influence of progesterone on gonadotropin release, *Endocrinology,* 90, 1168, 1972.
180. **Simpkins, J. W., Advis, J. P., Hodson, C. A., and Meites, J.,** Blockade of steroid-induced luteinizing hormone release by selective depletion of anterior hypothalamic norepinephrine activity, *Endocrinology,* 104, 506, 1979b.
181. **Simpkins, J. W. and Kalra, S. P.,** Blockage of progesterone-induced increase in hypothalamic LHRH and serum gonadotropin by intrahypothalamic implantation of 6-hydroxydopamine, *Brain Res.,* 170, 475, 1979.
182. **Weiner, R. I., Shryne, J. E., Gorski, R. A., and Sawyer, C. H.,** Changes in the catecholamine content of the rat hypothalamus following deafferentation, *Endocrinology,* 90, 867, 1972b.
183. **Donoso, A. O. and Stefano, F. J. E.,** Sex hormones and concentration of noradrenalin and dopamine in the anterior hypothalamus of castrated rats, *Experientia,* 23, 665, 1967.
184. **Anton-Tay, F., Anton, S. M., and Wurtman, R. J.,** Mechanism of changes in brain norepinephrine metabolism after ovariectomy, *Neuroendocrinology,* 6, 265, 1970.
185. **Bapna, J., Neff, N. H., and Costa, E.,** A method for studying norepinephrine and serotonin metabolism in small regions of the brain: effect of ovariectomy on amine metabolism in anterior and posterior hypothalamus, *Endocrinology,* 89, 1345, 1971.
186. **Crowley, V. R., O'Donohue, T. L., and Jacobowitz, D. M.,** Changes in catecholamine content in discrete brain nuceli during the estrous cycle of the rat, *Brain Res.,* 147, 315, 1978.

187. **Crowley, R., O'Donohue, T. L., Wachslicht, H., and Jacobowitz, D. M.,** Effects of estrogen and progesterone on plasma gonadotropins and on catecholamine levels and turnover in discrete brain regions of ovariectomized rats, *Brain Res.,* 154, 345, 1978.
188. **Simpkins, J. W., Huang, H. H., Advis, J. P., and Meites, J.,** Changes in hypothalamic NE and DA turnover resulting from steroid-induced LH and prolactin surges in ovariectomized rats, *Biol. Reprod.,* 20, 625, 1979.
189. **Zuspan, R. P. and Zuspan, K. J.,** Ovulatory plasma amine (epinephrine and norepinephrine) surges in women, *Am. J. Obstet. Gynecol.,* 117, 654, 1973.
190. **Rosner, J. M., Nagle, G. A., de LaBorde, N. P., Pedroza, E., Badano, A., Figuerosa Casas, P. R., and Carril, M.,** Plasma levels of norepinephrine (NE) during the periovulatory period and after LH-RH stimulation in women, *Am. J. Obstet. Gynecol.,* 124, 657, 1976.
191. **Simpkins, J. S., Kalra, P. S., and Kalra, S. P.,** Temporal alterations in luteinizing hormone-releasing hormone concentrations in several discrete brain regions: effects of estrogen-progesterone and norepinephrine synthesis inhibition, *Endocrinology,* 107, 573, 1980.
192. **Gallo, R. W. and Drouva, S. V.,** Effect of intraventricular infusion of catecholamines in LH release in ova and ova steroid primed rats, *Neuroendocrinology,* 29, 149, 1979.
193. **Schneider, H. P. G. and McCann, S. M.,** Possible rate of dopamine as transmitter to promote discharge of LH-releasing factor, *Endocrinology,* 85, 121, 1969.
194. **Schneider, H. P. G. and McCann, S. M.,** Mono and indolamines and control of LH secretion, *Endocrinology,* 86, 1127, 1970.
195. **Kamberi, I. A., Nical, R. S., and Porter, J. C.,** Luteinizing hormone-releasing activity in hypophysial stalk blood and elevation by dopamine, *Science,* 166, 388, 1969.
196. **Bennett, G. W., Edwardson, J. A., Holland, D., Jeffcoate, S. L., and White, H.,** Release of immunoreactive LHRH and TRH from hypothalamic synaptosomes, *Nature,* 157, 323, 1975.
197. **Rotsztejn, W. H., Charli, J. L., PaHou, E., Pelbarm, J. E., and Kordon, C.,** *In vitro* release of LHRH from rat mediobasal hypothalamus: effects of potassium, calcium and dopamine, *Endocrinology,* 99, 1663, 1976.
198. **Rotszteyn, W. H., Charli, J. L., PaHou, E., and Kordon, C.,** Stimulation by dopamine of LHRH release from the mediobasal hypothalamus in male rats, *Endocrinology,* 101, 1475, 1977.
199. **Leppaluoto, J. P., Mannisto, P., Ranta, T., and Linnoila, M.,** Inhibition of midcycle gonadotropin release in health women by pimozide and fusaric acid, *Acta Endocrinol.,* 81, 455, 1976.
200. **Beattie, C. W., Guckman, M. I., and Corbin, A.,** A comparison of alpha-butyrolactoe and pimozide on serum gonadotropins and ovulation in the rat, *Proc. Soc. Exp. Biol. Med.,* 153, 147, 1976.
201. **Ojeda, S. R., Harms, P. G., and McCann, S. M.,** Effect of blockage of dopaminergic receptors on prolactin and LH release: median eminence and pituitary sites of action, *Endocrinology,* 94, 1650, 1974.
202. **Cramer, O. M. and Porter, J. C.,** Input to releasing factor cells, *Prog. Brain Res.,* 39, 73, 1975.
203. **Miyachi, Y., Mecklenburg, R. S., and Lipsett, M. B.,** *In vitro* studies of pituitary-median eminence unit, *Endocrinology,* 93, 492, 1973.
204. **Beck, W. and Wuttke, W.,** Desensitization of the dopaminergic inhibition of pituitary LH release by prolactin in ovariectomized rats, *J. Endocrinol.,* 74, 67, 1977.
205. **Drouva, S. V. and Gallo, R. V.,** Further evidence of inhibition of episodic luteinizing hormone release in ovariectomized rats by stimulation of dopamine receptors, *Endocrinology,* 100, 792, 1977.
206. **Leblanc, H., Lachelin, G. C. L., Abu-Fadil, S., and Yen, S. S. C.,** Effects of dopamine infusion on pituitary hormone secretion in humans, *J. Clin. Endocrinol. Metab.,* 43, 668, 1976.
207. **Lachelin, G. C. L., Leblanc, H., and Yen, S. S. C.,** The inhibitory effects of dopamine agonists on LH release in women, *J. Clin. Endocrinol. Metab.,* 44, 728, 1977.
208. **Lofstrom, A.,** Catecholamine turnover alterations in discrete areas of the median eminence of the 4 and 5 day cyclic rat, *Brain Res.,* 120, 113, 1977.
209. **Simpkins, J. W., Mueller, G. P., Huang, H. H., and Meites, J.,** Evidence for depressed catecholamine and enhanced serotonin metabolism in aging male rats: possible relation to gonadotropin secretion, *Endocrinology,* 100, 1672, 1977.
210. **Hodson, C. A., Simpkins, J. W., Pass, K. A., Aylsworth, C. F., Steger, R. W., and Meites, J.,** Effects of a prolactin-secreting pituitary tumor on hypothalamic, gonadotropic and testicular function in male rats, *Neuroendocrinology,* 30, 7, 1980.
211. **McNeilly, A. S.,** Prolactin and the control of gonadotrophin secretion in the female, *J. Reprod. Fertil.,* 58, 537, 1980.
212. **Vijayan, E. and McCann, S. M.,** Re-evaluation of the role of catecholamines in control of gonadotropin and prolactin release, *Neuroendocrinology,* 25, 150, 1978.
213. **Fuxe, K. and Hökfelt, T.,** Participation of central monoaminergic neurons in the regulation of anterior pituitary secretion, in *The Hypothalamus,* Martini, L. and Meites, J., Eds., Academic Press, New York, 1973, 61.

214. **Wilson, C. A. and MacDonald, P. G.**, Inhibitory effect of serotonin on ovulation in adult rats, *J. Endocrinol.*, 60, 253, 1974.
215. **Kamberi, I. A.**, The role of brain monamines and pineal indoles in the secretion of gonadotropins and gonadotropin releasing factors, in *Progress in Brain Research*, Zimmermann, E., Gispen, W. H., Marks, B. H., and deWied, D., Eds., Elsevier, Amsterdam, 1973, 261.
216. **Chen, H. T.**, Role of Serotonin and Dopamine in Gonadotropin Release, Ph.D. dissertation, Michigan State Unversity, East Lansing, 1979.
217. **Kordon, C., Javoy, F., Vassent, G., and Glowinski, J.**, Blockade of superovulation in the immature rat by increased brain serotonin, *Eur. J. Pharmacol.*, 4, 169, 1968.
218. **Wheaton, J. E., Martin, S. K., Swanson, L. S., and Stormshak, F.**, Changes in hypothalamic biogenic amines and serum LH in the ewe during the estrous cycle, *J. Anim. Sci.*, 35, 801, 1972.
219. **Tonge, S. R. and Greengrass, P. M.**, The acute effects of oestrogen and progesterone on the monoamine levels of the brain of ovariectomized rats, *Psychopharmacologia*, 27, 374, 1971.
220. **Fuxe, K., Schubert, J., Hokfelt, T., and Jonsson, G.**, Some aspects of the interrelationship between central 5-hydroxytryptamine neurons and hormones, in *Advances in Biochemical Psychopharmacology*, Costa, E., Gessa, G. L., and Sandler, M., Eds., Raven Press, New York, 1974, 67.
221. **Hery, M., Laplante, E., and Kordon, G.**, Participation of serotonin in the phasic release of LH. I. Evidence from pharmacological experiments, *Endocrinology*, 99, 496, 1976.
222. **Markee, J. E., Everett, J. W., and Sawyer, C. H.**, The relationship of the nervous system to the release of gonadotropin and regulation of the sex cycle, *Rec. Prog. Horm. Res.*, 7, 139, 1952.
223. **Simonovic, I., Motta, M., and Martini, L.**, Acetylcholine and the release of the follicle-stimulating hormone-releasing factor, *Endocrinology*, 95, 1373, 1974.
224. **McCann, S. M. and Moss, R. L.**, Putative neurotransmitters involved in discharging gonadotropin-releasing neurohormones and the action of LH-releasing hormone on the CNS, *Life Sci.*, 16, 833, 1975.
225. **Synder, S. H., Brown, B., and Kuhar, M. J.**, The subsynaptosomal localization of histamine, histidine decarboxylase and histamine methyltransferase in rat hypothalamus, *Neurochemistry*, 23, 37, 1974.
226. **Libertun, C. and McCann, S. M.**, The possible role of histamine in the control of prolactin and gonadotropin release, *Neuroendocrinology*, 20, 110, 1976.
227. **Ondo, J.**, Gamma-aminobutyric acid effects on pituitary gonadotropin secretion, *Science*, 186, 738, 1974.
228. **Benson, B.**, Current status of pineal peptides, *Neuroendocrinology*, 24, 241, 1977.
229. **Meites, J., Bruni, J. F., VanVugt, D. A., and Smith, A. F.**, Relation of endogenous opioid peptides and morphine to neuroendocrine functions, *Life Sci.*, 24, 1325, 1979.
230. **Alder, M. W.**, Opioid peptides, (Mini Review), *Life Sci.*, 26, 497, 1980.
231. **McKnight, A. T. and Kosterlitz, H. W.**, Opioid peptides and pituitary function, *J. Reprod. Fertil.*, 58, 513, 1980.
232. **Quigley, M. E.**, The role of endogenous opiates on LH secretion during the menstrual cycle, *J. Clin. Endocrinol. Metab.*, 51, 179, 1980.
233. **Harms, P. G., Ojeda, S. R., and McCann, S. M.**, Prostaglandin involvement in hypothalamic control of gonadotropin and prolactin release, *Science*, 181, 760, 1973.
234. **Orczyk, G. P. and Behrman, H. R.**, Ovulation blockade by aspirin or indomethacin *in vivo* evidence for a role of prostaglandins in gonadotropin secretion, *Prostaglandins*, 1, 3, 1972.
235. **Roberts, J. S. and McCracken, J. A.**, Prostaglandin F_2 production by the brain during estrogen-induced secretion of luteinizing hormone, *Science*, 190, 894, 1975.
236. **Carrillo, A. J., Rabii, J., Carrer, H. F., and Sawyer, C. H.**, Modulation of the proestrous surge of luteinizing hormone by electrochemical stimulation of the amygdala and hippocampus in the unanesthetized rat, *Brain Res.*, 128, 81, 1977.
237. **Ellendorff, F.**, Evaluation of extrahypothalamic control of redproductive physiology, *Rev. Physiol. Biochem. Pharmacol.*, 76, 103, 1976.
238. **Kaplan, S. L. and Grumbach, M. M.**, The ontogenesis of human foetal hormones. II. Luteinizing hormone (LH) and follicle stimulating hormone (FSH), *Acta Endocrinol.*, 81, 808, 1976.
239. **Siler-Khodr, T. M. and Khodr, G. S.**, Studies in human fetal endocrinology. I. Luteinizing hormone-releasing factor content of the hypothalamus, *Am. J. Obstet. Gynecol.*, 130, 795, 1978.
240. **Groom, G. V. and Boyns, A. R.**, Gonadotrophin release from human foetal pituitary cultures induced by fragments of the luteinizing hormone-releasing hormone, *FEBS Lett.*, 33, 57, 1973.
241. **Gennser, G., Liedholm, P., and Thorell, J.**, Pituitary hormone levels in plasma of the human fetus after administration of LRH, *J. Clin. Endocrinol. Metab.*, 43, 470, 1976.
242. **Styne, D. M. and Grumbach, M. M.**, Puberty in the male and female, in *Reproductive Endocrinology*, Yen, S. S. C. and Jaffee, R. B., Eds., W.B. Saunders, Philadelphia, 1978, 189.
243. **Winters, A. J., Eskay, R. L., and Porter, J. C.**, Concentration and distribution of TRH and LRH in the human fetal brain, *J. Clin. Endocrinol. Metab.*, 39, 960, 1974.

244. **Faiman, C. and Winter, J. S. D.**, Gonadotropins and sex hormone patterns in puberty: clinical data, in *Control of the Onset of Puberty*, Grumbach, M. M., Grave, G. D., and Mayer, F. E., Eds., John Wiley & Sons, New York, 1974, 32.
245. **Judd, H. L., Parker, D. C., and Yen, S. S. C.**, Sleep-wake patterns of LH and testosterone release in prepubertal boys, *J. Clin. Endocrinol. Metab.*, 44, 865, 1977.
246. **Roth, J. C., Grumbach, M. M., and Kaplan, S. L.**, Effect of synthetic lutenizing hormone-releasing factor on serum testosterone and gonadotropins in prepubertal, pubertal and adult males, *J. Clin. Endocrinol. Metab.*, 37, 680, 1973.
247. **Kelch, R. P., Clemens, L. E., Markovs, M., Westhoff, M. H., and Hawkins, D. W.**, Metabolism and effects of synthetic gonadotropin-releasing hormone (GnRH) in children and adults, *J. Clin. Endocrinol. Metab.*, 40, 53, 1975.
248. **Dohler, K. D. and Wuttke, W.**, Serum LH, FSH, prolactin and progesterone from birth to puberty in female and male rats, *Endocrinology*, 94, 1003, 1974.
249. **Ramirez, V. D.**, Endocrinology of puberty, in *Handbook of Physiology, Section 7*, Vol. 4, Part 2, Knobil, E. and Sawyer, W. H., Eds., American Physiological Society, Washington, D.C., 1974, 1.
250. **VandeWiele, R., Bogumil, J., Dyrenfurth, I., Ferin, M., Jewelewicz, R., Warren, M., Rixkallah, T., and Mikhail, G.**, Mechanisms regulating the menstrual cycle in women, *Rec. Prog. Horm. Res.*, 26, 63, 1970.
251. **Smith, E. R., Bowers, C. Y., and Davidson, J. M.**, Circulating levels of plasma gonadotropins in 4 and 5 day cycling rats, *Endocrinology*, 93, 756, 1973.
252. **Butcher, R. L., Collins, W. E., and Fugo, F. W.**, Plasma concentration of LH, FSH, prolactin, progesterone and estradiol-17-beta throughout the 4-day estrous cycle of the rat, *Endocrinology*, 94, 1704, 1974.
253. **Terrill, C. E.**, Sheep, in *Reproduction in Farm Animals*, Hafez, E. S. E., Ed., Lea & Febiger, Philadelphia, 1974, 265.
254. **Hafez, E. S. E.**, Rabbits, in *Reproduction and Breeding Techniques for Laboratory Animals*, Hafez, E. S. E., Ed., Lea & Febiger, Philadelphia, 1970, 273.
255. **Reyes, F. L., Winter, J. S. D., and Faiman, C.**, Pituitary gonadotropin function during human pregnancy: serum FSH and LH levels before and after LHRH administration, *J. Clin. Endocrinol. Metab.*, 42, 590, 1976.
256. **MacDonald, G. J.**, Factors involved in maintenance of pregnancy in the rat. The temporal need for estrogen, pituitary prolacin and the ovary, *Biol. Reprod.*, 19, 817, 1978.
257. **Steger, R. W. and Peluso, J. J.**, Gonadotropin regulation in the lactating rat, *Acta Endocrinol.*, 88, 668, 1978.

PROLACTIN

Charles Hodson

INTRODUCTION

Numerous reviews concerning prolactin have appeared in the last ten years. The present chapter provides a general survey of the physiology of prolactin both in man and experimental animals. In many instances reviews rather than original papers are referenced. For a comprehensive review of prolactin physiology in man, the reader is referred to a discussion by Frantz.[1]

HISTORY

In 1928 Stricker and Grueter[2] isolated a lactogenic substance from the pituitary gland which stimulated milk secretion when given to pseudo-pregnant rabbits. This substance was named prolactin by Riddle et al.[3] who further purified the hormone and developed the pigeon crop-sac method of bioassay. In 1969, Li et al.[4] determined the primary structure of ovine prolactin. Although lactogenic activity independently of growth hormone had been demonstrated in man,[5] it was in 1972 that Friesen et al.[6] isolated human prolactin.

Many early studies on the function of prolactin were directed toward its lactogenic and gonadotropic properties. Prolactin, however, was found to have a wide variety of functions in the nonmammalian vertebrates. Riddle[7] suggested that prolactin is a general metabolic hormone. With the development of the prolactin radioreceptor assay,[8] receptors for prolactin were found in a variety of nonreproductive tissues.[9]

ASSAYS

The pigeon crop-sac test is the oldest bioassay for prolactin.[3] Prolactin stimulates the crop of pigeons and doves, causing the crop-sac wall to thicken and the apical cells to desquamate. The thick, milky secretion of desquamated cells is called crop milk. In the original crop-sac assay, prolactin was given by systemic injection and the increase in crop-sac weight was measured. More sensitive variations of this test have employed visual determination of the minimal amount of prolactin capable of stimulating the crop as an end point. In the "local" methods, prolactin is given by intradermal injection directly over the crop-sac and the area of crop-sac stimulated is measured.[10,11]

Other less specific bioassays for prolactin include the in vitro mouse mammary gland assays. In these tests, mammary tissue from mice in mid-pregnancy is incubated in insulin-rich culture media and the test agent or prolactin is administered. Some aspect of milk synthesis is examined, such as formation of casein, histologic changes, or lactose formation.[12,13] Weight gains by intraductal injections of prolactin,[15] or induction of lactation in estrogen-primed rats have also been used as in vivo bioassays of prolactin.[16]

Prolactin is commonly measured by radioimmunoassay (RIA) or by radioreceptor assay (RRA) and numerous methods and antibodies for various species are available.[8,9,17] Some investigators state that RRA's are the optimal method for prolactin assay because they measure the biologically active hormone.

The use of RIA to measure prolactin is criticized by Nicoll et al.[18] They note that there may be structural differences between prolactin in the pituitary gland and blood stream, and that bioassay or RRA's give a more accurate estimate of circulating prolactin concentration than do RIA's. The great sensitivity of RIA's and the speed at which these tests can be done, however, make the RIA the choice for routine serum prolactin assays.

CHEMISTRY OF PROLACTIN

The ovine prolactin molecule is the best characterized mammalian prolactin. It has a molecular weight of 24,000 and consists of 198 amino acids in the single chain. There are three disulfide bridges in the molecule which form two small and one large loop.[4] The primary structure of ovine, bovine, and human prolactin are very similar. Human placental lactogen and human growth hormone have structures similar to that of prolactin and produce similar biologic responses. It is likely that these compounds originated from a common ancestor.[1,4]

Human prolactin circulates in forms with different molecular size, as determined by elutions from Sephadex Tm columns. Small human prolactin has a molecular weight of 23,000 daltons (i.e., a monomer). Big human prolactin has a molecular weight of 56,000 daltons. A third, even larger molecule exists. It is not known whether the large forms of prolactin represent prolactin bound to a carrier molecule, secretory forms of the molecule, or aggregates of prolactin. All forms are biologically active.[19]

THE MAMMOTROPH

Prolactin is secreted by the anterior pituitary gland in acidophilic cells called mammotrophs. In the rat these cells are polygonal in shape and are uniformly distributed throughout the pituitary gland.[20,21,22] During pregnancy there is an increase in the number of these cells.

Mammotrophs have receptors for estrogens, dopamine, thyroid releasing hormone (TRH), and progesterone.[23,24,25] Estrogens act on the mammotrophs to promote prolactin synthesis.[23,26,27] Under estrogenic stimulation, there is proliferation of the endoplasmic reticulum and an initial increase followed by a decrease in the number of secretory granules in the cells.[20,21,22] Progesterone in part counteracts the stimulatory effects of estrogens on prolactin secretion.[28] Estrogens have mitogenic effects on the mammotrophs. During prolonged estrogenic stimulation, the number of mammotrophs is increased. In rodents, prolonged estrogen treatment results in the induction of pituitary adenomas.[29]

TRH acts on the mammotrophs to evoke prolactin release.[25,30] In contrast, dopamine inhibits the synthesis and secretion of prolactin and can counteract the stimulatory effects of TRH and estrogens upon the mammotrophs.[31]

PROLACTIN RELEASE IN MAMMALS

Prolactin is released in response to the suckling stimulus during lactation.[32] This response becomes conditioned in rodents after a litter has been nursed.[33] Prolactin is released in animals by a variety of stressful stimuli including heat, physical restraint, noise, and pain.[34] In man, physical stress also releases prolactin and psychogenic stress may evoke a tonic increase in prolactin secretion.[1] Prolactin is released during pseudopregnancy in the rat in diurnal and nocturnal surges and it is released in similar surges in the early stages of pregnancy in rodents.[35] Prolactin is released in response to an orgasm in women, but not in men.[1,36] Although the daily phasic nocturnal and diurnal surges of pseudo-pregnancy maintain the corpus luteum of the rat,[35] the function of prolactin release during orgasm in man is not known. Prolactin is released concurrently with the preovulatory LH surge during the estrous cycle of the rat and the menstrual cycle of primates.[35] Prolactin release can also be induced by hypoglycemia.[37]

PROLACTIN ACTION IN MAMMALS

The effects of prolactin in mammals are exerted primarily on the organs of reproduction. Prolactin stimulates the secretion of milk and causes growth of the mammary glands during pregnancy. In rodents, prolactin activates the corpus luteum and acts as part of a luteotropic complex with LH to maintain corpus luteum function. Prolactin acts on the testes, stimulating gonadotropin binding and increasing testosterone production. Prolactin acts on the prostate gland, and receptors in the prostate have been demonstrated.[38]

At high concentrations, prolactin is antigonadotropic.[39] Prolactin has a direct inhibitory effect on the hypothalamus and prevents gonadotropin secretion. Studies in rodents show that prolactin can prevent the release of gonadotropins in response to gonadectomy.[40] These results suggest that prolactin can prevent hypothalamic LHRH release.[41] Prolactin also has direct antigonadal effects. Thus, it is luteolytic in the rat.[42] At high levels, prolactin reduces 20 α-hydroxy steroid dehydrogenase activity in the ovary.[43] These antigonadotropic effects of prolactin occur both during lactation and disorders of prolactin secretion.

Prolactin has general metabolic effects in mammals similar to those of the growth hormone. Prolactin can promote nitrogen retention and can antagonize the action of insulin.[44] Receptors for prolactin have been found in mammalian kidneys and there are reports indicating that prolactin participates in salt regulation.[45,46,47] In other vertebrate classes, the actions of prolactin are very diverse and are briefly considered in a later section of this chapter.

CONTROL OF PROLACTIN SECRETION

In mammals, prolactin secretion is tonically inhibited by the hypothalamus. Prolactin secretion is increased when the pituitary is transplanted or when the median eminence of the hypothalamus is destroyed.[48,49]

Prolactin secretion is inhibited by dopamine or by an unidentified prolactin inhibiting factor (PIF).[26,50-53] These agents are carried from the median eminence to the mammotrophs in the hypophysial portal vessels where they prevent prolactin release. Dopamine has been detected and its concentration has been measured in hypophysial portal blood.[54] When dopamine is infused at the concentrations reported in portal blood vessels, prolactin secretion is inhibited.[55] The dopamine in the hypophysial portal vessels is released from the tuberoinfundibular system of the hypothalamus. The existence of a PIF distinct from dopamine is not established.[56,57]

Gamma-aminobutyric acid (GABA) and the catecholamines (epinephrine and norepinephrine) can directly inhibit prolactin secretion by the mammotrophs. However, the role of catecholamines as a physiologic PIF is doubtful because they are much less potent than dopamine in inhibiting prolactin secretion.[27,56,58]

When catecholamine synthesis is blocked by α-methyl-para-tyrosine (AMT), a prompt increase in prolactin secretion takes place.[27,50] When dopamine agonists like the ergots are administered, prolactin is decreased.

Prolactin acts on the hypothalamus to inhibit its own secretion. Prolonged hyperprolactinemia resulting from transplantable prolactin secreting tumors results in reduced in situ pituitary prolactin content. The reduction can be reversed by the blockade of hypothalamic catecholamine synthesis.[27,50]

Prolactin can increase dopamine turnover in the tuberoinfundibular system, and dopamine concentrations in hypophysial portal blood are increased when the tuberoinfundibular system is active.[59,60] Injections of ovine prolactin can prevent stress-induced prolactin release in rats.[61] Implants of prolactin in the median eminence in rats can interrupt pseudopregnancy.[52]

During conditions of stress, suckling during lactation, or pseudo-pregnancy, prolactin is rapidly secreted and surges in serum concentrations take place. It is not known whether inhibition of the tuberoinfundibular dopamine system or the release of a prolactin releasing factor (PRF) evokes these surges in prolactin secretion. The administration of dopamine agonists, however, can prevent prolactin release during these events. Existence of a PRF has been suggested, because blockade of dopamine receptors and prevention of synthesis in lactation augment the hormone surges induced by suckling.[62]

Thyrotropin releasing hormone (TRH) produces prolactin release in in vitro cultures of pituitary tissue and when given systemically. Since prolactin and TSH are not necessarily released concurrently (i.e., during conditions of heat and cold stress), it is not likely that TRH is the PRF.[63,64] The action of TRH on the mammotrophs is altered by estrogen and dopamine. TRH action is facilitated by estrogen and inhibited by dopamine or its agonists.[23,31]

Other hypothalamic neurotransmitters or putative neurotransmitters that influence prolactin secretion include acetylcholine, which probably inhibits prolactin secretion via the tuberoinfundibular dopamine system, and serotonin, melatonin, endorphins, and enkephalins, histamine, norepinephrine and GABA, all of which stimulate prolactin secretion via the hypothalamus, perhaps through PRF. The stated physiologic role of these neurotransmitters in the control of prolactin secretion is based largely on pharmacologic studies.

Acetylcholine injection into the ventricles of the brain or systemic injection of acetylcholine agonists reduces prolactin secretion. The inhibitory effects of acetylcholine or prolactin secretion are apparently mediated by catecholamines, because acetylcholine cannot prevent prolactin release when hypothalamic catecholamine activity is inhibited. A role of acetylcholine in the control of prolactin secretion is suggested because the acetylcholine agonist pilocarpine prevents stress and suckling-induced prolactin release.[64,65,66]

Serotonin, its precursors 5-hydroxytryptophan and tryptophan, or its metabolite melatonin stimulate prolactin release.[67,68,69] Blockade of serotonin receptors or of synthesis prevents the release of prolactin in response to the stimuli of suckling or estrogen injection.[68,70] Serotonin has no direct stimulatory effect on pituitary prolactin release, but whether serotonin releases PRF or inhibits the tuberoinfundibular dopamine system is not resolved. It is suggested that serotonergic neurons release a PRF, because serotonin agonists release prolactin more rapidly than does blockade of the brain catecholaminergic systems.[71,72]

The endogenous opiates (enkephalins and endorphins) and morphine cause a rapid increase in prolactin secretion when given by systemic or intraventricular injection.[73] Administration of opiate antagonists, such as naloxone or naltrexone, prevent prolactin release in response to stress or suckling and reduce basal prolactin secretion.[74,75] The endogenous opiates do not act directly on the pituitary gland. They may inhibit the activity of the tuberoinfundibular dopamine system,[75] perhaps through cholinergic neurons.[76]

Norepinephrine stimulation of prolactin release is different from the inhibitory effects of norepinephrine at the pituitary gland level. In the pituitary, norepinephrine binds to dopamine receptors on the mammotrophs and blocks prolactin release. In contrast, in vivo administration of L-dopa, which increases brain norepinephrine content, results in increased prolactin secretion.[77] Administration of clonidine (an α-2-adrenergic agonist) at high doses results in an increased prolactin secretion[78] as do intraventricular injections of norepinephrine.[79] Administration of disulfram,[80] (an inhibitor of norepinephrine synthesis and 6-hydroxydopamine),[81] which causes selective destruction of noradrenergic neurons, results in reduced prolactin secretion. Blockade of α-1 receptors with prazozine inhibits prolactin secretion.[82] Phenoxybenzamine increases prolactin secretion.[78] These results suggest that noradrenergic neurons stimulate prolactin release, although the role of these neurons is not resolved. The demonstration of α-1 and α-2 receptors in the brain makes interpretation of the drug studies and the role of noradrenergic neurons in the control of prolactin secretion difficult to resolve.[82]

Histamine given by intraventricular injection causes increased prolactin secretion[83] whereas blockade of histamine receptors inhibits release of prolactin in response to stress or suckling.[84] These effects suggest a stimulatory role of histamine-containing neurons in the regulation of prolactin secretion.

GABA has been reported both to stimulate and to inhibit prolactin secretion in the rat. Administration of GABA into the ventricular system of the rat brain stimulates prolactin secretion[85,86,87] whereas at very high concentrations, GABA can prevent prolactin release from pituitary glands in vitro. GABA is probably not a physiologic PIF because the concentrations of GABA required to inhibit prolactin release in vitro are higher than the known physiologic concentrations.[58] A role for GABA in the regulation of prolactin is not yet demonstrated.

Peptides are reported to stimulate prolactin release. The peptides include substance P, bombesin, neurotensin, and vasoactive intestinal polypeptide. The role of these peptides in the regulation of prolactin secretion is not clear.

Prostaglandins (PGs) influence prolactin secretion. Prolactin release is stimulated by PG E_1[88] and PG $F_2\alpha$.[89] Prostaglandins probably act as intracellular messengers within the hypothalamus.

MECHANISM OF PROLACTIN ACTION

Membrane bound receptor molecules for prolactin have been demonstrated in mammals in a variety of tissues, including liver, kidney, adrenal, ovary, testes, uterus, prostate, seminal vesicle, mammary gland, and in tumors. The number of receptors in these tissues varies in different mammalian species.[9,90,91,92] The prolactin receptor molecule of rabbit mammary gland has been isolated and antibodies to the receptor have been prepared.[8,93]

The binding of prolactin to its receptors is modulated by hormones. For example, in the rat liver, estrogens stimulate while ovariectomy results in decreased prolactin binding. Hypophysectomy reduces prolactin binding in the liver, an effect which can be reversed by prolactin injection.[91,92] Prolactin receptors in liver and mammary glands are both "up" and "down" regulated by prolactin. When prolactin is first dissociated from its receptors with $MgCL_2$, or if prolactin secretion is blocked by ergot treatment, receptor fields in the mammary gland and liver are opened. When prolactin is given, "down" regulation of the receptor field (i.e., reduction in prolactin receptors) takes place within 15 min. After this rapid "down" regulation, gradual "up" regulation (increased numbers of available prolactin receptors) takes place and within 24 hr the number of available prolactin receptors is restored.[92]

After the initial binding of prolactin to its receptor, prolactin is internalized in the target cells. Prolactin is found in the Golgi apparatus of rat livers, in mammary gland tissue, and in milk. Whether internalization of prolactin represents a degradation of the hormone receptor complex inside the cell or a control signal is unknown.[94,95] Studies on mouse mammary gland explants suggest that the intracellular effects of prolactin after its initial binding to membrane receptors are mediated by a variety of messengers, including cyclic nucleotides, prostaglandins, and polyamines.[96]

The stimulating effect of prolactin on milk synthesis is partially mediated by cyclic GMP (cCMP). Levels of cGMP rise and cyclic AMP levels decrease in the mammary gland when lactation is initiated.[97,98] Moreover, cGMP will mimic the effect of prolactin on mammary gland RNA synthesis.[99] In contrast, dibutyrl cAMP or theophylline treatment reduces DNA, RNA, and fat synthesis in mammary gland tissue.[100] Prostaglandin $F_2 \alpha$ stimulates the induction of lactation in the rat.[101] In tissue cultures, arachidonic acid and prostaglandins increase RNA synthesis, but do not increase casein synthesis.[102] Indomethacin, which blocks prostaglandin synthesis, reduces the stimulating effect of prolactin on both casein and RNA synthesis in mouse mammary gland explants.

Polyamine levels are elevated in the lactating mammary gland. Prolactin treatment promptly elevates ornithine decarboxylase activity in cultured mammary glands. Blockage of polyamine synthesis inhibits prolactin stimulated milk protein synthesis in vitro.[103,104]

COMPARATIVE ASPECTS OF PROLACTIN SECRETION AND PROLACTIN ACTION IN VERTEBRATES

Prolactin is found in all vertebrate classes and may have originated with growth hormone from a common ancestral molecule. Within the vertebrates there is no common mechanism by which prolactin secretion is controlled. In birds, prolactin secretion is stimulated by the hypothalamus,[105] but there may also be a prolactin inhibiting factor[106] in at least one species, the Peking duck. In amphibians, teleosts, and mammals, prolactin secretion is tonically inhibited by the hypothalamus.[107,108]

Of all pituitary hormones, prolactin has the most diverse actions. Attempts have been made to divide the various actions of prolactin into some basic categories. Nicoll and Bern[109] suggest that there are six distinct functional categories:

1. Control of water and electrolyte balance
2. Regulation of growth and development
3. Metabolic effects
4. Control of reproductive functions
5. Effects on integument and ectodermal structures
6. Actions that are synergistic with or antagonistic to the effects of steroid hormones

Within the above six categories prolactin may have at least 227 different effects.[45] These are not discussed here and only some examples in each of the categories are presented:

1. Prolactin treatment can prevent the death of hypophysectomized killi fish (*Fundulus heterclitus*) when they are moved from salt to fresh water. Prolactin prevents death by inhibiting sodium loss through the gills.[110]
2. In anuran larva (tadpoles) prolactin stimulates growth of the tail and tail fin. Prolactin treatment results in a doubling of body, weight and a five fold increase in the length of larval *Rana pipiens*.[111]
3. The concept that prolactin is a metabolic hormone was advanced by Riddle.[7] Prolactin has some of the effects attributed to growth hormone. Prolactin promotes the growth of the visceral organs of birds.
4. Production of crop milk and stimulation of brooding behavior are examples of the ability of prolactin to control reproductive function in birds.[2,7]
5. In 1980, Nicoll reported that there were 67 actions of prolactin on the integument.[45] Some examples are hair growth, sebaceous gland activity, and mammary gland alteration in mammals, pigmentation in amphibians, cornifications of the reptilian skin, and secretion of mucus by fish skin glands.[111]

6. The extensive work of Meier[112] shows that prolactin can act both synergistically and antagonistically with gluccocorticoids to promote deposition or depletion of body fat stores in birds. Similar interrelationships between prolactin and corticoids exist in other classes of vertebrates.

SUMMARY

Prolactin has more diverse actions than any other pituitary hormone. Progress has been made in understanding the mechanism of its action at the intracellular level. It remains to be demonstrated if unified mechanisms govern the effects of the hormone in the categories of the actions stated by Nicoll and Bern.[109]

Much progress has been made in understanding the physiology of prolactin receptors and their regulation. The actions of this hormone probably depend on both the concentration of hormone in the circulation and the available receptor field.

Progress has been made in understanding the hypothalamic regulation of prolactin secretion. While this picture is confusing because the number of neurotransmitters involved is very large, it is hoped that as the functional and anatomic relationships within the hypothalamus and between the hypothalamus and the rest of the brain are better understood, the role of these neurotransmitters in physiologic processes where prolactin is secreted can be placed in better perspective.

REFERENCES

1. **Frantz, A. G.,** Prolactin, in *Endocrinology,* Vol. 1, DeGroot, L. J., Ed., Grune & Stratton, New York, 1979, 153.
2. **Stricker, S. and Grueter, F.,** Action du lobe anterier de l'hypophyse sur la montee laiteuse, *C.R. Soc. Biol.,* 99, 1978, 1928.
3. **Riddle, O., Bates, R. W., and Dykshorn, S.,** The preparation, identification, and assay of prolactin, a hormone of the anterior pituitary, *Am. J. Physiol.,* 105, 191, 1933.
4. **Li, C. H.,** Chemistry of ovine prolactin, in *Handbook of Physiology,* Vol. 4, Part 2, Greet, R. O. and Astwood, E. B., Eds., Williams and Wilkins, Baltimore, Md., 1974, 103.
5. **Kleinberg, D. L. and Frantz, A. G.,** Human prolactin: measurement in plasma by in vitro bioassay, *J. Clin. Invest.,* 50, 1557, 1971.
6. **Hwang, P., Guyda, H., and Friesen, H.,** Purification of human prolactin, *J. Biol. Chem.,* 247, 1955, 1972.
7. **Riddle, O.,** Prolactin in vertebrate function and organization, *J. Natl. Cancer Inst.,* 31, 1039, 1963.
8. **Shiu, R. P. C. and Friesen, H. G.,** Solubilization and purification of a prolactin receptor from the rabbit mammary gland, *J. Biol. Chem.,* 249, 301, 1974.
9. **Fellows, R. E. and Soltysiak, R. M.,** Prolactin binding sites of rabbit mammary epithelial cells in culture, in *Central and Peripheral Regulation of Prolactin Function,* Macleod, R. M. and Scapagnini, U., Eds., Raven Press, New York, 1980, 159.
10. **Morris, C. J. O. R.,** The chemistry of gonadotropins, in *Marshall's Physiology of Reproduction,* Vol. 3, 3rd ed., Parkes, A. S., Eds., Little Brown, Boston, 1966, 379.
11. **Meites, J.,** Studies concerning the induction and maintenance of lactation. I. The mechanism controlling the initiation of lactation at parturition, *Missouri Agr. Exp. Stn. Res. Bull.,* 415, 1947.
12. **Elias, T.,** Cultivation of adult mouse mammary gland in hormone-enriched synthetic medium, *Science,* 126, 842, 1957.
13. **Turkington, R. W.,** Molecular biological aspects of prolactin, in *Lactogenic Hormones,* Wolstenholme, G. E. W. and Knight, J., Eds., Churchill Livingstone, London, 1972, 111.
14. **Turner, C. W.,** Hormones influencing intensity of milk secretion in the rat, *Missouri Agr. Exp. Stn. Res. Bull.,* 982, 1971.

15. **Lyons, W. R.**, The direct mammotrophic action of lactogenic hormone, *Proc. Soc. Exp. Biol. Med.*, 58, 308, 1942.
16. **Meites, J., Talwalker, P. K., and Nicoll, C. S.**, Induction of mammary gland growth and lactation in rabbits with epinephrine, acetylcholine and serotonin, *Proc. Soc. Exp. Biol. Med.*, 104, 192, 1960.
17. **Aubert, M. L.**, Radioimmunoassay for human prolactin, in *Handbook of Radioimunoassay*, Abraham, G. E., Ed., Marcel Dekker, New York, 1978, 179.
18. **Nicoll, C. S.**, Radioimmunoassay and radioreceptor assays for prolactin and growth hormone: a critical appraisal, *Am. Zool.*, 15, 881, 1975.
19. **Suh, H. K. and Frantz, A. G.**, Size heterogeneity of human prolactin in plasma and pituitary extracts, *J. Clin. Endocrinol. Metab.*, 39, 928, 1974.
20. **Costoff, A., Ed.**, *Ultrastructure of Rat Adenohypophysis: Correlation with Function*, Academic Press, New York, 1973, 130.
21. **Baker, B.**, Functional cytology of the hypophysial pars distalis and pars intermedia, in *Handbook of Physiology*, Vol. 4., Part 1, Greep, R. O. and Astwood, E. B., Eds., Williams and Wilkins, Baltimore, Md., 1974, 45.
22. **Kurosomi, K. and Fujita, H., Eds.**, *Functional Morphology, of Endocrine Glands*, Igaku Shoin, Tokyo, 1974, 48.
23. **McGuire, J. L. and Lisk, R. D.**, Estrogen receptors and their relation to reproductive physiology, in *The Sex Steroids*, McKerns, K. W., Ed., Meredith, New York, 1971, 53.
24. **Brown, G. M., Seeman, P., and Lee, T.**, Dopamine/neuroleptic receptors in basal hypothalamus and pituitary, *Endocrinology*, 99, 1047, 1976.
25. **Martin, T. F. T. and Tashjian, A. H., Jr.**, Cell culture studies of thyrotropin releasing hormone action, in *Biochemical Action of Hormones*, Vol. 4, Litwack, G., Ed., Academic Press, New York, 1977, 270.
26. **Meites, J. and Nicoll, C. S.**, Adenohypophysis: prolactin, *Ann. Rev. of Physiol.*, 28, 57, 1958.
27. **Macleod, R. M.**, Regulation of prolactin secretion, in *Frontiers in Neuroendocrinology*, Vol. 4, Martini, L. and Ganong, W. F., Eds., Raven Press, New York, 1976, 169.
28. **Chen, C. L. and Meites, J.**, Effect of estrogen and progesterone on serum and pituitary prolactin levels in ovariectomized rats, *Endocrinology*, 86, 503, 1970.
29. **Furth, J. and Clifton, K. H.**, Experimental pituitary tumors, in *The Pituitary Gland*, Vol. 2, Harris, G. W. and Donovan, B. T., Eds., Butterworths, London, 1966, 460.
30. **Tashjian, A. H., Jr., Barowsky, N. T., and Jensen, D. K.**, Thyrotropin releasing hormone: direct evidence for stimulation of prolactin production by pituitary cells in culture, *Biochem. Biophys. Res. Commun.*, 43, 516, 1971.
31. **Labrie, F., Ferland, L., Dipaolo, T., and Villeux, R.**, Modulation of prolactin secretion by sex steroids and thyroid hormones, in *Central and Peripheral Regulation of Prolactin Function*, Macleod, R. M. and Scapagnini, U., Eds., Raven Press, New York, 1980, 97.
32. **Reece, R. P. and Turner, C. W.**, The lactogenic and thyrotropic hormone content of the anterior lobe of the pituitary, *Mont. Agr. Exp. Stn. Res. Bull.*, 266, 1937.
33. **Grosvenor, C. E., Maiweg, H., and Mena, F.**, Observations on the development and retention during lactation of the mechanism for prolactin release by exteroceptive stimulation in the rat, in *Lactogenesis: The Initiation of Milk Secretion at Parturition*, Reynolds, M. and Folley, Jr., Eds., University of Pennsylvania Press, Philadelphia Press, Philadelphia, 1969, 181.
34. **Meites, J.**, Neuroendocrine control of prolactin in experimental animals, *Clin. Endocrinol.*, 6, (Suppl. 9S), 1977, 95.
35. **Neill, J. D.**, Prolactin: its secretion and control, in *Handbook of Physiology*, Vol. 4., Part 2, Greep, R. and Astwood, E. B. Eds., Williams and Wilkins, Baltimore, Md., 1974, 496.
36. **Stearns, E. L., Winter, J. S. D., and Faiman, C.**, Effects of coitus on gonadotropin, prolactin and sex steroid levels in man, *J.Clin. Endocrinol. Metab.*, 37, 687, 1973.
37. **Noel, G. L., Suh, H. K., Stone, G., and Frantz, A.**, Human prolactin release during surgery and other conditions of stress, *J. Clin. Endocrinol. Metab.*, 35, 840, 1972.
38. **Bartke, A.**, Role of prolactin in reproduction in male mammals, *Fed. Proc., Fed. Am. Soc. Exp. Biol.*, 39, 2577, 1980.
39. **Smith, M. S.**, Role of prolactin regulating gonadotropin secretion and gonad function in female rats, *Fed. Proc., Fed. Am. Soc. Exp. Biol.*, 39, 2571, 1980.
40. **Grandison, L., Hodson, C., Chen, H. T., Advis, J., Simpkins, J., and Meites, J.**, Inhibition by prolactin of post-castration rise in LH, *Neuroendocrinology*, 23, 312, 1977.
41. **Hodson, C. A., Simpkins, J. W., Pass, K. A., Aylsworth, C. F., Steger, R. W., and Meites, J.**, Effects of a prolactin secreting tumor on hypothalamic, gonadotropic and testicular function in male rats, *Neuroendocrinology*, 30, 7, 1980.
42. **Malven, P. V.**, Luteotrophic and luteolytic responses to prolactin in hypophysectomized rats, *Endocrinology*, 84, 1224, 1969.

43. **Zimgrod, A., Lindner, H. R., and Lamprecht, S. A.**, Reductive pathways of progesterone metabolism in the rat ovary, *Acta Endocrinol.*, 69, 141, 1972.
44. **Frantz, A. G.**, Prolactin, *New Engl. J. Med.*, 298, 201, 1978.
45. **Nicoll, C. S.**, Ontogeny and evolution of prolactin function, *Fed. Proc., Fed. Am. Soc. Exp. Biol.*, 39, 2563, 1980.
46. **Donatsch, P. and Richardson, B. P.**, Localization of prolactin in rat kidney tissue using a double antibody technique, *J. Endocrinol.*, 66, 101, 1975.
47. **Horrobin, D. F.**, Prolactin as a regulator of fluid and electrolyte metabolism in mammals, *Fed. Proc., Fed. Am. Soc. Exp. Biol.*, 39, 2567, 1980.
48. **Everett, J. W.**, Luteotropic function of autografts of the rat hypophysis, *Endocrinology*, 54, 685, 1954.
49. **McCann, S. M. and Friedman, H. M.**, The effect of hypothalamic lesions on the secretion of luteotrophin, *Endocrinology*, 67, 597, 1960.
50. **Macleod, R. M.**, Influence of norepinephrine and catecholamine-depleting agents on the synthesis and release of prolactin and growth hormone, *Endocrinology*, 85, 916, 1969.
51. **Birge, C. A., Jacobs, L. S., Hammer, C. T., and Daughaday, W. H.**, Catecholamine inhibition of prolactin secretion by isolated rat adenohypophysis, *Endocrinology*, 86, 120, 1970.
52. **Meites, J., Nicoll, C. S., and Talwalker, P. K.**, The central nervous system and the secretion and release of prolactin, in *Advances in Neuro-endocrinology*, Nalbandov, A. V., Ed., University of Illinois Press, Urbana, 1963, 238.
53. **Pasteels, J. L.**, Secretion de prolactin par l'hypophyse en culture de tissues, *C. R. Seances Soc. Biol. Paris*, 253, 2140, 1961.
54. **Ben-Jonathan, N., Oliver, C., Weiner, H. J., Mical, R. S., and Porter, J. C.**, Dopamine in hypophyseal portal plasma of the rat during the estrous cycle and during pregnancy, *Endocrinology*, 100, 452, 1977.
55. **Gibbs, D. M. and Neill, J. D.**, Dopamine levels in hypophysial stalk blood in the rat are sufficient to inhibit prolactin secretion *in vivo*, *Fed. Proc., Fed. Am. Soc. Exp. Biol.*, 37, 555, 1978.
56. **Shaof, C. J. and Clemens, J. A.**, The role of catecholamines in the release of anterior pituitary prolactin *in vitro*, *Endocrinology*, 95, 1202, 1974.
57. **Kordon, C. and Enjalbert, A.**, Prolactin inhibiting and stimulating factors, in *Central and Peripheral Regulation of Prolactin Function*, Macleod, R. M. and Scapagnini, U., Eds., Raven Press, New York, 1980, 69.
58. **Schally, A. V., Redding, T. W., Arimura, A., Dupont, A., and Linthicun, G. L.**, Isolation of gamma-aminobutyric acid from pig hypothalami and demonstration of its prolactin release inhibiting (PIF) activity *in vivo* and *in vitro*, *Endocrinology*, 100, 681, 1977.
59. **Gudelsky, G. A., Simpkins, J., Muller, G. P., Meites, J., and Moore, K. E.**, Selective actions of prolactin on catecholamine turnover in the hypothalamus and on serum LH and FSH, *Neuroendocrinology*, 22, 206, 1976.
60. **Perkins, N. A., Westfall, T. C., Paul, C. V., Macleod, R., and Rogol, D.**, Effect of prolactin on dopamine synthesis in medial basal hypothalamus: evidence for short-loop feedback, *Brain Res.*, 160, 431, 1979.
61. **Advis, J. P., Hall, T. R., Hodson, C. A., Muller, G. P., and Meites, J.**, Temporal relationship and role of dopamine in "short-loop" feedback of prolactin, *Proc. Soc. Exp. Biol. Med.*, 155, 567, 1977.
62. **Voogt, L. and Carr, L. A.**, Potentiation of suckling induced release of prolactin by inhibition of brain catecholamine synthesis, *Endocrinology*, 97, 891, 1975.
63. **Muller, G. P., Chen, H. T., Dibbet, J. A., Chen, H. J., and Meites, J.**, Effects of warm and cold temperatures on release of TSH, GH and prolactin in rats, *Proc. Soc. Exp. Biol. Med.*, 147, 698, 1974.
64. **Meites, J.**, Evaluation of research on control of prolactin secretion, in *Comparative Endocrinology of Prolactin*, Dellmann, H. D., Johnson, J. A., and Klanchko, D. M., Eds., Plenum Press, New York, 135, 1977.
65. **Grandison, L. and Meites, J.**, Evidence for adrenergic mediation of and cholinergic inhibition of prolactin release, *Endocrinology*, 99, 775, 1976.
66. **Enroth, P., Fuxe, K., Gustaffason, J. A., Hockfelt, T., Lofstrom, A., Skett, P., and Agnati, L.**, The effect of nicotine on central catecholamine neurons and gonadotropin secretion. III. Studies on prepubertal female rats treated with pregnant mare serum gonadotropin, *Med. Biol.*, 55, 167, 1977.
67. **Kamberi, L. A., Mical, R. S., and Porter, J. C.**, Effects of melatonin and serotonin on the release of FSH and prolactin, *Endocrinology*, 88, 1288, 1971.
68. **Kordon, C., Blake, C. A., Terkel, J., and Sawyer, C. H.**, Participation of serotonin-containing neurons in the suckling-induced rise in plasma prolactin levels in lactating rats, *Neuroendocrinology*, 13, 213, 1974.

69. **Mueller, G. P., Twohy, C. P., Chen, H. T., Advis, J. P., and Meites, J.,** Effects of 1-tryptophan and restraining stress on hypothalamic and brain serotonin turnover and pituitary TSH and prolactin release in rats, *Life Sci.*, 18, 715, 1976.
70. **Gallo, R. V., Rabii, J., and Moberg, G. P.,** Effect of methysergide, a blocker of serotonin receptors on plasma prolactin levels in lactating and ovariectomized rats, *Endocrinology*, 97, 1096, 1975.
71. **Clemens, J. A., Rousch, M. E., and Fuller, R. W.,** Evidence that serotonergic neurons stimulate secretion of prolactin releasing factor, *Life Sci.*, 22, 2909, 1978.
72. **Clemens, J. A. and Shaar, C. J.,** Control of prolactin secretion in mammals, *Fed. Proc., Fed. Am. Soc. Exp. Biol.*, 39, 2588, 1980.
73. **Van Vugt, D. A. and Meites, J.,** Influence of endogenous opiates on anterior pituitary function, *Fed. Proc., Fed. Am. Soc. Exp. Biol.*, 39, 2533, 1980.
74. **Bruni, J., Van Vugt, D. A., Marshall, S., and Meites, J.,** Effects of naloxone, morphine and methionine enkephalin on serum prolactin, luteinizing hormone, follicle stimulating hormone, thyroid stimulating hormone and growth hormone, *Life Sci.*, 21, 461, 1977.
75. **Van Vugt, D. A., Bruni, J. F., and Meites, J.,** Naloxone inhibition of stress-induced increase in prolactin secretion, *Life Sci.*, 22, 85, 1978.
76. **Shaar, C. R. and Clemens, J. A.,** The effects of opiate agonists on growth hormone and prolactin release in rats, *Fed. Proc., Fed. Am. Soc. Exp. Biol.*, 39, 2539, 1980.
77. **Donoso, A. O., Bishop, W., Fawcett, C. P., Krulich, L., and McCann, S. M.,** Effects of drugs that modify brain monoamine concentrations on plasma gonadotropin and prolactin levels in the rat, *Endocrinology*, 89, 774, 1971.
78. **Lawson, D. M. and Gala, R. R.,** The influence of adrenergic dopaminergic, cholonergic and serotonergic drugs on plasma prolactin levels in ovariectomized, estrogen-treated rats, *Endocrinology*, 96, 313, 1975.
79. **Vijayan, E. and McCann, S. M.,** Reevaluation of the role of catecholamines in the control of gonadotropin and prolactin release, *Neuroendocrinology*, 25, 150, 1978.
80. **Donoso, A. O., Bishop, W., and McCann, S. M.,** The effect of drugs which modify catecholamine synthesis on serum prolactin in rats with median eminence lesions, *Proc. Soc. Exp. Biol. Med.*, 143, 360, 1973.
81. **Fenske, M. and Wuttke, W.,** Effects of intraventricular 6-hydroxydopamine injections on serum prolactin and LH levels: absence of stress-induced pituitary prolactin release, *Brain Res.*, 104, 68, 1976.
82. **Clemens, J. A. and Shaar, C. J.,** Control of prolactin secretion in mammals, *Fed. Proc., Fed. Am. Soc. Exp. Biol.*, 39, 2588, 1980.
83. **Libertun, C. and McCann, S. M.,** The possible role of histamine in the control of prolactin and gonadotropin release, *Neuroendocrinology*, 20, 110, 1976.
84. **Arakelian, M. C. and Libertun, C.,** H_1 and H_2 histamine receptor participation in the brain control of prolactin secretion in lactating rats, *Endocrinology*, 100, 890, 1972.
85. **Mioduszewski, R., Grandison, L., and Meites, J.,** Stimulation of prolactin release in rats by GABA, *Proc. Soc. Exp. Biol. Med.*, 151, 44, 1976.
86. **Vijayan, E. and McCann, S. M.,** The effects of intraventricular injection of γ-aminobutyric acid (GABA) on prolactin and gonadotropin release in conscious female rats, *Brain Res.*, 155, 35, 1978.
87. **Pass, K. A. and Ondo, J. G.,** The effects of γ-aminobutyric acid on prolactin and gonadotropin secretion in the unanesthetized rat, *Endocrinology*, 106, 1437, 1977.
88. **Ojeda, S. R., Harms, R. G., and McCann, S. M.,** Central effects of prostaglandin (PG E1) on prolactin release, *Endocrinology*, 95, 613, 1974.
89. **Louis, T. M., Stellflug, N., Tucker, H. A., and Hafs, H. P.,** Plasma prolactin growth hormone, luteinizing hormone and glucocorticoids after prostaglandins $F_{2}\alpha$ in heifers, *Proc. Soc. Exp. Biol. Med.*, 147, 128, 1974.
90. **Aubert, M. L., Suard, Y., Sizonenko, P. C., and Kraehenbuhl, J. P.,** Receptors of lactogenic hormone: study with dispersed cells from rabbit mammary gland, in *Progress in Prolactin Physiology and Pathology*, Robyn, C. and Harter, M., Eds., Elsevier/North Holland, Amsterdam, 1978, 45.
91. **Kelly, P. A., Ferland, L., and Labrie, F.,** Endocrine control of prolactin receptors, in *Progress in Prolactin Physiology and Pathology*, Robyn, C. and Harter, M., Eds., Elsevier/North Holland, Amsterdam, 1978, 59.
92. **Kelly, P. A., Dijiane, J., and DeLean, A.,** Interaction of prolactin with its receptor: dissociation and down-regulation, in *Central and Peripheral Regulation of Prolactin Function*, Macleod, R. M. and Scapagnini, I., Eds., Raven Press, New York, 1980, 173.
93. **Shiu, R. P. C. and Freisen, H. G.,** Properties of prolactin receptor from the rabbit mammary gland, *Biochem. J.*, 140, 301, 1974.
94. **Josefsberg, Z., Posner, B. I., Patel, B., and Bergeron, J. M.,** The uptake of prolactin into female rat liver, *J. Biol. Chem.*, 254, 209, 1979.
95. **Nolin, J. M. and Witorsch, R. J.,** Detection of endogenous immunoreactive prolactin in rat mammary epithelial cells during lactation, *Endocrinology*, 99, 949, 1976.

96. **Rillema, J. A.**, Mechanism of prolactin action, *Fed. Proc., Fed. Am. Soc. Exp. Biol.*, 39, 2593, 980.
97. **Rillema, J. A.**, Cyclic AMP, adenylate cyclase and cyclic AMP phosphodiesterase in mammary glands from pregnant and lactating mice, *Proc. Soc. Exp. Biol. Med.*, 151, 748, 1976.
98. **Sapag-Hagar, M. and Greenbaum, A. L.**, Changes of the activity of adenylcyclase and cAMP-phosphodiesterase and of the level of 3′,5′-cyclic adenosine monophosphate in rat mammary gland during pregnancy and lactation, *Biochem. Biophys. Res. Commun.*, 53, 982, 1973.
99. **Rillema, J. A.**, Evidence suggesting that the cyclic nucleotides may mediate metabolic effects of prolactin in the mouse mammary gland, *Horm. Metab. Res.*, 7, 45, 1975.
100. **Sapag-Hagar, M., Greenbaum, A. C., Lewis, D. J., and Hallowes, R. C.**, The effects of di-butyryl cAMP on enzymatic and metabolic changes in explants of rat mammary tissue, *Biochem. Biophys. Res. Commun.*, 59, 261, 1974.
101. **Vermouth, N. T. and Deis, R. P.**, Inhibitory effect of progesterone on the lactogenic and abortive effect of prostaglandin $F_2\alpha$, *J. Endocrinol.*, 66, 21, 1975.
102. **Rillema, J. A.**, Effects of prostaglandins on RNA and casein synthesis in mammary gland explants of mice, *Endocrinology*, 99, 490, 1976.
103. **Oka, T., Perry, J. W., and Kano, K.**, Hormone regulation of spermine synthetase during the development of mouse mammary epithelium *in vitro*, *Biochem. Biophys. Res. Commun.*, 79, 979, 1977.
104. **Richards, J. F.**, Ornithine decarboxylase activity in tissues of prolactin-treated rats, *Biochem. Biophys. Res. Commun.*, 63, 292, 1975.
105. **Dodd, J. M., Follett, B. K., and Sharp, P. J.**, Hypothalamic control of pituitary function in submammalian vertebrate, *Adv. Comp. Physiol. Biochem.*, 4, 114, 1971.
106. **Tixner-Vidal, A. and Gourdji, D.**, Cellular aspects of the control of prolactin secretion in birds, *Gen. Comp. Endocrinol. Suppl.*, 3, 51, 1972.
107. **McKeown, B. A.**, Prolactin and growth hormone concentrations in the plasma of the toad *Bufo bufo* following ectopic transplantation of the pars distalis, *Gen. Comp. Endocrinol.*, 19, 167, 1972.
108. **Ball, J. N., Baker, B. I., Olvereau, M., and Peter, R. E.**, Investigations on hypothalamic control of adenohypophysial functions in teleost fishes, *Gen. Comp. Endocrinol.*, 3, 1, 1972.
109. **Nicoll, C. S. and Bern, H. A.**, On the actions of prolactin among the vertebrates: is there a common denominator, in *Lactogenic Hormones*, Wolstenholme, G. E. W., and Knight, J., Eds., Churchill Livingstone, London, 1971, 299.
110. **Pickford, G. E., Griffith, J., Torretti, E., Hendler, E., and Epstein, F. H.**, Bronchial reduction and renal stimulation of (Na^+K^+)-ATPase by prolactin in hypophysectomized killifish in freshwater, *Nature*, 228, 378, 1970.
111. **Dent, J. N.**, Integumentary effects of prolactin in the lower vertebrates, *Am. Zool.*, 15, 923, 1975.
112. **Meier, A. H.**, Chronophysiology of prolactin in the lower vertebrates, *Am. Zool.*, 15, 905, 1975.

THE OVARY

Varadaraj Chandrashekar

INTRODUCTION

It is a well known fact that the ovary produces both ova and hormones. There is interaction of the different ovarian compartments to produce fertilizable ova and ovarian steroids. The anterior pituitary gland participates in control of both these functions through its secretion of gonadotropins, follicle-stimulating hormone (FSH), and luteinizing hormone (LH) as well as prolactin. However, ovarian steroids, estrogens, progestins, and androgens can act on the hypothalamic regulatory hormones and influence the release of these pituitary hormones. Also, folliculostatin, a nonsteroidal ovarian substance, reduces the circulating levels of FSH, thus affecting ovarian function. The discussion in this chapter is directed primarily at the control of the ovarian endocrine function in some eutherian mammals; however, studies from a variety of vertebrate species are mentioned for comparative purposes when appropriate.

MORPHOLOGY

Development

In most of the vertebrates, ovaries are derived from the hypomere of the mesoderm. The undifferentiated primordial germ cells originate extra-gonadally and migrate to the genital ridge ventral to the embryonic mesonephros. Proliferation of nongerminal and germinal cells occur in the coelomic epithelium of the genital ridge leading to the formation of distinct gonadal primordia which are identical in both sexes. Further, there is the differentiation of two regions, outer cortex with secondary cords and inner medulla with primary cords. These two regions are separated by the primary *tunica albuginea*. Next, during sex differentiation, in the female, ovaries are developed from the cortex, and the medulla involutes. In the male fetus, the medulla differentiates into testes and the cortex becomes vestigial.

Location and Attachment

Usually the ovaries lie within the peritoneum. In mammals ovaries are located in the lumbar or pelvic region of the body cavity. The changes in the uterine size during gestation do not greatly alter the position of the ovaries.[1] Each ovary is attached to the middorsal body wall by a peritoneal fold called the mesovarium. An ovarian ligament connects the ovary with the uterus just below the opening of the fallopian tube.

Blood, Lymph and Nerve Supply

In all mammals the ovary has two blood vessels, the ovarian artery and vein. These vessels are the branches of the dorsal aorta and inferior vena cava, respectively.[2] The left ovarian vein drains into the left renal vein and the right ovarian vein drains into the vena cava. The ovarian vessels enter the mesovarium through its cephalic attachment and pass into the hilus of the ovary. Branches of the main ovarian artery and vein anastomose with the ovarian branches of the uterine vessels. In many species, including women, the ovarian vein forms a plexus near the ovary, which is similar to the pampiniform plexus of the testis. The veins converge from this plexus to form a common ovarian vein. The ovarian vein anastomoses with the uterine vein to form the uteroovarian vein.

Many large lymph vessels are found in the medulla of the ovary, where they anastomose with each other and with the branches from the cortex.[3] At the hilus region, the lymphatic plexuses converge to form main lymphatic vessels which follow the ovarian blood vessels and drain into the middle lumbar nodes. In women there is a secondary drainage to the sacral nodes.

The mammalian ovary has sympathetic innervation from the aortic and renal nerve plexuses. The ovarian preganglionic sympathetic fibers are present in the spinal cord segment at T-10 and T-11 levels. The ovarian parasympathetic fibers are from the vagus nerve.[4]

Comparative Morphology

Only one ovary is present in cyclostomes. However, the majority of fishes, amphibians, and eutherian mammals possess two ovaries. In most of the birds, the development of the right ovary is inhibited, hence the left ovary becomes functional in the adult birds. However, in some "birds of prey" both ovaries are functional in spite of the vestigial right oviduct.[5] It is interesting to note that in birds possessing a left functional ovary, if that is surgically removed, the right rudimentary ovary develops into a small testis.[6]

A lobular structure called Bidder's organ is present at the anterior end of each testis in male toads. This organ is histologically similar to an immature ovary. When the testes are removed, Bidder's organs transform into functional ovaries.[7]

The ovaries of fishes and amphibians are hollow and saccular. Among reptiles, saccular ovaries are present in snakes and lizards, whereas turtles and crocodiles possess solid ovaries. The ovarian follicles of birds are borne on stalks. Each ovarian stalk may carry many follicles in various phases of development. Mammalian ovaries are compact and somewhat solid in structure.

Microscopic Structure

A typical ovary of an eutherian mammal is made up of two regions (1) outer cortex; and (2) centrally located medulla. The cortex is covered by the germinal epithelium containing coelomic epithelial cells. In the cortex, ova, follicles at different stages of development, corpora lutea and corpora albicantia are imbedded in the stroma (Figure 1). The medulla contains supportive connective tissue, blood and lymph vessels, nerves as well as rudimentary structures like the rete ovarii, and medullary cords. The medulla also encloses the interstitial tissue.

Nerves, blood, and lymph vessels enter the ovary at a point called hilus. The hilus encloses steroid producing cells which are conspicuous during pregnancy and old age. In the human ovary these cells are morphologically similar to the Leydig cells of the testis, and they probably produce androgens.[8] In most ovaries, some cortical tissue may be found in the medulla and the medullary elements may extend into the cortex. There is no clear demarcation between the cortex and medulla.[2]

Normal Ovarian Follicular Complex

The most important organelles of the ovarian cortex are the follicular complex. The follicular complex of the mammalian ovary include follicles in four different stages of development. They are (1) primordial; (2) primary; (3) secondary; and (4) vesicular (antral or Graafian) follicles.

The primordial follicle consists of a layer of simple squamous epithelium which encloses the ovum. This simple squamous epithelium is transformed into simple low columnar epithelium and the follicle is then termed primary follicle. The cells of the primary follicles multiply to form multilayers of stratified cuboidal or columnar epithelium which are called granulosa cells,[2] or membrana granulosa.[8] This multilayered follicle is the secondary follicle. The secondary follicles develop a large fluid-filled cavity, the antrum. These vesicular follicles are also referred to as antral or Graafian follicles.

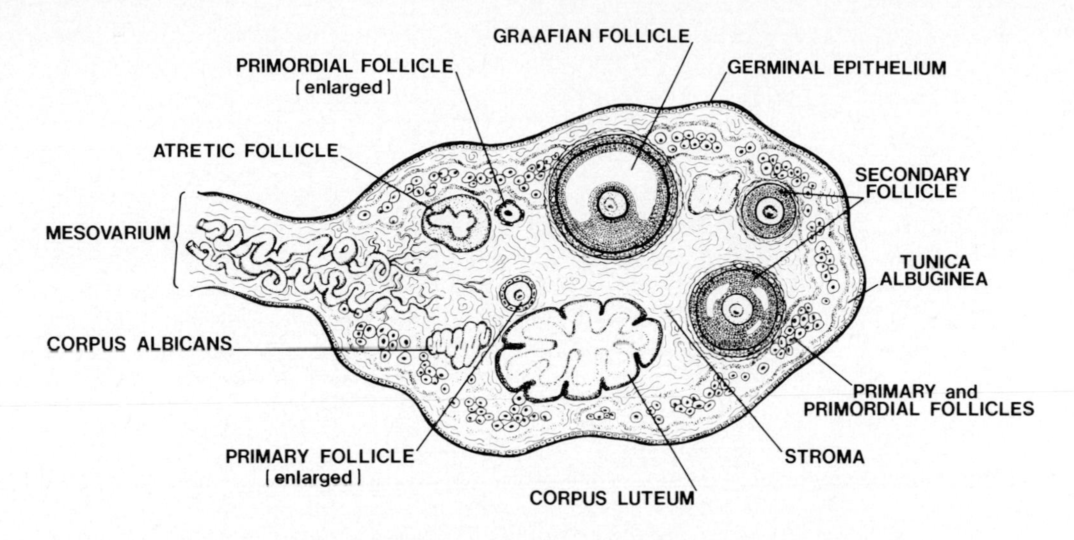

FIGURE 1. Microscopic anatomy of a mammalian ovary (Diagrammatic).

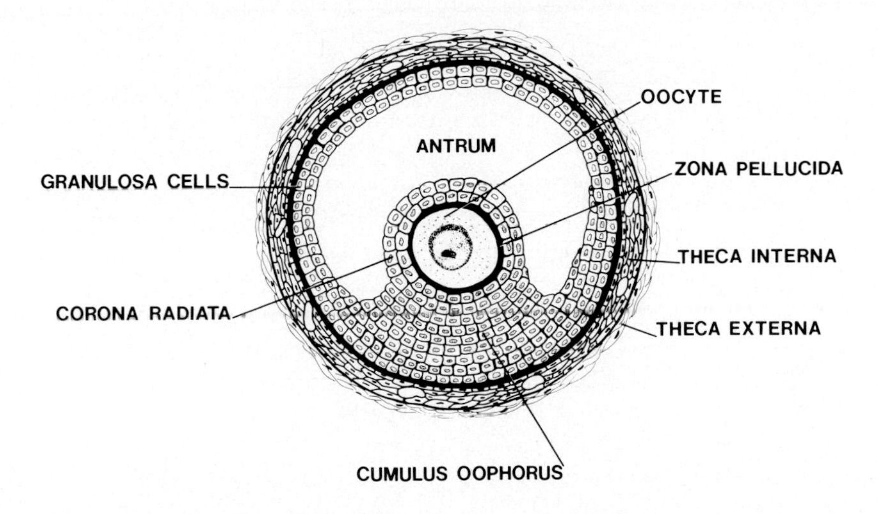

FIGURE 2. A Graafian follicle of a mammalian ovary (Diagrammatic).

The ovum in the Graafian follicle is surrounded by a translucent halo region made up of mucopolysaccharides secreted by the granulosa cells.[9] This region is the zona pellucida. The zona pellucida is surrounded by an irregular group of granulosa cells which become the corona radiata. The granulosa cells at the region of the ovum form a hillock like projection extending into the antrum. This region is termed the cumulus oophorus. The granulosa cell layers are followed by a basement membrane. Adjacent to the basement membrane is a layer of well vascularized, glandular cells, the theca interna. Spindle-shaped theca externa cells surround the theca interna. (Figure 2).

FOLLICULOGENESIS

The pituitary gonadotropins and ovarian steroids influence the development of the ovarian follicles. However, the stimulus that begins the growth of the follicles is unknown, but once they are stimulated, many follicles develop until the follicles ovulate or become atretic.[10] The major target for the gonadotropin action is the membrana granulosa and theca cells. The gonadotropins regulate the cell proliferation, hormone receptor content, adenyl cyclase — cAMP system and steroid production by these cells. Much of the present knowledge of follicular development in mammals is from extensive work on the laboratory rat and the rhesus monkey. Therefore, the major discussion in this section will be restricted to these two species.

Follicular Development During the Estrous Cycle

In the rat, some of the follicles grow during each estrous cycle and are exposed to various amounts of pituitary hormones and ovarian steroids. Therefore, it is necessary to give a brief description of the hormonal changes occurring during the estrous cycle. The follicles secrete little estrogen until the evening of diestrus 2. However, a significant increase in the levels of this steroid occurs at late diestrus 2. It continues to peak on the afternoon of proestrus, as the circulating levels of progesterone increase. At this time, gonadotropin as well as prolactin surges occur and follicles ovulate. The surge of FSH extends until early afternoon of estrus (Figure 3).[11]

It has been suggested that the follicles destined to ovulate are beginning to grow some 19 days earlier.[12] Therefore, it is conceivable that in the rat, the follicles complete their growth and maturation after they are exposed to at least three to four consecutive surges of FSH and LH. The follicles not selected or not capable of responding to gonadotropins fail to mature and become atretic. The follicle-stimulating hormone alone can induce follicular growth and antrum formation, but fails to induce growth of the preovulatory follicles in hypophysectomized rats.[13,14] However, LH and FSH act synergistically and stimulate the growth of these preovulatory follicles,[14] indicating the importance of both of these gonadotropins in follicular development.

The development of the follicles is probably associated with the responsiveness of the follicular cells to the gonadotropins, which may be related to their content of hormone receptors. In small follicles, LH receptors are present in the theca cells and FSH receptors are located in the granulosa cells.[15-19] Unlike the small follicles, granulosa cells of the preovulatory follicles also contain LH receptors.[17,19,20] There is evidence to show that FSH stimulates the 3-β-hydroxysteroid dehydrogenase activity and the appearance of LH receptors in the granulosa cells of the preantral follicles in mice.[21]

The role of estrogen in folliculogenesis came to light from the early observations that estrogen treatment increases the responsiveness of the ovaries.[22,23] Recent studies have revealed that estrogen stimulates granulosa cell proliferation and prevents follicular atresia in hypophysectomized rats.[24,25] Estrogen treatment also increases FSH binding in hypophysectomized rats.[24] It is known that estrogen is required for FSH to induce the appearance of LH receptor and this steroid increases the capability of FSH to induce cAMP accumulation in granulosa cells.[19,26] For estradiol synthesis, both granulosa and theca cells are required.[27] Androgen precursors are located in the theca cells and they are converted to estradiol. The aromatization enzymes are required for this conversion and they are present in the granulosa cells.[28-31]

Little is known about the role of LH on the growth of the follicles. In addition to induction of ovulation, LH luteinizes the antral follicles and depletes their contents of LH as well as of FSH receptors.[19,32] Thus ovarian cell response is reduced when ovulatory doses of LH are administered.[33]

There are indications that LH decreases the ovarian content of the hormone receptors associated with a loss or desensitization of hormone-induced adenyl cyclase activity.[33,34] These studies suggest that LH may act on some follicles which are not destined to ovulate and it induces the loss of gonadotropic hormone receptors. This in turn decreases the responsiveness of these follicles to gonadotropins and therefore may initiate atresia. However, LH can increase receptors for prolactin in preovulatory follicles, which in turn elevates luteal cell receptors for LH.[35] These investigations have clearly indicated that the ovarian follicular development is dependent on steroid and pituitary hormones, as well as hormone specific receptors.

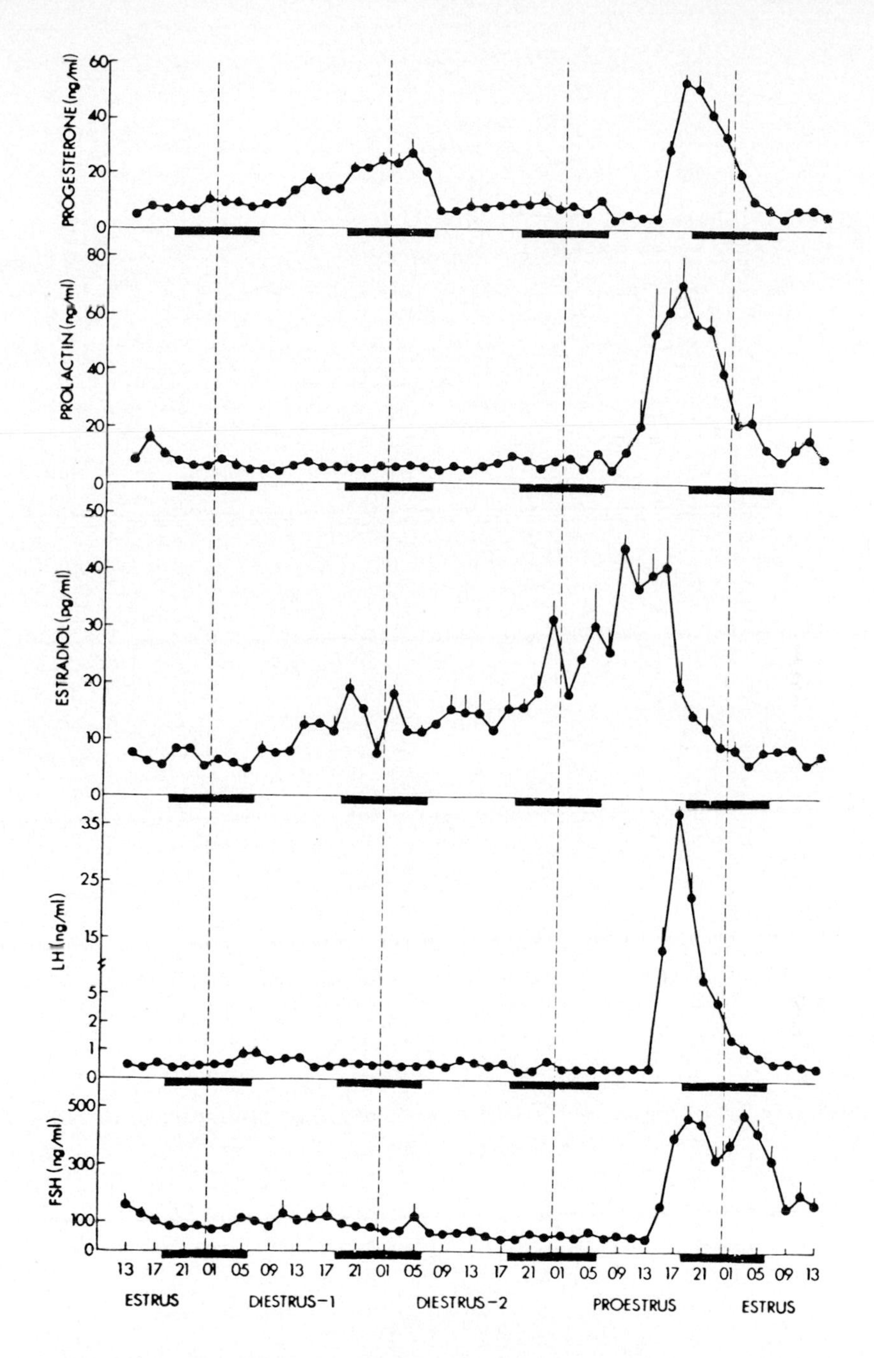

FIGURE 3. The pattern of progesterone, prolactin, estradiol, LH, and FSH levels throughout the estrous cycle of the rat. (From Smith, M. S., Freeman, M. E., and Neill, J. D., *Endocrinology*, 96, 219, 1975. With permission.)

Follicular Development During the Menstrual Cycle

The time course of the circulating gonadotropins and ovarian steroids during the menstrual cycle in rhesus monkeys is remarkably similar to that of normally cycling women,[36-39] (Figures 4 and 5). The duration of the menstrual cycle in both of these primates averages 28 days.

The reproductive cycle in the primates can be functionally divided into a follicular phase, an ovulatory phase, and a luteal phase. Unlike most of the nonprimates, in

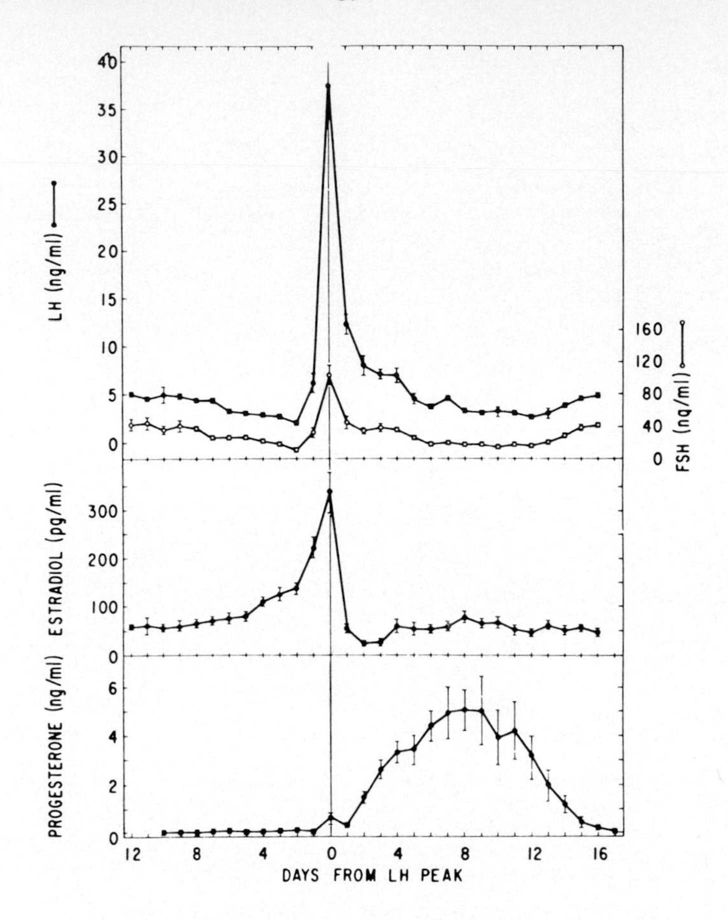

FIGURE 4. Plasma concentrations of LH, FSH, estradiol and progesterone throughout the normal rhesus monkey menstrual cycle normalized to the day of the midcycle LH peak (day 0). (From Knobil, E., *Rec. Prog. Horm. Res.*, 30, 1, 1974. With permission.)

higher primates during the follicular phase of each cycle, one follicle is selected for growth, maturation, and ovulation from a pool of nonproliferating primordial follicles formed during embryonic life. At mid-cycle, around day 13 or 14, gonadotropin surges occur followed by ovulation some 36 hr later. Following ovulation, follicular cells are luteinized and form into a corpus luteum (CL). The CL cells secrete progestins and estrogens throughout the luteal phase of the cycle. Extensive investigations in the rhesus monkey have suggested that the basal or tonic gonadotropin secretion of LH and FSH is controlled by the negative feedback action of estradiol and that the initiation of the mid-cycle, preovulatory gonadotropin surge is also due to the stimulatory effect of estradiol secreted by the growing follicle destined to ovulate.[36-40]

Studies involving removal of the preovulatory follicle or the active CL suggest that the follicular development of both ovaries are inhibited in the presence of a dominant follicle or an active CL.[40] Also, in the presence of the preovulatory, dominant follicle, the responsiveness of other follicles to gonadotropic stimulation is transiently attenuated.[41] However, ovulation was found to occur 12 days following ablation of the largest follicle during early follicular phase or the active CL at the early luteal phase of the cycle. Therefore, it may be inferred that the selection of the preovulatory follicle in the rhesus monkey takes place earlier than in the rat.[12,42] A recent study has suggested that the dominant follicle requires continued FSH stimulation, even in the immediate preovulatory interval.[43]

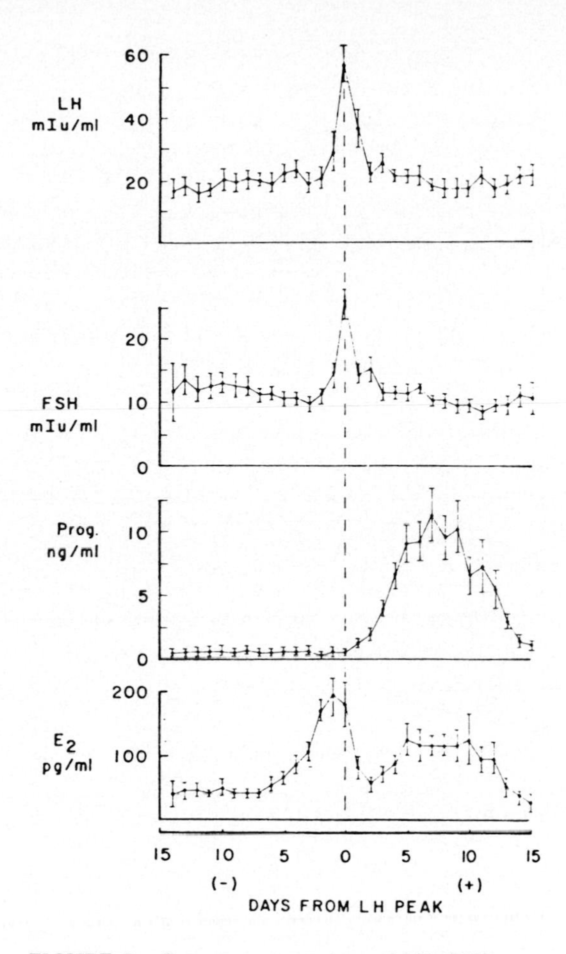

FIGURE 5. Serum concentrations of LH, FSH, progesterone and estradiol in the normal human menstrual cycle. The day of LH peak is designated day 0. (From Mishell, D. R. Jr., Nakamura, R. M., Crosignani, P. G., Stone, S., Kharma, K., Nagata, Y., and Thorneycroft, I. H., *Am. J. Obstet. Gynecol.*, 111, 60, 1971. With permission.)

The ovarian steroids may play an important role in folliculogenesis in the primates. In both women and rhesus monkeys, growth of the follicles to the preovulatory stages ceases during the luteal phase of the menstrual cycle, implying that progesterone secreted by the CL inhibits follicular growth.[44,45] Induction of the growth of a new follicle after lutectomy supports this concept.[40] However, a recent study has shown that progesterone does not inhibit gonadotropin induced follicular maturation in the nonhuman primate.[46] High concentrations of estrogen have deleterious effects on follicles since subcutaneous implantation of the silastic capsules containing crystalline estradiol-17β at the early follicular phase results in rapid degeneration of the follicle destined to ovulate.[47]

Follicular Development During Pregnancy

Little attention has been given to the follicular changes during pregnancy. The follicles are not quiescent during gestation. In the rat, if the ovulated eggs are fertilized, the ovulated follicular cells become functional corpora lutea and secrete progesterone until days 19 or 20 of gestation.[48,49] During this period the circulating levels of both

LH and FSH remain low.[50,51] In spite of low concentrations of gonadotropins, antral follicles capable of ovulating develop between days 3 and 5 as well as days 19 to 23 of gestation.[52] Ovulation does not occur during early pregnancy because progesterone may block LH surge. However, following parturition on day 23 of pregnancy, there are surges of gonadotropins and ovulation occurs 18 hr postpartum.[53,54] The growth of the follicles before the termination of pregnancy is associated with increased contents of LH and FSH receptors of the granulosa cells.[52] This probably increases the responsiveness of the follicles to gonadotropin surges, thus causing ovulation.

Very limited studies in pregnant women have revealed the presence of large, mature Graafian follicles during early gestation. Between 11 and 20 weeks of pregnancy, large antral follicles show increased features of atresia.[55] Large numbers of follicles show extensive luteinization.[55,56] The ovaries of preparturient women have been found covered with a dense population of small superficial follicles,[57] with a high incidence of atresia in these follicles. These investigations suggest that high concentrations of ovarian steroids during gestation,[58,59] does not prevent early follicular development but induces premature atresia in pregnant women.

In the rhesus monkey, the circulating levels of gonadotropins during the last three weeks of pregnancy are below the sensitivities of the radioimmunoassays,[60] indicating that the follicular development may be impaired during gestation. However, several primary and antral follicles in various stages of development and degeneration are present at early pregnancy,[61] suggesting that follicles may not be completely inactive during gestation.

In the pregnant pigtailed monkey, in spite of high serum concentrations of progesterone,[62] estradiol, and estrone,[63] the ovaries at both early and late pregnancy are packed with large and small antral follicles. Some of these follicles show various degrees of atresia. Although chorionic gonadotropin in circulation is undetectable after day 40 of pregnancy, moderate levels of FSH and detectable amounts of LH are present till and after parturition. It is conceivable that these pituitary gonadotropins may play important roles in the follicular activity during gestation in this primate species.

Folliculostatin

Administration of follicular fluid has an inhibitory effect on circulating levels of FSH, but it does not affect LH concentrations.[64-67] Follicular fluid also inhibits the growth of the follicles in mice,[68] cattle, and sheep.[69] Studies on the effect of follicular fluid have been extended to primates. Treatment of rhesus monkeys with charcoal-extracted porcine follicular fluid selectively suppresses serum FSH levels and folliculogenesis.[43,70]

The porcine follicular fluid FSH suppressing material is a nonsteroid, trypsin-labile substance and has a molecular weight in the range of 10,000 to 35,000 daltons.[71,72] It is an ''ovarian inhibin'',[73] termed folliculostatin.[64,71] The possible site of action of folliculostatin is at the level of the anterior pituitary.[64,74] The inhibin activity is also found in human follicular fluid.[73]

The role of folliculostatin in the physiologic control of circulating FSH has shown that FSH is essential for folliculogenesis in animals.[43,68-70] Additional clinical investigations may be helpful in understanding some of the causes for ovarian dysfunction in women. Since folliculostatin selectively inhibits serum FSH and folliculogenesis, this substance may have significance in the control of reproduction.

CORPUS LUTEUM

Luteal Function

The corpus luteum is a well studied structure of the mammalian ovary. In eutherian mammals the granulosa cells are transformed into luteal cells.[2,8] After rupture of the follicle and ovulation, the granulosa cells are vascularized. The blood vessels from the theca interna form a network among the enlarging granulosa lutein cells, which become part of the CL. The CL is a steroidogenic tissue and estrogens and/or progestins are its principle physiologic products.

The hormones that are essential to support the CL function varies among mammalian species. In the unmated rat, the CL in the estrous cycle is virtually nonfunctional. This may be the reason for the short 4 to 5 day cycle in this species. However, the CL becomes functional following mechanical stimulation of the cervix or by the female mating with an infertile male (at late proestrus or estrus stage) or when the rat becomes pregnant.

The condition in which the CL function is extended other than when due to pregnancy is referred to as "pseudo-pregnancy". During pseudo-pregnancy, the functional CL persists for 12 days, but in pregnancy, it stays functional for about 19 or 20 days.[48,49] The major luteotropic stimulus for the extension of the CL function during pseudopregnancy has been shown to be prolactin.[11]

The function of the CL during pregnancy varies during various stages of gestation. Investigation has shown that hypophysectomy on day 4 of pregnancy in the rat results in a failure of blastocyst implantation. Removal of the pituitary gland on any day between days 7 and 10 causes fetal resorption.[75] However, hypophysectomy on day 12 of gestation does not affect pregnancy,[76] implying that the pituitary hormones are required before day 12 of gestation for the secretion of progesterone by the CL. Progesterone is an important steroid hormone, in the rat, necessary for the maintenance of pregnancy.

Administration of LH antiserum to rats for one or more days, between days 8 and 11 of gestation results in fetal resorption.[77] However, the antiserum is ineffective in terminating pregnancy when administered on day 12. The termination of gestation by antiserum to LH prior to day 12 is prevented by the administration of LH or progesterone, but not by estrogen, nor by large doses of ovine prolactin, nor by homologous prolactin induced by pituitary homografts or placental extracts. Therefore, it is indicated that LH maintains pregnancy up to day 12 and LH is the specific stimulus for progesterone synthesis.[77] Since the CL secretes progesterone after day 12, even in the absence of LH, it is hypothesized that progesterone secretion is virtually "autonomous" during the second half of pregnancy. However, hysterectomy on day 12 of gestation leads to a precipitous decline in progesterone levels by day 16, but hypophysectomy on the same day does not affect this steroid secretion.[78] The combined effect of hypophysectomy-hysterectomy on day 12 is even greater in curtailing progesterone secretion in circulation. Also, CL growth stops or the CL slowly regresses soon after hypophysectomy-hysterectomy,[79] suggesting that the placenta plays a vital role in progesterone secretion by the CL. Therefore, the secretion of progesterone after day 12 of gestation does not appear to be autonomous. Placental luteotropin seems to be the factor necessary for the maintenance of the CL function.[80]

There are reports that LH is not essential for progesterone secretion throughout the first half of gestation.[79,80] Administration of LH antiserum to rats on the afternoon of day 7 does not terminate pregnancy.[80] However, ergocornine given on day 6 or 7 suppresses circulating concentrations of prolactin and causes abortion in the majority of rats, indicating that the prolactin is a luteotropin until day 7 of gestation.

Deprivation of prolactin shortens the duration of the diestrus in rats which have been hysterectomized on day 8 of pregnancy. Administration of day 12 pregnant rat serum (presumably containing placental luteotropin) to decidual tissue-bearing pseudopregnant rats on days 6 to 9 prevents the luteolytic effect of prolactin deprivation.[80] These and other findings,[79,81] indicate that during pregnancy in the rat, prolactin is a luteotropin through day 7. A "placental-luteotropin-LH complex" becomes essential from day 8 through day 11 for the production of progesterone by the CL.

Contrary to the suggestion that placental luteotropin plays a major role in maintaining the function of the CL during the second half of pregnancy, there is increasing evidence that estrogen exerts the luteotropic effect after day 12 of gestation.[78,82,83]

The mechanism of control of the CL function in other laboratory mammalian species with estrous cycles is less clear. In the hamster, the maintenance of functional CL requires a "luteotropic complex" of prolactin, FSH and small amounts of LH.[84] For the CL function in the guinea pig, pituitary support is essential for only the first 3 to 4 days of the cycle.[85] In the guinea pig, FSH may be an essential component of a luteotropic complex,[86] and the placental luteotropin may take part in continued function of the CL.[87] In the rabbit, estrogen is the "ultimate" luteotropic hormone that is required for progesterone secretion by the CL.[88] However, LH is required for estrogen production. Prolactin is the luteotropic hormone in the mouse at the beginning of gestation, but LH maintains the CL function after implantation.[89] Placental luteotropin may also sustain luteal function.[90]

The regulation of the CL function in primates seems to be less confusing than in other mammals. In women, surgical removal of pituitary adenoma and subsequent treatment with human gonadotropins result in ovulation as well as these patients have become pregnant.[91] Similarly, hypophysectomized women induced to ovulate by sequential treatment of FSH followed by human chorionic gonadotropin have become pregnant without further gonadotropin treatment. This implies that once the CL is formed after ovulation, it is essentially independent of pituitary support.[92] However, the CL formed in the hypophysectomized women produces subnormal amounts of progesterone and for no longer than 5 days.[92] In the nonhuman primate, LH is the luteotropin during the luteal phase of the menstrual cycle since administration of an antiserum to hCG, which neutralizes the endogenous LH, reduces circulating levels of progesterone and causes premature menstruation.[93]

There is a paucity of information about the influence of prolactin on luteal function during the menstrual cycle. The circulating levels of prolactin in women[94] and in monkeys[95,96] have been found to be relatively constant throughout the cycle. Progesterone levels are not modified following administration of prolactin during the luteal phase of the cycle.[97] These findings imply that normal luteal function can be achieved in the absence of prolactin.

In three species of monkeys and in women, the CL is functional during early pregnancy.[62,98-100] The activity of the CL in the rhesus monkey decreases before midgestation, but is subsequently "rejuvenated" before parturition.[101,102] Similarly, in pregnant pigtailed monkeys (Figure 6) and in pregnant women[103] the CL has been shown to be active near term. However, bilateral ovariectomy in the monkeys after initial establishment of gestation does not result in termination of pregnancy and a similar effect is observed in women.[62,104,105] Therefore, a functional CL is not required for maintenance of pregnancy during the major portion of gestation in these primates. A functional CL is indispensable before day 21 of gestation in the rhesus monkey, since ovariectomy before this time is followed by abortion and administration of progesterone maintains pregnancy.[98,105]

The patterns of circulating progesterone concentrations in pregnant rhesus monkeys are indistinguishable from those of the nonpregnant monkeys until days 9 to 11 of gestation. At that time, a significant rise of chorionic gonadotropin levels during gestation occurs concomitantly with an abrupt increase in progesterone concentration. This implies that CL of gestation is rescued by chorionic gonadotropin.[106,107]

Administration of a specific LH antiserum to pregnant rhesus monkeys during early gestation does not affect normal pregnancy.[108] Similarly, active immunization of female rhesus monkeys with ovine LH β-subunit, which induces development of antibodies to chorionic gonadotropins, causes a significant reduction in fertility.[109] These observations suggest that LH is not a luteotropic hormone and that chorionic gonadotropin is the luteotropic principle for the maintenance of the CL function during early pregnancy in the rhesus monkey.

Although chorionic gonadotropin is the luteotropin during early pregnancy in the rhesus monkey, this hormone does not appear to be involved in rejuvenation of the CL at late pregnancy since chorionic gonadotropin is nondetectable during mid and late gestation.[105,110,111] Unlike early pregnancy, chorionic somatomammotropin, and prolactin levels in the uterine vein as well as in the peripheral plasma are elevated at day 157.[112] However, it is interesting to note that the ovary containing the CL and the placenta continue to secrete progesterone during late pregnancy, even in hypophysectomized monkeys in which fetal death occurred. In these monkeys, circulating levels of chorionic somatomammotropin and prolactin were nondectable,[113] suggesting that the control of CL function in late pregnancy is more complex than in early pregnancy. Unlike the nonhuman primates, chorionic gonadotropin is present in the circulation throughout gestation in pregnant women[114] and this placental gonadotropin may have some influence on the functional activity of the CL during the late gestation.

Luteolysis

The termination of the CL function at the end of the cycle in some animals may be influenced by the luteolytic activity of the uterus. The nongravid uterus exerts the luteolytic action on the CL of the guinea pig,[115,116] hamster,[117,118] rat,[119,120] cow,[121,122] pig,[123,124] and sheep.[125,126] However, in monkeys and women, hysterectomy does not affect the normal luteal function,[127,128] indicating that the uterine luteolytic factor is not responsible for the involution of the primate CL.

Administration of prostaglandin $F_{2\alpha}$ causes luteal regression in a variety of animals.[129,130,131] At the beginning of the CL regression, the levels of prostaglandin in the endometrium[132] as well as in the uterine venous blood[130] increases. In vitro studies[133] have suggested that prostaglandin is the uterine luteolysin, hence hysterectomy extends the luteal function. It has been proposed that prostaglandin $F_{2\alpha}$ causes constriction of the ovarian vein,[119] reduces uteroovarian blood flow,[129] or releases a luteolytic level of LH.[134] However, there are studies implying that prostaglandin $F_{2\alpha}$ acts directly on the CL and the induction of luteolysis is by reduction of gonadotropin receptors in the luteal tissue.[135,136]

Although exogenous estrogen is known to support the CL function in the rat[78,82,83] and rabbit,[88] this steroid has a luteolytic effect in cyclic guinea pigs.[137] A luteolytic effect of estrogen has also been reported in the cow[138] and sheep.[139] Similarly, in the rhesus monkey as well as in women, administration of estrogen during the luteal phase of the menstrual cycle induces functional regression of the CL and premature menstruation.[140-143] Estrogen acts directly on the CL and induces luteolysis in primates.[144,145]

The ovaries of rat and rabbit secrete both progesterone and 20α-hydroxypregn-4-ene-3-one (20α-OHP). As the lifespan of the CL ends, ovarian vein progesterone concentration decreases, whereas levels of 20α-OHP increase.[146,147] The enzyme responsible for conversion of progesterone to 20α-OHP, 20α-hydroxysteroid dehydrogenase is found only in regressing CL.[148,149] Therefore, it is conceivable that 20α-hydroxysteroid dehydrogenase may also induce functional luteolysis in these two mammalian forms.

OVARIAN AGING

Decrease in the reproductive function with advancing age is due to alterations in the hypothalamus, pituitary, ovary, and uterus. The aging female rat shows a gradual reduction in the number of ovulations, irregularities in estrous cycles, with increased

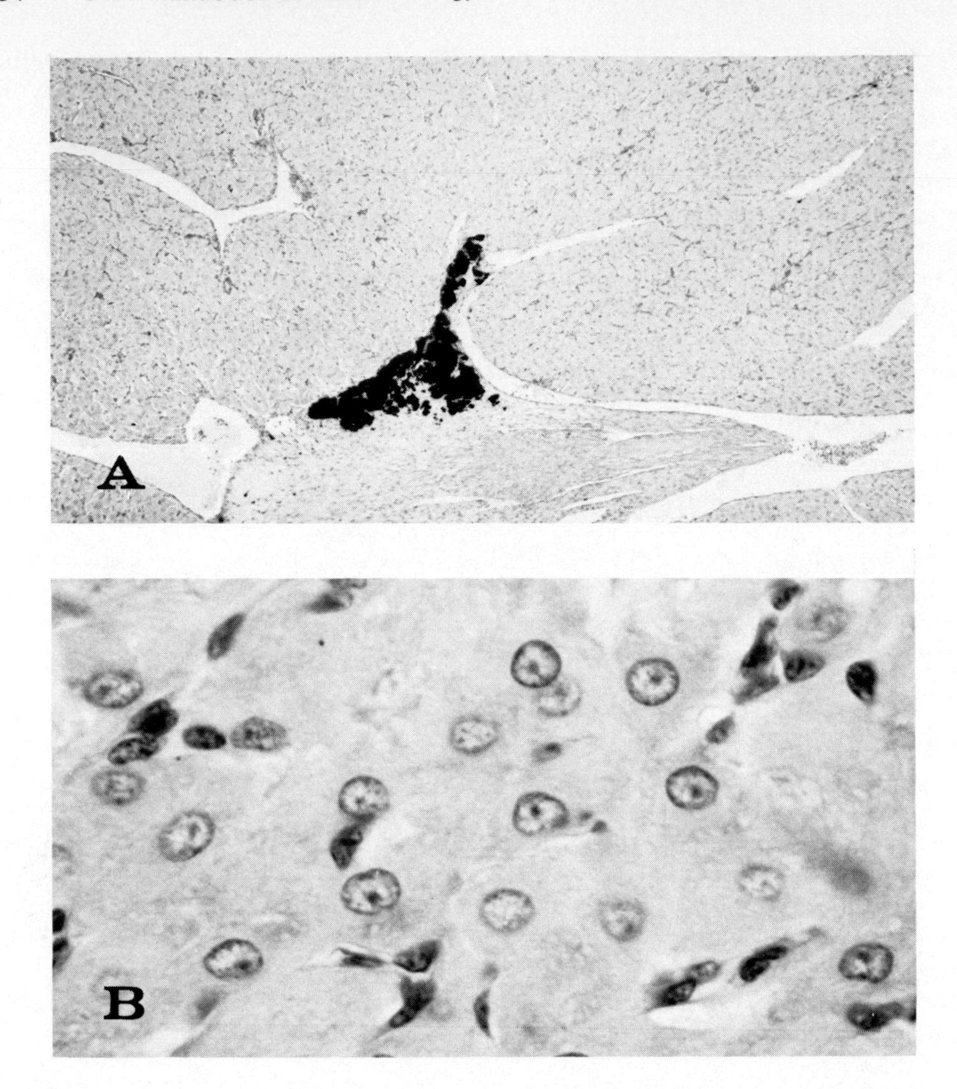

FIGURE 6. The corpus luteum of an ovary from a pigtailed monkey obtained at day 159 of pregnancy. The same CL was marked with India ink on day 25 of gestation. Note the presence of India ink (A) and active luteal cells (B). Chandrashekar, V., Wolf, R. C., and Dierschke, D. J., Unpublished.

incidence of constant estrus, followed by repeated pseudo-pregnancies and subsequent cessation of the cycle.[151,152] The rat loses normal reproductive function at 8 to 15 months of age[153,154] and the ovarian cycles cease at 2 to 3 years of age.[154] These changes in the estrous cycles do not appear to be due to the changes in the ovarian or pituitary function, since transfer of ovaries or pituitaries from old rats to young adult cycling rats do not alter the cyclicity in the young animals.[155] Hence, changes in hypothalamic function seem to be the major cause for the change in the reproductive function in the old female rat.

In the aging female rat, there seems to be a decrease in hypothalamic sensitivity to control inputs in relation to gonadotropin secretion by the pituitary gland. Following ovariectomy, elevation in FSH and LH levels in the circulation of old rats are lower than in young rats.[156,157] It has also been demonstrated that the negative feedback effect of ovarian steroids on the hypothalamic-hypophyseal axis is altered in aging female rats. Administration of estradiol benzoate to ovariectomized rats produces smaller decreases in serum levels of FSH and LH in old constant estrus and pseudopregnant rats than in young rats. However, the same treatment had no effect on gonadotropin levels in old anestrous rats.[157,158] Aging female rats also exhibit a reduction in LH release in response to the positive feedback effect on estrogen and progesterone.[154]

Ovulation can be induced in old constant estrus rats by electrical stimulation of the preoptic area of the hypothalamus or by treatment with progesterone or epinephrine.[159] Resumption of cyclicity in aging female rats occurs by daily administration of epinephrine.[160] This implies that there is a deficiency in hypothalamic catecholamine turnover.[154,161] Since catecholamines mediate the action of the gonadal steroids in releasing gonadotropins,[162] alterations in the catecholamine content of the hypothalamus in the aging female rats would be, at least in part, the reason for the altered ovarian function.

Ovaries of aged rats exhibiting constant estrus contained well developed and sometimes cystic follicles. These ovaries are without corpora lutea whereas the ovaries of pseudopregnant old rats contain many corpora lutea. Anestrous rats have small, atrophic ovaries with no follicles or corpora lutea.[151] Also, aged rat ovaries contain considerable numbers of oocytes throughout the lifespan of the animal.[163]

Histochemical studies of aging ovaries from rats as well as hamsters show no obvious change in Δ^5-3β-hydroxysteroid dehydrogenase activity,[164,165] suggesting that aging ovaries are steroidogenically active. However, serum concentrations of progesterone are lower in aging rats than in young animals, which may contribute to the decreased secretion of gonadotropins.[166] It appears that in the aging rat, the primary site of reproductive dysfunction does not arise in the ovary, but that the normal function of the hypothalamus is impaired.

In women after 40 years of age, the menstrual cycles become irregular with long or short cycles before cessation of vaginal bleeding during menopause. In the older women, short cycles are due to a shorter follicular phase. Prolonged cycles are attributed to an inadequate luteal phase or to anovulation.[167,168]

It is believed that the decline in the reproductive function in women is due to a reduction in ovarian function. One concept of the cause of menopause is that there is an exhaustion of oocytes and primordial follicles. This theory cannot be accepted since there are substantial numbers of primordial follicles present at the onset of menopause.[169] An ultrastructural study reveals that the primordial follicles and oocytes are normal in postmenopausal women,[170] although most of the follicles that advance from the primordial stage undergo atretic changes.

The ovarian steroid secretions change with age. During aging, the ovary secretes less estradiol.[167,168,171] Hence, there is less estradiol to inhibit the hypothalamus and the secretion of pituitary gonadotropins increases.[172,173,174] However, the number of ovarian stromal cells increases with age, and these cells contain well developed mitochondria, smooth endoplasmic reticulum, and abundance of lipid droplets, all indicative of secretory activity.[170]

In vitro studies reveal that the ovarian stromal tissue from postmenopausal women can synthesize androgenic steroid hormones, primarily dehydroepiandrosterone, androstenedione, and testosterone.[175,176] Furthermore, ovarian vein plasma concentrations of testosterone and androstenedione are more elevated than in peripheral vein samples.[177] Administration of human chorionic gonadtropin to postmenopausal women results in increased concentrations of testosterone and androstenedione in ovarian vein samples, whereas adrenocorticotropin fails to enhance androgen secretion significantly.[171] In all these investigations little or no estrogens have been found. These findings suggest that the menopausal ovary produces androgens and has less potentiality to secrete estrogens.

There is a paucity of information regarding ovarian aging in the subhuman primates.

Very limited study in rhesus monkeys has indicated that the aged ovary secretes less estrogen.[178] The circulating levels of both estradiol and progesterone are reduced whereas gonadotropins are elevated in older monkeys.[179] These reports suggest that the ovaries of aged rhesus monkeys are similar to the ovaries of menopausal women with regard to gonadotropin and steroid secretions.

The hypothalamo-hypophyseal system in aged women remains fully responsive to both the negative and positive feedback action of ovarian steroids. Administration of estrogens causes a prompt decline in both FSH and LH concentrations in postmenopausal women.[92,180,181] Infusion of ethinyl estradiol into postmenopausal women decreases gonadotropin levels. However, when these ethinyl-estradiol-treated women receive daily doses of medroxyprogesterone, a typical "ovulatory" release of both FSH and LH occurs.[182] The evidence strongly suggests that in women the hypothalamic-hypophyseal axis retains its functional capabilities during the aging process and that the primary functional alteration occurs in the ovary. It is the ovary that is responsible for the onset of the menopause.

DEDICATION

This chapter is dedicated to the memory of Dr. James H. Leathem, an outstanding teacher and researcher in reproductive endocrinology.

REFERENCES

1. **Hibbard, B. M.,** The position of the maternal ovaries in late pregnancy, *Br. J. Radiol.,* 34, 387, 1961.
2. **Mossman, H. W. and Duke, K. L.,** *Comparative Morphology of the Mammalian Ovary,* The University of Wisconsin Press, Madison, 1973.
3. **Morris, B. and Sass, M. B.,** The formation of lymph in the ovary, *Proc. R. Soc. London, Ser. B:,* 164, 577, 1966.
4. **Hill, R. T.,** Paradoxical effects of ovarian secretion, in *The Ovary,* Vol. 2, Zuckerman S., Ed., Academic Press, New York, 1962, 231.
5. **Stanley, A. J. and Witschi, E.,** Germ cell migration in relation to asymmetry in the sex glands of hawks, *Anat. Rec.,* 76, 329, 1940.
6. **Burns, R. K.,** Role of hormones in the differentiation of sex, in *Sex and Internal Secretion,* Vol. 1, 3rd ed., Young, W. C. and Corner, G. W., Eds., The William and Wilkins Co., Baltimore, Md., 76, 1967.
7. **Ponse, K.,** L'organe de Bidder et le déterminisme des caractéres sexuels sécondaires du crapaud *(Bufo vulgaris L.)., Rev. Suisse Zool.,* 31, 177, 1924.
8. **Harrison, R. J.,** The structure of the ovary, in *The Ovary,* Vol. 1, Zuckerman, S., Ed., Academic Press, New York, 1962, 143.
9. **Chiquoine, A. D.,** The development of the zona pellucida of the mammalian ovum, *Am. J. Anat.,* 106, 149, 1960.
10. **Pedersen, T.,** Follicle kinetics in the ovary of cyclic mouse, *Acta Endocrinol. (Kbh).,* 64, 304, 1970.
11. **Smith, M. S., Freeman, M. E., and Neill, J. D.,** The Control of progesterone Secretion during the estrous cycle and early pseudopregnancy in the rat: prolactin, gonadotropin and steroid levels associated with rescue of the corpus luteum of pseudopregnancy, *Endocrinology,* 96, 219, 1975.
12. **Richards, J. S. and Midgley, A. R., Jr.,** Protein hormone action: a key to understanding ovarian follicular and luteal cell development, *Biol. Reprod.,* 14, 82, 1976.
13. **Greep, R. O., Van Dyke, H. B., and Chow, B. F.,** Gonadotropins of the swine pituitary. I. Various biological effects of purified thylakentrin (FSH) and pure metakentrin (ICSH), *Endocrinology,* 30, 635, 1942.
14. **Lostroh, A. J. and Johnson, R. E.,** Amounts of interstitial cell-stimulating hormone and follicle-stimulating hormone required for follicular development, uterine growth and ovulation in the hypophysectomized rat, *Endocrinology,* 79, 991, 1966.

15. **Midgley, A. R., Jr.**, Autoradiographic analysis of gonadotropin binding to rat ovarian tissue sections, *Adv. Exp. Med. Biol.*, 36, 365, 1973.
16. **Channing C. P. and Kammerman, S.**, Binding of gonadotropins to ovarian cells, *Biol. Reprod.*, 10, 179, 1974.
17. **Zeleznik, A. J., Midgley, A. R. Jr., and Reichert, L. E. Jr.**, Granulosa Cell maturation in the rat: increased binding of human chorionic gonadotropin following treatment with follicle-stimulating hormone in vivo, *Endocrinology*, 95, 818, 1974.
18. **Amsterdam, A., Koch, Y., Liberman, M. E., and Lindner, H. R.**, Distribution of binding sites for human chorionic gonadotropin in the preovulatory follicle of the rat, *J. Cell. Biol.*, 67, 894, 1975.
19. **Richards, J. S., Ireland, J. J., Rao, M. C., Bernath, G. A., Midgley, A. R., Jr., and Reichert, L. E., Jr.**, Ovarian follicular development in the rat: hormone receptor regulation by estradiol, Follicle stimulating hormone and luteinizing hormone, *Endocrinology*, 99, 1562, 1976.
20. **Kammerman, S. and Ross, J.**, Increase in numbers of gonadotropin receptors on granulosa cells during follicular maturation, *J. Clin. Endocrinol. Metab.*, 41, 546, 1975.
21. **Eshkol, A and Lunenfeld, B.**, Gonadotropic regulation of ovarian development in mice during infancy, in *Gonadotropins*, Saxena, B. B., Beling, C. G., and Gandy, H. M., Eds., John Wiley & Sons, New York, 1972, 335.
22. **Pencharz, R. I.**, Effect of estrogens and androgens alone and in combination with chorionic gonadotropin on the ovary of the hypophysectomized rat, *Science*, 91, 554, 1940.
23. **Williams, P. C.**, Studies of the biological action of serum gonadotropin. I. Decline in ovarian response after hypophysectomy. 2. Ovarian response after hypophysectomy and estrogen treatment, *J. Endocrinol.*, 4, 127, 1945.
24. **Goldenberg, R. L., Reiter, E. O. and Ross, G. T.**, Follicle response to exogenous gonadotropins: an estrogen-mediated phenomenon, *Fertil. Steril.*, 24, 121, 1973.
25. **Harman, S. M., Louvet, J. P. and Ross, G. T.**, Interaction of estrogen and gonadotrophins on follicular atresia, *Endocrinology*, 96, 1145, 1975.
26. **Richards, J. S., Jonassen, J. A., Rolfes, A. I., Kersey, K. and Reichert, L. E., Jr.**, Adenosine 3′,5′-monophosphate, luteinizing hormone receptor and progesterone during granulosa cell differentiation: effects of estradiol and follicle-stimulating hormone, *Endocrinology*, 104, 765, 1979.
27. **Flack, B.**, Site of production of oestrogen in rat ovary as studied by microtransplants, *Acta. Physiol. (SC).*, (Suppl. 163), 47, 1959.
28. **Darlington, J. H., Moon, Y. S., and Armstrong, D. T.**, Estradiol-17β biosynthesis in cultured granulosa cells from hypophysectomized immature rats; stimulation by follicle-stimulating hormone, *Endocrinology*, 97, 1328, 1975.
29. **Erickson, G. F. and Ryan, K. J.**, Stimulation of testosterone production in isolated rabbit thecal tissue by FSH/LH dibutyl cyclic AMP, PGE 2α and PGE_2, *Endocrinology*, 99, 452, 1976.
30. **Fortune, J. E. and Armstrong, D. T.**, Androgen Production by theca and granulosa isolated from proestrous rat follicles, *Endocrinology*, 100, 1341, 1977.
31. **Makris, A. and Ryan, K. J.**, Aromatase activity of isolated and recombined hamster granulosa cells and theca, *Steroids*, 29, 65, 1977.
32. **Rao, M. C., Richards, J. S., Midgley, A. R., Jr., and Reichert, L. E. Jr.**, Regulation of gonadotropin receptors by LH in granulosa cells, *Endocrinology*, 101, 512, 1977.
33. **Conti, M., Harwood, J. P., Hsueh, A. J. W., Dufau, M. L., and Catt, K. J.**, Gonadotropin-induced loss of hormone receptors and desensitization of adenylate cyclase in the ovary, *J. Biol. Chem.*, 251, 7729, 1976.
34. **Hunzicker-Dunn, M. and Birnbaumer, L.**, Adenyl Cyclase activities in ovarian tissues. III. Regulation of responsiveness to LH, FSH and PGE_1 in prepubertal, cycling, pregnant and pseudopregnant rat, *Endocrinology*, 99, 198, 1976.
35. **Richards, J. S. and Williams, J. J.**, Luteal cell receptor content for prolactin (PRL) and luteinizing hormone (LH): regulation by LH and PRL, *Endocrinology*, 99, 1571, 1976.
36. **Knobil, E.**, On the control of gonadotropin secretion in the rhesus monkey, *Rec. Prog. Horm. Res.*, 30, 1, 1974.
37. **Ross, G. T., Cargille, C. M., Lipsett, M. B., Rayford, P. L. Marchall, J. R., Strott, C. A., and Rodbard, D.**, Pituitary and gonadal hormones in women during spontaneous and induced ovulatory cycles, *Rec. Progr. Horm. Res.*, 26, 1, 1970.
38. **Mishell, D. R., Jr., Nakamura, R. M., Crosignani, P. G., Stone, S., Kharma, K., Nagata, Y., and Thorneycroft, I. H.**, Serum gonadotropin and steroid patterns during the normal menstrual cycle, *Am. J. Obstet. Gynecol.*, 111, 60, 1971.
39. **Hodgen, G. D., Wilks, J. W. Vaitukaitis, J. L., Chen, H. C., Papkoff, H., and Ross, G. T.**, A new radioimmunoassay for follicle-stimulating hormone in macaques: ovulatory menstrual cycles, *Endocrinology*, 99, 137, 1976.
40. **Goodman, A. L., Nixon, W. E., Johnson, D. K., and Hodgen, G. D.**, Regulation of folliculogenesis in the cycling rhesus monkey: Selection of the dominant follicle, *Endocrinology*, 100, 155, 1977.

41. **diZerega, G. S. and Hodgen, G. D.**, The primate ovarian cycle: suppression of human menopausal gonadotropin-induced follicular growth in the presence of the dominant follicle, *J. Clin. Endocrinol. Metab.*, 50, 819, 1980.
42. **Richards, J. S.** Hormonal control of ovarian follicular development: 1978 perspective, *Rec. Prog. Horm. Res.*, 35, 343, 1979.
43. **diZerega, G. S., Turner, C. K., Stouffer, R. L., Anderson, L. D., Channing, C. P., and Hodgen, G. D.**, Suppression of follicle-stimulating hormone-dependent folliculogenesis during the primate ovarian cycle, *J. Clin. Endocrinol. Metab.*, 52, 451, 1981.
44. **Block, E.**, Quantitative morphological investigations of the follicular system in women, *Acta Endocrinol. (Kbh).*, 8, 55, 1951.
45. **Koering, M. J.**, Cyclic changes in ovarian morphology during the menstrual cycle in *Macaca mulatta, Am. J. Anat.*, 126, 73, 1969.
46. **Zeleznik, A. J. and Resko, J. A.**, Progesterone does not inhibit gonadotropin-induced follicular maturation in the female monkey, *(Macaca mulatta), Endocrinology*, 106, 1820, 1980.
47. **Clark, J. R., Dierschke, D. J. and Wolf, R. C.**, Estrogen-induced follicular atresia in rhesus monkeys, in *Ovarian Follicular Development and Function*, Midgley, A. R. and Sadler, W. A., Eds., Raven Press, New York, 1979, 71.
48. **Lacy, L. R., Knudson, M. M., Williams, J. J., Richards, J. S., and Midgley, A. R., Jr.**, Progesterone metabolism by the ovary of the pregnant rat: discrepancies in the catabolic regulation model, *Endocrinology*, 99, 929, 1976.
49. **Morishige, W. K., Pepe, G. J., and Rothchild, I.**, Serum Luteinizing hormone, prolactin and progesterone levels during pregnancy in the rat, *Endocrinology*, 92, 1527, 1973.
50. **Linkie, D. M. and Niswender, G. D.**, Serum levels of prolactin, luteinizing hormone, and follicle stimulating hormone during pregnancy in the rat, *Endocrinology*, 90, 632, 1972.
51. **Cheng, K. W.**, Changes in rat ovaries of specific binding for LH, FSH and prolactin during the oestrous cycle and pregnancy, *J. Reprod. Fertil.*, 48, 129, 1976.
52. **Richards, J. S. and Kersey, K. A.**, Changes in theca and granulosa cell function in antral follicles developing during pregnancy in the rat: gonadotropin receptors, cyclic AMP and estradiol-17β, *Biol. Reprod.*, 21, 1185, 1979.
53. **Hoffmann, J. C. and Schwartz, N. B.**, Timing of post-partum ovulation in the rat, *Endocrinology*, 76, 620, 1965.
54. **Rebar, R. W., Nakane, P. K., and Midgley, A. R., Jr.**, Post-partum release of luteinizing hormone (LH) in the rat as determined by radioimmunoassay, *Endocrinology*, 84, 1352, 1969.
55. **Govan, A. D. T.**, The human ovary in early pregnancy, *J. Endocrinol.*, 40, 421, 1968.
56. **Govan, A. D. T.**, Ovarian follicular activity in late pregnancy *J. Endocrinol.*, 48, 235, 1970.
57. **Guraya, S. S.**, Function of the human ovary during pregnancy as revealed by histochemical, biochemical and electron microscope techniques, *Acta Endocrinol. (Kbh.).*, 69, 107, 1972.
58. **Johansson, E. D. B. and Wide, L.**, Periovulatory levels of plasma progesterone and luteinizing hormone in women, *Acta Endocrinol. (Kbh.)*, 62, 82, 1969.
59. **Dhont, M., VandeKerchkhove, D., Vermeulen, A., and Vandeweghe, M.**, Daily concentrations of plasma LH, FSH, estradiol, estrone and progesterone throughout the menstrual cycle, *Europ, J. Obstet. Gynec. Reprod. Biol.*, 4(Suppl. 1), 154, 1974.
60. **Weiss, G., Butler, W. R., Hotchkiss, J., Dierschke, D. J. and Knobil, E.**, Periparturitional serum concentrations of prolactin, the gonadotropins and the gonadal hormones in the rhesus monkey, *Proc. Soc. Exp. Biol. Med.*, 151, 113, 1976.
61. **Bosu, W. T. K. and Johansson, E. D. B.**, Ovarian morphology and the plasma levels of estrogens and progesterone in rhesus monkeys in early pregnancy, *Fertil. Steril.*, 25, 443, 1974.
62. **Chandrashekar, V., Wolf, R. C., Dierschke, D. J. Sholl, S. A., Bridson, W. E., and Clark, J. R.**, Serum progesterone and corpus luteum function in pregnant pigtailed monkeys (*Macaca nemestrina*), *Steroids*, 36, 483, 1980.
63. **Chandrashekar, V., Dierschke, D. J. and Wolf, R. C.**, Unpublished data.
64. **Marder, M. L., Channing, C. P., and Schwartz, N. B.**, Suppression of serum follicle stimulating hormone in intact and acutely ovariectomized rats by porcine follicular fluid, *Endocrinology*, 101, 1639, 1977.
65. **Schwartz, N. B. and Channing, C. P.**, Evidence for ovarian "inhibin" suppression of the secondary rise in serum follicle stimulating hormone levels in proestrous rats by injection of procine follicular fluid, *Proc. Nat. Acad. Sciences, U.S.A.*, 74, 5721, 1977.
66. **DeJong, F. H. and Sharpe, R. M.**, Evidences for inhibin-like activity in bovine follicular fluid, *Nature*, 263, 71, 1976.
67. **Chappel, S. C.**, Cyclic fluctuation in ovarian FSH-inhibiting material in golden hamsters, *Biol. Reprod.*, 21, 447, 1979.
68. **Peters, H., Byskov, A. G., and Faber, M.**, Intraovarian regulation of follicle growth in immature mouse, in *The Development and Maturation of the Ovary and its Functions*, Peters, H., Ed., Excerpta Medica, Amsterdam, 1973, 20.

69. **Miller, K. F., Critser, J. K., Rowe, R. F., and Ginther, O. J.,** Ovarian effects of bovine follicular fluid treatments in sheep and cattle, *Biol. Reprod.,* 21, 537, 1979.
70. **Channing, C. P., Anderson, L. D., and Hodgen, G. D.,** Inhibitory effect of charcoal-treated porcine follicular fluid upon serum FSH levels and follicle development in the rhesus monkey, in *Ovarian Follicular and Corpus Luteum Function,* Channing, C. P., Marsh, J., and Sadler, W., Eds., Plenum Press, New York, 1979, 407.
71. **Lorenzen, J. R., Channing, C. P., and Schwartz, N. B.,** Partial characterization of FSH suppressing activity (folliculostatin) in porcine follicular fluid using the metestrous rat as an in vivo bioassay model, *Biol. Reprod.,* 19, 635, 1978.
72. **Williams, A. T., Rush, M. E., and Lipner, H.,** Isolation and preliminary characterization of inhibin-f, in *Ovarian Follicular and Corpus Luteum Function,* Channing, C. P., Marsh, J., and Sadler, W., Eds., Plenum Press, New York, 1979, 429.
73. **Channing, C. P.,** Follicular non-steroidal regulators, in *Ovarian Follicular and Corpus Luteum Function,* Channing, C. P., Marsh, J., and Sadler, W., Eds., Plenum Press, New York, 1979, 327.
74. **Shander, D., Anderson, L. D., Barraclough, C. A., and Channing, C. P.,** Modulation of pituitary responsiveness to LHRH by porcine follicular fluid: time and dose-dependent effects, in *Ovarian Follicular and Corpus Luteum Function,* Channing, C. P., Marsh, J., and Sadler, W., Eds., Plenum Press, New York, 1979, 423.
75. **Pencharz, R. I. and Long, J. A.,** Hypophysectomy in the pregnant rat, *Am. J. Anat.,* 53, 117, 1933.
76. **Deanesly, R.,** The endocrinology of pregnancy and foetal life, in *Marshall's Physiology of Reproduction,* Vol. 3, 3rd ed., Parkes, A. S. Ed. Little, Brown and Co., Boston, 1966, 891.
77. **Raj, H. G. M. and Moudgal, N. R.,** Hormonal control of gestation in the intact rat, *Endocrinology,* 86, 874, 1970.
78. **Takayama, M. and Greenwald, G. S.,** Direct luteotropic action of estrogen in the hypophysectomized-hysterectomized rat, *Endocrinology,* 92, 1405, 1973.
79. **Rothchild, I., Billiar, R. B., Kline, I. T. and Pepe, G.,** The persistence of progesterone secretion in pregnant rats after hypophysectomy and hysterectomy: a comparison with pseudopregnant, deciduomata-bearing pseudopregnant and lactating rats, *J. Endocrinol.,* 57, 63, 1973.
80. **Morishige, W. K. and Rothchild, I.,** Temporal aspects of the regulation of corpus luteum function by luteinizing hormone, prolactin and placental luteotrophin during the first half of pregnancy in the rat, *Endocrinology,* 95, 260, 1974.
81. **Akaka, J., O'Laughlin-Phillips, E., Antczak, E., Rothchild, I.,** The relationship between the age of the corpus luteum (CL) and the luteolytic effect of an LH-antiserum (LH-AS): comparison of hysterectomized pseudopregnant rats with intact pregnant rats for their response to LH-AS treatment at four stages of CL activity, *Endocrinology,* 100, 1334, 1977.
82. **Gibori, G., Antczak, E., and Rothchild, I.,** The role of estrogen in the regulation of luteal progesterone secretion in the rat after day 12 of pregnancy, *Endocrinology,* 100, 1483, 1977.
83. **Gibori, G. and Keyes, P. L.,** Role of intraluteal estrogen in the regulation of the rat corpus luteum during pregnancy, *Endocrinology,* 102, 1176, 1978.
84. **Greenwald, G. S. and Rothchild, I.,** Formation and maintenance of corpora lutea in laboratory animals, *J. Anim. Sci.,* 27, (Suppl. 1), 139, 1968.
85. **Nalbandov, A. V.,** Comparative aspects of corpus luteum function, *Biol. Reprod.,* 2, 7, 1970.
86. **Choudary, J. B. and Greenwald, G. S.,** Reversal by gonadotrophins of the luteolytic effect of oestrogen in the cyclic guinea pig, *J. Reprod. Fertil.* 19, 503, 1969.
87. **Bland, K. P. and Donovan, B. T.,** Control of luteal function during early pregnancy in the guinea pig, *J. Reprod. Fertil.,* 20, 491, 1969.
88. **Keyes, P. L., Yuh, K. M., and Miller, J. B.,** Estrogen action in the corpus luteum, in *Ovarian Follicular and Corpus Luteum Function,* Channing C. P., Marsh, J. M., and Sadler, W. A., Ed., Plenum Press, New York, 1979, 447.
89. **Robson, J. M., Sullivan, F. M., and Wilson, C.,** The maintenance of pregnancy during the preimplantation period in mice treated with phenelzine derivatives, *J. Endocrinol.,* 49, 635, 1971.
90. **Moor, R. M.,** Effect of embryo on corpus luteum function, *J. Anim. Sci.,* 27, 97, 1968.
91. **Gemzell, C.,** Induction of ovulation in patients following removal of pituitary adenoma, *Am. J. Obstet. Gynecol.,* 117, 955, 1973.
92. **Vande Wiele, R. L., Bogumil, J., Dyrenfurth, I., Ferin, M., Jeweiewicz, R., Warren, W., Rizkallah, T., and Mikhail, G.,** Mechanisms regulating the menstrual cycle in women, *Rec. Prog. Horm. Res.,* 26, 63, 1970.
93. **Moudgal, N. R., Macdonald, G. J., and Greep, R. O.,** Role of endogenous primate LH in maintaining corpus luteum function of the monkey, *J. Clin. Endocrinol. Metab.,* 35, 113, 1972.
94. **Hwang, P., Guyda, H., and Friesen, H.,** A radioimmunoassay for human prolactin, *Proc. Nat. Acad. Sci., U.S.A.,* 68,. 1902, 1971.
95. **Butler, W. B., Krey, L. C., Lu, K. H., Peckham, W. D., and Knobil, E.,** Surgical disconnection of the medial basal hypothalamus and pituitary function in the rhesus monkey. IV. Prolactin secretion, *Endocrinology,* 96, 1099, 1975.

96. **Quadri, S. K. and Spies, H. G.**, Cyclic and diurnal patterns of serum prolactin in the rhesus monkey, *Biol. Reprod.*, 14, 495, 1976.
97. **MacDonald, G. J. and Greep, R. O.**, Ability of luteinizing hormone (LH) to acutely increase serum progesterone levels during the secretory phase of the rhesus menstrual cycle. *Fertil. Steril.*, 23, 466, 1972.
98. **Meyer, R. K., Wolf, R. C., and Arslan, M.**, Implantation and maintenance of pregnancy in progesterone-treated ovariectomized monkeys (*Macaca mulatta*), *Rec. Advan. Primatology*, 2, 30, 1969.
99. **Hodgen, G. D., Stouffer, R. L., Barber, D. L., and Nixon, W. E.**, Serum estradiol and progesterone during pregnancy and the status of the corpus luteum at delivery in cynomolgus monkeys(*Macaca fascicularis*), *Steroids*, 30, 295, 1977.
100. **Tulsky, A. S. and Koff, A. K.**, Some observations on the role of the corpus luteum in early human pregnancy, *Fertil. Steril.*, 8, 118, 1957.
101. **Treloar, O. L., Wolf, R. C., and Meyer, R. K.**, The corpus luteum of the rhesus monkey during late pregnancy, *Endocrinology*, 91, 665, 1972.
102. **Koering, M. J., Wolf, R. C., and Meyer, R. K.**, Morphological and functional evidence for corpus luteum activity during late pregnancy in the rhesus monkey, *Endocrinology*, 93, 686, 1973.
103. **LeMaire, W. J., Conly, P. W., Moffett, A., and Cleveland, W. W.**, Plasma progesterone secretion by the corpus luteum of term pregnancy, *Am. J. Obstet. Gynecol.*, 108, 132, 1970.
104. **Melinkoff, E.**, Questionable necessity of the corpus luteum, *Am. J. Obstet. Gynecol.*, 60, 437, 1950.
105. **Tullner, W. W. and Hertz, R.**, Normal gestation and chorionic gonadotropin levels in the monkey after ovariectomy in early pregnancy, *Endocrinology*, 78, 1076, 1966.
106. **Neill, J. D., Johansson, E. D. B., and Knobil, E.**, Patterns of circulating progesterone concentrations during the fertile menstrual cycle and the remainder of gestation in the rhesus monkey, *Endocrinology*, 84, 45, 1969.
107. **Atkinson, L. E., Hotchkiss, J., Fritz, G. R., Surve, A. H., Neill, J. D., and Knobil, E.**, Circulating levels of steroids and chorionic gonadotropin during pregnancy in the rhesus monkey, with special attention to the rescue of the corpus luteum in early pregnancy, *Biol. Reprod.*, 12, 335, 1975.
108. **Chandrashekar, V., Meyer, R., Bridson, W. E. and Wolf, R. C.**, Circulating levels of chorionic gonadotropin and progesterone in the rhesus monkey treated with LH antiserum during early gestation, *Biol. Reprod.*, 20, 889, 1979.
109. **Sundaram, K., Chang, C. C., Laurence, K. A., Brinson, A. O., Atkinson, L. E., Segal, S. J., and Ward, D. N.**, The effectiveness in rhesus monkey of an antifertility vaccine based on neutralization of chorionic gonadotropin, *Contraception*, 14, 639, 1976.
110. **Hobson, W., Faiman, C., Dougherty, W. J., Reyes, F. I., and Winter, J. S. D.**, Radioimmunoassay of rhesus monkey chorionic gonadotropin, *Fertil. Steril.*, 26, 93, 1975.
111. **Hodgen, G. D., Niemann, W. H., and Tullner, W. W.**, Duration of chorionic gonadotropin production by placenta of the rhesus monkey, *Endocrinology*, 96, 789, 1975.
112. **Walsh, S. W., Wolf, R. C., Meyer, R. K., Aubert, M. L., and Friesen, H. G.**, Chorionic gonadotropin, Chorionic somatomammotropin and prolactin in the uterine vein and peripheral plasma of pregnant rhesus monkeys, *Endocrinology*, 100, 851, 1977.
113. **Walsh, S. W., Meyer, R. K., Wolf, R. C., and Friesen, H. G.**, Corpus luteum and fetoplacental functions in monkeys hypophysectomized during late pregnancy, *Endocrinology*, 100, 845, 1977.
114. **Braunstein, G. D., Rosor, J., Adler, D., Danzer, H., and Wade, M. E.**, Serum human chorionic gonadotropin levels throughout normal pregnancy, *Am. J. Obstet. Gynecol.*, 126, 678, 1976.
115. **Heap, R. B., Perry, J. S., and Rowlands, I. W.**, Corpus luteum function in the guinea-pig; arterial and luteal progesterone levels and the effects of hysterectomy and hypophysectomy, *J. Reprod. Fertil.*, 13, 537, 1967.
116. **Donavan, B. T.**, The control of ovarian function, *Acta Endocrinol. (Kbh).*, 66, 1, 1971.
117. **Caldwell, B. V., Mazer, R. S., and Wright, P. A.**, Luteolysis as affected by uterine transplantation in the Syrian hamster, *Endocrinology*, 80, 477, 1967.
118. **Orsini, M. W.**, Effect of hysterectomy on hamster corpora lutea, *Anat. Record.*, 163, 238, 1969.
119. **Pharriss, B. B., Tillson, S. A., and Erickson, R. R.**, Prostaglandins in luteal function, *Rec. Prog. Horm. Res.*, 28, 51, 1972.
120. **Anderson, L. L.**, Effects of hysterectomy and other factors on luteal function, in *Handbook of Physiology, Section 7*, Vol. 2 (Part 2), Greep, R. O. and Astwood, E. B., Eds., American Physiological Society, Washington, D.C., 1973, 69.
121. **Anderson, L. L., Neal, F. C., and Melampy, R. M.**, Hysterectomy and ovarian function in beef heifers, *Am. J. Vet. Res.*, 23, 794, 1962.
122. **Malven, P. V. and Hansel, W.**, Ovarian function in dairy heifers following hysterectomy, *J. Dairy Sci.*, 47, 1388, 1964.
123. **Anderson, L. L., Butcher, R. L., and Melampy, R. M.**, Subtotal hysterectomy and ovarian function in gilts, *Endocrinology*, 69, 571, 1961.

124. **Belt, W. D., Cavazos, L. F., Anderson, L. L., and Kraeling, R. R.**, Fine structure and progesterone levels in the corpus luteum of the pig during pregnancy and after hysterectomy, *Biol. Reprod.*, 2, 98, 1970.
125. **Kiracofe, G. H. and Spies, H. G.**, Length of maintenance of naturally formed and experimentally induced corpora lutea in hysterectomized ewes, *J. Reprod. Fertil.*, 11, 275, 1966.
126. **Moor, R. M., Hay, M. F., Short, R. V., and Rowson, L. E. A.**, The corpus luteum of the sheep: effect of uterine removal during luteal regression, *J. Reprod. Fertil.*, 21, 539, 1970.
127. **Neill, J. D., Johansson, E. D. B., and Knobil, E.**, Failure of hysterectomy to influence the normal pattern of cyclic progesterone secretion in the rhesus monkey, *Endocrinology*, 84, 464, 1969.
128. **Beling, C. G., Marcus, S. L., and Markham, S. M.**, Functional activity of the corpus luteum following hysterectomy, *J. Clin. Endocrinol. Metab.*, 30, 30, 1970.
129. **Behrman, H. R.**, Prostaglandins in hypothalamo-pituitary and ovarian function, *Ann. Rev. Physiol.*, 41, 685, 1979.
130. **McCracken, J. A., Carlson, J. C., Glew, M. C., Goding, J. R., Baird, D. T., Green, K., and Samuelson, B.**, Prostaglandin $F_{2\alpha}$ identified as a luteolytic hormone in the sheep, *Nat. N. Biol.*, 238, 129, 1972.
131. **Hansel, W., Concannon, P. W., and Kukaszewska, J. H.**, Corpora lutea of the large domestic animals, *Biol. Reprod.*, 8, 222, 1973.
132. **Wilson, L., Jr., Cenedella, R. J., Butcher, R. L., and Inskeep, E. K.**, Levels of prostaglandins in the uterine endometrium during the ovine estrous cycle, *J. Anim. Sci.*, 34, 93, 1972.
133. **Guthrie, H. D., Rexrod, C. E. Jr., and Bolt, D. J.**, *In vitro* release of progesterone and prostaglandin F and E by porcine luteal and endometrial tissue during induced luteolysis, in *Ovarian Follicular and Corpus Luteum Function*, Channing, C. P., Marsh, J. M., and Sadler, W. A., Eds., Plenum Press, New York, 1979, 627.
134. **Labhsetwar, A.**, Do prostaglandins stimulate LH release and thereby cause luteolysis?, *Prostaglandins*, 3, 729, 1973.
135. **Grinwich, D. L., Ham, E. A., Hichens, M., and Behrman, H. R.**, Binding of human chorionic gonadotropin and response of cyclic nucleotides to luteinizing hormone in luteal tissue from rats treated with prostaglandin $F_{2\alpha}$, *Endocrinology*, 98, 146, 1976.
136. **Grinwich, D. L., Hichens, M., and H. R. Behrman.**, Control of the LH receptor by prolactin and prostaglandin $F_{2\alpha}$ in rat corpora lutea, *Biol. Reprod.*, 14, 212, 1976.
137. **Choudary, J. B. and Greenwald, G. S.**, Luteolytic effect of oestrogen on the corpora lutea of the cyclic guinea-pig, *J. Reprod. Fertil.*, 16, 333, 1968.
138. **Wiltbank, J. N.**, Modification of ovarian activity in the bovine following injection of oestrogen and gonadotrophin, *J. Reprod. Fertil.*, Suppl. 1, 1, 1966.
139. **Stormshak, F., Kelley, H. E., and Hawk, H. W.**, Suppression of ovine luteal function by 17β-estradiol, *J. Anim. Sci.*, 29, 476, 1969.
140. **Auletta, F. J., Cadwell, B. V., vanWagenen, G., and Morris, J. M.**, Effects of postovulatory estrogen on progesterone and prostaglandin F levels in the monkey, *Contraception*, 6, 411, 1972.
141. **Johansson, E. D. B.**, Inhibition of the corpus luteum function in women taking large doses of diethylstilbestrol, *Contraception*, 8, 27, 1973.
142. **Gore, B. Z., Cadwell, B. V., and Speroff, L.**, Estrogen-induced human luteolysis, *J. Clin. Endocrinol. Metab.*, 36, 615, 1973.
143. **Karsch, F. J., Krey, L. C., Weick, R. W., Dierschke, D. J., and Knobil, E.**, Functional luteolysis in the rhesus monkey: the role of estrogen, *Endocrinology*, 92, 1148, 1973.
144. **Hoffmann, F.**, Untersuchungen uber die hormonale beeinflussung der lebensdauer des Corpus luteum in zyklus der frau, Geburtsh. *Frauenheilk.*, 20, 1153, 1960.
145. **Karsch , F. J., and Sutton, G. P.**, An intra-ovarian site for the luteolytic action of estrogen in the rhesus monkey , *Endocrinology*, 98, 553, 1976.
146. **Hashimoto, I., Henricks, D. M., Anderson, L. L., and Melampy, R. M.**, Progesterone and pregn-4-en-20α-01-3-one in ovarian venous blood during various reproductive states in the rat, *Endocrinology*, 82, 333, 1968.
147. **Hilliard, J., Spies, H. G., and Sawyer, C. H.**, Hormonal factors regulating ovarian cholesterol mobilization and progestin secretion in intact and hypophysectomized rabbits, in *The Gonads*, McKerns, K. W., Ed., Appleton-Century-Crofts, New York, 1969, 55.
148. **Wiest, W. G., Kidwell, W. R., and Balogh, K. Jr.**, Progesterone catabolism in the rat ovary: a regulatory mechanism for progestational potency during pregnancy, *Endocrinology*, 82, 844, 1968.
149. **Strauss, J. F. III , Foley, B., and Strambaugh, R.**, 20α-hydroxysteroid dehydrogenase activity in the rabbit ovary, *Biol. Reprod.*, 6, 78, 1972.
150. **Talbert, G. B.**, Effect of maternal age on reproductive capacity, *Am. J. Obstet. Gynecol.*, 102, 451, 1968.
151. **Huang, H. H. and Meites, J.**, Reproductive capacity of aging female rats, *Neuroendocrinology*, 17, 289, 1975.

152. **Aschheim, P.**, Aging in the hypothalamic-hypophyseal-ovarian-axis in the rat, in *Hypothalamus, Pituitary and Aging,* Everitt, A. V., and Burgess, Eds., Charles C Thomas, Springfield, Mass., 1976, 376.
153. **Miller, A. E., Wood, S. M., and Riegle, G. D.**, The effect of age on reproduction in repeatedly mated female rats, *J. Gerontol.,* 34, 15, 1979.
154. **Meites, J. Huang, H. H., and Simpkins, J. W.**, Recent studies in neuroendocrine control of reproductive senescence in rats, in *The Aging Reproductive System,* Schneider, E. L., Ed., Raven Press, New York, 1978, 213.
155. **Peng, M. T. and Huang, H. H.**, Aging of hypothalamic-pituitary-ovarian function in the rat, *Fertil. Steril.,* 23, 535, 1972.
156. **Howland, B. E. and Preiss, C**, Effects of aging on basal levels of serum gonadotropins, ovarian compensatory hypertrophy and hypersecretion of gonadotropins after ovariectomy in female rats, *Fertil. Steril.,* 26, 271, 1975.
157. **Huang, H. H., Marshall, S. S., and Meites, J.**, Capacity of old versus young female rats to secrete LH, FSH, and prolactin, *Biol. Reprod.,* 14, 538, 1976.
158. **McPherson, J. C., Costoff, A., and Mahesh, V. B.**, Effect of aging on the hypothalamic-hypophyseal-gonadal axis in female rats, *Fertil. Steril.,* 28, 1365, 1977.
159. **Clemens, J. A. Amenomori, Y., Jenkins, T., and Meites, J.**, Effects of hypothalamic stimulation, hormones and drugs on ovarian function in old female rats, *Proc. Soc. Exp. Biol. Med.,* 132, 561, 1969.
160. **Quadri, S. K., Kledzik, G. S., and Meites, J.**, Reinitiation of estrous cycles in old constant estrous rats by central acting drugs, *Neuroendocrinology,* 11, 807, 1973.
161. **Kamberi, I. A.**, Role of brain neurotransmitters in the secretion of hypothalamo-pituitary-gonadal principles, in *Neuroendocrine Regulation of Fertility,* Ananda Kumar, T. C., Ed., S. Karger, Basel, 141, 1976.
162. **Kalra, P. S., Kalra, S. P., Krulich, L., Fawcett, C. P., and McCann, S. M.**, Involvement of norepinephrine in transmission of the stimulatory influence of progesterone on gonadotropin release, *Endocrinology,* 90, 1168, 1972.
163. **Mandl, A. M. and Shelton, M.**, A quantitative study of oocytes in young and old nulliparous laboratory rats, *J. Endocrinol.,* 18, 444, 1959.
164. **Blaha, G. C. and Leavitt, W. W.**, Ovarian steroid dehydrogenase histochemistry and circulating progesterone in aged golden hamsters during the estrous cycle and pregnancy, *Biol. Reprod.,* 11, 153, 1974.
165. **Leathem, J. H. and Murono, E. P.**, Ovarian Δ^5-3β-hydroxysteroid dehydrogenase in aging rats, *Fertil. Steril.,* 26, 996, 1975.
166. **Miller, A. E. and Riegle, G. D.**, Temporal changes in serum progesterone in aging female rats, *Endocrinology,* 106, 1579, 1980.
167. **Sherman, B. M. and Korenman, S. G.**, Hormonal Characteristics of the human menstrual cycle throughout reproductive life, *J. Clin. Invest.,* 55, 699, 1975.
168. **Sherman, B.M., West, J. H., and Korenman, S. G.**, The menopausal transition: analysis of LH, FSH, estradiol and progesterone concentrations during menstrual cycles of older women, *J. Clin. Endocrinol. Metab.,* 42, 629, 1976.
169. **Block, E.**, Quantitative morphological investigation of follicular system in women, *Acta Anat.,* 14, 108, 1952.
170. **Costoff, A. and Mahesh, V. B.**, Primordial follicles with normal oocytes in the ovaries of postmenopausal women, *J. Am. Geriat. Soc.,* 23, 193, 1975.
171. **Greenblatt, R. B., Colle, M. L., and Mahesh, V. B.**, Ovarian and adrenal steroid production in the postmenopausal women. *Obstet. Gynecol.,* 47, 383, 1976.
172. **Wise, A. J., Gross, M. A., and Schlach, D. S.**, Quantitative relationships of the pituitary-gonadal axis in postmenopausal women, *J. Lab. Clin. Med.,* 81, 28, 1973.
173. **Yen, S. S. C., Martin, P. L. Burnier, A. M., Czekala, N. M., Greaney, M. O., and Callantine, M. R.**, Circulating estradiol, estrone and gonadotropin levels following administration of orally active 17β-estradiol in postmenopausal women, *J. Clin. Endocrinol. Metab.,* 40, 518, 1975.
174. **Reyes, F. I., Winter, J. S. D., and Faiman, C.**, Pituitary-ovarian relationships preceding the menopause. I. A cross-sectional study of serum follicle-stimulating hormone, luteinizing hormone, prolactin, estradiol and progesterone levels, *Am. J. Obstet. Gynecol.,* 129, 557, 1977.
175. **Mattingly, R. F. and Huang, W. Y.**, Steroidogenesis of the menopausal and postmenopausal ovary, *Am. J. Obstet. Gynecol.,* 103, 679, 1969.
176. **Monroe, S. E. and Menon, K. M. J.**, Changes in reproductive hormone secretion during the climacteric and postmenopausal periods, *Clin. Obstet. Gynecol.,* 20, 113, 1977.
177. **Judd, H. L., Judd, G. E., Lucas, W. E., and Yen, S. S. C.**, Endocrine function of the postmenopausal ovary: concentration of androgens in ovarian and peripheral vein blood, *J. Clin. Endocrinol. Metab.,* 39, 1020, 1974.

178. **Wortmann, W., Schenker, J., Wortmann, B., and Touchstone, J. C.,** Different aromatisation of ^{3}H-androstenedione in pre- and postmenopausal rhesus monkey ovaries, *Acta Endocrinol. (Kbh.).*, Suppl. 193, 60, 1975.
179. **Hodgen, G. D., Goodman, A. L., O'Connor, A., and Johnson, D. K.,** Menopause in rhesus monkeys: model for study of disorders in the human climacteric, *Am. J. Obstet. Gynecol.*, 127, 581, 1977.
180. **Tsai, C. C. and Yen, S. S. C.,** Acute effects of intravenous infusion of 17β-estradiol on gonadotropin release in pre- and postmenopausal women, *J. Clin. Endocrinol. Metab.*, 32, 766, 1971.
181. **Wise, A. J., Gross, M. A., and Schlach, D. S.,** Quantitative relationships of the pituitary-gonadal axis in postmenopausal women, *J. Lab. Clin. Med.*, 81, 28, 1973.
182. **Odell, W. D. and Swerdloff, R. S.,** Progestogen-induced luteinizing and follicle stimulating hormone surge in postmenopausal women: a stimulated ovulatory peak, *Proc. Nat. Acad. Sci. U.S.A.*, 61, 529, 1968.

THE TESTIS

Werner Leidl, Ulrich Braun, Joachim Braun, and Gerburg Buck

MORPHOLOGY AND FUNCTION

Developmental Aspects

Indifferent Stage and Sexual Differentiation

There is no morphologic difference between male and female individuals during the first stages of embryonic life. The testes as well as the ovaries develop from the genital ridge, a thickening at the medioventral side of the mesonephros. Primordial germ cells, originating from the yolk sac, invade the epithelium, which is later called germinal epithelium. Multiple invaginations of the germinal epithelium occur, forming the epithelial cords. The gonads become more compact and increase in size.[1] At this stage, sex differentiaton is initiated. The Y chromosome is responsible for the formation of the H-Y antigen, which determines the indifferent embryonic gonad to become a testis.[2]

The epithelial cords develop into seminiferous tubules. The tubules have a few germ cells in the center and a peripheral layer of supporting cells, which are the precursors of the Sertoli cells. The tubules remain in this stage without major changes until puberty.[3] Specialized mesenchymal cells in the connective tissue between the seminiferous tubules differentiate to interstitial cells called Leydig cells. These cells increase in size and number. Their maximum development is reached during fetal life and thereafter they regress to a certain extent.

Descent of the Testis

A rather unique aspect of the development of the testis in most mammals is the migration from its intraabdominal location to the extraabdominal site in the scrotum. This descent of the testis is achieved by several mechanisms. The posterior ligament of the testis, the gubernaculum testis, draws the testis to the ventral body wall. The increasing volume of the abdominal organs presses the testis towards the inguinal canal. The gubernaculum, which is connected to the newly formed processus vaginalis, draws the testis into the canal. Finally, the passage through the inguinal canal is achieved by contraction of the inguinal ring, by pressure from the abdominal cavity and pulling by the gubernaculum.

The descent of the testis is completed before or shortly after birth in most mammals, including man. Hormonal factors are involved in the descent, but no clear hormonal regulation has been defined.[4] Nevertheless, in individuals with certain forms of maldescended testis, therapy includes human chorionic gonadotropin (HCG) to bring the testis down into the scrotum.[5]

Testis

Location

In most mammals, the testes are located outside of the abdomen in the scrotum, either periodically during the time of reproductive activity, e.g., some seasonal breeders, or constantly, e.g., domestic mammals and man. The position of the scrotum in relation to the abdomen shows considerable species variation.

Blood and Nerve Supply

The testis is supplied with blood by the internal spermatic artery, which arises from the abdominal aorta. The artery runs directly into the testis and branches there in

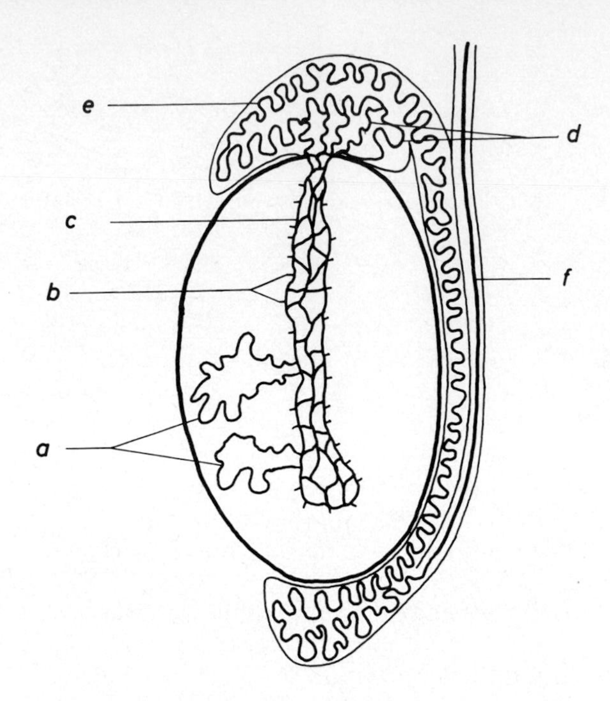

FIGURE 1. The efferent duct system of the testis and the epididymis (schematic): a. seminiferous tubules; b. tubuli recti; c. rete testis; d. ductuli efferentes; e. ductus epididymidis; f. ductus deferens.

animals with abdominal testes. In animals with scrotal testes, the artery runs along the body wall, passes through the inguinal canal and coils before it reaches the testicular surface. The veins leaving the testis form the pampiniform plexus, which surrounds the coils of the artery.

The nerve supply is derived from the superior spermatic nerve of lumbosacral origin and consists mainly of sympathetic fibers. The nerves follow the spermatic arteries to the surface of the testis, where they branch into the testicular parenchyma. Intact nerve supply is important, as denervation causes dilatation of testicular blood vessels and degeneration of germ cells in the seminiferous tubules.[6]

Function of the Scrotum

The scrotum is part of a temperature regulating mechanism, maintaining the temperature of the gonads several degrees lower than that of the body. This is important because in species with a scrotum, spermatogenesis is particularly sensitive to temperature.[7] Additional parts of this temperature controlling system are the venous pampiniform plexus (acting as a counter-current cooler), the smooth muscle fibers in the skin of the scrotum and the external cremaster muscle.

Structure of the Testis

The testis has an ovoid shape and is encased by a tough capsule, the tunica albuginea. There are relatively few blood vessels and smooth muscle fibers in the tunica albuginea. The testicular parenchyma consists mainly of the seminiferous tubules which are cylindrical, highly convoluted and densely packed, leaving only small interstitial spaces. The spermatozoa are produced inside the seminiferous tubules. Usually both ends of the tubules open into the rete testis via the short tubuli recti (Figure 1).

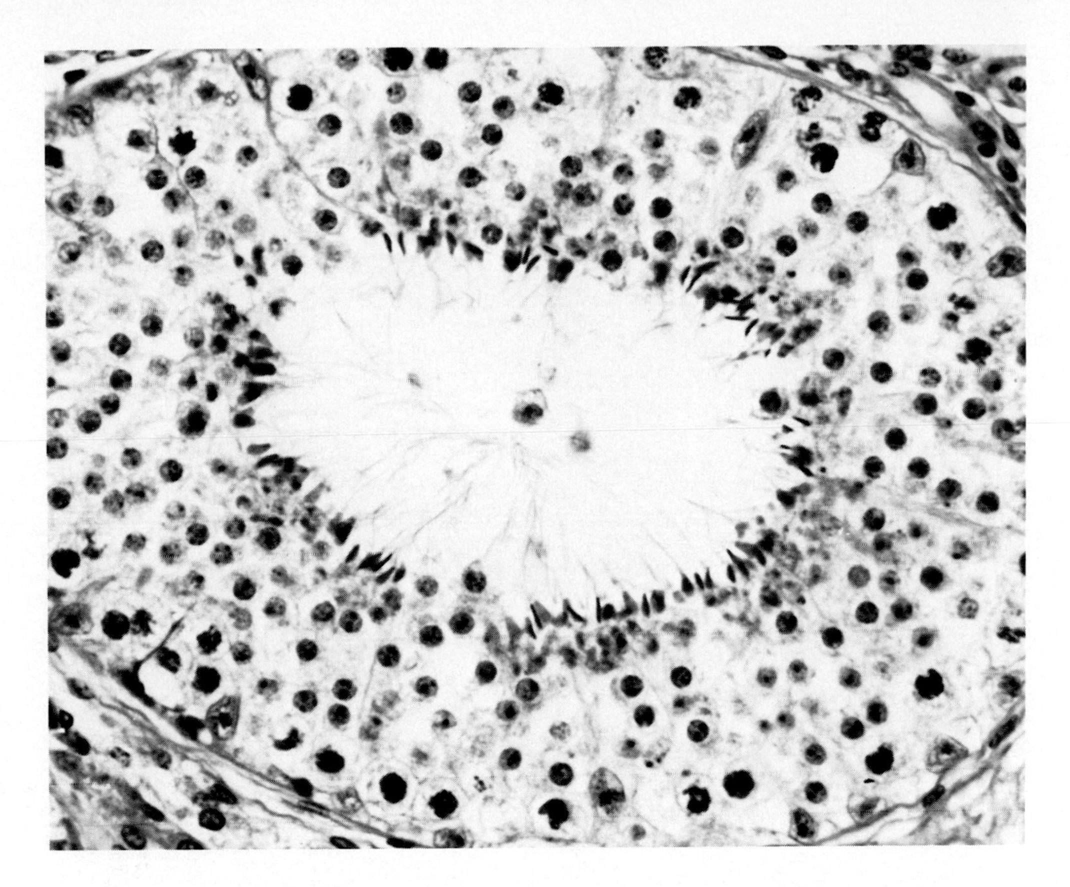

FIGURE 2. Cross section of seminiferous tubules in the bull.

Seminiferous Tubules

Inside the tubules, there are somatic cells called Sertoli cells and also germinal cells in various stages of maturation (Figure 2). The Sertoli cells lie immediately inside the tubule wall, their cytoplasm extending from the tubule wall to the lumen. They are diploid and do not divide after puberty.

The remaining space between the tubule wall and the lumen is occupied by the germinal cells, the spermatogonia along the tubule wall and the more mature germ cells towards the lumen. In the final stages of the maturation process, they are embedded in the luminal cytoplasm of the Sertoli cells. The Sertoli cells are therefore thought to have a nutritive function. They are involved in fluid secretion into the tubules, phagocytosis, maturation, release of spermatozoa, and in the synthesis of the intratubular androgen-binding protein, which is under the control of FSH and testosterone.[8] Inhibin may be produced by the Sertoli cells.[9]

It is presumed that the mature germ cells, the spermatozoa, are carried to the rete testis by the tubular fluid after they are liberated from the Sertoli cells.

Interstitial Tissue

The interstitial tissue occupies the space between the seminiferous tubules (Figure 3). It consists of connective tissue, blood and lymph vessels, nerves, and the interstitial cells (Leydig cells). Depending on the Leydig cell content, the amount of interstitial tissue in relation to total testicular volume varies from about 10% in the rat to about 60% in the boar.[10]

The Leydig cells are relatively large, polyhedral epitheloid cells. They are the main production site for steroid hormones in the testis.[11] In most adult mammals, including

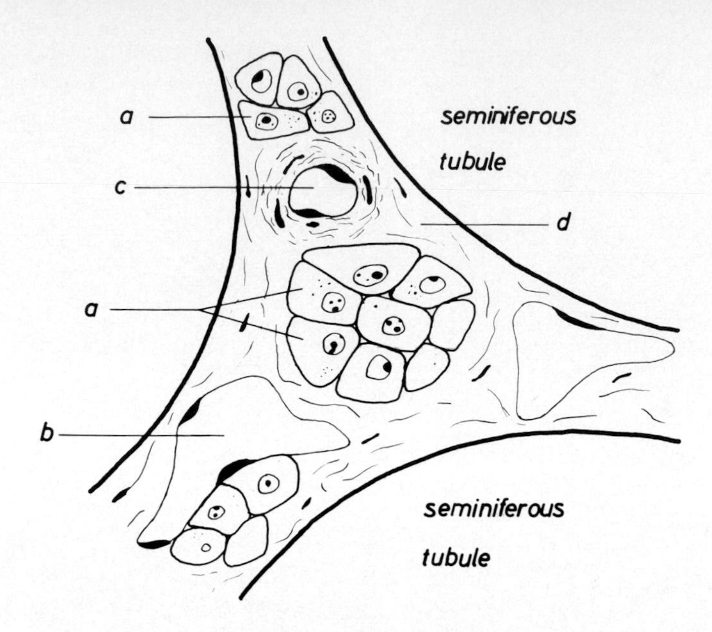

FIGURE 3. The interstitial tissue (schematic): a. Leydig cells; b. lymphatic sinusoid; c. artery; d. connective tissue.

man, the Leydig cells are arranged in clusters, with many junctions between the cells. They are rich in smooth endoplasmatic reticulum and mitochondria. Both contain enzymes necessary for steroidogeneis.[12] It is not known how testosterone from the Leydig cells is transported into the blood.

The development and differentiation of new generations of Leydig cells begin between birth and puberty. The main source of new Leydig cells seems to be mesenchymal or fibroblastic cells, since cellular division of Leydig cells is rarely found. In old age, Leydig cells may become less numerous and somewhat irregular in their appearance.[13]

Spermatogenesis

The spermatogenic process is a series of complex cellular changes, which results in the formation of the male haploid gamete, the spermatozoon.[14] Sperm cells are produced continuously from puberty to senescence.

During spermatogenesis, four basic cell types can be recognized: the spermatogonia, the spermatocytes (primary and secondary), the spermatids, and the spermatozoa (Figure 4). Spermatogonia multiply by mitotic division. The last generation produces the primary spermatocytes. DNA is synthesized for the last time during spermatogenesis by these primary spermatocytes. The first meiotic division results in secondary spermatocytes.

The second meiotic division gives rise to the spermatids which undergo a transformation leading to the mature sperm cells with their characteristic form.

Spermatogenesis follows principally the same rules in all mammals, including man. Since the division and the transformation of cells during the spermatogenesis are well coordinated, the germ cells are always found in special associations. The associations may be classified into stages, according to all cells of an association or according to the characteristics of the acrosome of the spermatids only. At any one part of a tubule, spermatogenesis goes through all stages until the initial association reappears. A complete set of cell associations forms the germinal epithelial cycle. The duration of the germinal epithelial cycle is species specific, e.g., 16 days in man,[15] 13 days in the bull,[16] 10 days in the ram,[16] 8.6 days in the boar,[17] and 12 days in the rat.[18]

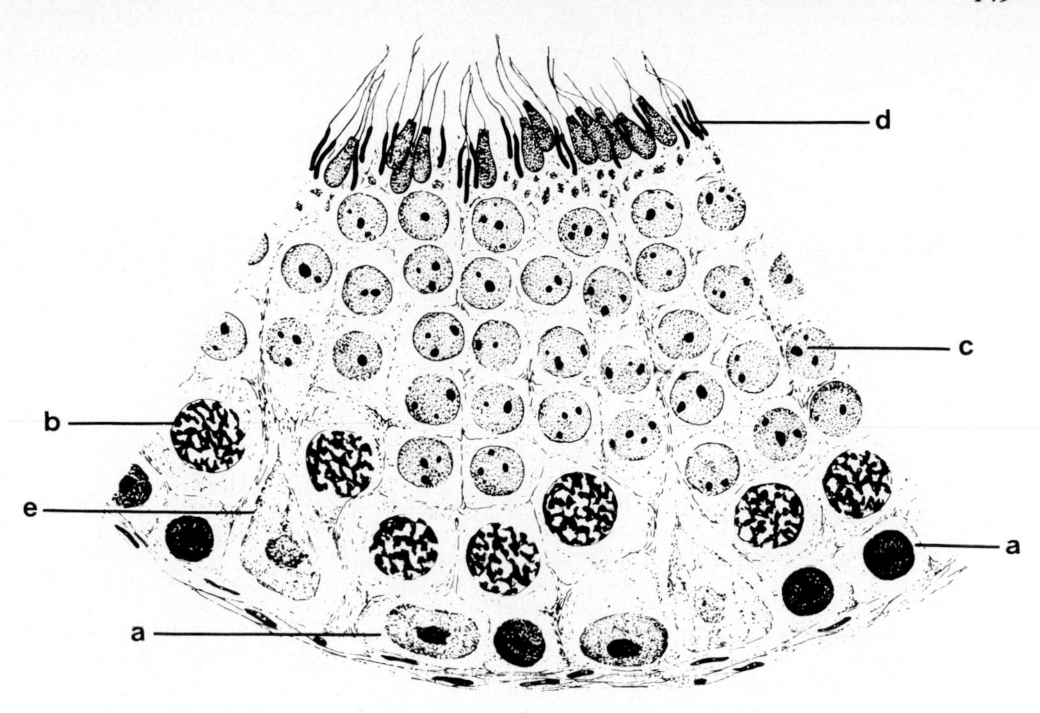

FIGURE 4. Spermatogenesis in the bull (schematic): a. spermatogonia; b. spermatocytes; c. spermatids; d. spermatozoa; e. Sertoli cells.

In most mammals, large parts of the tubule walls are covered by cells in the same stage of the germinal epithelial cycle, but in man one stage covers only a relatively small area. Therefore, cross sections of seminiferous tubules in mammals, other than man, show a regular pattern.

Epididymis

Structure

Firmly connected to the testis is the epididymis, a compact organ consisting of a single extremely convoluted duct (see Figure 1). The efferent ducts from the rete testis leave the gonad and join to form the epididymal duct. The first part of the epididymis, the head, is attached to the cranial pole of the testis. The elongated body of the epididymis extends to the caudal pole of the testis, where the rather prominent tail is formed. The deferent duct arises from the tail of the epididymis and through it the spermatozoa are expelled at ejaculation. The ductus deferens connects the epididymis with the urethra.

Function

The epididymis fulfills three main functions. One is the reabsorption of most of the fluid leaving the rete testis. This takes place in the first part of the epididymis, which is furnished with a resorptive epithelium. The spermatozoan suspension leaving the testis becomes concentrated during passage through the epididymis.[19]

The second function of the epididymis concerns sperm maturation. Morphologic changes of the sperm cells have been described, e.g., migration and detachment of the cytoplasmic droplets, then modifications of the acrosome and of the sperm plasma membrane.[20] The spermatozoa become motile and potentially fertile during their passage through the epididymis.

The third function is the storage of spermatozoa in the tail of the epididymis.

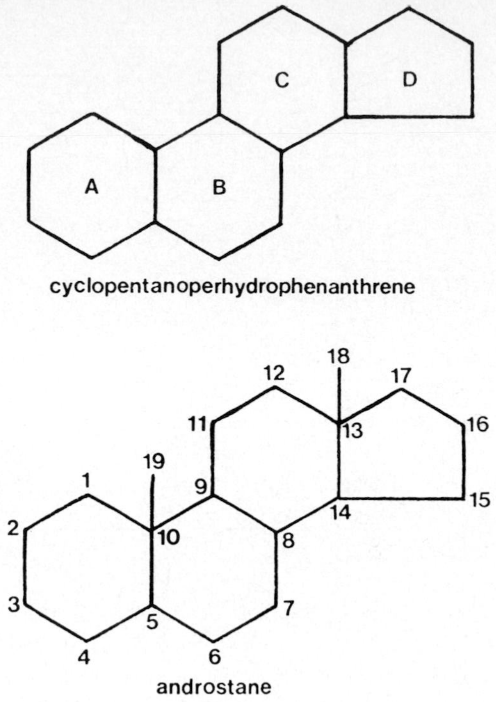

cyclopentanoperhydrophenanthrene

androstane

FIGURE 5. Basic structure of androgens.

HORMONES OF THE TESTIS

Introduction

One of the first experiments in endocrinology was performed by Berthold in 1849.[21] He demonstrated that castration of the cock was followed by regression of the comb and that the size of the comb was maintained after transplantation of the testes to a new site. Interest in steroid compounds developed in the 1920s and 1930s, when a series of steroids with androgenic activity was isolated. In 1935, testosterone was isolated[22] and synthesized.[23,24]

Considerable progress has been made in elucidating the mechanism of action of androgens as specified methods for measuring androgens became available. It is also known that there are other hormones of testicular origin besides the androgens.

Androgens

Biochemistry of Androgens

Basic Structure

All steroid hormones have a common cyclopentanoperhydrophenanthrene nucleus (Figure 5). This is a completely reduced structure with 17 carbon atoms arranged in three six-membered rings (A, B, and C) and a five-membered ring (D). Androgens are named systematically by reference to a parent structure, androstane, a steroid with methyl groups (CH_3) on carbon atoms 10 and 13 (Figure 5). Naturally occurring androgens possess additional substitutions on carbon atoms 3 and 17 in the form of a hydroxy (OH) or oxy (=O) group.

The formula of a steroid hormone cannot adequately represent its structure because the carbon atoms are oriented in space in the so-called chair form and the substituents may be above the ring (β-form) or below the ring (α-form). The conformation determines the relative physiologic activities of androgens on target organs.[25]

Cholesterol Synthesis

All steroid hormones, including androgens, are derived from cholesterol.

Cholesterol production is located mainly in the liver and to a certain degree in the gastro-intestinal tract and the testis. Cholesterol is synthesized from acetyl-CoA, either derived from the blood or formed during metabolism of glucose. Synthesis is thought to occur primarily in the smooth endoplasmic reticulum.

The first step during biosynthesis of cholesterol is the formation of a C_6-compound, mevalonic acid, from three molecules of acetyl-CoA. Coupling of six molecules of mevalonic acid produces the C_{30}-hydrocarbon squalene, which is transformed by cyclization to lanosterol, the first cyclic cholesterol precursor. Cholesterol is formed after removal of three methyl groups.[26]

Cholesterol for androgen production comes from the blood and from synthesis in the testis. The contribution of each source differs from species to species. By feeding ^{14}C-cholesterol the contribution of plasma cholesterol to the production of testicular androgens is found to be 13% in the guinea-pig[27] and approximately 40% in the rat.[28] In vitro incorporation of ^{14}C-acetate into testosterone occurs in rabbit but not in rat testis.[29,30] These findings suggest that the relative contributions of testicular and plasma cholesterol to the synthesis of androgens may also vary under different conditions.

Conversion of Cholesterol to Pregnenolone

The conversion of cholesterol to pregnenolone is referred to as the "side-chain cleavage of cholesterol" (Figure 6). It is thought that cholesterol is hydroxylated first at C_{20} or C_{22}. In both cases the resulting compound is hydroxylated further to form 20α,22-dihydroxy-cholesterol. The side-chain is then cleaved between C_{20} and C_{22}, producing the side-chain fragment isocaproic aldehyde and the C_{21}-steroid pregnenolone. This process requires cytochrome P-450, NADPH, and oxygen and occurs in the mitochondria of the Leydig cells.[31]

The conversion of cholesterol to pregnenolone appears to be the site of action of LH on steroidogenesis.[32] The LH-molecule activates adenylate cyclase to form cAMP from ATP. There are several ways by which cAMP may influence the transformation of cholesterol to pregnenolone, via an increase of a cofactor such as NADPH, transport of cholesterol into the mitochondria, or by enhancing the transport of an end-product inhibitor, such as pregnenolone, out of the mitochondria.[33]

Conversion of Pregnenolone to Testosterone

The conversion of pregnenolone, a key intermediate compound in steroidogenesis, to androgens takes place in the smooth endoplasmic reticulum of Leydig cells. There are several alternative pathways from pregnenolone to testosterone. The preferred pathway may vary from species to species.

Two principal pathways have been discovered. One involves 5-en-3β-hydroxysteroid metabolites and is called the "5-en-3-hydroxy" pathway. The other involves 4-en-3-oxosteroid metabolites and is called the "4-en-3-oxo" pathway. These pathways are also referred to as the Δ^5 and Δ^4 pathways, respectively. Both require the same three enzymes, 17α-hydroxylase, C_{17}-C_{20}-lyase, and 17β-hydroxy-steroid dehydrogenase. Isomerization from the "5-en-3-hydroxy" to the "4-en-3-oxo" pathway can take place at any stage of the reaction and requires 3β-hydroxysteroid dehydrogenase and hydroxysteroid isomerase (Figure 7).[34,35]

Secretion, Transport and Catabolism of Androgens

Androgens are released from the testes into the seminiferous tubules, into the testicular lymph, and via the bloodstream to the rest of the body. The concentration of androgens in the lymph and in the rete testis fluid is higher than in the spermatic

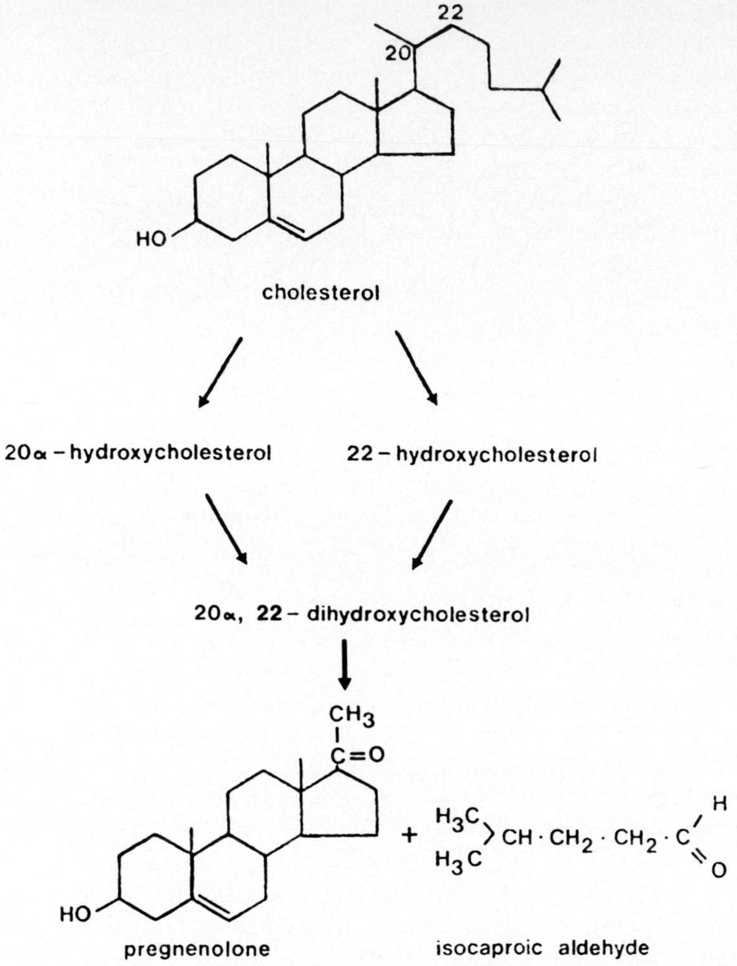

22

20

HO

cholesterol

20α – hydroxycholesterol

22 – hydroxycholesterol

20α, 22 – dihydroxycholesterol

CH_3

C=O

HO

+ H_3C H_3C > $CH \cdot CH_2 \cdot CH_2 \cdot C$ H O

pregnenolone

isocaproic aldehyde

FIGURE 6. Conversion of cholesterol to pregnenolone. (Modified from Gower, D. B., *Biochemistry of Steroid Hormones*, Makin, H. L. J., Ed., Blackwell Scientific, Oxford, 1975, 47.)

venous blood. However, the flow rate of blood exceeds that of the other fluids mentioned above by approximately a hundredfold. Therefore, the major portion of androgens leaves the testis via the spermatic venous blood.

The concentration of testosterone in peripheral blood in different species such as man, monkey, dog, rat, rabbit, ram, bull, and boar is 2 to 5 ng/mℓ.[36] Testosterone concentrations in peripheral blood show a circadian rhythm, with the lowest concentrations around midnight and the highest values in the morning. This can be demonstrated in man,[37] rhesus monkey,[38] pig,[39] and horse.[40] In other species such as the bull[41] and the ram,[42] there are irregular fluctuations of testosterone concentration, but no consistent diurnal rhythm.

Testosterone is transported in the blood plasma attached to carrier proteins by a weak and reversible binding. In man, some 60% is bound to the so-called testosterone-binding globulin (TeBG), 38% to albumin, and a mere 2% is free or bound to cortisol-binding globulin.[43] TeBG also binds 5α-dihydrotesterone (5α-DHT) and 17β-estradiol to some extent.[44] The TeBG is formed in the liver and is chemically and immunologically indistinguishable from the androgen-binding protein produced by Sertoli cells.

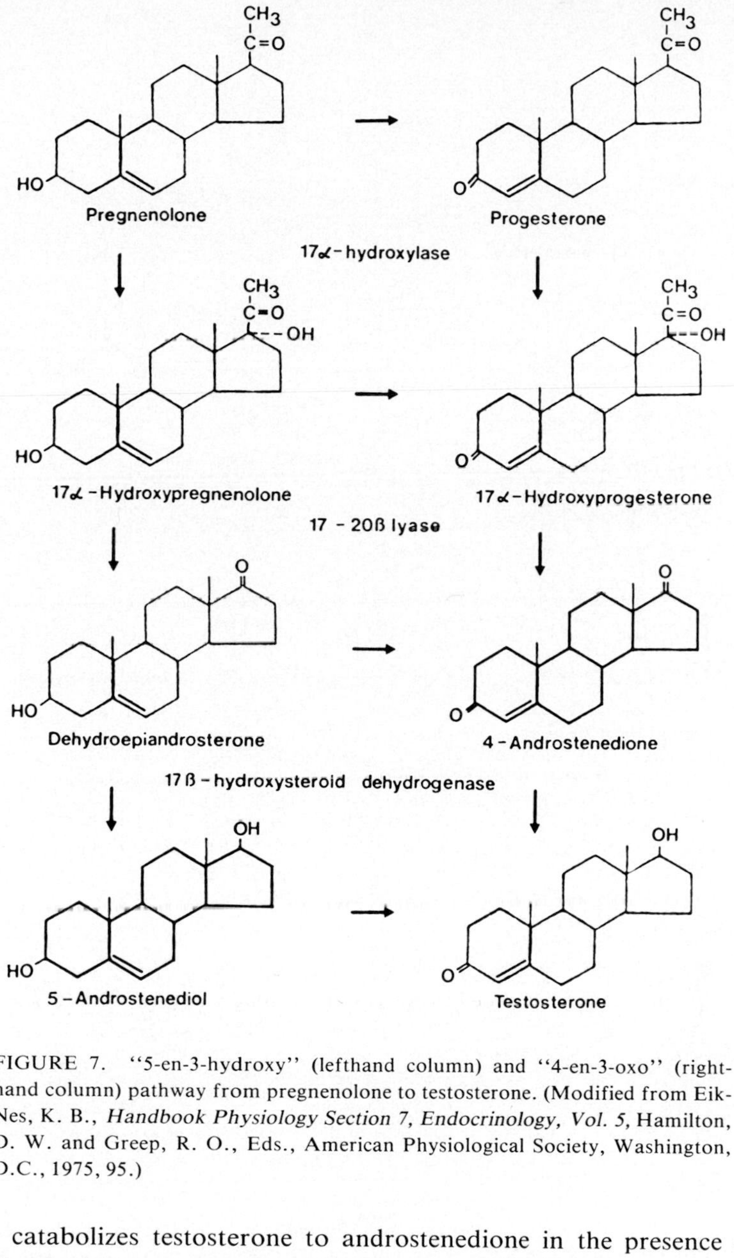

Pregnenolone → Progesterone

17α-hydroxylase

17α-Hydroxypregnenolone → 17α-Hydroxyprogesterone

17 - 20β lyase

Dehydroepiandrosterone → 4-Androstenedione

17β-hydroxysteroid dehydrogenase

5-Androstenediol → Testosterone

FIGURE 7. "5-en-3-hydroxy" (lefthand column) and "4-en-3-oxo" (righthand column) pathway from pregnenolone to testosterone. (Modified from Eik-Nes, K. B., *Handbook Physiology Section 7, Endocrinology, Vol. 5,* Hamilton, D. W. and Greep, R. O., Eds., American Physiological Society, Washington, D.C., 1975, 95.)

The liver catabolizes testosterone to androstenedione in the presence of 17β-hydroxysteroid dehydrogenase by the oxidation of the 17β-hydroxy group. Further reduction of this compound leads to the A-saturated steroids, 5α- and 5β-androstane-3,17-diones. The two androstanediones are converted to four isomeric 17-oxosteroids: androsterone, epi-androsterone, aetiocholanolone, and epiaetiocholanolone. These are conjugated as sulfates or glucuronides and excreted in the urine or feces. In a similar way, testosterone can be reduced to isomeric androstanediols, which are conjugated to glucuronides prior to excretion (Figure 8)[45]

The clearance of testosterone by the liver is not as complete as that of many other steroids. The binding of circulating testosterone to the TeBG prevents it from being inactivated completely during one passage through the liver. Androstenedione, which is only nonspecifically bound to albumin, is cleared more effectively.[44]

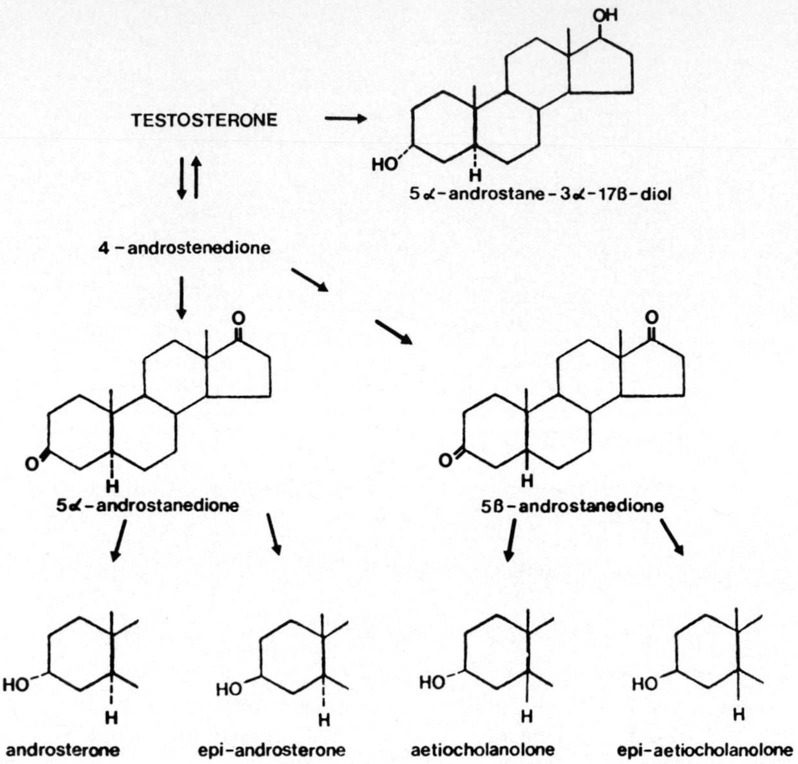

FIGURE 8. Catabolic pathway of testosterone (Modified from Gower, D. B., *Biochemistry of Steroid Hormones*, Makin, H. L. J., Ed., Blackwell Scientific, Oxford, 1975, 47.)

Effects of Androgens

Sexual Differentiation

The differentiation of the gonads into ovaries or testes takes place at an early stage of gestation, e.g., on day 12 in mice, day 13 to 14 in rats, day 41 to 42 in cattle, and day 42 to 45 in humans.[46]

In the case of a developing ovary, no gonadal hormones appear to be required for the development of the female phenotype. The testis produces two principal hormones which are responsible for the formation of the male phenotype, the anti-Mullerian-hormone (AMH) and androgens.[47]

Anti-Müllerian Hormone (AMH)

The pioneer work of Jost[48] demonstrated that a testicular product other than testosterone is responsible for regression of the Müllerian duct. It is now known that this hormone is produced by the fetal testis of several mammalian species, e.g., rat, rabbit, cattle, and man. Production begins shortly after testicular differentiation. The active fraction has been shown to be protein or glycoprotein. Responsivity of the Mullerian duct to this substance is limited to a short period: until day 15 of embryonic life in the rat, day 62 in the calf, and day 60 in the human. AMH is detectable in testicular tissue throughout fetal life and for a short period after birth.[46]

AMH acts independently of testosterone as demonstrated in castrated fetuses, in which the Müllerian duct persists and the Wolffian duct does not develop. Development of the Wolffian duct can be induced by injections of testosterone but this treatment leaves the Müllerian duct unaffected and the two systems develop side by side.

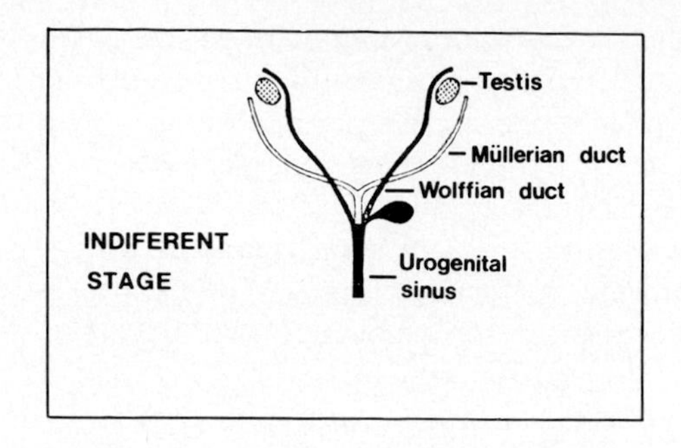

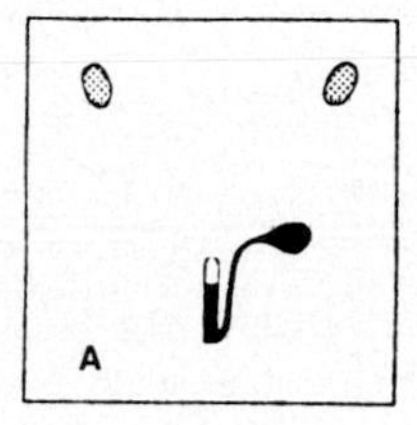

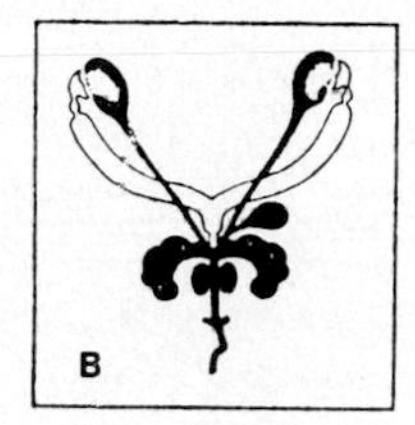

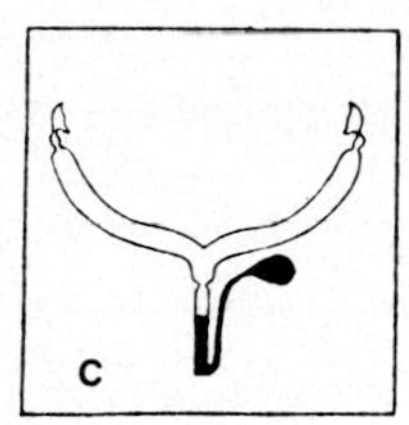

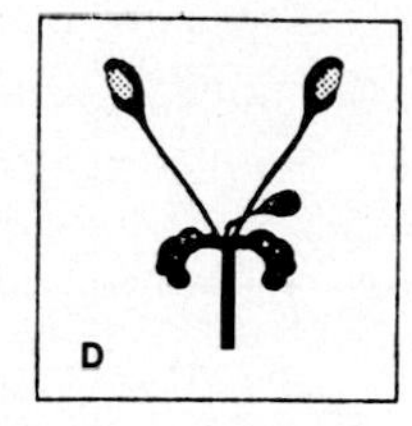

FIGURE 9. Hormonal effects on sexual differentiation. (Adapted from Neumann, F., Elger, W., and Steinbeck, H., *J. Reprod. Fert. Suppl.*, 7, 9, 1969, and Wilson, J. D., Griffin, J. E., and George, F. W., *Biol. Reprod.*, 22, 9, 1980.) A. (Intact fetus): treatment with anti-androgens prevents development of the Wolffian duct but does not affect regression of the Müllerian duct; B. (Castrated fetus): testosterone induces development of the Wolffian duct, the Müllerian duct is unaffected; C. (Castrated fetus): in the absence of androgens, the Wolffian duct does not develop, the Müllerian duct persists; D. (Intact fetus): 5a-reductase deficiency leads to normal Wolffian duct development and failure of external virilization.

In intact fetuses treated with cyproteron-acetate, a potent antiandrogen, the Wolffian duct does not develop due to the lack of androgen effects, but the Müllerian duct regresses normally. These individuals have testes, but no other sexual organs (Figure 9).[49]

Androgens

The fetal testis synthesizes androgens in large amounts. In the rat, rabbit, and human, testosterone is the only androgen produced in significant quantities whereas in the mouse, sheep, pig, and cattle additional androstenedione is synthesized. The onset of androgen production is closely correlated with the differentiation of Leydig cells.[46]

In the male fetus, the first step in development of the genital tract is the regression of the Müllerian duct. As this regression begins, the Wolffian duct undergoes differentiation. The cranial part of the Wolffian duct connects with the seminiferous cords to form the rete testis. The remainder of the duct gives rise to epididymis, vas deferens, seminal vesicles, and the ejaculatory duct.[47]

Development of the urethra, the accessory organs, and the external genitalia begins shortly after the virilization of the Wolffian duct. This process takes place under the influence of 5α-dihydrotestosterone, which is formed in target tissues by 5α-reduction. Deficiency of 5α-reductase leads to failure of external virilization (Figure 9.)[50]

Sexual Differentiation of the Central Nervous System

The hypothalamus shows a cyclic pattern of activity charcteristic of the female unless it is exposed to androgens during a critical period. This effect is most easily studied in the rat because changes can be produced by treatment after birth. If testes of fetal rats are transplanted to infant female rats, they do not ovulate when they reach maturity. It is possible to induce ovulation in such animals by hypothalamic stimulation after progesterone priming. Thus, these females are able to secrete LH at a steady rate like the male but cannot produce the distinct LH-peak necessary for ovulation.[51] Similarly, castration of male neonates induces definite alterations in the ultrastructure of the pituitary whereas ovariectomy does not.[52]

The early exposure of the brain to hormones also determines the pattern of sexual behavior that develops after puberty. The effects of androgens on sexual behavior are mediated by estrogens, formed by local conversion of androgens in the brain.[53]

In primates, the pattern of gonadotropin secretion is not changed by administration of androgens.[51] Sexual behavior of female primates is not influenced by fetal exposure to androgens.[54]

From Birth to Puberty

During postnatal maturation, testosterone production shows a slow rise at the beginning with a sharp increase in the immediate prepuberal period. This abrupt increase is evidently related to changes in pituitary function. It is presumed that maturation of hypothalamic, androgen-sensitive tissue is involved. The maturation probably takes the form of a decrease in sensitivity to androgen-negative feedback, which allows increased gonadotropin secretion.[31]

Spermatogenesis

LH stimulates the Leydig cells to produce the androgens required for maintaining spermatogenesis. Two lines of evidence suggest that testosterone is important for spermatogenesis. Testosterone can qualitatively maintain spermatogenesis and production of ABP in the adult hypophysectomized rat if treatment begins immediately following surgery.[55] However, once atrophy inside the tubules has occurred, spermatogenesis cannot be reinitiated by testosterone alone. Testosterone appears to act during prophase on primary spermatocytes.[56]

The effects of testosterone on the germ cells are exerted directly and via Sertoli cells. Evidence for a direct influence is the presence of androgen receptors in germ cells. The possibility of in vivo stimulation of testicular ABP-production by testosterone implies that androgens also act on Sertoli cells, since ABP-synthesis is thought to occur only in Sertoli cells. Thus, testosterone, with FSH, triggers its own specific transport system.[55]

Epididymis

The most important functional change which the spermatozoa undergo in the epididymis is the acquisition of the ability to fertilize ova. This functional maturation and the ability of the epididymis to store spermatozoa in a mature state are androgen dependent. It was shown in rat, rabbit, and hamster that castration or hypophysectomy impairs the survival of spermatozoa in the epididymis. This can be counteracted by testosterone.

Androgens stimulate the secretory activity of the epididymis. The products interact with spermatozoa to bring about changes required for their maturation and survival. Studies on the composition of fluid removed from various sites along the epididymis suggest that carnitine, glycerylphosphorylcholine, and inositol play a role in this mechanism.[57]

Testosterone can enter the epididymis in two ways, directly by a luminal pathway bound to ABP and from the circulating blood. The initial segment of the epididymis reabsorbs most of the fluid secreted by the seminiferous tubules. This function is probably regulated by the androgens in the fluid.[58] The succeeding segments depend to a higher degree on the effects of androgens transported by the blood. There is evidence that testosterone is converted to 5α-DHT by epididymal tissue.[59]

Accessory Organs and External Genitalia

The main actions of androgens on male accessory organs are detected by changes following castration in adults or by the failure to develop particular characteristics after prepuberal castration. Normal development of the accessory organs of the male reproductive tract is closely correlated with physical and testicular growth. The increased androgen secretion before and during puberty influences the size of penis and scrotum as well as growth and functional maturation of the accessory glands.[60] Testosterone is the most important factor for the formation and secretion of some chemical compounds by the accessory glands, e.g., fructose and citric acid.[61] While most of these actions are produced by androgens transported by the blood, the ampulla the glandular portion of the vas deferen may also be affected by androgens in the luminal fluid.[62]

Sexual Behavior

Individuals castrated before puberty fail to develop adult patterns of sexual behavior unless given androgens. After castration of adults, sexual activity may persist for a variable time. The duration depends on the involvement of psychic elements in libido.[60] In intact males, high blood concentrations of androgens are not necessarily reflected in the libido and administration of androgens in cases of impotence is usually ineffective.[63] Castration also produces more general changes in behavior such as reduced aggression and this effect was probably the main reason for introducing castration in male domestic animals.[60]

General Effects

Androgens exert anabolic effects like increase of muscle protein. This is reflected in a higher level of urinary creatinine and a decrease in urinary nitrogen excretion. The anabolic activity of androgens is not related to their androgenic potency. The mechanism of action of androgens on muscle is not definitely clarified because an androgen receptor protein probably does not exist in ordinary muscle.[64] Small doses of androgens accelerate growth of the long bones and large doses appear to terminate their growth. Therefore, prepuberal castration results in continued growth, a phenomenon well known in humans and in animal husbandry. In human males, androgens control the pattern of hair growth and lengthening of the vocal chords, which contribute to the secondary male sex characteristics.[60]

Molecular Aspects of Androgen Action

Binding of steroids to receptors in target tissues or cells is an essential intermediate step in the molecular expression of steroid-induced responses. There are two main types of androgen receptors in target tissue, a cytoplasmic and a nuclear receptor. It has not been clarified whether they are of separate origin or whether the cytoplasmic receptor is modified when the receptor-hormone complex enters the nucleus and becomes the nuclear receptor.

Physicochemical properties of the receptor proteins show only slight differences, such as a different sedimentation coefficient in a linear glycerol-stabilized sucrose gradient (nuclear-receptor 3S; cytoplasmic receptor at 4-5S or 8-10S). Molecular weight estimations result in 100,000 daltons for the nuclear receptor and about 200,000 for the cytoplasmic receptor.[65]

Most of our knowledge about the mechanism of actions of androgens is derived from studies on the ventral prostate gland of the rat. Testosterone probably enters the cell by passive diffusion. In the cell, testosterone can combine either directly with a receptor protein or first be reduced to 5α-DHT. Receptors in the testis appear to bind testosterone and 5α-DHT with approximately the same affinity. In other target organs, especially the prostate, testosterone is transformed by a 5α-reductase to 5α-DHT, which binds to the cytoplasmic receptor. 5α-DHT is therefore considered to be the major form of "active" androgens. The hormone-receptor complex is translocated to the nucleus, where it is either modified or the steroid hormone binds to the nuclear receptor. This nuclear receptor-hormone complex interacts with acceptor sites of nuclear genes, resulting in a changed chromatin activity. This activation involves stimulation of a RNA-polymerase, which in turn increases RNA-synthesis. Ultimately new messenger-RNA reaches the cytoplasm of the cell and new proteins are synthesized.[66]

Inactivation of testosterone or 5α-DHT probably takes place in the cytoplasm by further reduction to 5α-androstane-3α,17β-diol and 5α-androstane-3,17β-diol. Both these compounds possess less androgenic potency than 5α-DHT.[45]

Other Testicular Hormones

16-Unsaturated C_{19}-Steroids

The testes of the boar produce 16-unsaturated C_{19}-steroids, which are concentrated in the body fat and in the salivary glands. They act as pheromones. Pheromones are agents used for communication among individuals of the same species. The most active compounds in the boar are 5α-androst-16-en-3-on, 5α-androst-16-en-3α-ol, and 5-androst-16-3β-ol. These steroids are definitely not derived from testosterone or its direct precursors, but are formed from pregnenolone or progesterone (Figure 10). They do not possess any detectable androgenic potency.[67]

Estrogens

The ability of the mammalian testis to secrete estrogens is well established, although the cellular source has been controversial. Production of estrogens by the testis has been demonstrated in several animals, e.g., dog,[68] rat,[69] pig,[67] cattle,[70] and horse.[71] In man, about 20% of total estradiol produced is secreted by the testis.[68]

In vitro studies in the rat suggest that the site of estrogen formation lies inside the seminiferous tubules. Cultured Sertoli cells in a medium containing testosterone respond to FSH with extensive 17β-estradiol synthesis whereas pregnenolone is ineffective as a substrate.[72] However, more recent experiments indicate that 17β-estradiol synthesis occurs in cultured Leydig cells, but not in Sertoli cells.[73]

In vivo, the main products of estrogen synthesis are 17β-estradiol and estrone. In the stallion, where the testis contains appreciable amounts of estrogens in comparison to other species, the major parts of estradiol and estrone are conjugated with sulfate groups. Conjugation may be a mechanism to protect the testis from undesirable effects of the estrogens produced.[35]

A pathway of testosterone to estrogens probably requires NADPH as well as oxygen and is cytochrome P-450 dependent (Figure 11).[34]

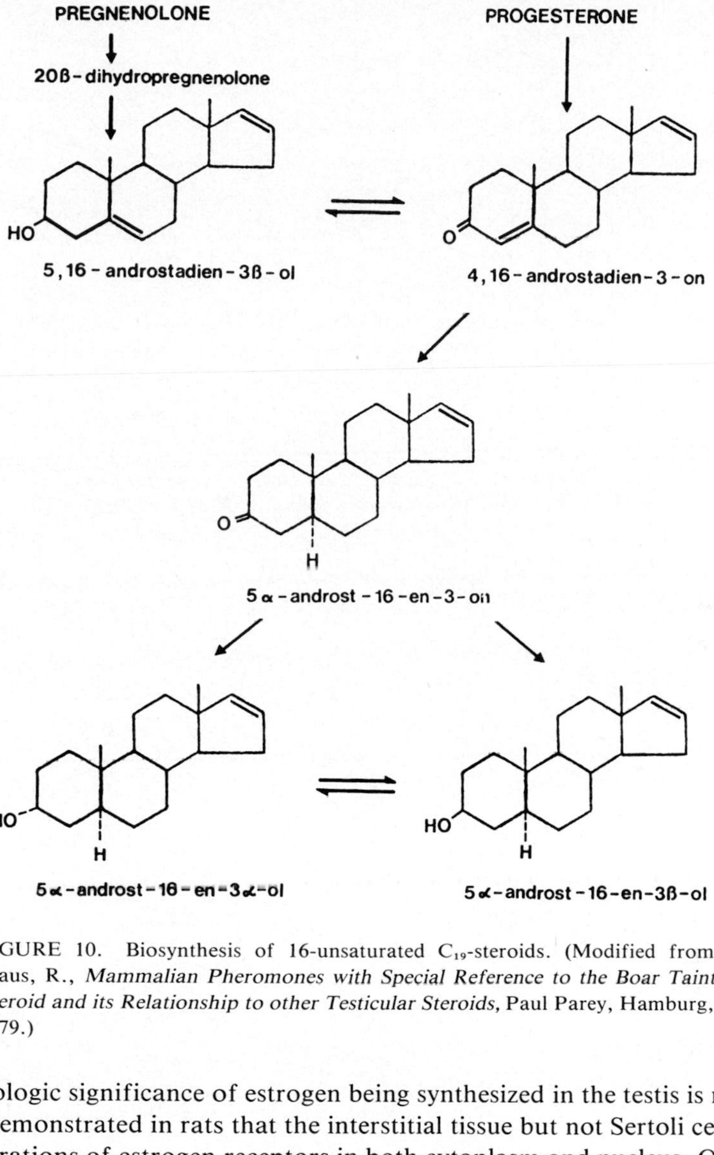

PREGNENOLONE

20ß-dihydropregnenolone

PROGESTERONE

5,16-androstadien-3ß-ol

4,16-androstadien-3-on

5α-androst-16-en-3-on

5α-androst-16-en-3α-ol

5α-androst-16-en-3ß-ol

FIGURE 10. Biosynthesis of 16-unsaturated C_{19}-steroids. (Modified from Claus, R., *Mammalian Pheromones with Special Reference to the Boar Taint Steroid and its Relationship to other Testicular Steroids*, Paul Parey, Hamburg, 1979.)

The physiologic significance of estrogen being synthesized in the testis is not known. It has been demonstrated in rats that the interstitial tissue but not Sertoli cells contains high concentrations of estrogen receptors in both cytoplasm and nucleus. One possible function of estrogens is to exert a local regulatory effect on the metabolism of interstitial cells. A second possible role is a short feedback loop to modulate testicular function. A high transfer of estradiol from venous to arterial blood in the pampiniform plexus occurs in bulls.[70]. These findings suggest a cooperation between Leydig cells and Sertoli cells.

Inhibin

In the 1930s the existence of a nonsteroidal inhibitor of FSH was proposed and called inhibin.[74] A modern statement of its "inhibin hypothesis" in its simplest form is as follows: two pituitary gonadotropins act as the testis. FSH stimulates the seminiferous tubules whereas LH stimulates the Leydig cells. The Leydig cells produce androgens, which control LH secretions by negative feedback and the Sertoli cells produce inhibin, which controls FSH secretion also by negative feedback.[75] Inhibin-like activity has been found in rete testis fluid, seminal plasma, testis extracts, and spermatozoa.[76] Sertoli cells in culture secrete a factor which selectively suppresses FSH release by pi-

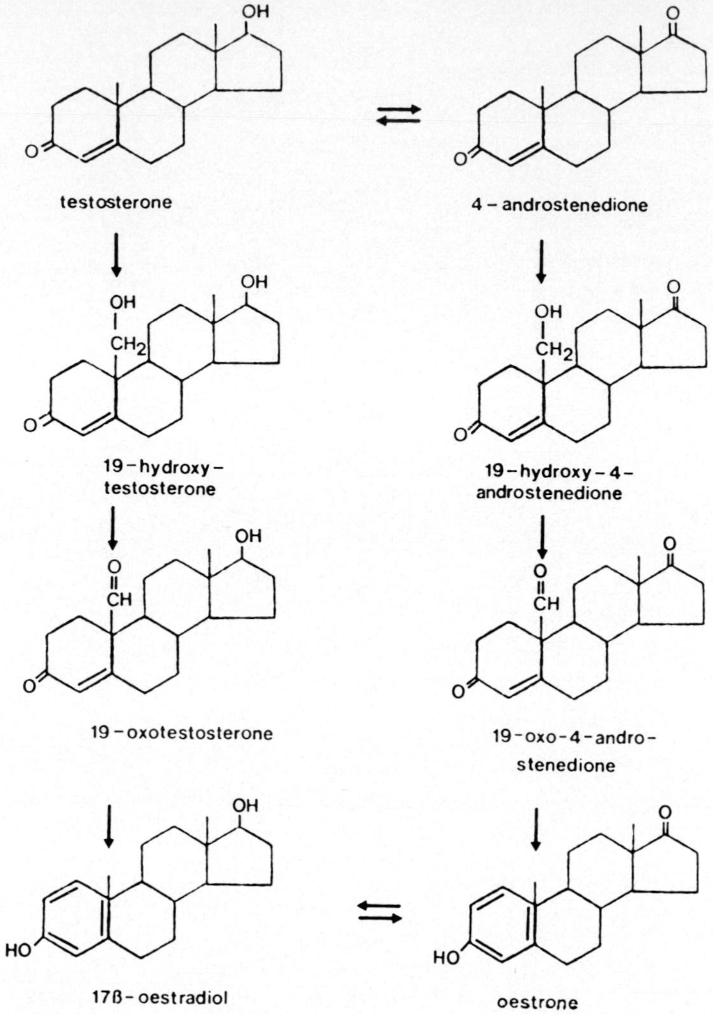

FIGURE 11. Possible pathways of testosterone to estrogens. (Modified from Gower, D. B. and Fotherby, K., *Biochemistry of Steroid Hormones*, Makin, H. L. J., Ed., Blackwell Scientific, Oxford, 1975, 77.)

tuitary cells in vitro whereas the LH release is not affected.[77] Although inhibin has not yet been isolated and purified, intensive experiments have shown that it must be a nonsteroidal factor of protein nature and of low molecular weight.

Prostaglandins

The testes contain appreciable amounts of prostaglandins (PG), although the levels are much lower than in other parts of the male reproductive system. The testis itself may be able to produce PGs. Histochemical localization of PG-synthetase activity in the male rat reproductive tract shows that spermatozoa do not produce large amounts of PGs in the testis. Maximal synthesis occurs in the interstitial tissue and in the capsule.[78]

There are a number of ways in which PG-synthesis may interfere with androgen production. One is competition for NADPH during lipid peroxidation, because the enzymes for this step of the PG-synthesis are related to the steroid transforming enzymes. Furthermore, lipid peroxidation is also gonadotropin dependent like androgen synthesis.[79]

A possible function of PGs produced by the testes is to act on the contractility of the testis capsule and seminiferous tubules. In the capsule, concentrations of PGE_2 and $PGF_{2\alpha}$ are about 100 times higher than in decapsulated testes.[80] An indirect effect of PGs could be modulation of gonadotropin secretion. Although PGs diminish testicular blood flow, it is unlikely that this effect is a regulating factor.[79]

NEUROENDOCRINE REGULATION OF TESTICULAR FUNCTIONS

The nervous system is involved to a varying degree in almost every aspect of the physiology of reproduction. A major part of neural involvement is the regulation of gonadal function by the brain through hypothalamic control of anterior pituitary gonadotropin secretion. Current ideas regarding hypothalamic control of reproduction are based on the discovery of neurosecretion and of the functional significance of the hypophyseal portal vasculature. The terms LH-RH and FSH-RH are used to describe "factors" in the hypothalamus which stimulate the release of LH and FSH from the pituitary.

The target tissues for FSH and LH are different components of the testes. FSH exerts an effect primarily on the Sertoli cells and on the seminiferous tubules whereas LH influences the Leydig cells. Gonadotropins are secreted by the pituitary in amounts relative to the function of the gonads.

The quantity and types of steroids secreted by the gonads act as feedback signals. The signals are mediated by specific steroid binding proteins or by steroid receptors present in certain hypothalamic neurons and in pituitary cells. The steroids bound by these receptors influence FSH and LH secretion and thereby maintain a state of dynamic equilibrium between the secretions of hypothalamic gonadotropin-releasing hormones (LH-RH, FSH-RH), pituitary gonadotropins (LH, FSH), and gonadal steroids. This system of interdependent endocrine organs forms the hypothalamo-pituitary-gonadal axis.

Hypothalamic Gonadotropin-Releasing Hormones

The release of pituitary gonadotropins is controlled by hypothalamic neurosecretion. Experiments were therefore performed to detect gonadotropin-releasing hormones in hypothalamic extracts. Schally,[81] using porcine hypothalamus, and Guillemin,[82] using ovine hypothalamus, isolated a decapeptide with combined LH-RH and FSH-RH activity and having the sequence p-Glu-His-Trp-Ser-Tyr-Gly-Leu-Arg-Pro-Gly-NH_2. Neither was able to separate a substance with only LH-RH or FSH-RH activity. The decapeptide, called gonadotropin hormone releasing hormone (Gn-RH), was synthesized and found to release FSH and LH as effectively as the natural product.[83]

Because Gn-RH releases LH more readily than FSH, it has been suggested that there may be a second gonadotropin-releasing hormone which releases FSH more readily than LH. A chemically defined FSH-RH has yet to be confirmed. The theory that only one releasing hormone controls the secretion of both gonadotropins is also supported by immunologic studies.

Localization and Transport of Gn-RH to the Pituitary

It can be demonstrated, using either bio- or radioimmuno-assay to measure Gn-RH in different regions of the hypothalamus, that releasing hormones are synthesized in the hypophysiotropic area.[84] The hypophyseal portal vessels, a vascular connection between the hypothalamus and the pituitary, transport Gn-RH from the hypothalamus to the pars distalis of the pituitary.[85] Gn-RH is taken up into the hypophyseal portal vessels by modified ependymal cells, called tancyctes, which cover the superficial surface of the median eminence.

Effects on Gonadotropin Secretion

Gn-RH does not release FSH as readily as LH.[86] The maximum incremental change in plasma concentration is always less than that of LH. Following an injection of Gn-RH, plasma FSH levels rise slower than LH levels, but remain elevated longer.

Gn-RH stimulates the synthesis of gonadotropins. The pituitary LH and FSH concentrations in rats actively immunized against Gn-RH are low. This indicates that gonadotropin synthesis is impaired when Gn-RH activity is inhibited.[87] If ^{3}H-glucosamine is added to a rat pituitary cell culture, then the addition of Gn-RH results in the incorporation of the labeled substance into FSH and LH. Addition of Gn-RH to rat pituitary cell culture also causes an increase in the concentrations of LH and FSH in both the culture tissue and the medium.[88]

Gonadotropins

The gonadotropic hormones FSH (follicle-stimulating hormone) and LH (luteinizing hormone) also known as ICSH (interstitial cell-stimulating hormone) are synthesized in and released from the anterior pituitary under the influence of the hypothalamic-releasing hormones. Both hormones are glycoproteins and are produced in the basophil cells of the pars distalis. The importance of the anterior pituitary for the maintenance of testicular function has been known a long time. Much knowledge about the effects of the gonadotropins has been acquired with experiments on hypophysectomized animals. The extensive testicular atrophy that occurs following hypophysectomy can partly be prevented by treating such animals with gonadotropins, which act synergistically.

If mature hypophysectomized male rats are grafted with anterior pituitaries under the kidney capsule one or two days after hypophysectomy, testicular atrophy can be prevented to a certain extent and spermatids are present in numerous seminiferous tubules.[89] No detectable levels of LH and FSH can be measured in the serum of hypophysectomized rats whereas transplantation of anterior pituitary grafts leads to inconsistently detectable serum levels of LH and FSH. The study provides evidence that pituitary grafts can secrete small but significant amounts of LH and FSH, which are believed to be responsible for the partial maintenance of spermatogenesis. It is supposed that the pituitary grafts are stimulated by the presence of Gn-RH in the systemic circulation.

Luteinizing Hormone (LH)

Site of Action

LH is responsible for the morphologic appearance of the Leydig cell. It also stimulates androgen production in the Leydig cells, thus indirectly promoting spermatogenesis.

Mechanism of Action

The first step of the mechanism is to bind LH to the surface of the Leydig cells. The binding can be demonstrated in rats by injection of the labeled hormone or with testis homogenates.[90,91] Binding most likely occurs on the cell membrane, not inside the cell,[92] (Figure 12). Much more luteinizing hormone can be bound than is necessary for maximal stimulation of testosterone synthesis. However, no significance can be ascribed to this phemonenon.

Stimulation by LH enhances adenylate cyclase activity and the formation of cAMP.[93] A response in cAMP synthesis can be detected in less than 1 min whereas the response of testosterone synthesis requires at least 20 min.[92,94,95] This suggests that a complex series of metabolic events is interposed between the formation of cAMP and the release of testosterone. The involvement of a protein kinase is probable.[96] The protein kinase presumably catalyzes the formation of a messenger protein which then activates the conversion of cholesterol to pregnenolone.

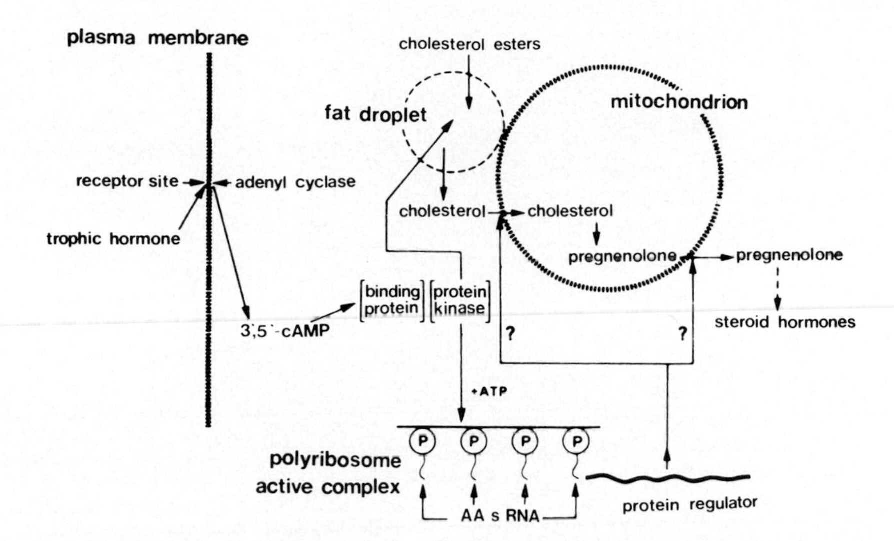

FIGURE 12. Control of steroidogenesis. (From Rommerts, F. F. G., Cooke, B. A., and van der Molen, H. J., *J. Steroid Biochem.*, 5, 279, 1974. With permission.)

Follicle-Stimulating Hormone (FSH)

Site of Action

FSH is important in the initiation of the spermatogenic process and may be important in the mature animal for the maintenance of optimal testicular function. The major target for FSH within the testis is the Sertoli cell. An effect on spermatogonia is also possible as are indirect effects on the other germinal cells via the Sertoli cells. Evidence that FSH acts on the Sertoli cells was demonstrated by the effect of FSH on the tubules of rats containing Sertoli cells only but no germ cells[97] and on Sertoli cells in culture.[98,99] The precise mechanism by which FSH exerts its effect on the spermatogenic process is still unknown.

Membrane Receptors for FSH

The incubation of testes with a highly purified preparation of tritiated human FSH was shown to result in a significant binding to Sertoli cells.[100] Binding is tissue specific, time and temperature dependent, and hormone specific, since only FSH is found to effectively compete with the (^{3}H) FSH.

Following separation of testes into seminiferous tubules and interstitial cells, only the seminiferous tubules bind FSH.[100,101] The main radioactivity is associated with the plasma membrane fraction after subcellular fractionation of the tubular cells and incubation with (^{3}H) FSH. The binding component of the plasma membrane appears to be at least partially protein in nature, since the preincubation of seminiferous tubules with trypsin abolishes the ability to bind FSH.

The amount of labeled FSH bound per testis in rats increases with age until about 15 days postnatally and then remains constant.[102] This corresponds with the division of Sertoli cells in the testis. Thereafter, little if any cell division occurs.[103]

Metabolic Effects

Following binding to membrane receptors, FSH stimulates adenylate cyclase. This results in an increased intracellular accumulation of cAMP and stimulates the catalytic activity of a cAMP-dependent protein kinase.[101,102,104]

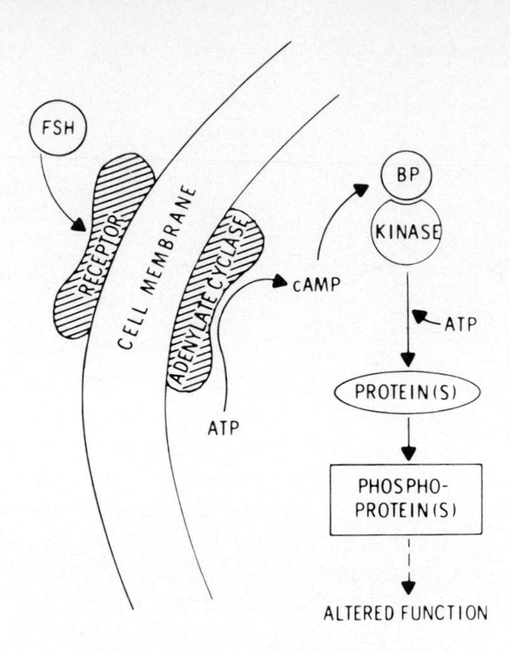

FIGURE 13. Effects of FSH on the Sertoli cell. (From Means, A. R., Fakunding, J. L., Huckins, C., Tindall, D. J., and Vitale, R., *Rec. Prog. Horm. Res.*, 32, 478, 1976. With permission.)

The activation of protein kinase is thought to result in phosphorylation of enzymes or structural proteins, which leads to an alteration of function (Figure 13).

The effects of FSH on protein synthesis are age dependent. It is not possible to stimulate cAMP levels to a significant degree in mature animals.[105] The mechanism responsible for the decrease in receptivity to FSH with age is not known. Fractionation of testis cytosol demonstrates the existence of two peaks of cAMP-dependent protein kinase activity.[106] The levels of peak I and peak II protein kinase were quantified during testicular development in the Sertoli cell-enriched rat model. The ratio of peak I to peak II is greater than two during the early stages of testicular development. The ratio drops to approximately 0.85 with increasing age. The decline corresponds with the decline in FSH sensitivity. These data suggest that FSH results only in the activation of peak I protein kinase and may be an explanation for the age-dependent stimulation of protein synthesis by FSH.

The increased testicular protein synthesis following injection of FSH can be determined by amino acid incorporation. There is an accelerated transport of amino acids into testicular cells and a greater activity of testicular polyribosomes.[107-109] Therefore, FSH stimulates testicular protein synthesis by increasing the synthesis of RNA as was shown in rats.[102,110] The effect of FSH on RNA synthesis seems to be of a quantitative rather than a qualitative nature.

Modulation of Androgen-Binding Protein Activity

The meaning of events induced by FSH could be better elucidated if a specific product regulated by FSH was found. Androgen-Binding Protein (ABP) is assumed to be a FSH-regulated protein.[111] It is produced by Sertoli cells, secreted into the lumen of the seminiferous tubules and transported via the ductuli efferentes into the caput epididymis. ABP disappears following hypophysectomy but reappears after long-term administration of FSH. It is therefore of interest to determine whether ABP can be used as a specific product to measure FSH effects on the Sertoli cell. An FSH injection into immature or hypophysectomized rats results in an increased activity of ABP within 30 min.[102,107,110] Experiments testing the specificity of ABP stimulation by FSH produce unexpected results. Highly purified human FSH shows no effect on ABP synthesis. But testosterone and hormones which activate the production of testosterone produce a distinct stimulation. The ABP activity and testis testosterone concentration are closely correlated following a single injection of LH.[112] These data suggest that testosterone itself might be the primary hormone responsible for the regulation of ABP. The stimulation by FSH seen previously might have been due to impurities in the FSH preparations used.[112]

Other Pituitary Hormones

Prolactin

Effects on the Testis

The physiologic role of prolactin in the male is obscure. In mice and rat testis, prolactin supposedly induces the activity of some enzymes required for testosterone metabolism.[114] It seems important in maintaining a pool of hormone precursors on which LH can act to stimulate testosterone production. Prolactin alone has only a small effect on plasma testosterone levels, but treatment with prolactin and LH elevates plasma concentrations above those seen in control animals.[115] The fact that blood concentrations of prolactin and testosterone in adult men are correlated supports the suggestion that prolactin has an effect on steroidogenesis.[116] On the other hand, very high levels of blood prolactin concentration can be associated with hypogonadism and impotence.[117] There is some evidence that prolactin acts on the prostate. Investigations indicate that prostate growth and secretion depend on the combined action of prolactin and androgens.[118]

Prolactin and Reproductive Behavior

There are only few studies on the role of prolactin in reproductive behavior in male mammals. In male rabbits, exogenous administration of prolactin has been reported to have a marked inhibitory effect on the copulatory activity.[119] In bulls, a transitory increase of blood prolactin concentration occurs following mounting a cow[120] and ejaculation.[121] This is also observed in billy goats following copulation.[122]

Oxytocin

The oxytocin content in the male neurohypophysis is the same as in the female. Several workers failed to demonstrate a stimulating effect of oxytocin on the male genital tract. On the other hand, it could be shown that oxytocin causes contractions of the seminiferous tubules in the rat[123] and increases the output of fluid and spermatozoa from the ram testis.[124] The contractility of the ductus epididymidis and of the vas deferens can be stimulated by oxytocin in male rabbits[125] and rams.[126]

Injection of oxytocin shortly before ejaculation increases the number of spermatozoa in semen in rabbits, rams,[126] and bulls.[127] In rats and rabbits a long-term treatment with oxytocin results in an increase in testicular weight and Leydig cell population.[128]

Stimulation of the male genital tract can induce secretion of oxytocin from the neurohypophysis, e.g., it was demonstrated in the boar that ejaculation is accompanied by an increased oxytocin blood concentration.[129]

Hypothalamic and Extrahypothalamic Control Mechanism

The secretion of Gn-RH from the hypothalamus is influenced by various control mechanisms (Figure 14). It is governed directly or indirectly by higher nerve centers sensitive to changes in the internal and external environment. These include time-dependent rhythms, peripheral nerve reflexes, hormonal as well as chemical, and physical changes in cerebrospinal fluid and blood and external stimuli such as stress, season, light, and temperature.

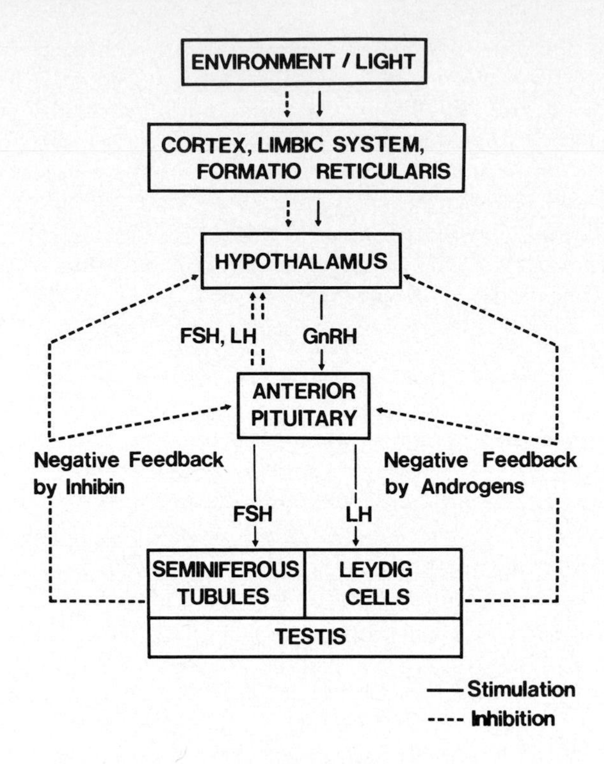

FIGURE 14. Neuroendocrine regulation of testicular function.

Levels of Control

Hypothalamic Neuron Autonomy

The hypothalamic neurons are capable of certain autonomous functions. This has been shown by experiments in which the hypothalamo-pituitary complex has been isolated from the rest of the brain.[113] The pulsatile rhythm of basal FSH and LH release remains unaffected.

Basal Gonadotropin Secretion

The hypophysiotropic area, containing the mediobasal hypothalamus, is responsible for the basal gonadotropin secretion. The rates of FSH and LH secretion are more or less constant in males and sufficient to maintain the basic integrity of the gonadal steroids. In females, a cyclic rhythm superimposed on a steady secretion is necessary.

Extrahypothalamic Areas

Stimulatory and inhibitory inputs from higher nerve centers are necessary for the full functioning of the hypothalamus, although some function can occur in isolation. The anterior pituitary is probably controlled at two levels. One regulates the basal secretion and a second higher level, which includes all other hypothalamic and extrahypothalamic structures, exerts stimulatory or inhibitory effects.

The limbic system is probably the most important among the nerve centers which influence the hypothalamic control of the gonadotropin secretion. Structures of the mesencephalon, especially the formatio reticularis, are also involved. Stimulatory and inhibitory effects are mediated by components of a complex system of fiber tracts, which connect the limbic system, the preoptic area, the medial basal hypothalamus, and the midbrain. Depending upon which area is stimulated, gonadotropin release can be facilitated or inhibited.[130]

Neurotransmitters

The chemical nature of the mediators involved in transferring information from extra-hypothalamic areas to the Gn-RH-synthesizing neurons of the hypothalamus has not been fully elucidated. There is evidence that the neurotransmitters acetylcholine (ACh), noradrenalin (NA), and γ-aminobutyric acid (GABA) are concerned with different aspects of gonadotropin release and 5-hydro-xytryptamine (5-HT) with its inhibition.[131,132] The release of anterior pituitary hormones, regulated by feedback action of steroid hormones, may also be mediated by neurotransmitter activity. Some internal and external influences known to alter the secretion of gonadotropins, e.g., diurnal rhythm, castration, steroid administration, and stress, change neurotransmitter activity in the hypothalamus. This is determined by alteration in content, turnover, and rate of synthesis from labelled precursors.[133,134] Different forms of hypothalamic stimulation or inhibition may involve different transmitters.

Some pathways of mediators in the brain can be localized by fluorescent antibody and enzyme-isotopic techniques. The mediators influence the hypothalamic control at several sites,[135,136] e.g., at a synapse of a nerve tract from an extra-hypothalamic region to the Gn-RH-synthesizing neurons or at a direct synapse of extrahypothalamic fibers with the cell body of the hypothalamic neuron. The complexity of the neural arrangements and the indirectness of the evidence prevent firm conclusions about the role of specific transmitters in the various parts of the hypothalamo-pituitary system. All transmitters probably have multiple effects.

Feedback Mechanisms

Feedback mechanisms may take place at the levels of the pituitary, the hypothalamus, or at extra-hypothalamic sites. The evidence is conclusive that the hypothalamus is the major site for feedback. Plasma gonadotropins and gonadal steroids are maintained in a state of dynamic equilibrium.

Negative Feedback

Estrogens and androgens are the main steroids responsible for the negative feedback control of the basal gonadotropin secretion. Because androgens are principally produced by the testis and estrogens by the ovary, it is concluded that androgens are the main negative feedback steroids in the male and estrogens are the main negative feedback steroids in the female. Increase in the plasma steroid concentration inhibits the gonadotropin secretion and a decrease stimulates production and secretion. Thus, gonadotropin concentrations of the pituitary and blood plasma increase after castration. This effect can be suppressed to a certain degree by administration of sex steroids. The length of time required for an increase in FSH and LH concentrations after castration or semicastration is different.[137,138] This lead to the assumption that separate control mechanisms for FSH- and LH regulation exist.

Positive Feedback

The positive feedback effect, that is the stimulation of the gonadotropin secretion by increasing steroid concentrations, plays an important role in the female in the induction of ovulation. There is no clear evidence of a positive feedback between the testis and the hypothalamo-pituitary system.

Short Loop Effect

The gonadotropins can inhibit their own release by feedback effects at the hypothalamic level. How the short loop effect functions is not known. One way may be to change the production of the releasing hormones or gonadotropins, another is to influence the sensitivity of the hypothalamus or the anterior pituitary to internal and external inputs.

Episodic Release

Gonadotropins are released episodically in castrated male animals. Each discharge lasts about 10 min and occurs at approximately hourly intervals. In intact males, LH is also released episodically although the frequency and the amplitude of the discharge are less. The episodic LH release is associated with pulsatile discharges of testosterone. It is thought that episodic LH release is controlled by a central α-adrenergic nervous mechanism since it can be inhibited with α- but not with β-adrenergic blocking agents.[139]

Environment and Reproduction

Environmental influences on reproduction can be classified into inanimate factors (photoperiodism, season, and stress) and animate factors (pheromones and sexual stimuli).

Photoperiodism

Photoperiodism is a major factor regulating reproduction. It is important in moderate and high latitudes with the distinct differences in seasons. The seasonal, photoperiodically dependent variation of gonadal activity is responsible for the parturition of many species at a time of year offering the optimal chance of survival for offspring. Species sensitive to photoperiodism can be divided into two groups. Those responding to increasing day length are called ''long-day species'' because the onset of the breeding season is controlled by increasing light periods. Those responding to short day length are ''short-day species''.[140] In both groups the onset of the breeding season is hastened by diminishing the photoperiod and ended by increasing it. Many mammals are long-day species (e.g., horse, mink, cat, and ferret), others are short-day species (e.g., sheep, goat, and deer), and for some species photoperiodism is of little or no importance (e.g., cow, dog, and rabbit).

The effects of light are mediated by the hypothalamus and the anterior pituitary, but the mechanisms which translate photoperiodic changes at the hypothalamus are not well understood. The retina of the eye may act as a photometer and register the small daily changes in increasing or decreasing day length. Impulses are then transmitted to the hypothalamus. The anterior pituitary is in turn stimulated to release gonadotropins which then stimulate the gonadal steroid secretion.

The pineal gland is probably involved in the transmission of photoperodic effects on the gonadotropin secretion. Pineal hormones exert pro- and anti-gonadotropic activities. In sheep, gonadotropin peaks, mainly of LH, become more frequent from August to December with the progression of the breeding season. This is accompanied by an increased frequency and amplitude of testosterone peaks, followed by an increased mating activity and increased ejaculate volume.[141]

The red deer is a short-day breeder species. Histologic study of the testes of stags shot in autumn (sexual season) and spring (quiescent period) indicate that the threefold increase in testicular size in the autumn is due to proliferation of intertubular tissue and germinal epithelium.[142]

In the stallion, secretion of LH and testosterone is influenced by season.[143,144] This finding is consistent with the seasonal variations in libido (mounts per ejaculate, reaction time).

Pheromones

Pheromones are endogenous compounds released by animals into the urine (mouse and rat), into the secretions of the anal glands (dog and fox), into the prepuce, into the salivary glands,[145] or into the secretions of the cervix and vagina. Pheromones cause specific physiologic and behavioral reactions in members of the same or of closely related species. They play an important role for recognition of partners in estrus and for inducing readiness and standing reflex for copulation. The effects of the pheromones are well known among animal breeders and they are well documented since ancient times by authors like Vergil:[146] "Nonne vides, ut tota tremor pertemptet equorum corpora, si tantum notas odor attulit auras?" (Don't you see how trembling overcomes the stallion's bodies as soon as they smell the well known odor?). There are indications that pheromones are also involved in regulating hypothalamo-pituitary activity. Investigations are limited because the exact chemical structure of most pheromones is not known.

Sexual Stimuli

Sexual stimuli of various kinds have a notable influence on the hypothalamo-pituitary-gonadal axis in both sexes. In female cats and rabbits a coital stimulus is required for ovulation. In these species the coital stimulus is thought to induce FSH and LH secretion from the anterior pituitary by a neurohormonal reflex, thereby provoking ovulation. In male rabbits, the act of copulation, or merely the presence of a doe, results in a substantial rise in the level of testosterone in the peripheral blood within 30 min,[147] possibly due to a reflex release of LH. In men, sexual activity may result in an increase in urinary testosterone excretion.[148] It has been demonstrated that there is an increase in beard growth in anticipation of sexual activity. This is thought to be a reflection of increased androgen secretion.[149] In the bull, sexual stimulation, such as the sight of a cow or "teasing", causes an immediate release of a large amount of LH, followed by a testosterone peak.[150]

Stress Stimuli

Stress serves as one example for external stimuli affecting the hypothalamo-pituitary-gonadal axis. Surgical stress in human male patients causes a transitory rise, then a fall in plasma LH and a sustained fall in plasma testosterone.[151] A depressing effect of opiates may be involved.[152] In the chicken, the stress caused by repeated handling results in an immediate fall in plasma LH.[153]

Puberty

The onset of sexual function, puberty, coincides with a definite state of body development.[154] It is retarded by a delay in growth. This seems to be a safety measure preventing reproduction before a certain size is reached. Puberty is well defined in its timing and its occurrence is predictable within the boundaries of each species. This has led to the supposition of a puberty-inducing mechanism.

The gonadotropic function develops during fetal life before the differentiation of the central nervous system leads to the control of hypothalamic regulation. Shortly after birth, it decreases abruptly and only minute quantities of gonadotropins are produced. This damping of the neonatal gonadotrophic function appears as a basic process in development, independent of steroids, but controlled by a central nervous mechanism. The onset of puberty is marked by a change in the secretion of gonadotropic hormones. The gradual rise in the mean gonadotropin level, especially in LH, is related to a gradual lessening of the central nervous system damping mechanism observed in man, rams, and rats. In puberal bulls no consistent changes in serum FSH or LH occur although serum testosterone increases markedly at about 5 months of age.[155]

During puberty there is a gradual adjustment between gonadotropin concentration and the gonadal steroid secretions which they induce. The rise in testicular testosterone secretion is characteristic of prepuberty. When steroid production increases, the mean rate of circulating gonadotropin decreases.

REFERENCES

1. **Gier, H. T. and Marion, G. B.,** Development of the mammalian testis, in *The Testis I,* Johnson, A. D., Gomes, W. R., and Vandemark, N. L., Eds., Academic Press, New York, 1970, 1.
2. **Wachtel, S. S.,** The dysgenetic gonad: aberrant testicular differentiation, *Biol. Reprod.,* 22, 1, 1980.
3. **Abdel-Raouf, M.,** The postnatal development of the reproductive organs in bulls with special reference to puberty, *Acta Endocrinol.,* Suppl. 49, 109, 1960.
4. **Attanasio, A. and Gupta, G.,** Hormonal events related to the process of normal testicular descent, in *Cryptorchidism,* Bierich, J. R. and Giarola, A., Eds., Academic Press, New York, 1979, 239.
5. **Bierich, J. R.,** Clinical treatment of maldescensus testis, in *Cryptorchidism,* Bierich, J. R. and Giarola, A., Eds., Academic Press, New York, 1979, 375.
6. **Hodson, N.,** Sympathetic nerves and reproductive organs in the male rabbit, *J. Reprod. Fertil.,* 10, 209, 1965.
7. **Steinberger, E. and Dixon, W. G.,** Some observations on the effect of heat on the testicular germinal epithelium, *Fertil. Steril.,* 10, 578, 1959.
8. **Fawcett, D. W.,** Ultrastructure and function of the Sertoli cell, in *Handbook of Physiology, Section 7,* Vol. 5, Hamilton, D. W. and Greep, R. O., Eds., American Physiological Society, Washington, D.C., 1975, 21.
9. **Setchell, B. P., Davies, R. V., and Main, S. J.,** Inhibin, in *The Testis IV,* Johnson, A. D. and Gomes, W. R., Eds., Academic Press, New York, 1977, 190.
10. **Fawcett, D. W., Neaves, W. B., and Flores, M. D.,** Comparative observations on intertubular lymphatics and the organization of the interstitial tissue of the mammalian testis, *Biol. Reprod.,* 9, 500, 1973.
11. **Bubenik, G. A., Brown, C. M., and Grota, L. J.,** Localization of immunoreactive androgen in testicular tissue, *Endocrinology,* 96, 63, 1975.
12. **Murota, S., Shikita, M., and Tamaoki, B-I.,** Intracellular distribution of the enzymes related to androgen formation in the mouse testis, *Steroids,* 5, 409, 1965.
13. **Hooker, C. W.,** The postnatal history and function of the interstitial cells of the testis of the bull, *Am. J. Anat.,* 74, 1, 1944.
14. **Ortavant, R., Courot, M., and Hochereau de Reviers, M. T.,** Spermatogenesis in domestic mammals, in *Reproduction in Domestic Animals,* Cole, H. H. and Cupps, P. T., Eds., Academic Press, New York, 1977, 203.
15. **Heller, C. G. and Clermont, Y.,** Spermatogenesis in man: an estimate of its duration, *Science,* 140, 184, 1963.
16. **Hochereau, M. T., Courot, M., and Ortavant, R.,** Labelling of the germinal cells of the ram and bull by the injection of triated thymidine into the spermatic artery, *Ann. Biol. Anim. Biochim. Biophys.,* 4, 157, 1964.
17. **Swierstra, E. E.,** Cytology and duration of the cycle of the seminiferous epithelium of the boar; duration of spermatozoon transit through the epididmyis, *Anal. Rec.,* 161, 171, 1968.
18. **Clermont, Y., Leblond, C. P., and Messier, B.,** Duration of spermatogenesis in the rat, as shown by radioautography after thymidine-H^3 injection, *Anat. Rec.,* 133, 261, 1959.
19. **Crabo, B.,** Studies on the composition of epididymal content in bulls and boars, *Acta Vet. Scand.,* 6, Suppl. 5, 1, 1965.
20. **Bedford, J. M.,** Maturation, transport and fate of spermatozoa in the epididymis, in *Handbook of Physiology, Section 7,* Vol. 5, Hamilton, D. W. and Greep, R. O., Eds., American Physiological Society, Washington, D.C., 1975, 303.
21. **Berthold, A. A.,** Transplantation der Hoden, *Arch. Anat. Physiol. Wissench. Med.* 16, 42, 1849.
22. **David, K., Dingemanse, E., Freud, J., and Laqueur, E.,** Über Krystallinisches Männliches Hormon aus Hoden (Testostron), Wirksamer als aus Harn oder aus Cholesterin, *Z. Physiol. Chem.,* 233, 281, 1935.
23. **Butenandt, A. and Harrisch, G.,** Ein Weg zur Testosteron-Umwandlung des Dehydroandrostendions in Androstendiol und Testosteron, *Z. Physiol. Chem.,* 237, 89, 1935.
24. **Ruzicka, L. and Wettstein, A.,** Über die Künstliche Herstellung des Testikelhormones Testosteron (Androsten-3-on-17-ol), *Helv. Chem. Acta,* 18, 1264, 1935.
25. **Kellie, A. E.,** Structure and nomenclature, in *Biochemisry of Steroid Hormones,* Makin, H. L. J., Ed., Blackwell Scientific Publications, Oxford, 175, 1.
26. **Goad, L. J.,** Cholesterol biosynthesis and metabolism, in *Biochemistry of Steroid Hormones,* Makin, H. L. J., Ed., Blackwell Scientific Publications, Oxford, 1975, 17.
27. **Werbin, H. and Chaikoff, I. L.,**Utilization of adrenal gland cholesterol for synthesis of cortisol by the intact normal and the ACTH-treated guinea pig, *Arch. Biochem. Biophys.,* 93, 476, 1961.
28. **Morris, M. D. and Chaikoff, I. L.,** The origin of cholesterol in liver, small intestine, adrenal gland and testis of the rat: dietary versus endogenous contributions, *J. Biol. Chem.,* 234, 1095, 1959.

29. **Hall, P. F. and Eik-Nes, K. B.,** The action of gonadotrophic hormones upon rabbit testis in vitro, *Biochem. Biophys. Acta,* 63, 411, 1962.
30. **Brady, R. O.,** Biosynthesis of radioactive testosterone in vitro, *J. Biol. Chem.,* 193, 145, 1951.
31. **Gower, D. B.,** Biosynthesis of the corticosteroids, in *Biochemistry of Steroid Hormones,* Makin, H. L. J., Ed., Blackwell Scientific Publications, Oxford, 1975, 47.
32. **Hall, P. F.,** On the stimulation of testicular steroidogenesis in the rabbit by interstitial cell-stimulating hormone, *Endocrinology,* 78, 690, 1966.
33. **Marsh, J. M.,** The role of cyclic AMP in gonadal steroido-genesis, *Biol. Reprod.,* 14, 30, 1976.
34. **Gower, D. B.and Fotherby, K.,** Biosynthesis of the androgens and oestrogens, in *Biochemistry of Steroid Hormones,* Makin, H. L. J., Ed., Blackwell Scientific Publications, Oxford, 1975, 77.
35. **Eik-Nes, K. B.,** Biosynthesis and secretion of testicular steroids, in *Handbook Physiology Section 7, Endocrinology,* Vol. 5, Hamilton, D. W. and Greep, R. O., Eds., American Physiological Society, Washington, D.C., 1975, 95.
36. **Setchell, B. B.,** *The Mammalian Testis,* Paul Elek, London, 1978.
37. **Nieschlag, E.,** Circadian rhythm of plasma testosterone, in *Chronobiological Aspects of Endocrinology,* Aschoff, J., Ceresa, F., and Halberg, F., Eds., Schattauer, Stuttgart, 1974, 117.
38. **Goodmann, R. L., Hotchkiss, J., Karsch, P. J., and Knobil, E.,** Diurnal variations in serum testosterone concentrations in the adult male rhesus monkey, *Biol. Reprod.,* 11, 624, 1974.
39. **Ellendorff, F., Parvici, N., Pomerantz, D. K., Hartjen, A., König, A., Smidt, D., and Elsaesser, F.,** Plasma luteinizing hormone and testosterone in the adult male pig: 24 hours fluctuations and the effect of copulation, *J. Endocrinol.,* 67, 403, 1975.
40. **Kirkpatrick, J. F., Vail, R., Devous, S., Schwend, S., Baker, C. B., and Wiesner, L.,** Diurnal variations of plasma testosterone in wild stallions, *Biol. Reprod.,* 15, 98, 1976.
41. **Katangole, C. B., Naftolin, F., and Short, R. V.,** Relationship between blood levels of luteinizing hormone and testosterone in bulls and the effect of sexual stimulation, *J. Endocrinol.,* 50, 45, 1971.
42. **Katangole, C. B., Naftolin, F., and Short, R. V.,** Seasonal variations in blood luteinizing hormone and testosterone levels in rams, *J. Endocrinol.,* 60, 101, 1974.
43. **Vermeulen, A.,** The physical state of testosterone in plasma, in *The Endocrine Function of the Human Testis,* Vol. 1, James, V. H. T., Serio, M., and Martini, L., Eds., Academic Press, New York, 1973, 157.
44. **Corvol, P. and Bardin, C. W.,** Species distribution of testosterone-binding globulin, *Biol. Reprod.,* 8, 277, 1973.
45. **Gower, D. B.,** Catabolism and excretion of steroids, in *Biochemistry of Steroid Hormones,* Makin, H. L. J., Ed., Blackwell Scientific Publications, Oxford, 1975, 149.
46. **Gondos, B.,** Development and differentiation of the testis and male reproductive tract, in *Testicular Development, Structure and Function,* Steinberger, A. and Steinberger, E., Eds., Raven Press, New York, 1980, 3.
47. **Gondos, B.,** Testicular development, in *The Testis,* Vol. 4, Johnson, C. A. D. and Gomes, W. R., Eds., Academic Press, New York, 1977, 1.
48. **Jost, A.,** Recherches sur la differenciation sexuelle de l'embryon de lapin. III. Rôle des gonades foetales dans la différenciation sexuelle somatique, *Arch. Anat. Microsc. Morphol. Exp.,* 36, 271, 1947.
49. **Neumann, F., Elger, W., and Steinbeck, H.,** Drug induced intersexuality in mammals, *J. Reprod. Fert. Suppl.,* 7, 9, 1969.
50. **Wilson, J. D., Griffin, J. E. and George, F. W.,** Sexual differentiation: early hormone synthesis and action, *Biol. Reprod.,* 22, 9, 1980.
51. **Ganong, W. F.,** Role of the nervous system in reproductive processes, in *Reproduction in Domestic Animals,* 3rd ed., Cole, H. H. and Cupps, P. T., Eds., Academic Press, New York, 1977, 49.
52. **Shiino, M. and Rennels, E. G.,** Ultrastructural observations on pituitary gonadotrophs following gonadectomy or administration of LH/FSH-releasing hormone in neonatal rats, *Tex. Rep. Biol. Med.,* 32, 561, 1974.
53. **Plapinger, L. and McEwen, B.S.,** Gonadal steroid-brain interactions in sexual differentiation, in *Biological Determinations of Sexual Behaviour,* Hutchinson, J. B., Ed., John Wiley & Sons, New York, 1978, 153.
54. **Goy, R. W. and Resko, J. A.,** Gonadal hormones and behaviour of normal and psuedohermaphroditic non-human female primates. *Recent Progr. Horm. Res.,* 28, 707, 1972.
55. **Sanborn, B. M., Elkington, J. S. H., Steinberger, A., Steinberger, E., and Meistrich, M. L.,** Androphilic proteins in the testis, in *Regulatory Mechanisms of Male Reproductive Physiology,* Spilman, C.H., Lobl, T. J., and Kirton, K. T., Eds., Excerpta Medica, Amsterdam, 1976, 13.
56. **Lostroh, A. J.,** Hormonal control of spermatogenesis, in *Regulatory Mechanisms of Male Reproductive Physiology,* Spilman, C. H., Lobl, T. J., and Kirton, K. T., Eds., Excerpta Medica, Amsterdam, 1976, 13.

57. **Orgebin-Christ, M. C., Danzo, B. J., and Davies, J.**, Endocrine control of the development and maintenance of sperm fertilizing ability in the epididymis, in *Handbook Physiology Section 7, Endocrinology*, Vol. 5, Hamilton, D. W., and Greep, R. O., Vol. Eds., American Physiological Society, Washington, D.C., 319, 1975.
58. **Fawcett, D. W. and Hoffer, A. P.**, Failure of exogenous androgens to prevent regression of the initial segment of the rat epididymis after efferent duct ligation or orchidectomy, *Biol. Reprod.*, 15, 162, 1979.
59. **Hammerstedt, R. H. and Amann, R. P.**, Interconversions of steroids by intact bovine sperm and epididymal tissue, *Biol. Reprod.*, 15, 686, 1976.
60. **Parkes, A. S.**, The internal secretions of the testis, in *Marshall's Physiology of Reproduction*, Vol. 3, Parkes, A. S., Ed., Longman, London, 1966, 412.
61. **Mann, T.**, *Biochemistry of Semen and of the Male Reproductive Tract*, Methuen, London, 1964.
62. **Skinner, J. D. and Rowson, L. E. A.**, Effects of testosterone injected unilaterally down the vas deferens on the accessory glands of the ram, *J. Endocrinol.*, 42, 355, 1968.
63. **Benkert, O.**, *Sexuelle Impotenz*, Springer-Verlag, Berlin, 1973.
64. **Voss, H. E. and Oertel, G.**, *Androgene I*, Springer-Verlag, Berlin, 1973.
65. **Wagner, R. K. and Hughes, A.**, Current view on androgen receptors and mechanism of androgen action, in *Androgens II and Antiandrogens*, Eichler, O., Farah, A., Herken, H., and Welch, W. D., Eds., Springer-Verlag, Berlin, 1974, 1.
66. **Hiipakka, R. A., Loor, R. M., and Liao, S.**, Receptors and factors regulating androgen action in the rat ventral prostate, in *Gene Regulation by Steroid Hormones*, Roy, A. K. and Clark, J. H., Eds., Springer-Verlag, Berlin, 1980, 194.
67. **Claus, R.**, *Mammalian Pheromones with Special Reference to the Boar Taint Steroid and its Relationship to Other Testicular Steroids*, Paul Parey, Hamburg, 1979.
68. **Kelch, R. P., Jenner, M. R., Weinstein, R., Kaplan, S. L., and Gumbach, M. M.**, Estradiol and testosterone secretion by human, simian and canine testes, in males with hypogonadism and in male pseudohermaphrodites with feminizing testes syndrome, *J. Clin. Invest.*, 51, 824, 1972.
69. **DeJong, F. H., Hey, A. H., and van der Molen, H. J.**, Effects of gonadotropins on the secretion of oestradiol-17β and testosterone by the rat testis, *J. Endocrin.*, 57, 277, 1973.
70. **Amann, R. P. and Ganjam, V. K.**, Steroid production by the bovine testis and steroid transfer across the pampiniform plexus, *Biol. Reprod.*, 15, 695, 1976.
71. **Savard, K. and Goldzieher, J. W.**, Biosynthesis of steroids in stallion testes tissue, *Endocrinology*, 66, 617, 1960.
72. **Dorrington, J. H., Fritz, I. B., and Armstrong, D. T.**, Control of testicular estrogen synthesis, *Biol. Reprod.*, 18, 55, 1978.
73. **Tcholakian, R. K. and Steinberger, A.**, In vitro metabolism of testosterone by Sertoli cells and interstitial cells and the effect of FSH, in *Testicular Development, Structure and Function*, Steinberger, A. and Steinberger, E., Eds., Raven Press, New York, 1980, 177.
74. **McCullagh, D. R.**, Dual endocrine activity of testis, *Science*, 76, 19, 1932.
75. **Main, S. J., Davies, R. V., and Setchell, B. P.**, The evidence that inhibin must exist, *J. Reprod. Fert., Suppl.*, 26, 3, 1979.
76. **Setchell, B.P., Davies, R. V., and Main, S. J.**, Inhibin, in *The Testis IV*, Johnson, A. D. and Gomes, W. R., Eds., Academic Press, New York, 1977, 190.
77. **Steinberger, A. and Steinberger, E.**, Inhibition of FSH by a Sertoli cell factor in vitro, in *The Testis in Normal and Infertile Men*, Troen, P. and Nankin, H. R., Eds., Raven Press, New York, 1977, 271.
78. **Johnson, J. M.**, The Histochemical Localization of Prostaglandin Synthetase in the Male Reproductive System of the Rat, M. S. thesis, Utah State University, Logan, 1976.
79. **Ellis, L. C. and Hargrove, J. L.**, Prostaglandins, in *The Testis*, Vol. 4, Johnson, C. A. D. and Gomes, W. R., Eds., Academic Press, New York, 1977, 289.
80. **Gerozissis, K. and Dray, F.**, Prostaglandins in the isolated testicular capsule of immature and young adult rats, *Prostaglandins*, 13, 777, 1977.
81. **Schally, A. V., Arimura, A., Baba, Y., Nair, R. M. G., Matsuo, H., Redding, T. W., Debeljuk, L., and White, W. F.**, Isolation and properties of the FSH and LH-releasing hormone, *Biochem. Biophys. Res. Commun.*, 43, 393, 1971.
82. **Amoos, M., Burgus, R., Blackwell, R., Vale, W., Fellows, R., and Guillemin, R.**, Purification, amino-acid composition and N-terminus of the hypothalamic luteinizing hormone-releasing factor (LRF) of ovine origin, *Biochem. Biophys. Res. Commun.*, 44, 205, 1971.
83. **Schally, A. V., Arimura, A., Kastin, A. J., Matsuo, H., Baba, Y., Redding, T. W., Nair, R. M. G., Debeljuk, L., and White, W. F.**, Gonadotrophin-releasing hormone: one polypeptid regulates secretion of luteinizing and follicle stimulating hormones, *Science (New York)*, 173, 1036, 1971.
84. **Palkovits, M., Arimura, A., Brownstein, M., Schally, A. V., and Saavedra, J. M.**, Luteinizing hormone-releasing hormone (LR-RH) content of the hypothalamic nuclei in rat, *Endocrinology*, 95, 554, 1974.

85. **Porter, J. C., Kamberi, I. A., and Grazia, Y. A.**, Pituitary blood flow and portal vessels, in *Frontiers in Neuroendocrinology,* Martini, L. and Ganong, W. F., Eds., Oxford University Press, New York, 145, 1971.
86. **Franchimont, P., Becher, H., Ernould, C. Thys, C., Demoulin, A., Bourgiurgon, J. P., Legros, J. J., and Valcke, J. C.**, The effect of hypothalamic luteinizing hormone releasing hormone (LH-RH) on plasma gonadotrophin levels in normal subjects, *Clin. Endocrinol.,* 3, 27, 1974.
87. **Fraser, H. M., Gunn, A., Jeffcoate, S. L., and Holland, D. T.**, Effect of active immunization to luteinizing hormone-releasing hormone on serum and pituitary gonadotrophins, testes and accessory sex organs in the male rat, *J. Endocrinol.,* 63, 399, 1974.
88. **Redding, T. W., Schally, A. V., Arimura, A., and Matsuo, H.**, Stimulation of release and synthesis of luteinizing hormone (LH) and follicle stimulating hormone (FSH) in tissue culture of rat pituitaries in response to natural and synthetic LH and FSH releasing hormone, *Endocrinology,* 90, 764, 1972.
89. **Lu, K. H., Grandisch, L., Huang, H. H., Marshall, S., and Meites, J.**, Relation of gonadotropin secretion by pituitary grafts to spermatogenesis in hypophysectomized male rats, *Endocrinology,* 100, 380, 1977.
90. **Kretser, D. M. de, Catt, K. J., and Paulsen, C. A.**, Studies on the in vitro testicular binding of iodinated luteinizing hormone in rats, *Endocrinology,* 88, 332, 1971.
91. **Catt, K. J., Tsuruhara, T., and Dufau, M. L.**, Gonadotrophin binding sites of the rat testis, *Biochem. Biophys. Acta,* 279, 194, 1972.
92. **Catt, K. J., Tsuruhara, T., Mendelson, C., Ketelslegers, J.-M., and Dufau, M. L.**, Gonadotrophin binding and activation of the interstitial cells of the testis, *Curr. Top. Molec. Endocrinol.,* 1, 1, 1974.
93. **Dorrington, J. H., Vernon, R. G., and Fritz, I. B.**, The effect of gonadotrophins on the 3′,5′-AMP levels of seminiferous tubules, *Biochem. Biophys. Res. Commun.,* 46, 1523, 1972.
94. **Rommerts, F. F. G., Cooke, B. A., Kemp, J. W. C. M. van der, and Molen, H. J. van der,** Effect of luteinizing hormone on 3′,5′-cyclic AMP and testosterone production in isolated interstitial tissue of rat testis, *FEBS Lett.,* 33, 114, 1973.
95. **Cooke, B. A., Rommerts, F. F.G., Kemp, J. W.C. M. van der, and Molen, H. J. van der,** Effects of luteinizing hormone, follicle stimulating hormone, prostaglandin E_1 and other hormones on adenosine-3′5′-cyclic monophosphate and testosterone production in rat testis tissues, *Mol. Cell. Endocrinol.,* 1, 99, 1974.
96. **Cooke, B. A., Janszen, F. H. A., Clotscher, W. F., and Molen, H. J. van der,** Effect of protein-synthesis inhibitors on testosterone production in rat testis interstitial tissue and Leydig-cell preparations, *Biochem. J.,* 150, 413, 1975.
97. **Means, A. R., Fakunding, J. L., Huckins, C., Tindall, D. J., and Vitale, R.**, Follicle-stimulating hormone, the Sertoli cell and spermatogenesis, *Rec. Prog. Horm. Res.,* 32, 477, 1976.
98. **Fritz, I. B., Rommerts, F. G., Louis, B. G., and Dorrington, J. H.**, Regulation by FSH and dibutyryl cyclic AMP of the formation of androgen-binding protein in Sertoli cell-enriched cultures, *J. Reprod. Fertil.,* 46, 17, 1975.
99. **Fritz, I. B., Louis, G. B., Tung, P. S., Griswold, M., Rommerts, F. G., and Dorrington, J. H.**, Biochemical responses of cultured Sertoli cell-enriched preparations to follicle stimulating hormone and dibutyryl cyclic AMP, *Curr. Top. Mol. Endocrinol.,* 2, 367, 1975.
100. **Means, A. R. and Vaitukaitis, J.**, Peptide hormone receptors specific binding of ^{3}H-FSH to testis, *Endocrinology,* 90, 39, 1972.
101. **Means, A. R.**, Specific interaction of ^{3}H-FSH with rat testis binding sites, *Adv. Exp. Med. Biol.,* 36, 431, 1973.
102. **Means, A. R., Fakunding, J. L., Huckins, C., Tindall, D. J., and Vitale, R.**, Follicle-stimulating hormone, the Sertoli cell and spermatogenesis, *Rec. Progr. Horm. Res.,* 32, 477, 1976.
103. **Steinberger, A., Heindel, J. J., Lindsey, J. N., Elkington, J. S. H., Sanborn, B. M., and Steinberger, E.**, Isolation and culture of FSH responsive Sertoli cells, *Endocrinol. Res. Commun.,* 2, 261, 1975.
104. **Means, A. R. and Huckins, C.**, Coupled events in the early biochemical actions of FSH on the Sertoli cells of the testis, in *Hormone Binding and Target cell Activation in Testis,* Dufau, M. L. and Means, A. R., Eds., Plenum Press, New York, 1974, 1945.
105. **Dorrington, J. H. and Fritz, I. B.**, Effects of gonadotropins on cyclic AMP production by isolated seminiferous tubule and interstitial cell preparations, *Endocrinology,* 94, 395, 1974.
106. **Means, A. R., Fakunding, J. L., and Tindall, D. J.**, Follicle stimulating hormone regulation of protein kinase activity and protein synthesis in testis, *Biol. Reprod.,* 14, 54, 1976.
107. **Fakunding, J. L., Tindall, D. J., Dedman, J. R., Mena, C. R., and Means, A. R.**, Biochemical actions of follicle stimulating hormone in the Sertoli cell of the rat testis, *Endocrinology,* 98, 392, 1975.
108. **Means, A. R. and Hall, P. F.**, Protein biosynthesis in the testis: the nature of stimulation by follicle stimulating hormone, *Biochemistry,* 8, 4293, 1969.

109. **Means, A. R. and Hall, P. F.**, Protein biosynthesis in the testis. VI. Action of follicle stimulating hormone on polyribosomes in immature rats, *Cytobios*, 3, 17, 1969.
110. **Means, A. R. and Tindall, D. J.**, FSH-induction of androgen binding protein in testis of Sertoli cell only rats, in *Hormonal Regulation of Spermatogenesis*, French, F. S., Hansson, V., Ritzen, E. M. and Nayfeh, S. N., Eds., Plenum Press, New York, 1975, 383.
111. **Hansson, V., Reusch, E., Trygstad, O., Torgersen, O., French, F. S., and Ritzen, E. M.**, FSH stimulation of testicular androgen binding protein (ABP), *Nat. New Biol.*, 246, 56, 1973.
112. **Tindall, D. J. and Means, A. R.**, Concerning the hormonal regulation of androgen binding protein in the rat, *Endocrinology*, 99, 809, 1976.
113. **Krey, L. C., Butler, W. R., and Knobil, E.**, Surgical disconnection of the medial basal hypothalamus and pituitary function in the Rhesus monkey. I. Gonadotropin Secretion, *Endocrinology*, 96, 1073, 1975.
114. **Hafiez, A. A., Philpott, J. E., and Bartke, A.**, The role of prolactin in the regulation of testicular function: the effect of prolactin and luteinizing hormone on 3β-hydroxy-steroid dehydrogenase activity in the testes of mice and rats, *J. Endocrinol.*, 50, 619, 1971.
115. **Hafiez, A. A., Lloyd, C. W., and Bartke, A.**, The role of prolactin in the regulation of testis function: the effects of prolactin and luteinizing hormone on the plasma levels of testosterone and androstendione in hypophysectomized rats, *J. Endocrinol.*, 52, 327, 1972.
116. **Rubin, R. T., Gonin, P. R., Lubin, A., Poland, R. E., and Pirke, K. M.**, Nocturnal increase of plasma testosterone in men: relation to gonadotropins and prolactin, *J. Clin. Endocrinol. Metab.*, 40, 1027, 1975.
117. **Boyar, R. M., Kapen, S., Finkelstein, J. W., Perlow, M., Sassin, J. F., Fukushima, D. K., Weitzman, E. D., and Hellman, L.**, Hypothalamic-pituitary function in diverse hyper-prolactinemic states, *J. Clin. Invest.*, 53, 1588, 1974.
118. **Horrobin, D. F.**, *Prolactin: Physiology and Clinical Significance*, MTP Medical and Technical Publishing, St. Leonhardgate, Lancaster, 1973, 45.
119. **Hartmann, G., Endroczi, E., and Lissak, K.**, The effect of hypothalamic implantation of 17-β oestradiol and systemic administration of prolactin on sexual behavior in male rabbits, *Acta Physiol. Acad. Sci. (Hungary)*, 30, 53, 1966.
120. **Schams, D.**, Untersuchunger über Prolaktin beim Rind, in *Advances in Animal Physiology and Animal Nutrition, Suppl. J. Anim. Phys. Anim. Nutr., No. 5*, Breirem, K., Brüggemann, J., Lenkeit, W., Schürch, A., and Wöhlbier, W., Eds., Paul Parey, Berlin and Hamburg, 1974, 50.
121. **Convey, E. M., Bretschneider, E., Hafs, H. D., and Oxender, W. D.**, Serum levels of LH, prolactin and growth hormone after ejaculation in bulls, *Biol. Reprod.*, 5, 20, 1971.
122. **Bryant, G. D., Linzell, J. L., and Greenwood, F. C.**, Plasma prolactin in goats measured by radioimmunoassay: the effect of teat stimulation, mating behavior, stress, fasting and of oxytocin, insulin and glucose injections, *Hormones*, 1, 26, 1970.
123. **Niemi, M. and Kormano, M.**, Contractility of the seminiferous tubule of the postnatal rat testis and its response to oxytocin, *Ann. Med. Exp. Biol. Fenn.*, 43, 40, 1965.
124. **Voglmayr, J. K.**, Output of spermatozoa and fluid by the testis of the ram and its response to oxytocin, *J. Reprod. Fert.*, 43, 119, 1975.
125. **Melin, P.**, Effects in vivo of neurohypophysial hormones on the contractile activity of accessory sex organs in male rabbits, *J. Reprod. Fert.*, 22, 283, 1970.
126. **Knight, T. W.**, A qualitative study of the factors affecting the contractions of the epididymis and vas deferens of the ram, *J. Reprod. Fert.*, 40, 19, 1974.
127. **Klenner, A. and Boryczko, Z.**, Beeinflussung der Spermienejektion beim Bullen durch Prostaglandin $F_{2\alpha}$ and Oxytocin, *Zuchthygiene*, 15, 21, 1980.
128. **Armstrong, D. T. and Hansel, W.**, Effects of hormone treatment on testes development and pituitary function, *Int. J. Fertil.*, 3, 296, 1958.
129. **Ewy, Z., Wȯjcik, K., Barowicz, T., Kolczak, T., and Wierzchoś, E.**, Veränderungen in der Oxytocinaktivität in Blutplasma und Hämatokritwerte beim Eber während der Samenentnahme, *Proc. VII. Int. Kongr. tier. Fortpflanz. Haustierbes. III*, Munchen, June 6 to 9, 1972, 2267.
130. **Carrer, H. F. and Taleisnik, S.**, Effects of mesencephalic stimulation of release of gonadotropins, *J. Endocrinol.*, 48, 527, 1970.
131. **Ganong, W. F.**, Role of catecholamines and acetyl-choline in the regulation of endocrine function: review, *Life Sci.*, 15, 1401, 1974.
132. **Reichlin, S.**, Regulation of the hypophysiotropic secretion of the brain, *Arch. Intern. Med.*, 135, 1350, 1975.
133. **de Wied, D. and de Jong, W.**, Drug effects and hypothalamic-anterior pituitary function, *Ann. Rev. Pharmacol.*, 14, 389, 1974.
134. **Porter, J. C. and Ben-Jonathan, N.**, Neuroendocrine mechanisms involved in biorhythms, in *Biorhythms and Human Reproduction*, Ferin, M., Hallberg, F., Richart, R. M., and Vande Wiele, R. L., Eds., John Wiley & Sons, New York, 1974, 607.

135. **Wurtman, R. J.**, Brain catecholamines and the control of secretion from the anterior pituitary gland, in *Hypophysiotropic Hormones of the Hypothalamus: Assay and Chemistry,* Meites, J., Ed., Williams & Wilkins, Baltimore, 1970, 184.
136. **Gay, V. L.**, The hypothalamus: physiology and clinical use of releasing factors, *Fertil. Steril.*, 23, 50, 1972.
137. **McCann, S. M.**, Regulation of follicle stimulating hormone and luteinizing hormone, in *Handbook of Physiology, Endocrinology,* Vol. 4, (Part 2), Knobil, E. and Sawyer, W. H., Eds., American Physiological Society, Washington D.C., 1974, 489.
138. **Leidl, W., Braun, U., Stolla, R., and Schams, D.**, Effects of hemicastration and unilateral vasectomy on the remaining gonad and on the FSH, LH and testosterone blood concentration in bulls, *Theriogenology,* 14, 173, 1980.
139. **Knobil, E.**, On the control of gonadotrophin secretion in the rhesus monkey, *Rec. Prog. Horm. Res.*, 30, 1, 1974.
140. **Turner, C. D. and Bagnara, J. T.**, *General Endocrinology,* W. B. Saunders, Philadelphia, 1971, 480.
141. **Sanford, L. M., Palmer, W. M., and Howland, B. E.**, Changes in the profiles of serum LH, FSH and testosterone, and in mating performance and ejaculate volume in the ram during the ovine breeding season, *J. Anim. Sci.*, 45, 1382, 1977.
142. **Hochereau-de Revier, M. T. and Lincoln, G. A.**, Seasonal variation in the histology of the testis of the red deer, *Cervus elaphus, J. Reprod. Fert.*, 54, 209, 1978.
143. **Thompson, D. L., Pickett, B. W., Berndtson, W. E., Voss, J. L., and Nett, T. M.**, Reproductive physiology of the stallion. VIII. Artificial photoperiod, collection interval and seminal characteristics, sexual behavior and concentrations of LH and testosterone in serum, *J. Anim. Sci.*, 44, 656, 1977.
144. **Pickett, B. W., Faulkner, L. C., and Sutherland, T. M.**, Effect of month and stallion on seminal characteristics and sexual behavior, *J. Anim. Sci.*, 31, 713, 1970.
145. **Claus, R.**, Mammalian pheromones with special reference to the boar taint steroid and its relationship to other testicular steroids, *Advances in Animal Physiology and Animal Nutrition, Suppl. J. Anim. Phys. Anim. Nutr., No. 10,* Günter, K. -D., Kirchgessner, M., Lenkeit, W., and Schürch, A., Paul Parey, Berlin and Hamburg, 1979, 32.
146. **Vergilius, M.**, Georgica, in *Bucolica-Georgica-Catolepton,* Gölle, J., and Gölle, M., Eds., Heimeran-Verlag, Munchen, 1970, 136.
147. **Haltmeyer, G. C. and Eik-Nes, K. B.**, Plasma levels of testosterone in male rabbits following copulation, *J. Reprod. Fert.*, 19, 273, 1969.
148. **Ismail, A. A. A. and Harkness, R. A.**, Urinary testosterone excretion in men in normal and pathological conditions, *Acta Endocrinol. (Copenhagen),* 56, 469, 1967.
149. **Anon.**, Effects of sexual activity on beard growth in man, *Nature (London),* 226, 869, 1970.
150. **Katangole, C. B., Naftolin, F., and Short, R. V.**, Relationship between blood levels of leuteinizing hormone and testosterone in bulls, and the effects of sexual stimulation, *J. Endocrinol.*, 50, 457, 1971.
151. **Aono, T., Kurachi, K., Mizutani, S., Hamanata, Y., Vozumi, T., Nakasima, A., Koshiyama, K., and Matsumoto, K.**, Influence of major surgical stress of plasma levels of testosterone, luteinizing hormone and follicle stimulating hormone in male patients, *J. Clin. Endocr. Metab.*, 35, 535, 1972.
152. **Steger, R. W., Sonntag, W. E., Van Vugt, D. A., Forman, L. J., and Meites, J.**, Reduced ability of naloxone to stimulate LH and testosterone release in aging male rats; possible relation to increase in hypothalamic met^5-enkephalin, *Life Sci.*, 27, 747, 1980.
153. **Wilson, S. C. and Sharp, P. J.**, Episodic release of luteinizing hormone in the domestic fowl., *J. Endocrinol.*, 64, 77, 1975.
154. **Levasseur, M. C.**, Thoughts on puberty, Initiation of the gonadotrophic function, *Ann. Biol. Anim. Bioch. Biophys.*, 17, 345, 1977.
155. **Karg, H., Gimenez, T., Hartl, M., Hoffman, B., Schallenberger, E., and Schams, D.**, Testosterone, luteinizing hormone (LH) and follicle stimulating hormone (FSH) in peripheral plasma of bulls: levels from birth through puberty and short term variations, *Zbl. Vet. Med. A.*, 23, 793, 1976.

THE POSTERIOR PITUITARY

George H. Gass and Warren E. Finn

INTRODUCTION

The hypophysis (pituitary) was known to ancient and medieval anatomists, but was considered unimportant until about the present century. Its essential importance is evidenced, however, by its presence throughout the vertebrate phylum.

Galen, the early Greek physician, thought that the pituitary gland was a secretory organ which filtered moisture and waste from the brain into the nasopharynx.[13]

Its name is thus derived from the Latin "pituita" (slime or phlegm). The term "hypophysis" from the Greek (under and growth) is an appropriate alternate term.

Oliver and Schäfer in 1895[23] found that pituitary extracts increased arterial blood pressure in dogs. Howell in 1898[24] ascribed this effect to the posterior pituitary. The responsible hormone was termed vasopressin. Magnus and Schäfer in 1901[25] found vasopressin to have an antidiuretic effect as well. By 1913 the antidiuretic hormone (ADH) was being used in the therapy of diabetes insipidus. By 1928 ADH was found to be different from oxytocin. The reader is referred to Heller[26] for an excellent detailed review of the history of posterior pituitary research.

GLAND MORPHOLOGY

The hypophysis cerebri, or pituitary gland, is an ovoid structure, weighing 600 mg in man, the gland being slightly heavier in the female than in the male.[12] It measures less than 1 cm anteroposteriorly and just greater than 1 cm transversely.

The anterior and posterior lobes of the pituitary are anatomically and functionally distinct, although they are seated together in the sella turica of the middle cranial fossa of the skull (sphenoid bone).[31,32]

The posterior pituitary is an integral extension of the hypothalamus and serves essentially as a storage and release area for certain hormones synthesized by the hypothalamus. In the secretory sense, the posterior pituitary is not an endocrine gland.

The anterior pituitary can independently synthesize at least six discrete hormones (discussed elsewhere in this text), but the hypothalamus is involved in regulating the pituitary secretions by sending down releasing (hypophysiotropic) hormones.

Terminology and Relationships

In standard nomenclature, the complex including the pituitary gland is divided into adenohypophysis and neurohypophysis (Figure 1). The former is a glandular portion and the latter is a neural portion. The adenohypophysis occupies about three fourths of the entire gland.

The adenohypophysis includes the (1) pars tuberalis; (2) pars intermedia, not well defined in man; and (3) pars distalis (pars anterior).

The neurohypophysis includes the (1) median eminence portion of the tuber cinereum; (2) infundibular stem; and (3) infundibular process, which is the neural lobe of the pituitary (pars nervosa).

Parts of the pars tuberalis of the adenohypophysis and the infundibular stem constitute a hypophyseal stalk.

Crafts[28] emphasizes the importance of the relationships of the pituitary to surrounding structures. Tumors of the gland occur, which can be followed by considerable

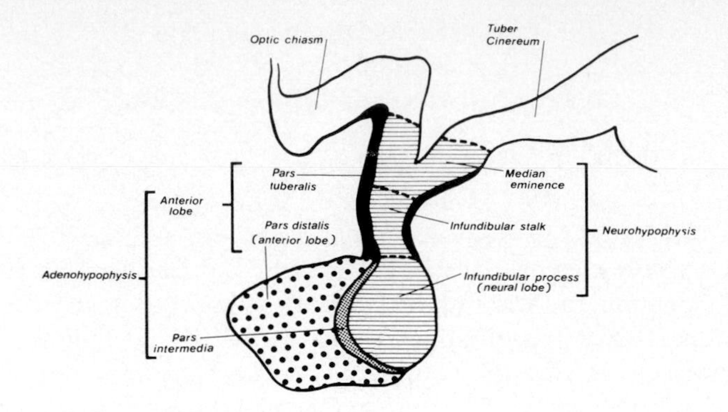

FIGURE 1. Midsagittal section of human pituitary gland and parts of hypothalamus.

enlargement. Since the pituitary is related superiorly to the optic chiasm and optic tracts, tumors may produce visual disturbances. The pituitary is related laterally to the internal carotid artery as well as other structures in the cavernous sinus, tumors thus causing pressure on these structures. The bony skull prevents extension of a tumor anteriorly, posteriorly and inferiorly.

If the stalk, which includes the tracts, is interrupted at any level, the axons and nerve cells suffer retrograde degeneration. An interruption below the median eminence does not cause diabetes insipidus because axons ending in the median eminence remain intact and are fully secretory. A lesion above this level will usually be associated with diabetes insipidus.

Blood Supply

The superior and inferior hypophyseal arteries branch off the internal carotid arteries. The superior vessels supply the stalk and adjacent parts of the anterior lobe while the inferior arteries supply the posterior lobe.

The pars distalis (pars anterior) portion of the anterior lobe derives its blood supply mainly from a portal venous system. In this arrangement, capillaries of the pars tuberalis section of the anterior lobe and nearby stalk send blood into veins that traverse the stalk and form sinusoidal capillaries of the pars distalis.[34,38]

From the above descriptions, it is seen that the anterior lobe has a supply of both arterial and venous blood. The neurohypophysis, apparently as a result of a primary vascular supply, is less vulnerable to hypoxia than is the adenohypophysis.[29]

Hypophyseal veins are called the lateral hypophyseal veins. They empty into the cavernous and intercavernous sinuses.

Nerve Supply

The pars distalis (glandular) cells have an uncertain innervation. Green[33] identified sympathetics traveling cranially away from the superior cervical ganglion along the blood vessels.

The neural innervation of the neurohypophysis involves (1) the supraoptical hypophyseal tract, located in the ventral part of the median eminence; and (2) the tuberohypophyseal tract, found in the dorsal wall of the median eminence and the stalk.

Both of the tracts listed are contained within the main hypothalamo-hypophyseal tract. The origin is the hypothalamus.

Microscopic Anatomy

The neurohypophysis includes the median eminence of the tuber cinereum, the infundibular stalk, and the infundibular process. There are a large number of cells called pituicytes and the terminals of axons whose cell bodies are in the hypothalamus. Most of the mass is unmyelinated nerve fibers which compose the hypothalamo-hypophyseal tract. The tract begins mainly in hypothalamic supraoptic nucleus and in the paraventricular nucleus in the third ventricle wall. After funneling into the median eminence, the fibers use the infundibular stalk to reach the infundibular process where they terminate and intertwine with the plexus of posterior lobe vessels. Discrete masses of neurosecretory material, called Herring bodies, can be traced down from hypothalamic nuclei and are especially concentrated in the infundibular process. Herring bodies represent secretory material that has originated in the supraoptic and paraventricular regions and which has traveled through the stalk to be stored in the infundibular process. There are also granular vesicles, of unknown function.

The pituicytes are supportive, but are possibly concerned with metabolic events in the endocrine secretion; the pituicytes do not secrete hormones as such.

The supraoptic nuclei primarily form vasopressin while the paraventricular nuclei primarily form oxytocin. However, both hormones are synthesized by each of these nuclei.

Developmental Anatomy

The hypothalamic floor develops several structures, some of which have relationship to the hypophysis of the hypothalamic structures which include the infundibulum, tuber cinereum, and mammillary bodies. The infundibulum specializes into the stalk and neural lobe of the hypophysis.

The hypophysis has a double origin. A glandular part originates from an ectodermal pocket, or sac, called Rathke's pouch, a diverticulum of the stomodeum. The pouch elongates and meets the second progenitor of the hypophysis, that is a sac-like extension of the infundibulum which is the forerunner of the neural lobe. Rathke's pouch loses its connection with the oral epithelium at the end of the second month. The pouch differentiates into the glandular cords of the anterior lobe, in the third and fourth months of development.

The original apex of Rathke's pouch remains thin and becomes the pars intermedia.

There is an additional glandular part called the pars tuberalis, which stretches forward along the infundibulum. This portion develops by fusion of two lateral lobes which have budded away from Rathke's pouch at a point where the stalk of the pouch has fused with the stomodeum.

The neural lobe, which has originated in the floor of the third ventricle, retains its connection by the infundibular stalk to the diencephalon. The lobe is transformed into a solid mass of neuroglia tissue and spindle-shaped cells.

In most vertebrates, the neurohypophysis differentiates into two subdivisions, the neural or posterior lobe (pars nervosa) and the median eminence. In some species, as in man, where the infundibulum evaginates sufficiently so that the neural lobe is distinct from the brain, the connecting region is called the stalk. The stalk contains nerve fibers and blood vessels.

CHEMISTRY OF THE NEUROHYPOPHYSEAL HORMONES

There are two active hormones in the posterior pituitary, oxytocin (pitocin), and vasopressin (pitressin; antidiuretic hormone, ADH). Both have been isolated, purified, and their structure determined. They are cyclic octapeptides (consisting of eight different amino acids) and both are similar in structure (Figure 2). These hormones have been synthesized.[27] In vasopressin, arginine and phenylalamine replace leucine and isoleucine of oxytocin. This similarity explains the frequent functional similarities.

The hormones in question are actually nonapeptides. However, because two of the amino acids are cysteine which are joined by a disulfide bond to produce one molecule of cystine, the hormones may be regarded as octapeptides.

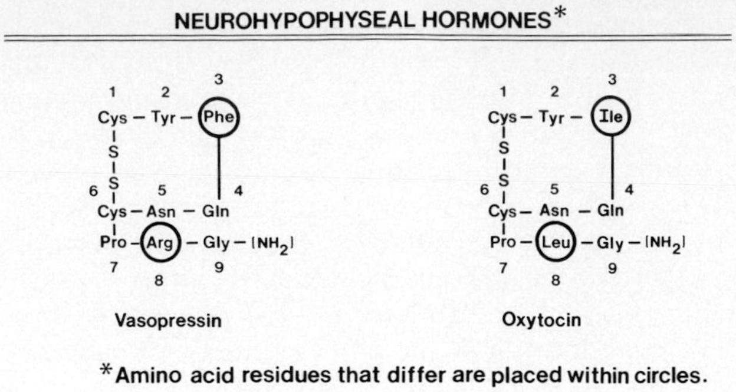

NEUROHYPOPHYSEAL HORMONES*

Vasopressin: Cys(1) – Tyr(2) – (Phe)(3) – Gln(4) – Asn(5) – Cys(6) – Pro(7) – (Arg)(8) – Gly(9) – (NH_2); S–S bridge between Cys 1 and Cys 6

Oxytocin: Cys(1) – Tyr(2) – (Ile)(3) – Gln(4) – Asn(5) – Cys(6) – Pro(7) – (Leu)(8) – Gly(9) – (NH_2); S–S bridge between Cys 1 and Cys 6

*Amino acid residues that differ are placed within circles.

FIGURE 2. Neurohypophyseal hormones.*

In mammals, there is a single form of oxytocin, but there are two vasopressins.[36] Figure 2 represents an ''arginine vasopressin'' found in man and some other species. In the pig a second form is seen as an 8-lysine vasopressin, in which lysine is present instead of arginine as the eighth amino acid. There is also a synthetic vasopressin, suitable for therapeutic use in man.

PHYLOGENY

In cyclostomes the neurohypophysis is just a thickened part of the floor of the diencephalon. There is no differentiation to median eminence and neural lobe.[14] In fish, a nonglandular saccus vasculosus, of unknown function, is added to the median eminence and posterior lobe.

In elasmobranchs a ventral lobe, homologous to the pars tuberalis, grows downward from the pituitary. Because it secretes gonadotropins, it is the equivalent to the pars distalis cells seen in other vertebrates.

In birds and a few species of mammals, the intermediate lobe is absent.[14]

In regard to the secretions, neurohypophyseal octapeptides are seen in all classes of vertebrates, the most widely distributed being arginine vasotocin (AV). This was first identified in the chicken and it contains isoleucine at position 3 and arginine at position 8.[12] AV is the only neurohormone in the cyclostome, the most primitive vertebrate. Thereafter, it appears among other neurohormones in all vertebrates. Thus AV may be the single ancestral molecule from which all other posterior pituitary hormones evolved.[12]

AV performs the antidiuretic function in amphibians, reptiles, and birds which arginine and lysine vasopressins performs in mammals. Vasotocin appears to have been discarded as mammals evolved, and a separation developed between an octapeptide involved in uterine contractility and milk ejection (oxytocin) and that promoting water conservation (vasopressins or ADH). The presence of these hormones in aquatic vertebrates is puzzling. Antidiuresis is an adaptation to terrestrial existence and the pituitary hormones are not concerned with water conservation in fishes. They are active, however, in renal sodium regulation.

The reader is referred to reviews by Maetz and Lahlou[40] on posterior pituitary hormones in fishes, and by Bentley[39] for neurohypophyseal peptides in amphibians, reptiles, and birds.

The two important posterior pituitary hormones in mammals are oxytocin and vasopressin. In most mammals the molecule is arginine vasopressin, although arginine and lysine vasopressin appear to be functionally equivalent.[14]

BIOSYNTHESIS OF HYPOPHYSEAL HORMONES

Vasopressin (antidiuretic hormone, ADH) and oxytocin are synthesized in a secretory system that acts as a neuron. The sites of origin include the paraventricular and supraoptic nuclei, although there is specialization of cells for each hormone. The supraoptic nucleus is especially secretory for vasopressin and the paraventricular nucleus for oxytocin. Other hypothalamic areas may also be sites of biosynthesis.[18]

The matured hormones are bound with neurophysins and transported for storage into the posterior pituitary.

The pituicytes were once thought to be the sources of the hormones. This is now denied. Pituicytes are neuroglia. They may be involved in the release mechanism or in the separation of the hormones from their carrier.

REGULATION OF VASOPRESSIN SECRETION

Vasopressin is secreted in response to changes in plasma osmolality. An increase in osmolality of only a few milliosmoles per kg excites the hormonal release. A small decrease in osmolality inhibits vasopressin release.

The osmolality (and osmotic pressure) of the plasma are determined markedly by the concentrations of sodium and chloride. There are osmoreceptors to sense the resulting osmolality in the endothelium of the carotid arteries. These receptors may be connected by autonomic afferents to the neurohypophysis. The hypothalamus is also said to have osmoreceptors which are located in the supraoptic nuclei.

A rise in osmotic pressure of the plasma results in the release of ADH. The reabsorption of water in the renal tubules decreases the urinary volume, while correcting the high salt concentration in the plasma.

Other stimuli can affect vasopressin secretion. A large loss of plasma volume stimulates hormone release even though the toxicity may not be changed. There are volume receptors in the walls of the atria and the large veins.

Severe stress can act as a stimulus for ADH release. Stress probably acts via the hypothalamus.

Drugs affect release. Thus nicotine enhances release, whereas alcohol suppresses it.

Thirst centers of an excitatory or inhibitory nature within the hypothalamus radiate their impulses to the neurohypophyseal nuclei. Disorders of the thirst centers thus have an influence of a corrective nature on ADH release.

REGULATION OF OXYTOCIN SECRETION

Since the actions of oxytocin are evident during parturition and lactation, it is expected that oxytocin release would be triggered by stimuli associated with early pregnancy, late pregnancy, and also with lactation.

In lactation, the suckling or milking process is adequate stimulation to excite sensory receptors in the nipples. Impulses pass to the paraventricular nuclei of the hypothalamus. In turn, oxytocin is released from its storage sites in the neurohypophysis.

The milk-ejection reflex is vital for milk removal in most species. In some ruminants, however, milk removal is achieved in the absence of the reflex.

Oxytocin levels in the blood vary with the particular organ that is stimulated.[46] Distention of the human female genital tract during parturition is probably the most effective stimulus. This is not true for the mammary gland, where suckling or milking rather than nonspecific stimulation triggers the milk-ejection reflex.

TRANSPORT OF THE HORMONES

The hormones exist within the hypothalamus in a protein linkage. This complex, when released, is sent via the hypothalamo-hypophyseal tract to the posterior pituitary. The latter area serves for storage, releasing the hormones into the general circulation upon demand.

In the stalk, the hormones are transmitted by two proteins, neurophysins 1 and 2. Oxytocin is associated with 1 and vasopressin with 2. The neurophysin 2 relationship is weak and the complex dissociates fully when the pituitary releases ADH (vasopressin) into the blood stream.

The nature of the neurophysins is discussed elsewhere.[35,44] Their molecular weights are about 1×10^4 daltons. Neurophysin 2 has 97 amino acids, is globular, and has some alphahelical segments. Neurophysin 2s tertiary structure is maintained by seven disulfide bridges.

Transport of the hormones from the hypothalamic nuclei to the pituitary is relatively rapid. It was found in the rat that after a stimulus such as hemorrhage, hormones can be detected in the pituitary in about 30 min.[17]

The transport mechanism in the blood may involve binding with a plasma globulin. Neither oxytocin nor vasopressin bind or enter into erythrocytes.[45] Data on protein binding for vasopressin are inconsistent, but they indicate that less than one-third may be bound. For oxytocin, less than two-thirds may be bound in human plasma, but the evidence for that is conflicting. There are no data on the binding of oxytocin or vasotocin to proteins in the plasma of submammalian species.[45]

DEGRADATION OF THE HORMONES

The hormones are enzymatically degraded in organs such as the liver, muscle, kidney, and uterus. These organs contain the enzymes vasopressinase and oxytocinase. The kidney may be the chief site of degradation.

There is a capacity to inactivate oxytocin and vasopressin in blood or plasma of women during pregnancy.[41] Oxytocinase is present in abundance in pregnant women. It is probable function is to prevent a premature abortion due to the presence of oxytocin.

The half-life of circulating vasopressin is about 10 min. The kidney clears up to 50% of it, both by glomerular filtration and tubular secretion. Very little remains for passage into the urine. The clearance median of oxytocin in man was estimated by Fabian and coworkers[42] to be about 20 mℓ/kg/min. Saameli[43] estimated the half-life of oxytoxin in pregnant women near term to be 3 to 4 min.

Four sites of cleavage are identified for natural hormones. The very important ones occur at positions 7 to 8 and 8 to 9 in the linear section of the peptide. There is also modification at the disulfide bond and position 1 to 2.[16]

PHYSIOLOGIC EFFECTS OF OXYTOCIN

Some hormones, such as growth hormone and thyroxine have most of the cells of the body as their target. Others have a relatively small number of target cells. Oxytocin is at another extreme, apparently acting solely or primarily on the uterine muscle and the myoepithelial cells of the lactating mammary glands.

Oxytocin appears to be important in initiating and maintaining contractions of the uterus at parturition. The uterus becomes especially sensitive at full term of pregnancy. The effect involves changes in the axon potentials of the myometrium. There is a dependence upon the presence of estrogen and the immature uterus is resistant to contractile activity.[21]

Oxytocin initiates lactation, this effect being mechanical. The hormone stimulates the myoepithelial cells and milk is ejected from the alveoli in the ducts. In domestic animals this is called milk let-down. There is no neural autonomic control.

Oxytocin can cause contraction of smooth muscles other than those of the uterus and breast. ADH is even more powerful in exciting contractions of the other smooth muscles.

The effects are of a relaxing nature on vascular smooth muscle when large doses of oxytocin are administered. Associated cardiac effects include decreased systolic and diastolic pressures, tachycardia and increased cardiac output. The vasodilator effects do not depend upon autonomic receptors.[15]

It is claimed that oxytocin promotes fertilization of the ovum. The mechanism involved causes uterine propulsion of the sperm cranially in the oviducts.

There is a third effect related to the hypothalamic areas controlling the pituitary hormone output. If the anterior region of the hypothalamus is stimulated, there may be milk ejection (oxytocin effect), decreased production of urine (ADH effect), and also polydipsia. The diversity of response is due to the functional interrelationship between the hypothalamic thirst nuclei and those of the supraoptic and paraventricular nuclei.

Suprisingly, there is no known deficiency syndrome of oxytocin. Parturition and lactation proceed normally in diabetes insipidus, showing either that oxytocin is independently released as a distinct hormone or that possibly other oxytocic factors elsewhere are brought in to maintain labor and expression of milk. ADH can stimulate the pregnant uterus, but less than 1/100 as potently as oxytocin. The latter has 1/100 the vasopressor activity of ADH and is 100 times more effective in facilitating milk ejection.

ADH and oxytocin are released independently.[30] Suckling in women soon after delivery induces marked oxytocin-like and milk-ejecting activities, but negligible antidiuresis. Also, hypertonic saline produces marked antidiuresis, but negligible oxytocin-like or milk-ejecting activities.

The effects of oxytocin are related to binding sites in the myometriuses.[20] The receptors are on the plasma membrane of the smooth muscle cells and they display specificity.

The effects of oxytocin and also vasopressin are influenced by prostaglandins.[11] The prostaglandins enhance the activity of oxytocin, but antagonize those of vasopressin. Both E and F prostaglandins stimulate uterine contractions and are possible intermediates in oxytocin-induced labor. The prostaglandins have been found in amniotic fluid and unbilical cord at full term.[9,10] Oxytocin is produced in males where its functions are unknown. Also, it has no proven function in the nonpregnant female.

PHYSIOLOGIC EFFECTS OF ADH (VASOPRESSIN)

Reabsorption of Water from the Kidneys

ADH causes increased reabsorption of water in the distal convoluted tubules and collecting ducts of the kidney. ADH combines specifically with a receptor on the basal surface of the tubule epithelium and excites the production of cyclic AMP. It is the cAMP that increases the permeability of the membranes, which may involve enlargement of the pores. Water is allowed to diffuse freely into the peritubular fluids. The process is one of osmosis.

Through fluctuations in the plasma ADH one can change the specific gravity of the urine osmolality from 40 to 1400 milliosmols/ℓ. or vary the volume of urine from 0.5 to 20 ℓ/day.

The mechanism of these controls may not be limited to regulation of membrane permeability. A second action may be to vasoconstrict arterioles passing to the vasa recta (vessels) of the renal medulla. By reducing local flow in this region, the hypertonic fluid within the medullary peritubular space is prevented from being washed out. A third mechanism is to facilitate the transport of sodium ions into the hypertonic medullary fluid.

It should be emphasized that water homeostasis involves not only ADH, but also mineralocorticoids and glucorticoids of the adrenal cortex, thyroid hormones, and estrogen.

B. Regulation of Sodium Ion Concentration

ADH helps regulate the osmolality of the extracellular fluids. Its effect is exerted not only because of water reabsorption, but more importantly because of its influence on sodium ion resorption. The sodium concentration in the plasma determines about 95% of the prevailing osmotic pressure.

C. Contraction of Smooth Muscles

In a secondary action, ADH in large doses can excite contraction of smooth muscles throughout the body. This may be of little physiologic importance because of the large quantities of ADH needed.

D. Involvement in Blood Pressure Regulation

ADH can have a vasoconstrictive effect on arterioles, if present in moderate to high concentrations. The stimulus is a severe loss in blood volume. This excites not only atrial receptors but also baroreceptors elsewhere in the arterial vasculature.

The question of the importance of the role of vasopressin in the homeostasis of arterial pressure is not resolved, however. Padfield and co-workers[22] found that in patients with malignant hypertension, vasopressin levels ae elevated but they do not correlate with arterial pressure. Also, blood pressure in normal persons does not rise when vasopressin is considerably increased by infusion. In patients with inappropriate ADH secretion, blood pressure is not raised, but vasopressin is elevated and does not correlate with systolic or diastolic pressure. These data indicate that an acute or chronic excess of vasopressin does not make an important contribution to the normal regulation of blood pressure.

E. Effects on Blood Coagulation

Vasopressin is effective in the treatment of moderate hemophilia and von Willebrand's disease, apparently by enhancement of the level of factor 8.[19] The hormone can be given to prevent bleeding in surgery. The mechanism is yet to be elucidated.

ASSAYS FOR OXYTOCIN

Methods for assay of oxytocin are discussed adequately by Kagan and Glick[6] and Chard and Forsling.[5]

Bioassays for oxytocin are cumbersome, subjective, and lacking in specificity. Wheeler et al.[2] produced antibodies of adequate titer and affinity to allow the development of a sensitive radioimmunoassay. This method does not detect oxytocin in unextracted plasma nor is it simple or free from interfering factors. A radioimmunoassay procedure by Chard et al.[3] presents similar problems.

Chard[3] reported oxytocin concentrations as follows: normal males, nonpregnant women, women in third trimester of pregnancy, and in both first and second stages of labor, less than 1.5 pg/mℓ of plasma.

Cord venous blood plasma, 0 to 200 pg/mℓ; cord arterial blood plasma, 7 to 290 pg/mℓ.

The finding by Chard and associates[4] that human maternal oxytocin levels during labor are very low suggests that oxytocin may be less important than thought in that period.

Chad and Forshing[5] state that it is uncertain whether there is a normal value of circulating oxytocin. There is a relase in a series of spurts, so that frequency of release rather than plasma concentration may be the important parameter.

ASSAYS FOR VASOPRESSIN

Glick and Kagan[6] and Chard and Forsling[5] present concise reviews of assays for vasopressin. A radioimmunoassay for vasopressin was developed early by Permatt et al.[7] and Robertson et al.[8] but there were difficulties with cross-reacting plasma artifacts.

Glick and Kagan[6] list their own and other values: plasma level in healthy, recumbent males, 1.5 pg/mℓ or less; after dehydration, 5 to 10 pg/mℓ.

Vasopressin excretion into urine, 0 to 0.35 mIU/hr (120IU/mg) in water-loaded normal males; 1.2 to 6.5 mIU/hr in dehydrated normals.

REFERENCES

1. **Kagan, A. and Glick, S. M.**, Oxytocin, in *Methods of Hormone Radioimmunoassay*, Jaffe, B. M. and Behrman, H. R., Eds., Academic Press, New York, 1974, 173.
2. **Wheeler, M., Kagan, A., and Glick, S. M.**, Radioimmunoassay of oxytocin, *Clin. Res.*, 14, 479, 1966.
3. **Chard, T., Forsling, M. L., Kitan, M. H. R., and Landon, J.**, The development of a radioimmunoassay for oxytocin: specificity and the dissociation of immunological and biological activity, *J. Endocrinol.*, 46, 533, 1970.
4. **Chard, T., Boyd, N. R. H., Forsling, M. L., McNeilly, A. S., and Landon, J.**, The development of a radioimmunoassay for oxytocin: the extraction of oxytocin from plasma and its measurement during parturition in human and goat blood, *J. Endocrinol.*, 48, 223, 1970.
5. **Chard, T. and Forsling, M. L.**, Bioassay and radioimmunoassay of oxytocin and vasopressin, in *Hormones in Human Blood: Detection and Assay*, Antoniades, H. N., Ed., Harvard University Press, Cambridge, 1976, 488.
6. **Glick, S. M. and Kagan, A.**, Vasopressin, in *Methods of Hormone Radioimmunoassay*, Jaffe, B. M. and Behrman, H. R., Eds., Academic Press, New York, 1974, 187.
7. **Permutt, M. A., Parker, C. W., and Utiger, R. D.**, Immunochemical studies with lysine vasopressin, *Endocrinology*, 78, 809, 1966.
8. **Robertson, G. L., Klein, L. A., Roth, J., and Gorden, P.**, Immunoassay of plasma vasopressin in man, *Proc. Natl. Acad. Sci. U.S.A.*, 66, 1298, 1970.
9. **Karim, S. M. M.**, The identification of prostaglandins in human umbilical cord, *Br. J. Pharmacol.*, 29, 230, 1967.
10. **Karim, S. M. M. and Devlin, J.**, Prostaglandin content of amniotic fluid during pregnancy and labour, *J. Obstet. Gynaecol. Br. Commonw.*, 74, 230, 1967.
11. **Pharriss, B. B.**, Interactions of prostaglandins and hormones, in *The Action of Hormones*, Foa, P. O., Ed., Charles C Thomas, Springfield, Ill., 1971, 262.
12. **Turner, C. D. and Bagnara, J. T.**, *General Endocrinology*, 5th ed., W. B. Saunders, Philadelphia, 1971, 74.
13. **Grollman, A.**, *Essentials of Endocrinology*, J. B. Lippincott, Philadelphia, 1947, 17.
14. **Waterman, A. J., Frye, B. E., and Johansen, K.**, *Chordate Structure and Function*, Macmillan, New York, 1971.
15. **Hays, R. M.**, Agents affecting the renal conservation of water, in *Goodman and Gilman's The Pharmacological Basis of Therapeutics*, 6th ed., Gilman, A G., Goodman, L. S., and Gilman, A., Eds., Macmillan, New York, 1980, 916.

16. **Walter, R. and Simmons, W. H.,** Metabolism of neurohypophyseal hormones: considerations from a molecular viewpoint, in *Neurohypophysis: International Conference on the Neurophyophysis,* Moses, A. M., and Share, L., Eds., S. Karger, Basel, 1977, 167.
17. **Norstron, A. and Sjostrand, J.,** Effect of haemorrhage on the rapid axonal transport of neurohypophysial proteins of the rat, *J. Neurochem.,* 18, 2017, 1971.
18. **George, J. M.,** Immunoreactive vasopressin and oxytocin: concentration in individual human hypothalamic nuclei, *Science,* 200, 342, 1978.
19. **Manucci, P. M., Pareti, F. I., Ruggeri, Z. M., and Capitano, A.,** 1-Deamino-8-0-arginine vasopressin: a new pharmacological approach to the management of haemophilia and von Willebrand's disease, *Lancet,* 1, 869, 1977.
20. **Soloff, M. S., Alexandrova, M., and Fernstrom, M. J.,** Oxytocin receptors: triggers for parturition and lactation?, *Science,* 204, 1313, 1979.
21. **Csapo, A.,** Function and regulation of the myometrium, *Am. Acad. Sci. (New York),* 75, 790, 1959.
22. **Padfield, P. L., Brown, J. J., Lever, A. F., Morton, J. J., and Robertson, J. I.,** Blood pressure in acute and chronic vasopressin excess, *N. Engl. J. Med.,* 304, 1067, 1981.
23. **Oliver, G. and Schäfer, E. A.,** On the physiological action of extracts of the pituitary body and certain other glandular organs, *J. Physiol. (London),* 18, 277, 1895.
24. **Howell, W. H.,** The physiological effects of extracts of the hypophysis cerebri and infundibular gocy, *J. Exptl. Med.,* 3, 245, 1898.
25. **Magnus, R. and Schäfer, E. A.,** The action of pituitary extracts upon the kidney, *J. Physiol. (London),* 27, 9, 1901.
26. **Heller, H.,** History of neurohypophyseal research, in *Handbook of Physiology, Section 7, Endocrinology, Vol. 4, The Pituitary Gland and its Neuroendocrine Control,* Greep, R. O., Astwood, E. B., Knobil, E., Sawyer, W. H., and Geiger, S. R., Eds., American Physiological Society, Washington, D.C., 1974, 103.
27. **du Vigneaud, V., Lalwer, H. C., and Popenoe, E. A.,** The synthesis of an oxypeptide amide with the hormonal activity of oxytocin, *J. Am. Chem. Soc.,* 75, 4879, 1953.
28. **Crafts, R. C.,** *A Textbook of Human Anatomy,* Ronald Press, New York, 1966, 462.
29. **Ezrin, C., Godden, J. O., Volpe, R., and Wilson, R., Eds.,** *Systematic Endocrinology,* Harper & Row, New York, 1973, 15.
30. **Gaitan, E., Cobo, E., and Mizrachi, M.,** Evidence for the differential secretion of oxytocin and vasopressin in man, *J. Clin. Invest.,* 43, 2310, 1964.
31. **Gardner, E., Gray, D. J., and O'Rahilly, R.,** *Anatomy,* 3rd ed., W. B. Saunders, Philadelphia, 1969, 612.
32. **Goss, C. M., Ed.,** *Gray's Anatomy of the Human Body,* 28th ed., Lea & Febiger, Philadelphia, 1966, 1347.
33. **Green, J. D.,** The comparative anatomy of the hypophysis, with special reference to its blood supply and innervation, *Am. J. Anat.,* 88, 225, 1951.
34. **Green, H. T.,** The venous drainage of the human hypophysis cerebri, *Am. J. Anat.,* 100, 435, 1947.
35. **Montgomery, R., Dryer, R. L., Conway, T. W., and Spector, A. A.,** *Biochemistry, a Case-Oriented Approach,* C. V. Mosby, St. Louis, 1974, 528.
36. **Montgomery, D. A. D. and Welburn, R. B.,** *Medical and Surgical Endocrinology,* The Williams & Wilkins Company, Baltimore, 1975, 55.
37. **Stanfield, J. P.,** The blood supply of the human pituitary gland, *J. Anat. (London),* 94, 257, 1960.
38. **Bentley, P. J.,** Actions of neurohypophyseal peptides in amphibians, reptiles and birds, in *Handbook of Physiology, Section 7, Endocrinology,* Greep, R. O. and Astwood, E. B., Eds., American Physiological Society, Washington, D.C., 1974, 545.
39. **Maetz, J. and Lahlou, B.,** Actions of neurohypophyseal hormones in fishes, in *Handbook of Physiology, Section 7, Endocrinology,* Greep, R. O. and Astwood, E. B., Eds., American Physiological Society, Washington, D.C., 1974, 521.
40. **Tuppy, H.,** The influence of enzymes on neurohypophyseal hormones and similar peptides in *Handbuch der Experimentellen Pharmakologie,* Berde, B., Ed., Springer-Verlag, Berlin, 1968, 67.
41. **Fabian, M., Forsling, M. L., Jones, J. J., and Pryor, J. S.,** The clearance and antidiuretic potency of neurohypophyseal hormones in man, and their plasma binding and stability, *J. Physiol. (London),* 204, 653, 1969.
42. **Saameli, K.,** An indirect method for the estimation of oxytocin blood concentration and half-life in pregnant women near term, *Am. J. Obstet. Gynecol.,* 85, 186, 1963.
43. **Hope, D. B. and Pickup, J. C.,** Neurophysins, in *Handbook of Physiology, Section 7, Endocrinology,* Vol. 4, (Part 1), Greep, R. O. and Astwood, E. B., Eds., American Physiological Society, Washington, D.C., 1974, 173.
44. **Lawson, H. D.,** Metabolism of the neurohypophyseal hormones, in *Handbook of Physiology, Section 7, Endocrinology,* Vol 4, (Part 1), Greep, R. O. and Astwood, E. B., Eds., American Physiological Society, Washington, D.C., 1974, 287.

45. **Tindal, J. S.,** Stimuli that cause the release of oxytocin, in *Handbook of Physiology, Section 7, Endocrinology,* Vol. 4, (Part 1), Greep, R. O. and Astwood, E. B., Eds., American Physiological Society, Washington, D.C., 1974, 257.

THE ADRENAL CORTEX

William T. Allaben

INTRODUCTION

The adrenal glands are endocrine organs that lie at the cranial pole of each kidney. The glands are frequently referred to as the suprarenal glands and in the older literature as suprarenal bodies, suprarenal capsules, and anatomically as glandula suprarenalis. The glands consist of two parts which differ by origin, structure and function. Functionally, the organs are divided into two major chemical categories (1) the cortex, which is involved in the biosynthesis of steroids (steroidogenesis); and (2) the medulla, which is involved in the biosynthesis of catecholamines (catechologenesis).

The cortex is the outer most tissue of the adrenal gland, lying between the capsule (covering of the gland and the adrenal medulla. This chapter deals only with the adrenal cortex, its development, anatomy, biochemistry, function, and pathology.

HISTORICAL

The adrenal glands were first described by B. Eustacchio in a document entitled "Tabulae Anatomicae", dated 1563, in which he termed them *glandulae Renibus incumbentes.* However, his work was not published until 1714 when Lancisi, an Italian scientist, published Eustacchio's drawings with his (Lancisi's) own captions added to the illustrations.[1] The secrets of the adrenal gland remained intact for many more decades. It wasn't until Addison published his first observations of the adrenals in disease, in a paper in 1849, and later his monograph in 1855, describing the symptoms displayed from individuals who had been discovered to have diseased adrenals at autopsy,[2] that any significant scientific data was published. From that time forward, the research efforts on the adrenal gland increased as did the controversies regarding the significance and biological role of that organ. Early experimentation with animals showed that removal of the adrenals led to certain clinical symptoms followed by death.[3] However, numerous other reports stated that adrenalectomy did not always lead to death. The controversy, especially arising from Philipeaux's work,[4] was the result of his use of the rat as an experimental animal, now known to possess accessory adrenal bodies that serve as functional adrenal cortical tissue when the adrenal glands are removed.

Few papers of significance were published concerning the split functions of the adrenal gland until the early 1900s. A paper by Biedl[5] implied that in fish, which have separate cortical and cromaffin tissue, destruction of the cortical tissue alone was responsible for the observed adrenal failure symptomatology. Others, such as Hartman,[6] Houssay,[7] and Wheeler[8] contributed to the literature by defining the separation of function between cortical and medullary tissue and establishing the importance of the adrenal cortex in maintaining life. The reason that the adrenal cortex was necessary for life eluded scientists for years. Many thought that it had a detoxifying function, primarily because the glands are so richly supplied with blood vessels. By the early 1930s clues were uncovered showing that the adrenal cortical tissue contained a substance that, when extracted and administered to adrenalectomized animals, prolonged the life of these animals indefinitely.[9-13] The observed symptoms of adrenalectomized animals was dramatically reversed with the administration of the cortical tissue extracts. It wasn't long before the extract was used clinically with equally successful results. Rountree et al. treated a patient with Addison symptoms in 1930, using the extracts prepared by Swingle and Pfiffner.[14] Gradually the adrenal cortical extract was recognized as a hormone. With the progress in chemical methodology developing in the third decade of the 20th century, many steroid compounds were isolated from adrenal cortical extracts. These isolated steroids were a curiosity and the importance of their biological effects would wait several years before being uncovered.[15-17] Besides the steroids isolated, the aqueous fraction contained another important factor which seemed to have a vital function. This compound, today known as aldosterone, is a potent mineralocorticoid.

Even before the chemistry of the adrenal cortex was being uncovered, many facts about the physiology that the adrenal gland controls were recorded. The fact that the adrenal gland influenced the kidney was suggested in 1916 with a report by Marshall and Davis.[18] Some 10 years later two reports were published noting that there was a lower serum sodium concentration but an elevated serum potassium concentration in adrenalectomized cats, and that sodium salts and glucose administration would prolong the life of these animals.[19,20] Clinically, Loeb was the first to demonstrate that sodium chloride administration to an Addison disease patient would benefit the patient.[21] This type of therapy was not life sustaining however. Some years later Allers and Kendall[22] discovered that a diet high in sodium and low in potassium, administered to adrenalectomized dogs, would prolong the life of the animal for indefinite periods of time. While the importance of the adrenal gland in the regulation of electrolyte metabolism was being established by the efforts of many, Britton published two papers in 1932 stating the significance of the adrenal glands in regulating carbohydrate metabolism,[23] and the importance of the adrenal cortex in that regulation.[24] Additional evidence that the adrenal cortex was involved in gluconeogenesis was collected during the next few years and in 1940 Long[25] published a paper which convinced the majority of the adrenal gland investigators of the importance of this gland in glucose metabolism.

Early in the 20th century some investigators were observing and reporting an apparent relationship of the adrenal gland to the gonads.[26-27] These observations were further substantiated some years later when it was noted that pregnant dogs survived adrenalectomy much longer than nonpregnant ones.[28] The key to the pregnancy effect noted in pregnant adrenalectomized dogs became apparent when Gaunt in 1938 administered progesterone to adrenalectomized ferrets.[29] His animals survived quite well with progesterone, here substituting for corticosteroids. Similarly, pseudopregnancy maintained the life and health of adrenalectomized ferrets.

The early literature suggests that pituitary trauma or disease was often accompanied by adrenal atrophy. These observations were reinforced in 1930 when P.E. Smith[30] noted that pituitary destruction resulted in retrogressive changes in the adrenal cortical tissue and that administrating fresh pituitary implants after such an operation generally prevent such changes in the cortex. The inference was there. There must be a substance which is secreted from the pituitary which controls the adrenal cortex and its secretions.

Ingle and Kendall, in 1937, reported that cortin, the major substance produced by the adrenal cortex, would also cause an atrophy of the adrenal cortex when administered continuously over a period of time.[31] Thus there was established a biofeedback system between the adrenal cortex and the pituitary gland. As we now know the adrenocorticotropin hormone (ACTH) is a relatively small polypeptide released by the anterior pituitary gland. Work continued through the 1940s on the pituitary-adrenal functions and control. Some papers contributed significantly to the understanding of the relationship of the adrenal gland and the normal physiological responses of many organ systems. Such was the report by Sayers[32] and his description of the adrenal cortex's control of homeostasis.

Though crystalline material isolated from adrenal cortex extracts was prepared by

Kendall[33] and by Grollman[34] in 1933, it wasn't until Reichstein ioslated a substance which had corticosteroid activity that the name corticosterone appeared.[35] In 1937, Steiger and Reichstein synthesized deoxycorticosterone acetate, the first synthetic cortical steroid duplicated from a laboratory.[36] Further advances in steroid biochemistry in the 1940s and 1950s enabled the relationship between glucocorticosteroids and mineralocorticord, their physiological and pharmacological effects, and controlling factors regulating them to be identified.

DEVELOPMENT

Human

The adrenal cortical cells appear very early in the development of the fetus. By the sixth week cells from the splanchnic mesoderm aggregate to become recognizable as primodial cortical tissue. There is an accelerated local proliferation of cells beginning from the splanchnic mesoderm around the notch on either side of the dorsal mesentery near the cephalic pole of the mesonephros, usually when the embryo is between 9 to 12 mm in size.

Cells which are located near the bottom of a groove (in the coelom) form a mass in the mesenchyme which extends towards the developing aortic artery. In the eighth week of embryonic life these cells become cord shape with spaces between which contain blood. Shortly after this, as the connection with the coelomic mesothelium is lost, a capsule of connective tissue begins to encompass these cells. Cells which are destined to become medullory, (ectodermal in origin) have by this time infiltrated the cortical tissue. The fetal adrenal cortex continues to grow rapidly and now can be histologically differentiated into two distinct layers. The outer layer is a more diffuse layer with no apparent pattern. The inner layer is more differentiated and cord like in appearance and is active in secretion. At birth the adrenals are about one third the size of the kidney. However, towards the end of fetal life the inner cortical layer begins to regress and is completely resorbed about two months after birth. The outer cortical layer begins to differentiate into the three layers which are typical of the adult adrenal cortex.

Nonhuman

In many of the lesser animals the "cortical" and "medullary" glands are entirely separate, not only in origin and function, but also in their anatomical location. Both are, however, always closely associated with the kidneys.

The cortical tissue arises from the gonadal ridge and underlying nephrogenic mesoderm (mesodermal origin) while the medullary tissue springs from the neural crest and is of ectoderm origin.

Examples of animals where the "medulla" and "cortex" are separate organs include the lampreys, elasmobranchs, and some teleosts. In reptiles, there is frequent mating of the chromaffin and steroidogenic bodies forming one complex. This complex differs from most mammalians, however, in that the chromaffin bodies frequently encapsulate the steroidogenic bodies. Some mammals exhibit variations in the position of chromaffin and steroidogenic cells. The sea lion, for example, has adrenal glands which intertwine with chromaffin and steroidogenic tissue.

ANATOMY (HUMAN)

Description

The adrenals are located at the cranial pole of each of the two kidneys. The weight of the adrenals varies but averages 4 to 6 gms in the adult. The appearance of the gland is somewhat nodular and the glands are dark yellow in color. They are usually surrounded by areola tissue rich in fat and covered by a thin fibrous capsule. Both glands are located extraperitoneally and each is distinct in size and shape.

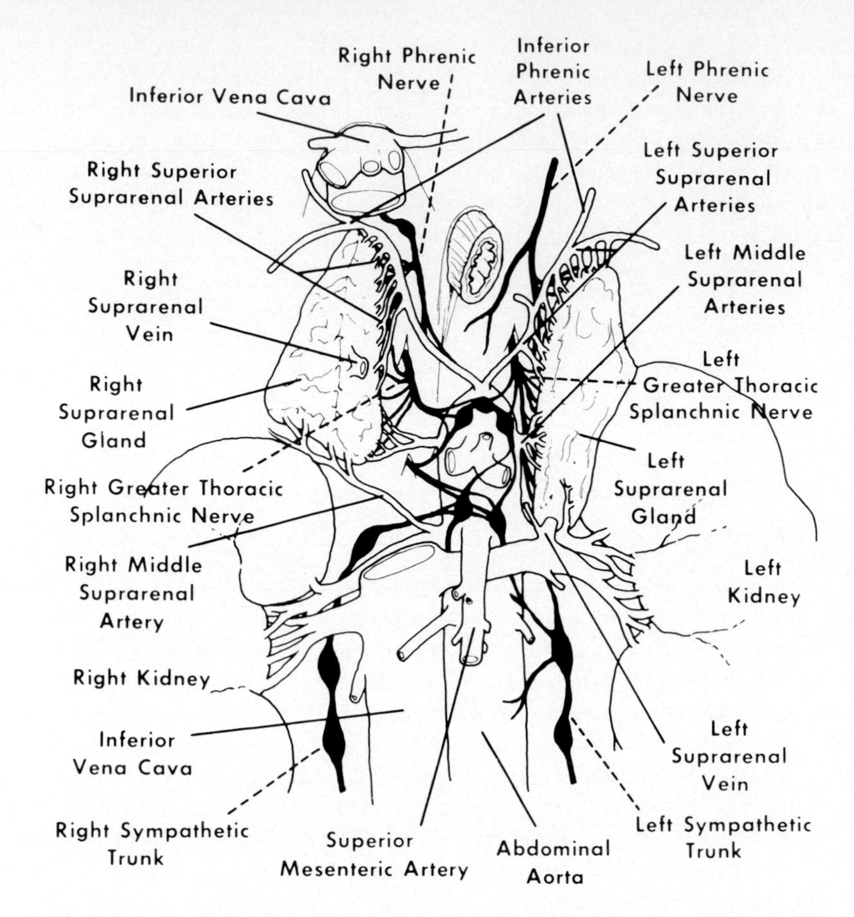

FIGURE 1. The anatomical position of the right and left suprarenal glands with blood and nerve supply. (Adapted from original paintings by Netter, F. H., from THE CIBA COLLECTION OF MEDICAL ILLUSTRATIONS, CIBA Pharmaceutical Co., Division of CIBA-GEIGY Corporation. With permission.)

The glands are located on the posterior wall at the level of the 11th thoracic rib, but lateral to the 18th lumbar vertebra. The adrenal glands have their own fascial supports independent of the kidney (Figure 1).

The left adrenal gland is elongated, crescent shaped with a concavity which conforms to the medial border of the cranial pole of the left kidney. It appears more centrally and somewhat lower than the right adrenal gland. Posteriorly the gland lies close to the diaphragm and splanchnic nerves. The ventral surface is bordered by the omental bursa above and the pancreas, renal artery, and splenic vein below and is not covered by peritoneum. Dorsally the gland is near the crus of the diaphragm medially and borders the ventral surface of the left kidney. Near the caudal portion there is a furrow from which the suprarenal vein emerges.

The right adrenal gland is pyramidal in shape and is located more lateral than the left gland. Posteriorally the surface is in close opposition to the right diaphragmatic curs. It is dorsal to the inferior vena cava and right lobe of the kidney. Ventrally the medial surface borders the inferior vena cava. Laterally and cranially the bare liver lies above.

The caudal portion is covered by peritoneum reflected from the inferior layer of the coronary ligament. Slightly below the apex is a small furrow (hilum) from which the suprarenal vein emerges.

Blood Vessels

Arterial

The adrenal cortex is richly supplied with blood through a series of short and intermediate arterioles which branch from the inferior phrenic artery superiorly and the superior suprarenal artery supramedially. Medially and inferiorly the arterial blood is supplied from the middle suprarenal artery and the inferior suprarenal artery. Additional branches come from the decending aorta itself. Occasionally branches from the ovarian artery and internal spermatic artery may contribute to the blood supply.

Venous

Blood is returned from the right suprarenal gland through the right suprarenal vein, a short (4 to 5 mm) vein emptying into the inferior vena cava. The left suprarenal vein empties into the left renal vein. This vein frequently junctions with the left inferior phrenic vein before reaching the left renal vein. The left suprarenal vein is several millimeters long. In addition to the major venous return there are numerous small surface veins accompanying adjacent arteries which also assist in venous return.

Internal Branching

Arterioles

Arteries reaching the capsule (arteriae capsulae) branch many times before entering the body of the adrenal gland.[37] Arteriolar anastomoses may occur just beneath the capsule of the gland.[38] While some arteries entering the adrenal gland branch to the arteriole stage where they may be "end arterioles,"[39] others form cortical capillaries and feed the parenchymal elements. There are also large capillary beds which may be termed sinusoids.[40] Some arteries entering the cortical tissue continue unbranched to the adrenal medulla (arteriae medullae)[39] where they form arterioles and capillary networks.

Venous

At the corticomedullary border capillaries widen to form the peripheral radicles of the venous tree.[41] Large channels form terminal veins which drain into the central vein. The central vein of the adrenal gland is very large compared to the size of the gland. In addition, this vein contains some bands of smooth muscle.[42,43] The presence of smooth muscle bundles in the venous drainage of the adrenal suggests: (1) the restriction of venous return leading to eventual engorgement of the adrenal gland with blood so that ACTH or other necessary nutrients may reach the inner areas of the cortex,[43] and (2) possible control of the release of various hormones from the adrenal gland.

Innervation

The suprarenal glands are innervated by nerves which are autonomic in origin. There are large variations according to the species studied. In man the sympathetic preganglionic fibers reaching these glands are axons of nerve cells located in the last two thoracic and first lumbar section of the spinal cord. The corresponding spinal nerves branch forming the greater, lesser, and least thoracic nerves and the first lumbar splanchnic nerves. These branches pass through the celiac, corticorenal, and renal ganglia where some fibers end. Numerous nerves leave the celiac plexus after being joined from parts of the greater and lesser thoracic splanchnic nerves and enter the suprarenal glands. Near the medial border of the suprarenal gland there lies a suprarenal plexus which is comprised of many smaller nerves. Nerve filaments form a lattice work in the subcapsularis area from which fascicles penetrate the cortex reaching the medulla without supplying cortical tissue. They do, however, supply both cortical arteries, arterioles, and veins. Many more nerves forming the suprarenal plexus enter the gland near

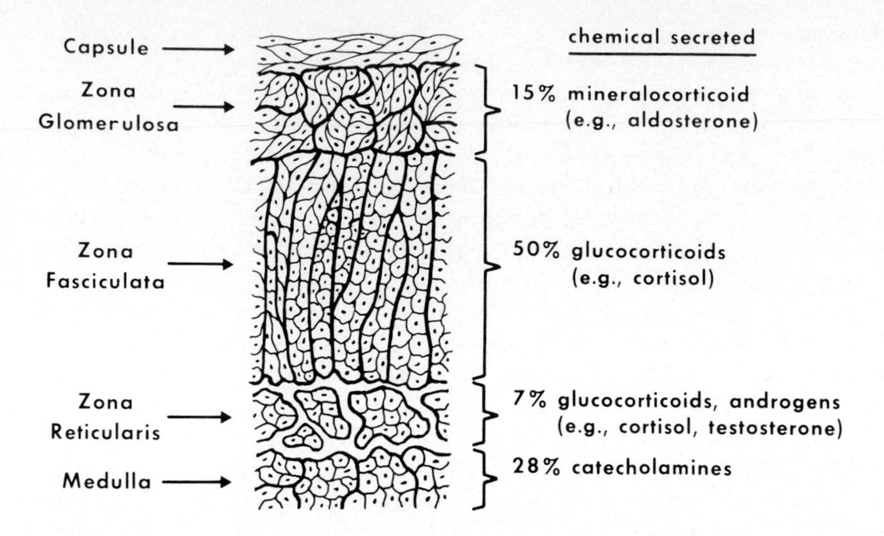

FIGURE 2. Representative zonation found in the human adrenal cortex. See text for explanation of chemical function by zones. Percentages are approximate and vary according to health status.

the hilus in the form of bundles. These nerves go to the medulla, where once reaching the medullary tissue, ramify and terminate in synoptic-type endings around the medullary chromaffin cells.

The nerves entering the adrenal gland are primarily regulating the medullary tissue, except as noted where smooth muscle control exist for cortical arteries, arterioles, and veins.

Histology

Functional

The zones of the adrenal cortex were first described by Arnold in 1866.[44] In his description of the zones, i.e., the zona glomerulosa, zona fasciculata, and zona reticularis, he named the three now commonly known layers according to the complex arrangement of connective tissue and the vascular supplies to each of these layers (Figure 2). In the adrenals of man the cortical tissue contains an abundance of lipid, making the three zones easily recognized microscopically.

Species variation does occur; for example there is a zona intermedius present in the rat, cat, dog, rabbit, and horse.[45] A so-called X zone has been described in the mouse,[46] and as noted earlier, a diffuse cortical layer exists in the fetal adrenal cortex termed the fetal zone.[47]

One of the most interesting theories regarding the histologically distinct layers of the adrenal cortex was that proposed by Gottschau.[48] He suggested a cell migration theory in which cells would rise at the level of the capsule, migrate inward, and degenerate at the medullary zona reticularis border. However, in 1940 Swann proposed the theory of functional zonation, i.e., because the zona glomerulosa is essentially independent of ACTH control and secretes mineralocorticoid hormones (aldosterone, Na^+ retaining), while the zona fasciculata and zona reticularis depend on ACTH and secrete glucocorticoids (cortisal-gluconogenesis), the histologically distinct zones in the adrenal cortex must be distinct developmentally also.[49] Jonutti[50] and Chester Jones[51] have supported a theory that the zona fasciculata is the actively secreting part of the gland being supported by the zona glomerulosa and zona reticularis only when stimulated by high ACTH blood levels. Others believe that remnants of the zona glomerulosa proliferate to form the histologically and functionally normal adrenal cortex.[52-54]

The zonal theory as proposed by Swann[49] and named by Chester Jones[51] is the most supported theory scientifically. Hypophysectomy in the rat can lead to the atrophy of the two inner zones leaving the zona glomerulosa relatively unchanged histologically.[55,56] The zona glomerulosa nuclei increase in size after spironolactone injections (increases aldosterone secretion) but decrease in size following deoxycorticosterone acetate injection (decreases aldosterone secretion).[57]

There have been a number of studies where artificial alteration of the sodium/potassium ratio in animals has resulted in histological changes in the zona glomerulosa with little or no change noted in the zona reticularis or zona fasciculata.[58-63] Others have injected renin or angiotensin and noted an increase in zone width of the zona glomerulosa but no change in the inner two zones histologically.[55,64-66]

Other means have been utilized to determine the functional role of the zones of the adrenal cortex. Removing the capsula of the adrenal gland removes most of the zona glomerulosa, leaving the decapsulated zona fasiculata, zona reticularis, and the medullary tissue. Experiments in which capsulated and decapsulated tissues were incubated (and incubation mixture extracted) have shown that aldosterone is the primary steroid produced by the capsular tissue,[67] whereas the decapsular tissue produces primarily cortisol and cortisone.[68]

Addition of ACTH only enhanced the production of cortisol and cortisone but did not affect the aldosterone levels. Further studies of the steroid specificity of the various zones of the adrenal cortex suggest that androgen production is carried out primarily by the zona reticularis.[69-71] Some researchers suggest that estrogenic steroids are also produced by the adrenal cortex.[72,73]

Microscopic

The cells which make up the adrenal cortex are generally epitheloid in appearance having a centrally located nucleus. Within the cytoplasm there are usually many lipid vacuoles in addition to mitochondria and Golgi apparatus. There is a fibrous capsule from which many trabeculae rise and extend into the cortex to form septa between cell rows. The zona glomerulosa, the outermost zone, is narrow and made up of smaller cells, forming groups resembling a kidney glomerulus. The zona fasciculata, the widest zone, is next and makes up the bulk of the adrenal cortex (75 to 80%). It is comprised of cells in column which are arranged in long cords, radials, or fascicles. The inner zone, the zona reticularis, which lies next to medullary tissue, is a loose mesh of pigmented and compact cells irregularly arranged with cell cords entwined to form a reticulum. As mentioned earlier the two inner zones are under ACTH control while the outer zone responds to changes in the Na^+/K^+ ratios and the renin/angiotensin levels.

Subcellular Morphology

Histologically the tissue of the adrenal cortex is not unique except for the abundance of lipid vacuoles which are distributed throughout the cytoplasm. Yet metabolically this structure is one of the most active and dynamic tissues known. There are, however, certain subcellular organelles which deserve special attention.

In man the endoplasmic reticulum is made up mostly of the smooth type.[74] The network of tubules comprising the endoplasmic reticulum is very extensive and contains many of the steroidogenic enzymes necessary for the production of mineralocorticoids and glucocorticoids secreted by the cortex.

One of the more unique features of the subcellular organelles is the appearance of the mitochondria. Whereas the mitochondria of other cells are divided internally by a folding of the inner membrane forming cristae, most adrenal cortical mitochondria have tubular finger like projections formed by the inner membranes and free floating vesicles formed from the finger like projections may occur.[75] Mitochondrial morphology also shows zonal differences.[76] In the rat and other species, the cell type may be identified by observing the mitochondrial morphology. The mitochondria are probably functionally unique also.

Lipid droplets (liposomes) are distributed extensively throughout the cytoplasm in all three zones of the adrenal cortex. In man the liposomes are in higher concentration in the zona glomerulosa and the zona reticularis.[74,76] The lipid droplet is a storage site for cholesterol and it can frequently be seen in contact with both mitochondria and smooth endoplasmic reticulum in electron micrographs.[77]

There are few if any ultrastructure changes in the zona glomerulosa after hypophysectomy or ACTH administration.[78,79] The ultrastructure of the zona glomerulosa does however, show modification after Na^+ deprivation, K^+ injection or Na^+ excess whereas the inner two zones remain relatively unchanged.[74,78,80] In contrast, ACTH administration or hypophysectomy does alter the appearance of the ultrastructure of the zona fasciculata and zona reticularis. ACTH administration causes an increase in liposomes size and number.[79] Hypophysectomy causes a general atrophy accompanied by an increased number of lysosomes.[80]

It is obvious that ultrastructure changes will occur commensurate with procedures that alter the controlling chemical levels in the circulation. What is uncertain is just how the ultrastructural organelles participate in the actual biochemical events leading to steroidogenesis and the eventual packaging and release of the hormones synthesized.

ADRENALCORTICAL HORMONES

Steroid Chemistry

Steroid hormones are derivatives of a phenanthrene core to which a cyclopentane group is attached, i.e., a sterane. The resulting structure is termed a cyclopentanophenanthrene nucleus. This series of ringed structures are labeled (from left to right) ring A, B, C, and D (Figure 3). Most of the naturally occurring steroids are plannar. If the molecule was viewed as lying horizontally, structures which projected below the plane of the ring structure would be alpha (α) while those that projected above the plane of the ring would be beta (β). However, if viewing steroid molecules in the conventional way in which they are drawn, alpha structures would project away from the viewer or behind the plane of the molecule while beta structures would project in front of the plane of the molecular or toward the viewer. Alpha structures are drawn with a dotted/dashed valance line while beta structures are drawn with a solid valance line (Figure 4). The α-position is *trans*, while the β-position is *cis*. The term "epi" generally refers to the unnatural occurring steroids, such as 11-epicortisal = 11α, cortisal.

Steroids, though planar, still exist in a three-dimensional plane. Because of bond restriction angles created by ring fusions at positions 5 to 10, 8 to 9, and 13 to 14, the "chair" form becomes the most stable position for rings B and C while ring A could theoretically exist in either a "chair" or "boat" form. However, with the adrenal corticoids, the conformational arrangement for ring A is the "chair", due to steric properties of the C-3 hydroxyl and the C-10 methyl groups. These molecules are therefore, *trans* (Figure 4).

The structural restrictions of the steroid molecules give them a shape recognized only by specific cell receptors, thus depending on key angular groups (e.g., C-10, C-13 methyls and C-3 hydroxyl, C-4 double bond); allowing for molecular specificity.

Double bonds are usually designated by the delta symbol (Δ). A double bond between positions 4 and 5 would be shown as Δ^4 or as 4-ene-, indicating the double bond starts at position C-4 and goes to position C-5 in a sterene molecule. Cortisol, for example, is 11β, 17α, 21-trihydroxy-Δ^4-pregnene-3,20-dione. The name pregnone designates the parent nucleus from which all corticosteroids are derived. The suffix (ane)

A. Sterane

B. Sterane

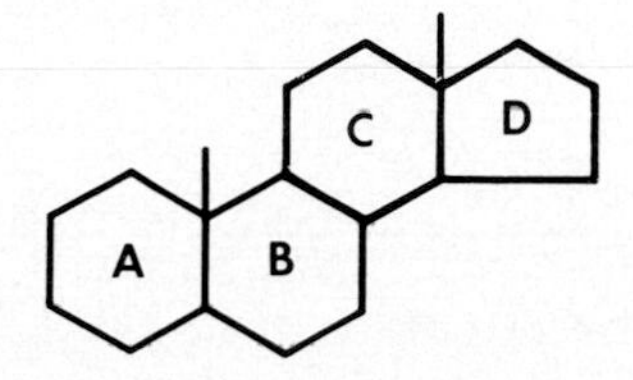

C. Cyclopentanophenathrene Steroid Nucleus

FIGURE 3. A. Structure of sterane, showing the lettering of the 4 rings and the numbering of each carbon. B. The typical presentation of alpha (α) hydrogens (away from viewer) and beta (β) hydrogens (towards viewer). C. Presentation of the steroid molecules as typically drawn; ring hydrogen atoms are not shown and the C-18, C-19 methyl groups are represented by a straight line from C-10 and C-13, respectively.

means carbon saturation (no double bonds) while (ene) refers to the presence of a double bond. In the above example, 3,20-dione refers to two keto groups at positions C-3 and C-20, while 11β, 17α,21-trihydroxy signifies the presence of three hydroxyl groups, at positions C-11, C-17, and C-21. The C-11 hydroxyl is beta (projected towards the viewer) and the C-17 hydroxyl is alpha (projected away from the viewer) (Figure 4).

Cholesterol is the most abundant steroid in the body. A normal 70-kg man would contain about 230 to 250 gm of cholesterol. It is a monounsaturated sterol having the formula $C_{27}H_{45}OH$ and was so named because it was the predominant constituent of human gallstones (viz., chole-bile, and stereos-solid). Cholesterol is present in all normal tissue in part as a free alcohol and in part as an ester.

Biosynthesis of Cholesterol

The biosynthesis of cholesterol occurs by a series of reductive addition reactions. This work was eloquently worked out by Rittenberg and Schoenheimer[81] in 1937 and Bloch and Rittenberg[82] in 1942 and confirmed by others.[83-87] The major events in this biosynthetic pathway are (1) conversion of acetate molecules to squalene; (2) the conversion of squalene to lanosterol; and (3) lanosterol's conversion to cholesterol (Figure 5).

The steroid is linked in a head-to-head, tail-to-tail fashion in a steriospecific manner. Acetyl coenzyme A (acetyl CoA) adds and condenses in a series of reactions and is reduced by NADPH to mevalonic acid. Mevalonic acid is phosphorylated by ATP and decarboxylated liberating 3-isopentenyl pyrophosphate, the major biological isoprene unit.[88-90] A 3-isopentenyl pyrophosphate unit condenses in a head-to-head fashion with 3,3′dimethyl-allyl leading to the C_{10} intermediate, geranyl pyrophosphate. This molecule combines with another molecule of 3,3′-dimethylallyl pyrophosphate (the protonated form of 3-isopentyl pyrophosphate) to form farnesyl pyrophosphate, a C_{15} compound.[91] This reaction can continue due to the regeneration of the protonated form

A. Normal Presentation of Cortisol
11β,17α, 21-trihydroxy-pregn-4-ene-3,20-dione

B. Pregnane - the Corticosteroid Nucleus

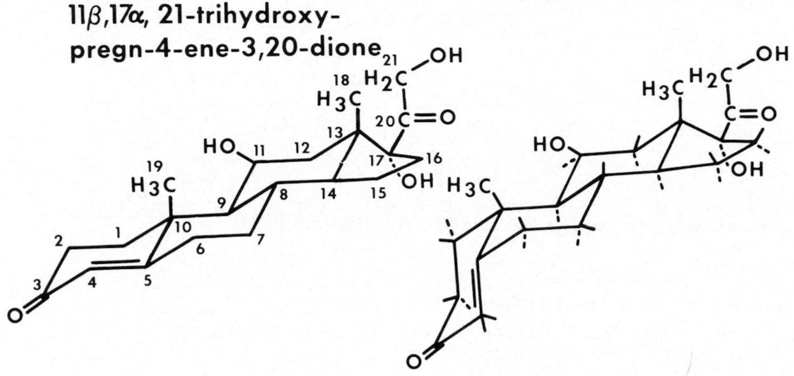

C. Cortisol - In the Naturally Occurring 'trans' - Configuration

D. Cortisol - In a hypothetical 5-10 (A/B) 'cis' configuration. alpha (α) is a dotted valence line, beta (β) is a solid valence line.

FIGURE 4. Examples of the standard way a steroid molecule is drawn (A, B) and the "chair/boat" stereochemical presentation. (C, D) Cortisol appears in the 'trans' form (C), i.e. ring fusion is such that the C-19 methyl group and the C-5 hydrogen group (of the parent compound pregnane) are on opposite sides of the plane. In D, the C-19 methyl and the C-5 hydrogen would be on the same side of the plane being *cis*. The parent corticosteroid nucleus is shown in B.

of 3-isopentyl pyrophosphate. Each condensation follows a stereospecific manner.[92-93] The next step in the synthesis is a tail-to-tail union of farnesyl pyrophosphates which yields squalene, a C_{30} compound.[98-100] Lanosterol is next formed through a series of specific oxidative cyclization, utilizing molecular O_2, resulting in the hydroxylation at C-3 and the formation of four condensed rings. Then through a series of reductions, double bond migrations and the oxidative removal of three methyl groups, lanosterol is transformed to zymosterol, to desmosterol and finally to cholesterol.

Cholesterol to Cortical Hormones

Cholesterol is the principle precursor of all adrenal cortical hormones, although desmosterol can be converted to pregnenolone should problems in the conversion of desmosterol to cholesterol develop.[97] Cholesterol, through a series of hydroxylations requiring molecular O_2 and NADPH, is converted to pregnenolone (rate limiting).

The research efforts of many have led to the elucidation of the biochemical pathways by which pregnenolone is converted to all the known adrenal cortical hormones that are produced in significant amounts (Figure 6). Pregnenolone is converted to (1) 17α-hydroxypregnenolone (17-hydroxylase + NADPH + H^+ + O_2); or 2) Δ^5-pregnenedione (3β-hydroxydehydrogenase + NAD^+). In man, 17-hydroxypregnenolone appears

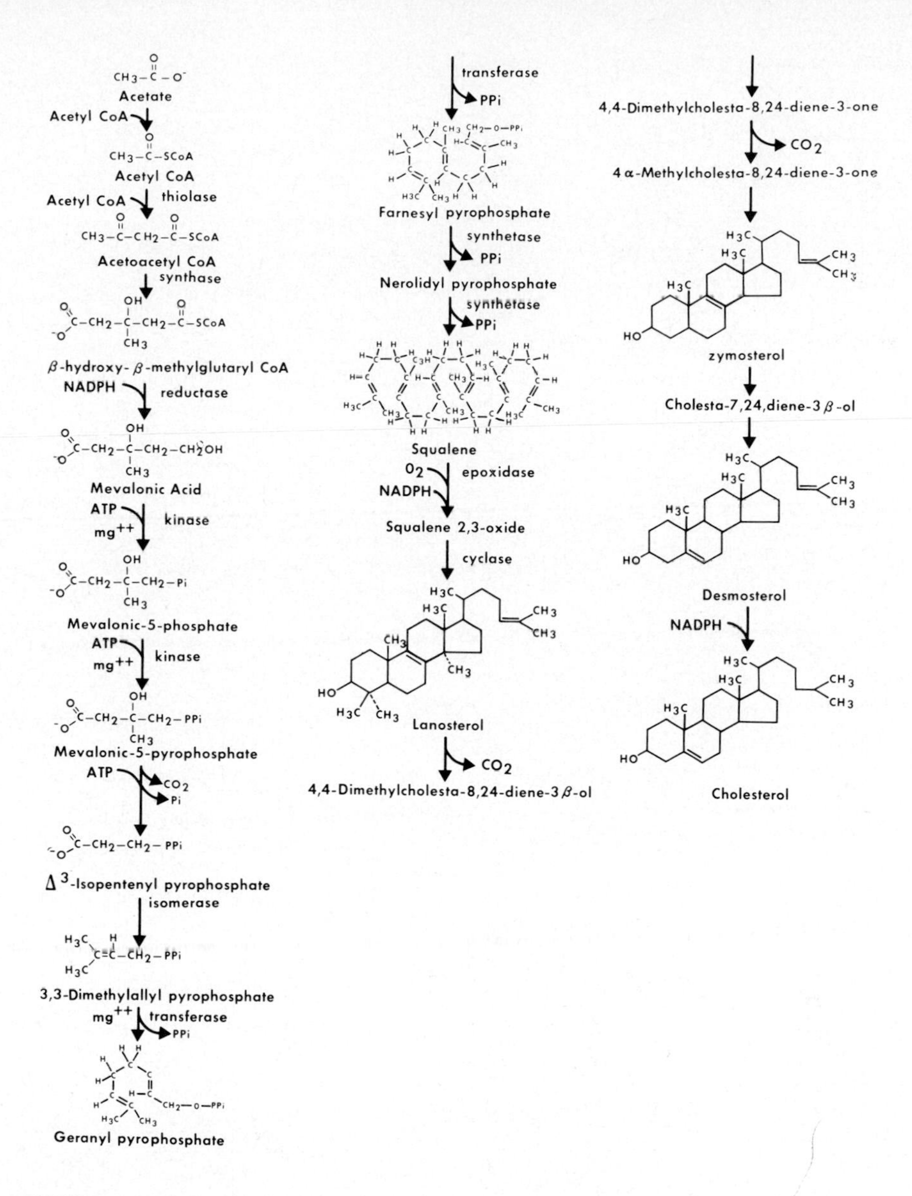

FIGURE 5. The synthetic pathway for the synthesis of cholesterol. The smooth endoplasmic reticulum synthesizes cholesterol from acetate. Only about 10% of the cholesterol pool is synthesized by adrenal cortex. The rest reaches the cortical tissue via the HDL transport system. The hydrogens attached to ring carbons are not shown after squalene; Pi = Phosphate, PPi = Pyrophosphate.

to be the major pathway.[98,99] Δ^5-Pregnenedione, by the action of a Δ^4-Δ^5-isomerase, is converted to pregn-4-ene-3,20-dione (progesterone). 17-hydroxypregnenolone goes to 17-hydroxy-Δ^5-pregnenedione (3β-hydroxy-dehydrogenase + NAD^+) and is converted to 17-hydroxyprogesterone by the action of a Δ^5-Δ^4-isomerase.

Progesterone can be converted to 17-hydroxyprogesterone by the action of a 17α-hydroxylase and NADPH + H^+ + O_2. Dehydroepiandrosterone, the most abundant C-19 steroid produced by the adrenal cortex, is a product of the action of a 17,20-lyase (requiring NADPH + H^{2+} + O_2) on 17-hydroxy-pregnenolone. This product is usually found as the 3-sulfate conjugate.[100] In the fetus, 16α-hydroxy-dehydroepiandrosterone has also been isolated from adrenal cortical tissue.[101] This steroid is also sulfated (3β-sulfokinase) and excreted.

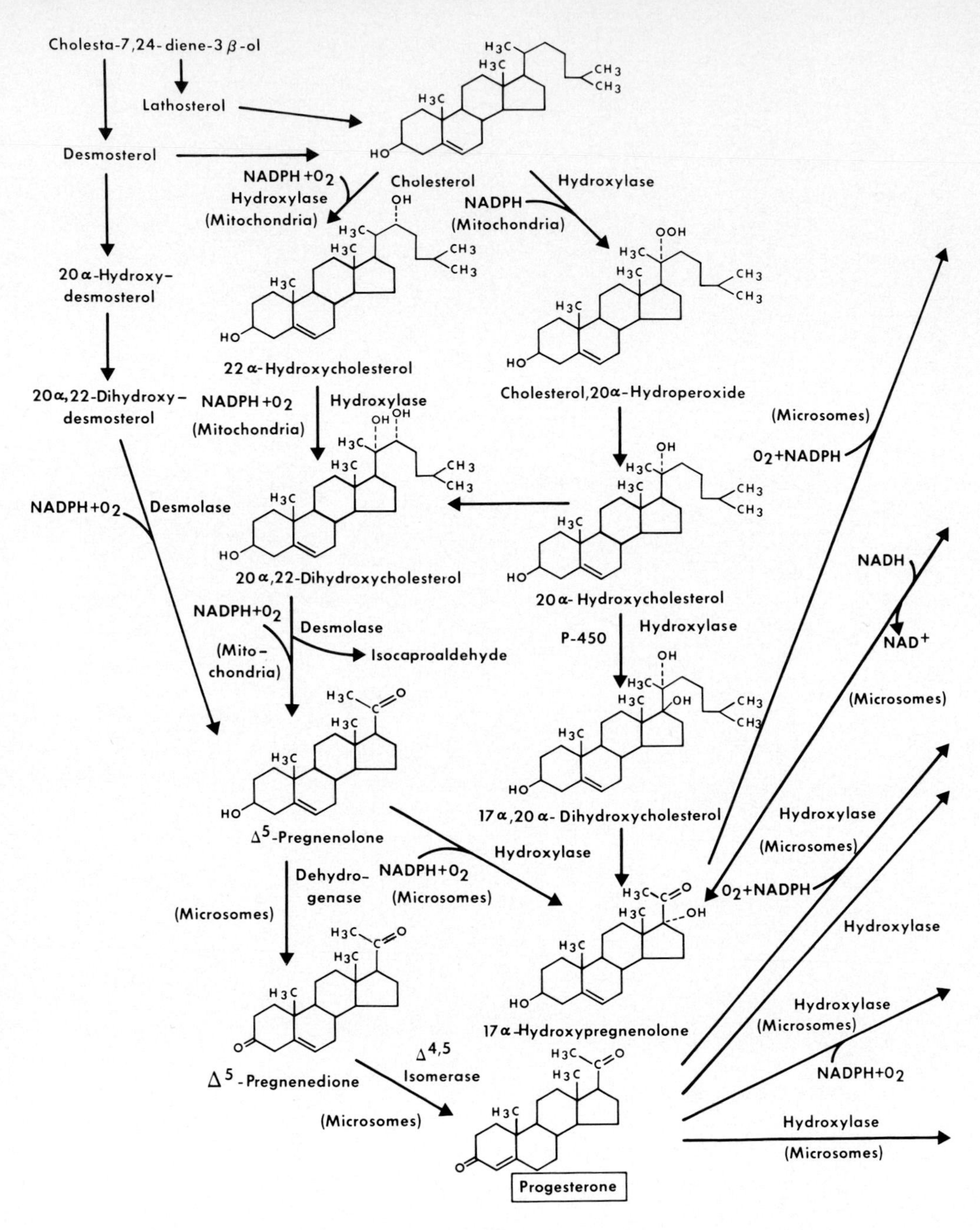

Cholesta-7,24-diene-3 β-ol
Lathosterol
Desmosterol
Cholesterol
NADPH +O2
Hydroxylase
(Mitochondria)
Hydroxylase
NADPH
(Mitochondria)
20 α-Hydroxy-desmosterol
22 α-Hydroxycholesterol
Cholesterol,20α-Hydroperoxide
20α,22-Dihydroxy-desmosterol
NADPH +O2
(Mitochondria)
Hydroxylase
(Microsomes)
O2+NADPH
NADPH+O2
Desmolase
20 α,22-Dihydroxycholesterol
20α- Hydroxycholesterol
NADH
NAD+
NADPH+O2
Desmolase
(Mito-chondria)
Isocaproaldehyde
P-450
Hydroxylase
(Microsomes)
Δ5-Pregnenolone
17 α,20 α- Dihydroxycholesterol
Hydroxylase
(Microsomes)
Hydroxylase
Dehydro-genase
NADPH+O2
(Microsomes)
(Microsomes)
O2+NADPH
Hydroxylase
17 α-Hydroxypregnenolone
Hydroxylase
(Microsomes)
Δ4,5
Isomerase
Δ5 - Pregnenedione
NADPH+O2
(Microsomes)
Hydroxylase
(Microsomes)
Progesterone

FIGURE 6A.

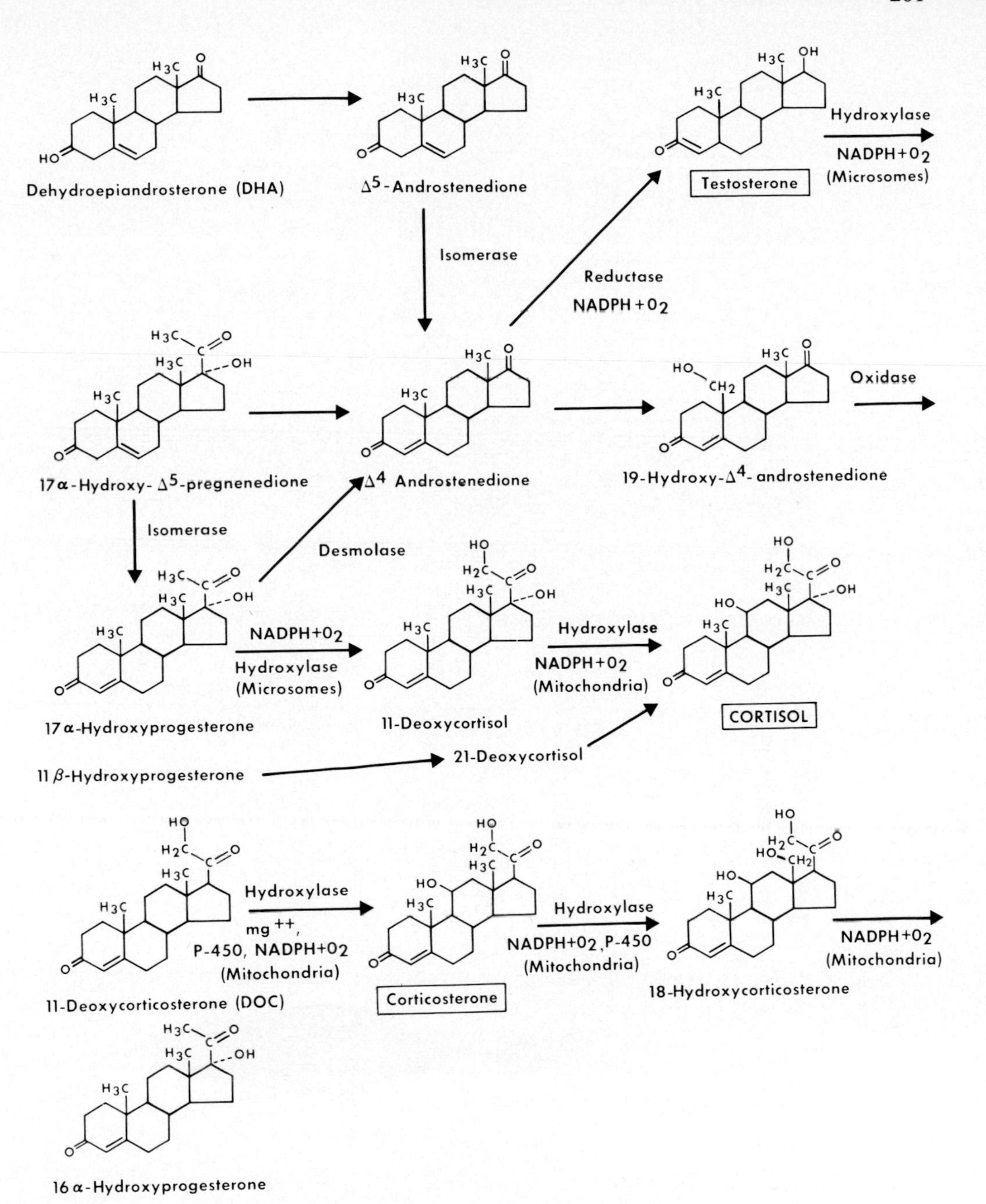

H3C
HO
Dehydroepiandrosterone (DHA)
Δ5-Androstenedione
Isomerase
Reductase
NADPH+O2
Testosterone
Hydroxylase
NADPH+O2
(Microsomes)
17α-Hydroxy-Δ5-pregnenedione
Δ4 Androstenedione
19-Hydroxy-Δ4-androstenedione
Oxidase
Isomerase
Desmolase
NADPH+O2
Hydroxylase
(Microsomes)
17α-Hydroxyprogesterone
11-Deoxycortisol
Hydroxylase
NADPH+O2
(Mitochondria)
CORTISOL
11β-Hydroxyprogesterone
21-Deoxycortisol
Hydroxylase
mg++,
P-450, NADPH+O2
(Mitochondria)
11-Deoxycorticosterone (DOC)
Corticosterone
Hydroxylase
NADPH+O2,P-450
(Mitochondria)
18-Hydroxycorticosterone
NADPH+O2
(Mitochondria)
16α-Hydroxyprogesterone

FIGURE 6B.

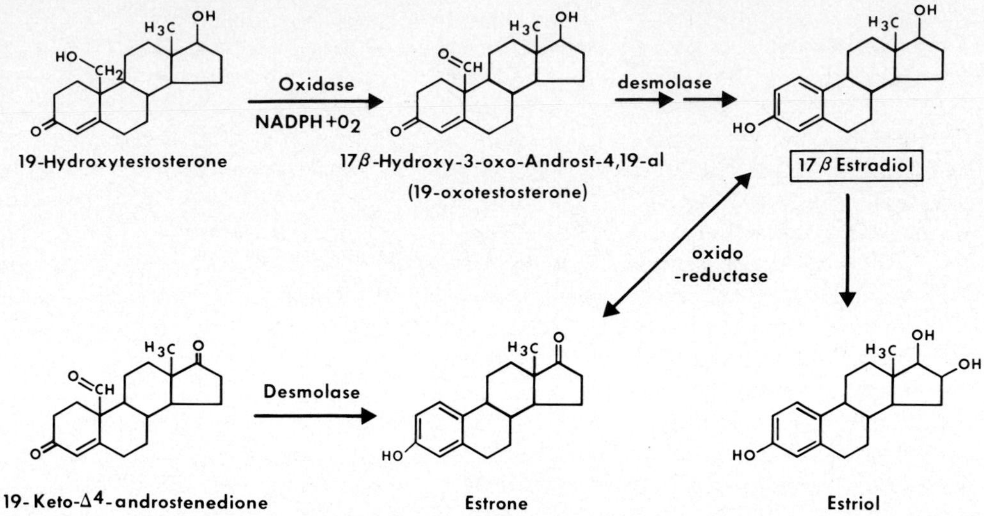

19-Hydroxytestosterone

Oxidase

NADPH+O_2

17β-Hydroxy-3-oxo-Androst-4,19-al
(19-oxotestosterone)

desmolase

17β Estradiol

oxido
-reductase

19-Keto-Δ^4-androstenedione

Desmolase

Estrone

Estriol

Trivial Name	Chemical Name
Aldosterone	11 β, 21-dihydroxy-20-oxopregn-4-en-18-ol-3-one, 18, 11-hemiacetal
Cholesterol	5-cholesten-3-β-ol
Corticosterone	11 β, 21-dihydroxy-4-pregnene-3, 20-dione
Cortisol	11 β, 17 α, 21-trihydroxy-4-pregnene-3, 20-dione
Deoxycorticosterone	21-hydroxy-4-pregnene-3, 20-dione
Estradiol-17 β	1, 3, 5 (10)-estatriene-3, 17 β-diol
Progesterone	4-pregnene-3, 20-dione
Testosterone	17 β-hydroxy-4-androsten-3-one

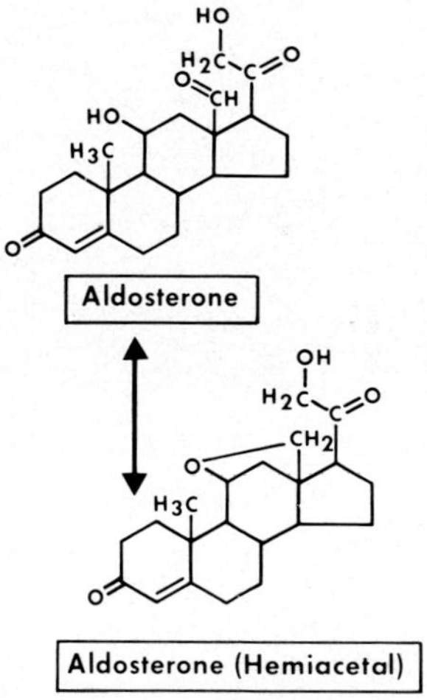

Aldosterone

Aldosterone (Hemiacetal)

FIGURE 6. Biosynthetic pathway to the adrenal cortical steroids. Hydrogens attached to ring carbons are not shown. Area of enzyme activity shown in brackets ( ), if known.

Progesterone, by the action of a 21-hydroxylase and NADPH + H^+ + O_2 forms 11-deoxycorticosterone. 11-Deoxycorticosterone (DOC), is hydroxylated in the 11 position (Cofactor: NADPH + H^+ + O_2) forming corticosterone. Corticosterone is the pivotal steroid for the production of aldosterone. Even though DOC can undergo C-18 hydroxylation, corticosterone is a much more efficient substrate for the C-18 hydroxylation reaction. The C-18 methyl group of corticosterone is hydroxylated by an 18-hydroxylase (requiring NADPH + H^+ + O_2 as cofactors) to form 18-hydroxy-corticosterone, which is then oxidized to an aldehyde to form aldosterone.

Cortisol is apparently formed only from 17-hydroxyprogesterone, which is the substrate for a C-21 hydroxylase requiring NADPH + H^+ + O_2. 11-Deoxycortisol is then hydroxylated in the C-11 position (requiring NADPH + H^+ + O_2) forming cortisol (hydrocortisone). The only difference between the two major glucocorticords is the 17-hydroxyl group of cortisol.

The androgenic steroids produced by the adrenal cortex are largely the result of a scission at the C-17 position of 17-hydroxyprogesterone giving rise to Δ^4-androstenedione. Δ^4-Androstenedione converts readily to testosterone, 19-hydroxytestosterone and finally to estradiol 17β. Δ^4-androstenedione can also be acted on by a C-19 hydroxylase converting it to 19-hyroxy-Δ^4-adrostenedione which gives rise to estrone. Estriol, which is at high concentrations in the urine of pregnant women, is formed through a biochemical symbiotic relationship between fetal adrenal cortex and the placenta. 16α-Hydroxy-dehydroepiandrosterone sulfate, produced by the fetal adrenal cortex, is desulfated by placental enzymes and converted to estriol by way of 16α-hydroxy-testosterone.[102] In addition, the placenta forms large amounts of progesterone and pregnenolone which enters the fetal blood supply. The fetal adrenal cortex utilizes progesterone to form 11-deoxycorticosterone, corticosterone and cortisol. Pregnenolone, however, is the pathway by which the fetal adrenal cortex forms dehydroepandrosterone sulfate, which is returned to the placenta via maternal veins and desulfated, leaving dehydroepiandrosterone as a substrate to be converted to estradiol and estrone.

Metabolism of Corticosteroids

The major metabolic pathways of the corticosteroids are (1) conjugation reactions; (2) hydrogenation reactions (reductions of unsaturated bonds; and (3) oxidation reactions. Most of these metabolic events take place in the liver although the kidney plays a minor functional role in metabolic regulation (Figure 7). In pregnancy, the placenta is also metabolically active.

Steroids which contain a 3-keto group and a double bond at C-4 are metabolized in the liver. The keto group is reduced to a hydroxyl group and the double bond at C-4 is hydrogenated. After these reactions the steroid is conjugated with glucuronic acid or sulfate, which enhances its aqueous solubility and is excreted via the urine and to some extent the bile. The C-4 double bond reduction requires a 4-ene-5α-reductase (endoplasmic reticulum) or a 4-ene-5β-reductase (cytosol) and NADPH. The second reduction is accomplished with a 3 α-hydroxy-dehydrogenase and NADPH.

Cortisol is metabolized first to dihydrocortisol and then to tetrahydrocortisol. Once at the tetrahydrocortisol stage it becomes a substrate for a 3α-glucuronidation reaction which yields a 3α-tetrahydroglucuronide, the major metabolite of cortisol. A similar reaction can occur with cortisone yielding a hexahydroglucuronide. Dihydrocortisol will not, however, act as a substrate for the glucuronidation reaction. Cortisol can also be converted to cortisone (11-keto instead of 11-hydroxy) by a mechanism that is largely regulated by thyroxin, i.e., thyroxin has a regulatory effect on 11β-hydroxy-dehydrogenase, the enzyme responsible for that conversion.[103] About 5% of cortisol metabolized may yield 17-keto-steroids, by the cleavage of its side chain, although the majority of 17-ketosteroid production results from steroids present in the urine before

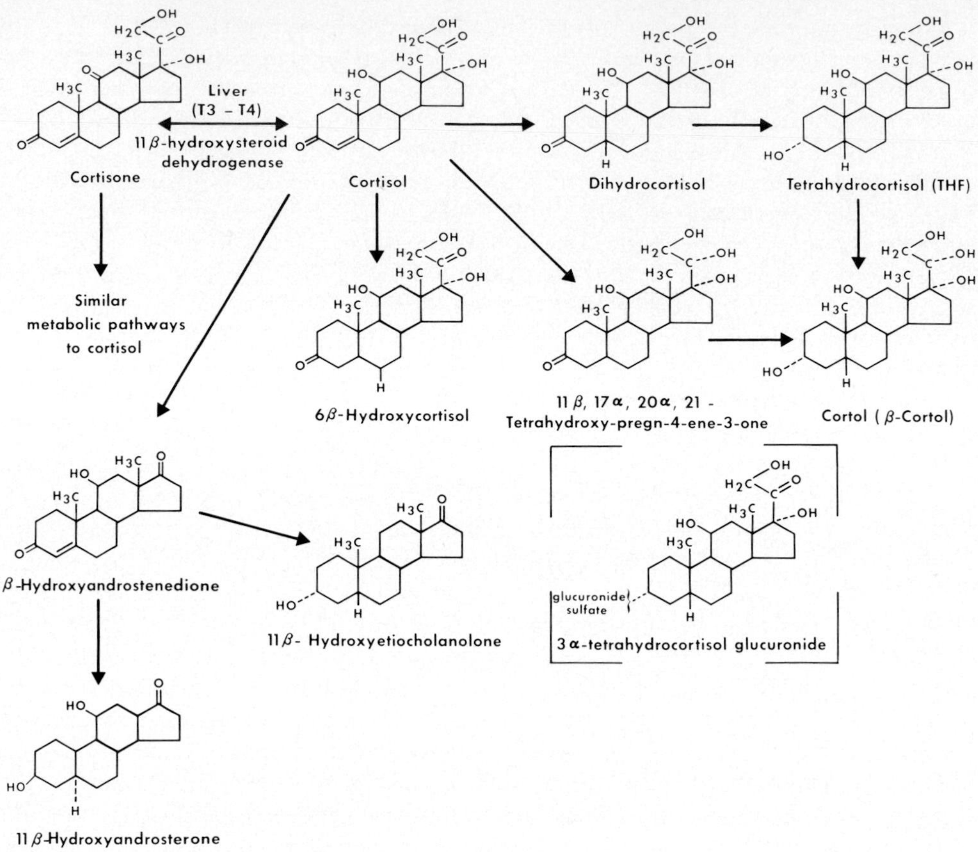

FIGURE 7. Metabolism of cortisol and cortisone. Cortisol is converted to cortisone in the liver by the action of 11β-hydroxysteroid dehydrogenase. This reaction is reversible. About 30% of the tetrahydro derivatives appear in the urine. Cortic acids may account for 10%. Conjugation reactions can occur with the tetrahydrocorticosteroids in the 3α position forming the sulfate or glucuronide conjugates. Aldosterone and corticosterone are metabolized in a similar manner. Aldosterone can form a C-18 conjugate. A small percentage of cortisol contributes to the 17-ketosteroid pool.

oxidative side chain cleavage is performed, i.e., primarily C-19 androgens. Cortisol can also be excreted unchanged in small quantities (< 0.5%) and through a minor metabolic pathway, 6β-hydroxycortisol is formed by the action of 6β-hydroxylase and NADPH.

Cortisol and cortisone can also be metabolized to cortols and cortolones (Figure 7). Cortols and cortolones are formed by a reduction of the keto group at carbon-20, a reaction catalyzed by 20 (α or β)-hydroxy-steroid dehydrogenase. Two isomeric hydroxyl groups give rise to α or β cortol (from cortisol) and α or β cortolone (from cortisone).

Acidic metabolites are also formed from cortisol or cortisone. These compounds, plus their tetrahydro metabolites, can be converted to an isoderivative where the C-21 carbon has a keto function. Further oxidative reactions occur forming an acid function at the C-21 carbon, a compound called cortolic acid (from cortisol), or cortolonic acid (from cortisone).

The metabolism of most other corticosteroids also occurs primarily by reductive reactions. Corticosterone, for example, appears as the glucuronide of tetrahydrocorticosterone and a small amount is excreted as unconjugated corticosterone.

Progesterone is excreted as 5β-pregnone-3α,20α-diol (pregnonediol) and 17α-hydroxy-progesterone is excreted as 5β-pregnone-3α,17α,20α,-triol (pregnonetrial). Both appear as the glucuronide.

Aldosterone metabolism is similar to cortisol in that there is a hydrogenation reaction of the C-4 double bond followed by the 3-keto function yielding 4 tetrahydroandrosterones epimeric at C-3. The major site of metabolism is the liver. In addition, aldosterone is reduced at the C-20-keto function producing two hexahydro metabolites, 3,21-dihydroxypregnane (11β,18) or (11,20α) dioxide.[104] In contrast to cortisol metabolism, oxidation of the 11β-hydroxy group does not apparently occur due to the C-11 to C-18 hemiacetal link that persists in recovered metabolites[105] About 0.1% of aldosterone is excreted unchanged whereas about 5% is excreted as the C-18, O-glucuronide. The major metabolites of aldosterone are tetrahydroaldosterone epimeric forms, linked by the 3-oxygen forming the glucuronide. The 3α-5β-predominates, as was the case with cortisol. During pregnancy, the C-18, O-glucuronide increases dramatically.

Most of the metabolism of the androgens results in the production of 17-ketosteroids in the urine. The urinary 17-ketosteroid group is quite complex, having been produced by the adrenal cortex (70%) and the gonad (30%), secreted at various concentrations, depending on the time of day (17-ketosteroids analysis is at least a 24 hr urine collection) and on pathological conditions. Testosterone is generally secreted as the glucuronide, of testosterone itself (17-oxyglucuronic acid-1%) or after having been metabolized via androstenedione and glucurionidated or sulfated. In addition, dehydroepiandrosterone is sulfated and excreted. A very small amount of 11-hydroxyandrostenedione is glucuronidated or sulfated and excreted, adding to the 17-ketosteroid pool. Androsterone, epiandrosterone, and eticholanolone are also metabolic products of testosterone or androstenedione, all of which undergo conjugation reactions.

Synthetic Corticosteroids

Modification of the structural confluent of naturally occurring corticoid or synthesis of a new compound with similar structural characteristics can result in increased potency of these steroids, often with decreased adverse biological side effects. Prednisolone has an added double bond at C-1 (Figure 8). This addition results in an increased anti-inflammatory response with a decrease in the sodium-retaining capability. Another example of increased potency is the addition of a 9α-fluorine in cortisol. The resulting compound has both increased anti-inflammatory and sodium retention ability. Dexamethasone is a powerful synthetic glucocorticoid. Besides a 9α-fluorine group and a double bond at C-1, there is a 16-methyl group. The double bond at C-1 interferes with the rate of reductive metabolism of the A ring plus, dexamethasone is not bound to cortical binding protein (CBG) in the plasma, allowing higher concentrations to reach extravascular compartments. The increased anti-inflammatory effect is largely due to some stereo specific characteristic of this compound.[106] There are many new synthetic steroids that exhibit glucocorticoid or mineralocorticoid type responses (Figure 8).

Most all synthetic anti-inflammatory molecules have, in addition to the normal cortisol groups, i.e., the 3,20-keto, 4 to 5 double bond, and the C-11, C-17, C-21 hydroxyls, a 9α-fluoro, a 1-2 double bond, a 6α-methyl, and a 16-methyl or hydroxyl group.

Some of the synthetic glucocorticoids have been implicated in the development of cleft palate and other teratogenic problems.[107,108] They have also been used in cases of infertility and for the maintenance of pregnancy.[109] In cases so documented, the offspring were smaller than others from matched controls.[109] Administration of the synthetic corticosteroid triamcinolone to pregnant monkeys early in gestation caused craniofacial malformations and when given during the middle to late gestation produced thymic involution in the newborn.[110]

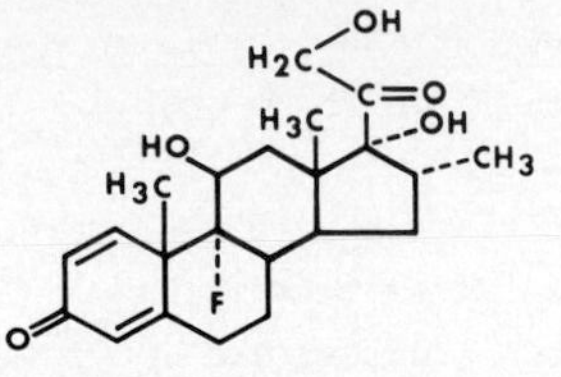

16 α-methyl-9 α-fluoro-Δ'-cortisol
(Dexamethasone)

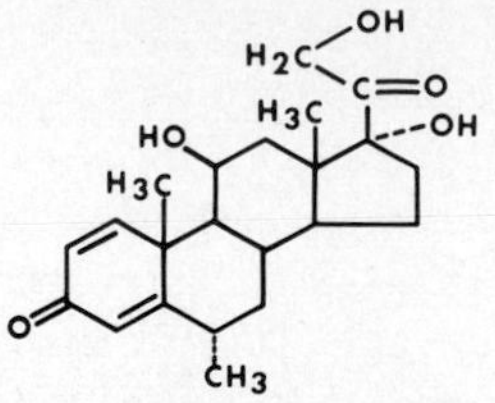

6 α-methylprednisolone

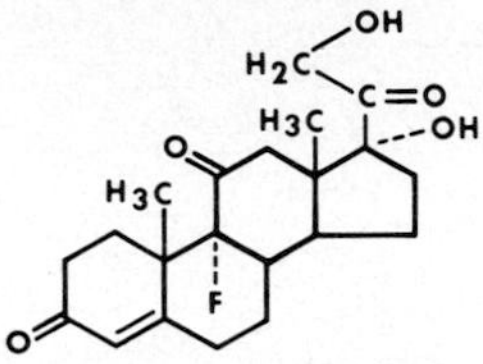

9 α-fluorocortisone
(Fludrocortisone)

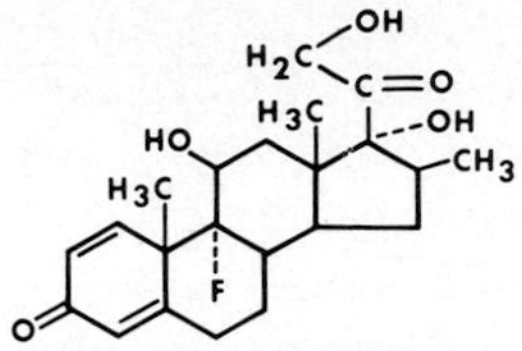

16 β-methyl-9 α-fluoro-Δ'-cortisol
(Betamethasone)

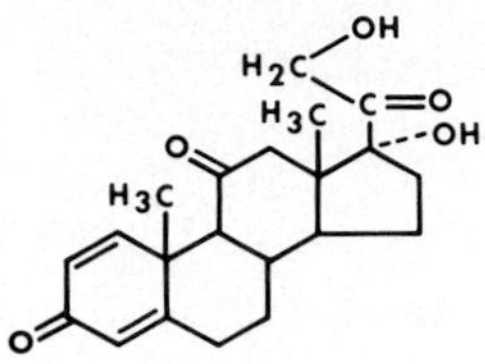

Δ'-cortisone
(Prednisone)

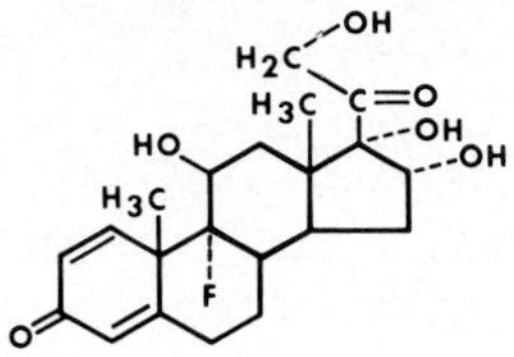

16 α-hydroxy-9 α-fluroprednisolone
(Triamcinolone)

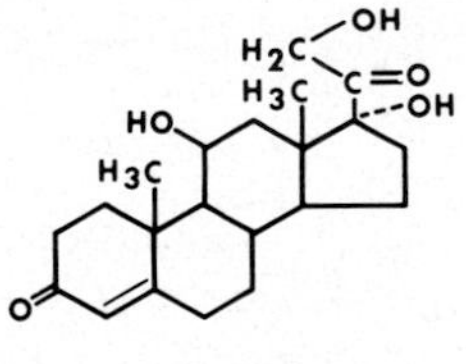

Cortisol

FIGURE 8. Examples of synthetic corticosteroids. Dexamethasone and Betamethasone, while having good anti-inflammatory properties, have little mineralocorticoid activity. Fluorocortisone, however, has excellent anti-inflammatory and mineralocorticoid properties. Comparison of structures can be made with the naturally occurring glucocorticoid, cortisol.

While the use of both naturally occurring and synthetic glucocorticoids has beneficial effects, there are also side effects that could cause serious teratogenic or other toxicologic problems.

REGULATION OF ADRENAL CORTICOL STEROIDOGENESIS

ACTH - Glucocorticoids

Adrenocorticordtropic hormone (ACTH) is secreted by the adenohypophysis after receiving chemical stimulation by corticotropic releasing factors (CFRs). The amount of ACTH released fluctuates over a 24 hr period of time, accounting for the circadian variations observed when measuring cortical plasma concentrations.

Adrenocorticotropic hormone release, after transportation, reception, and transmission of the chemical signal, elicits a response from the adrenal cortex in about 2 to 3 min.[111] Since there is little glucocorticoid stored in the adrenal cortex, the increased

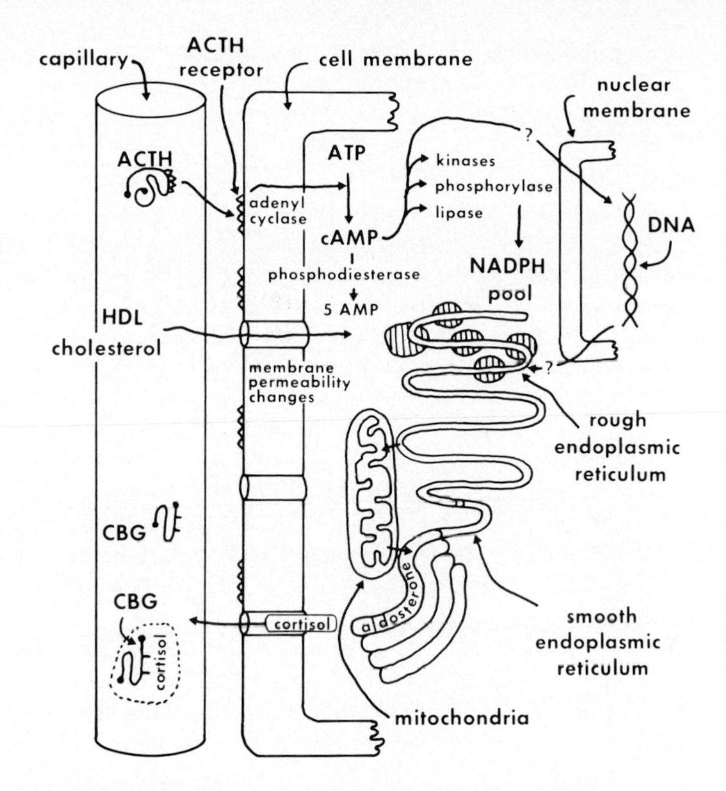

FIGURE 9. Example of how ACTH may activate cellular mechanisms to elicit the production of corticosteroids. ACTH is caught by the cell membrane receptor activating membrane responses resulting in the production of adenyl cyclase, which in turn increases the production of cellular enzymes. ACTH also initiates the uptake of circulating cholesterol, may alter cell membrane permeability or even cause changes at the level of the nucleus. The NADPH pool increases allowing the action of hydrolases to progress. The result is the production of various steroids packaged and released to the circulation. There they are bound by corticosteroid-binding globulin or albumin and transported to sites throughout the body.

cortisol released, as measured in the adrenal vein, must, therefore, represent an increase in steroidogenesis. ACTH is thought to act by binding to a receptor in the cell membrane, thus setting off a series of events resulting in the activation of adenyl cyclase (Figure 9). Cyclic AMP is enhanced resulting in the activation of various cellular kinases, which in turn activate steroidogenic enzymes. Cholesterol, through side chain cleavage, is then converted to Δ^5-pregnenolone and the other enzymatic steps of glucocorticoid steroidogenesis progress rapidly resulting in the release of cortisol[112] (Figure 9).

There are other hypotheses regarding the mode of action of ACTH. Some researchers have proposed that ACTH acts by (1) increasing NADPH; (2) increasing mitochondrial permeability, thus controlling substrate and cofactor entrance and product removal; and (3) controlling protein synthesis directly (enzyme synthesis).[113] The probable mechanism likely involves the activation of cellular kinases through cyclic-AMP resulting in a combination of reactions culminating in the release of cortisol.

Concentrations of ACTH as low as 10^{-16} M will cause a significant increase in steroidogenesis in the adrenal cortex.[114] This is thought possible because of the high number of receptors which are located on the plasma membrane of cortical cells. The adrenal cortical receptor also has high affinity for ACTH. These combined effects aid in capturing the ACTH molecule and assures that a response will result.

ACTH is a polypeptide which has 39 amino acid residues. The importance of the sequence and the active site of the molecule has been reported.[115-120] There are relatively few amino acids which apparently make up the active site for receptor activation (His^6-Phe^7-Arg^8-Trp^9), leaving the rest of the peptide to function in receptor capture or in other, as yet undefined, functions.[120,121]

The N terminal 30 amino acids (AA) are the same for the human, pig, ox, and sheep. The amino acids 25 to 39 apparently have little to do with biological activity as a 24 amino acid fragment has equipotent activity with the 39 amino acid parent.[122] Further shortening of the peptide to AA-19 decreases a biological activity slightly, but removal of AAs 18 to 15 causes a dramatic decrease in biological potency.[123] The amino acid sequence 1 to 10 has been found to possess slight biological functions.[124]

ATCH is metabolized relatively quickly having a biological half-life of about 10 min. There is apparently a cleavage between position 16 and 17 leaving two peptide segments with little biological potency.[125]

ACTH synthesis and release is regulated by corticotropic releasing factors (CRF), as demonstrated in 1949 by Green and Harris[126] and in 1950 by Harris and Jacobson.[127] There is a hypothalamic-pituitary adrenal cortical neuroendocrine axis formed which is under a complex array of controlling mechanisms. Excitation impulses from both the somatic and autonomic nervous system travel afferent fibers reaching the hypothalamus, where neurotransmitters are released and stimulate the synthesis and release of CRF.[128-130] There are many neural pathways converging in the hypothalamus. Tracts traverse the brain stem via oligosynaptic or multisynaptic connections to enter the hypothalamus from the spinal cord. The cerebral cortex, basal ganglia, rhinencephalon, and thalamus, are extensively linked to the hypothalamus. The hypothalamus is thus the focal point at which impulses arriving can signal release or inhibition of CRF.[131]

Stressful situations can result in high plasma concentrations of glucocorticoid and to a lesser degree cortical androgens. There are two major types of stress stimuli (1) emotional (higher brain centers); and (2) physical (traumatic). Both are equally capable of causing very high ACTH and cortisol synthesis and release.[132]

In addition to the release of CRF in stressful situations, there is a normal pattern of ACTH secretion resulting in higher plasma cortisol levels. This release occurs intermittently with several peaks during sleep.[133] The neuro-transmitters acetylcholine and 5-hydroxytryptamine have been implicated in the control of circadian release of ACTH.[134,135] In addition, catecholamines (e.g., norepinephrine) may have some control of cortical secretion by inhibiting ACTH release.[136] Melatonin as well has been shown to inhibit the release of CRF from the rat hypothalamus in vitro in response to 5-hydroxytryptamine or acetylcholine stimulation.[130,137] Some authors have suggested that variations in 5-hydroxytryptamine and melatonin levels may account for the episodic nature of CRF release from the hypothalamus.[131] In addition, others have suggested that vasopressin can act as a CRF.[138-140] However, whether the release of ACTH observed after vasopressin administration is due directly to vasopressin or whether vasopressin is acting as a synergist resulting in increased sensitivity to CRF is not yet understood. It is possible that more than one CRF is synthesized and released from other than one centrally located area in the hypothalamus.[141]

Adrenocorticotropic hormone release is also controlled by a negative feedback mechanism implemented by corticosteroids. Ingle and Kendall were first to show that corticosteroids inhibited ACTH release.[31] Glucocorticoid control is mediated both at the level of the anterior pituitary[142-144] and at the level of the hypothalamus.[141,145,146] Thus, corticosteroids can inhibit both the synthesis and release of ACTH by acting directly at the level of the anterior pituitary or possibly by inhibiting CRF synthesis and release in the hypothalamus. In addition, it has been suggested that ACTH can feed back directly on the hypothalamus influencing CRF release in a so-called short loop mechanism.[147-149] The major controlling site is, however, at the level of the anterior pituitary.

Another possible controlling site of the corticosteroids was suggested to be located in higher centers in the brain. Thus, by stimulating a neural inhibitory system, there would be a decrease in CRF release or synthesis.[150,151] However, that theory has been disputed.[152,153]

The feedback mechanism that is initiated by the glucocorticoids has both a fast, rapidly-acting component[154] and a longer, slower-acting component.[155-157] The fast-acting feedback occurs when there is a rapid rise in the plasma concentrations of corticosteroids. However, after the plasma concentration plateaued (20 min or longer), the feedback response to corticosteroids was greatly diminished until about 2 hr later when there was an even greater feedback inhibition than noticed in the early fast-acting phase. The fast and delayed feedback by glucocorticoid acts both at the level of the hypothalamus and the anterior pituitary. The fast-acting feedback mechanism has been shown to inhibit the release but not the synthesis of CRF,[152,158] while the delayed feedback mechanism in the hypothalamus may be primarily initiated by corticosterone influence on the inhibition of CRF synthesis.[140,159] In the anterior pituitary, the delayed feedback mechanism is believed to act at the level of protein synthesis, i.e., ACTH production, thereby reducing ACTH availability.[160]

Adrenal corticoandrogens are also under the control of ACTH and are secreted episodically and concurrently with cortisol.[157] Besides the adrenal corticoandrogens there are also 18-hydroxylated corticosteroids synthesized and released by the adrenal cortex. Two of these are 18-hydroxy-11-deoxycorticosterone (18-hydroxy-DOC), and 18-hydroxycorticosterone.[162] The control of 18-hydroxy-deoxycorticosterone secretion is largely under ACTH influence while 18-hydroxy-11-corticosterone appears to be regulated by fluid, sodium and potassium balance much the same way that aldosterone is controlled.[163]

Adrenocorticotropic hormone is under the direct control of CRF synthesized and released from the hypothalamus though extrahypothalamic sites have been suggested.[164,165]

Renin/Angiotensin-Aldosterone

The zona glomerulosa synthesizes and releases aldosterone and this release is, as is cortisol, episodic in nature.[161] Whereas episodic glucocorticoid secretion is under the control of ACTH, episodic mineralocorticord secretion is not (dexamethasone pretreatment abolishes cortisol episodic release but not aldosterone episodic release).[161]

It is likely that the CNS is responsible for stimulating both hypothalamic CRF release and juxtaglomerular renin release, resulting in the episodic nature of glucocorticoid and mineralocorticoids plasma concentrations though through different biochemical mechanisms.[166]

Early work with sodium imbalance, deoxycorticosterone acetate and the juxtaglomerular cells in the kidney suggested a relationship between the kidney and the adrenal glands.[167-170] It was later determined that a aldosterone stimulating hormonal agent, different from ACTH, was present in the blood.[171] This agent, called aldosterone stimulating hormone (ADH), was reported to have extrapituitary origin.[172-174] Davis reported that ADH was located in the kidney and suggested it was renin.[172,175,176] While the importance of renin in controlling the synthesis and release of aldosterone was being determined, Taragh reported that angiotensin 2, after infusion to humans, increased the output of aldosterone from the adrenal cortex.[177] Similar findings were reported in animal studies.[178] The working relationship between renin, angiotensin, and aldosterone synthesis and release has been determined through the efforts of many investigators (Figure 10).

Renin is synthesized and released from the juxtaglomerular cells lining the afferent

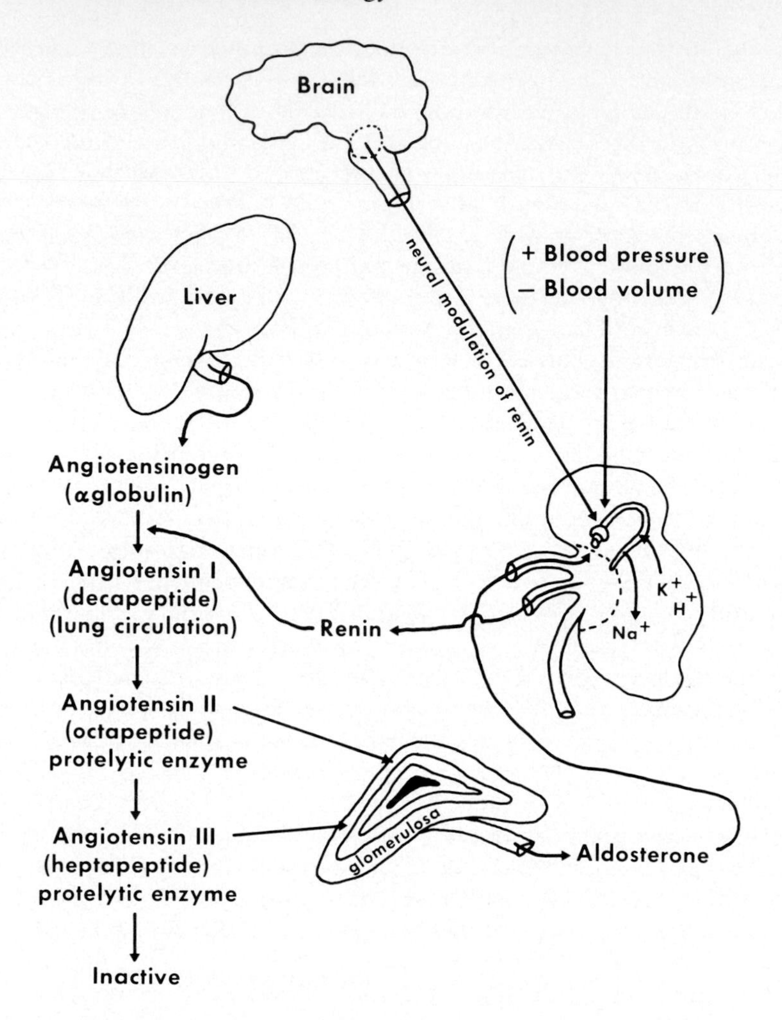

FIGURE 10. Control of aldosterone synthesis and release. Renin is secreted by the juxtaglomerular cells near the glomerulus. It is modulated by direct neural control, Na^+ depletion, blood loss and other extrinsic factors. Renin converts angiotensinogen to angiotensin 1, which is con verted to angiotensin 11 by lung enzymes. Angiotensin 11 is converted to angiotensin 111. Both can act on the zona glomerulosa of the adrenal cortex to increase the output of aldosterone. Aldosterone, a potent hormone, acts back on the kidney to increase Na^+ retention. ACTH can also increase the production of aldosterone, but this mechanism accounts for a minor controlling factor.

arterioles leading to the glomerulus. The release of renin is under the influence of several stimuli (1) a change in the flux of sodium across the distal tubule (macula densa cells), i.e., an increase in the rate of Na^+ loss across the tubule increases renin release; (2) a fall in renal perfusion pressure (baroreceptor); (3) an increase in pressure in the right atrium (decreases renin output); (4) an increased sympathetic response to the kidney (endogenous catecholamines, α and β-receptors); (5) a change in plasma potassium ion concentration; (6) the action of angiotensin 2 (indirect, decreasing hemodynamics in renal arterioles); (7) the action of vasopressin; and (8) by the action of aldosterone (negative feedback).[179,180]

While renin release and synthesis may be modulated by many factors, the response of the vascular "baroreceptors" located in the macula densa and the renal afferent arterioles are likely the major controlling influence for the release of renin.[180]

Once renin is released to the blood it acts on an α-globulin (a tetradecapeptide) which is synthesized released by the liver (angiotensinogen or renin substrate). This reaction results in the formation of the decapeptide angiotensin 1. It circulates through the lung (high concentrations of converting enzyme) and is catalyzed to an octapeptide, angiotensin 2. Angiotensin 2 (a powerful vasoconstrictor) stimulates aldosterone synthesis and release in the zona glomerulosa, where it is believed to promote the biochemical conversion of cholesterol to Δ^5-pregnenolone.[181,182] Angiotensin 2 can be further metabolized to an active state, angiotensin 3 by the action of an angiotensin 2 aminopeptidase, which removes the N terminal aspartic acid residue. [183] The specific importance of angiotensin 3 awaits further investigation.

Angiotensin 2 is a potent vasoconstrictor and acts at the level of the brain to increase blood pressure,[184] increase the thirst response, [185] and to release vasopressin. The functions of the angiotensins, other than for aldosterone production and release, are speculative at best. However, the primary control system for aldosterone synthesis and release appears to be the renin-angiotensin mechanism. Other factors, e.g., sympathic neural fibers at the juxtaglomerular cells, certainly can modulate renin release and thus aldosterone levels but they do not represent a major controlling mechanism.

Besides the angiotensin mechanism, ACTH can also stimulate the synthesis and release of aldosterone. The mean plasma levels of ACTH probably maintain the zona glomerulosa in a ready state so that it can respond to increases in angiotensin 2 and 3.[180] Plasma potassium may also influence the production of aldosterone directly in the zona glomerulosa; presumably necessary for the activation of enzymes or cofactors required for aldosterone synthesis.[179]Growth hormone and β-MSH have also been suggested to be involved with aldersterone secretion but in vitro and in vivo data conflict. [186,187]

Aldosterone serves as the principal corticosteroid in the bullfrog, though corticosterone is also secreted. Because 17β-hydroxylase is absent in adrenal tissues, cortisol is not formed.[172] Fish more primitive than the elasmobranchis do not produce aldosterone though the lungfish may have aldosterone concentrations as high as in the amphibians.[179]

The principal corticosteroid of the rat is corticosterone and 18-hydroxy, 11-deoxycorticosterone. Like the human, aldosterone is produced in the zona glomerulosa of the rat adrenal cortex.

TRANSPORTATION-PLASMA PROTEINS

The adrenal corticosteroids complex with proteins in the plasma. These complexes dissociate easily and the association/dissociation equilibrium is governed by the Law of Mass Action.[188] The types of chemical bonds that form these association complexes are primarily hydrophobic and hydrogen, and lower energy bonds. The affinity corticosteroids have for their binding globulin depends on the structure of the steroid and the polarity the steroid exhibits. An increase in the number of polar groups generally results in a decrease in binding affinity, at least with serum albumin.

Plasma proteins which form corticosteroid complexes are (1) human serum albumin; (2) α-acid glycoprotein (AAG); and (3) corticosteroid-binding globulin (CBG or transcortin). While these proteins have similar molecular weights, they differ in their availability to form steroid/protein complexes and in their affinity for binding the corticosteroids.[188] Albumin, which is a 1000-fold higher in serum concentration than CBG, has the lowest affinity for cortisol (highest capacity) while CBG, which is in low serum concentrations (34 to 38 mg/ℓ), has the highest affinity (lowest capacity) for the cortisol.[189] Cortisol binds CBG readily, but progesterone has an even higher degree of binding affinity than cortisol, while corticosterone binds CBG only slightly more efficiently than cortisol. About 75% of serum cortisol is bound to CBG, serum albumin binds about 14% and α-acid glycoprotein binds only about 2%. The remainder is available as free cortisol (about 10%). While aldosterone, a hemiacetal structure, binds CBG, it does so much less efficiently. The role of α-acid glycoprotein binding to the corticosteroids is likely insignificant biologically since its binding is not significantly higher than albumin and it is present in relatively low concentrations. The corticosteroids bound to plasma albumin represent about 8 to 10% of total plasma cortisol. However, only about 10% of total plasma cortisol is represented as free cortisol, the biologically active form, the remainder bound to CBG, and other plasma proteins. The bound cortisol is biologically inactive and represent a "reserve" of cortisol constantly present in the circulation. The cortisol bound to albumin, through biologically inactive, is metabolized by the liver and thus can reduce the cortisol reserve.[189] This is not the case for CBG bound cortisol, which is not metabolized by the liver and is released as stated earlier, i.e., by the Law of Mass Action. Aldosterone, which is transported primarily by serum albumin, has a relatively short biological half-life (about 30 min) as compared to cortisol (4 to 5 hr).

The reason for the shorter half-life is the availability of serum albumin bound steroids for metabolism, whereas cortisol, bound primarily to CBG, is not available for metabolic conversion.

Corticosteroid binding globulin itself is under the control of the sex steroids. During pregnancy or when estrogen is administered, there is an increase in both the corticosteroid and sex steroid binding globulins, though CBG concentrations are the same for men and nonpregnant women.[188] Testosterone has a modulatory effect on CBG synthesis in male rats. Castration resulted in a 70% increase in CBG plasma levels while administration of testosterone reduced these concentrations back to precastration levels. The same testosterone administration to noncastrated males does not reduce the CBG levels further.[190]

The function of the high affinity binding globulin (CBG) is predictive in that it affords the biological system a reserve for the corticosteroids (cortisol), readily available for use should the free circulating form, i.e., the biologically active one, be reduced. In addition, the corticosteroids bound to CBG are unavailable for metabolism, thus lengthening the biological half-life of the reserve and increasing biological efficiency.

BIOLOGICAL FUNCTIONS OF THE CORTICOSTEROIDS

Glucocorticoids

The glucocorticoids formed by the adrenal cortex influence virtually every biochemical and physiological function involved in the maintenance of homeostatis. These steroids are essential as chemical modulators of cellular biochemistry enabling the organism to operate under normal as well as stressful conditions.

Cortisol is the major glucocorticoid secreted by man. About 20 to 25 mg is released by the adrenals each day. Though a major glucocorticoid, cortisol does have slight mineralocorticoid properties.

The mechanism of action of the glucocorticoids involves the presence of receptors in the cytosol of cells under glucocorticoid influence (Figure 11). These receptors recognize the specific steroid (e.g., cortisol) and because of a high affinity exhibited for this molecule, binds it readily. Once cortisol, which apparently moves freely into the cell, is bound to the receptor, this complex is believed to migrate through the cytoplasm and into the nucleus where it binds the chromatin with a high degree of specificity. There follows transcription, transportation of resultant mRNA to the cytoplasm and the translation of the message into enzymes and substrates necessary for cellular func-

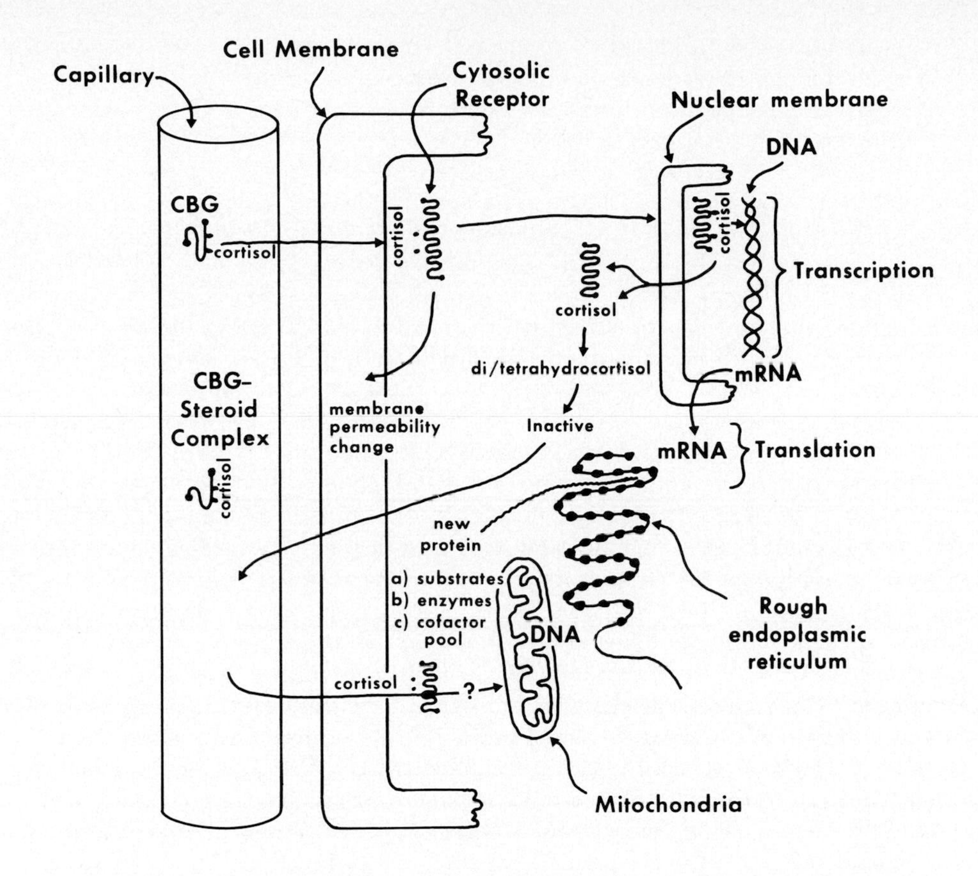

FIGURE 11. Example of steroid hormone (cortisol) activation of cellular processes. This process is believed to involve cytosolic receptor capturing the cortisol molecule, the translocation of the complex to the nucleus where transcription occurs. Message is sent back to the cytoplasm where translation leads to new protein synthesis. The length of time the receptor complex occupies the chromatin may be important in determining specific cellular responses.

tion. One cannot exclude, however, the possibility that direct local effects may also occur (change in membrane permeability) and that the cyclic AMP-kinase system of cellular activation may also be involved in glucocorticoid control of cellular processes.[191]

The control of glucocorticoids on cellular processes is both catabolic and anabolic in nature, depending on what specific message has been transcribed in the cell type activated by the glucocorticoid.

The glucocorticoids regulate or modulate alone or in concert with other hormones and cellular stimuli, the following processes:

1. Carbohydrate metabolism
2. Protein metabolism
3. Lipid metabolism
4. Bone and cartilage metabolism
5. Maintenance of the cardiovascular system
6. Maintenance of the hemopoeitic system
7. Maintenance of the skin, connective tissue, and mesenchymal tissue
8. Maintenance of CNS responsiveness
9. Maintenance of the immune system
10. Maintenance of the striated muscles

11. Growth hormone
12. The inflammatory responses to injury or disease
13. Maintenance of the gastrointestinal system
14. The response to olfaction, audition, and gustation.

The glucocorticords, as the name implies, increase the production of glucose, thereby augmenting the concentration of hepatic glucogen by stimulating gluconeogenesis. Muscle glycogen is also under cortisol control.

Mobilization of protein and amino acids requires cortisol. Hepatic uptake of amino acids is maintained and an anti-anabolic or protein catabolic effect is caused by glucocorticoid administration, initiated by the modulation of mRNA regulating protein synthesis.

Both thymic and lymphoid tissues are under the influence of the glucocorticoids. These tissues retrogress with excessive cortisol loads. The site of action appears to be at the level of mRNA thereby controlling protein synthesis within these cells, i.e., protein synthesis is reduced. In addition, glucocorticoids influence the resistance one has for disease. Hypersensitivity reactions (allergic responses) can be decreased with cortisol treatment, probably by blocking the synthesis of proteins necessary to convert histidine to histamine, as tissue histamine stores become depleted after cortisol administration.

Cortisol also slows the ossification and cartilaginous synthesis and proliferation at the epiphysis. This is accomplished by regulating protein synthesis, calcium absorption from the gut and modulating the action of parathyroid hormone and vitamin D.

Gut mucosa integrity is controlled by the glucocorticoids. Control of HCl secretion by the parital cell and mucus production are two important functions of the glucocorticoids. Decrease in cortisol levels causes a breakdown of the mucosa. These steroids also influence smooth muscle activation but have a significant effect on striated muscle. Muscle weakness is typical in cases of Addison's disease (adrenocortical insufficiency), corrected only with treatment of glucocorticoid.

Individuals on chronic cortisol therapy frequently have psychic changes, such as depression with irritability and schizoid manifestations. These changes seem to be reversible. As mentioned earlier, glucocorticoids inhibit the transmission rates through the nerves in signals coming from the ears (hearing), tongue (taste), and olfactory area (smell). In contrast, adrenalcorticoid insufficient patients have an increased sensitivity for the detection of smell, taste, and hearing.[192]

Glucocorticoid, in pharmacological doses, can also modulate the inflammatory processes. This is accomplished by decreasing the tissue responses to inflammation. Regulation in the production of tissue kinins, prevention of lysone disruption, suppression of vascular permeability, depression of lymphocyte and leucocyte migration and infiltration, alteration of phagocytosis ability, inhibition of fibroblastic proliferation, and decrease in collagen production have all been implicated as processes which have been modified by the presence of glucocorticoids.[193]

Mineralocorticoids

Though some of the glucocorticoids have mineralocorticoid properties, the primary steroid responsible for water and electrolyte metabolism is aldosterone. Aldosterone is secreted at a rate of about 100 ug/day in normal adults. The main action of aldosterone in the kidney is at the level of the distal tubule, causing sodium reabsorption and potassium loss (Figure 10). The mechanism of action is believed to involve the synthesis of a protein which increases sodium transport by altering cell permeability and by increasing the amount of ATP necessary for the "Na^+ pump" to operate.[194-196] In this system Na^+ ions are exchanged for both H^+ and K^+ ions.

This same mechanism occurs in the salivary glands, the gastrointestinal tract, and the sweat glands. Thus, Na^+ is retained at the expense of K^+ and H^+ ions, increasing blood and extracellular fluid volumes. Glucocorticoids have been implicated in the regulation of water metabolism by modulating the release of vasopressin (ADH), and by having a direct effect on the distal nephron, thereby decreasing water excretion. Aldosterone probably has a less important role in regulating water excretion and/or retention.

Adrenocorticoandrogens

The effects of the adrenocorticoandrogens are typical of all the sex steroids. They regulate cellular function in the typical steroid fashion, i.e., by the receptor-transcription-translation mechanism. Target tissues are those that have the specific receptor for each sex steroid. The mechanism of action of these steroids is addressed elsewhere in this reference book.

ADRENALCORTICAL DISORDERS

Adrenalcortical Insufficiency

Adrenalcortical insufficiency is commonly referred to as Addison's disease, as named by Wilds in 1862.[197] The disease may be idiopathic (cytotoxic/autoimmune) or caused by other disease, such as tuberculosis, neoplasia, etc. In addition, acute adrenal cortical insufficiency may occur due to trauma, infection, hemorrhage, thrombosis, or stress in individuals already in a tenuous adrenal cortical state. Other areas of cause may be secondary to the adrenal gland, i.e., pituitary ACTH or hypathalamic CRF disorders. In addition, inborn errors in metabolism (enzymatic deficiency) can also account for corticosteroid insufficiency.

Symptoms of the disease include a general weakness and fatigue with muscle strength impaired. Hyperpigmentation, especially in the gingiva area, is common due to elevated levels of MSH and ACTH in the plasma. There is general weight loss, anorexia, a capricious appetite, nausea, and a general distaste for food. Diarrhea and hypochlorhydria are common. Postural hypotension, low blood pressure, and faintness are common. Hypoglycemia would, of course, be expected. Other symptoms include apathy, reduced mental activity, and drowsiness. ACTH plasma levels distinguish primary from secondary adrenal atrophy.

The treatment of adrenal cortical insufficiency requires replacement therapy. Where a patient diagnosed with Addison's Disease between 1855 and 1930 died within 24 months, today the prognosis is much improved. Cortisol is the drug of choice, and is usually administered 20 to 30 mg/24 hr divided into three doses. In severe cases, a mineralocorticoid must be supplemented, such as fluorocortisone, at 0.05 to 0.1 mg/24 hr.

Adrenalcortical Excess

Adrenal cortical excess or Cushing's syndrome, is an uncommon disease usually affecting women between the ages of 30 and 50 years. The symptoms are caused by sustained and elevated plasma levels of free (unbound) cortisol. These elevated cortisol levels are induced by (1) ACTH producing tumors in the anterior pituitary; (2) CRF increase due to pathophysiological disorders in the hypothalamus; (3) cortisol producing tumors of the adrenal cortex; and (4) ectopic ACTH syndrome. The net result is an elevated plasma cortisol level resulting in the disease.

Symptoms include weight gain with resulting obesity, characterized by the pendulous abdomen and buffalo hump fat pad of the cervico-dorsal area and a rounding of the face. There is an accompanying moderate hypertension and a general muscular weakness. Typical are the red striae which accompanies obesity and the "thin-skin" and friable integument. Fatigue, weakness, and asthenia are typical complaints. Hirsutism is common in women, menses is irregular, and fertility rare.

The truncal skeletal system undergoes osteoporesis resulting in compressed vertebrae. Mental outlook is poor with depression and periods of irritability. There is generally a hyperglycemia and abnormal response to glucose, elevated hemoglobin, and neutrophilia. The plasma 17-hydroxy-corticoids are elevated and there is no observed diurnal variation in cortisol levels.

Treatment is by surgical removal of tumors or by radio-therapy. If the tumors are nonmalignant, prognosis is good.

Adrenal Cortical Androgenic Excess

Adrenal cortical androgenic excess (adrenogenital syndrome) is the expression of excessive androgen release from the adrenal cortex. There are two types (1) infantile; and (2) adult. In the infantile type, the syndrome is the result of faulty biosynthesis of the adrenal cortical steroids (Figure 12). The clinical form of the syndrome depends on the location of the enzyme block.

Enzyme defects involved in this syndrome are (1) cholesterol "desmolase"; (2) 3β-hydroxysteroid dehydrogenase; (3) 17α-hydroxylase; (4) 21-hydroxylase; (5) 11β-hydroxylase; and (6) 18-hydroxysteroid dehydrogenase (Figure 11).

Cholesterol Desmolase Defect

This type of infantile adrenogenital syndrome is called lipoid type adrenal hyperplasia. There is no steroid production so the individual lacks cortisol, aldosterone, and the related androgenic steroids. The genitalia of the male fail to develop normally but the female is unaffected. Neither sex develops normally at puberty. There is severe sodium wastage, volume depletion, and hypotension.

3β-Hydroxysteroid Dehydrogenase Defect

A similar clinical pattern develops as seen above. However, dehydroepiandrosterone is produced in high concentrations due to CRF/ACTH release. Females may have ambiguous genitalia at birth and both males and females lose sodium. Gonadal steroids are not produced. There is hypotension, volume depletion, and hypoatremia.

17α-Hydroxylase Defect

This type syndrome produces excessive deoxycorticosterone which leads to sodium retention, volume increase, and hypertension. There is also hypokalemia (low potassium) and a decrease renin output. Males have ambiguous genitalia (no androgens) but females are not affected. Both males and females develop hypertension because of ACTH aldosterone production.

21-Hydroxylase Defect

This is the most common type of infantile adrenogenital syndrome, accounting for about 95% of all cases. Cortisol and aldosterone are lacking, but androgen and estrogens are produced. The symptoms are similar to adrenal cortex insufficiency, accompanied by precocious puberty in males and ambiguous genitalia in females. There may be mild forms where a partial block will allow sufficient aldosterone synthesis for the maintenance of normal blood pressure and sodium balance. There is usually elevated plasma 17α-hydroxyprogesterone and testosterone levels and elevated urinary pregnonetriol levels.

11β-Hydroxylase Defect

Again there is a deficiency in cortisol and aldosterone production but not for androgens or estrogens. Increased testosterone secretion results in precocious puberty in males with ambiguous genitalia in females. There is also hypertension and hypokalemia with this syndrome due to the accumulation of deoxycorticosterone.

18-Hydroxysteroid Dehydrogenase Defect

Sodium wasting occurs due to the lack of aldosterone synthesis. There is also hypoatremia, hyperkalemia, and dehydration. Deoxycorticosterone levels are elevated but not sufficiently high to correct the sodium wasting. Plasma cortisol and ACTH levels remain normal.

Treatment of Adrenogenital Syndrome

Treatment of this disease is by replacement therapy. It is geared to the type of enzyme defect found and whether or not virilization has occurred. Corticosteroid has to continue indefinitely. The prognosis is good if the disease is recognized early and treatment initiated.

The adult type syndrome is frequently the result of tumor formation or bilateral adrenal hyperplasia. There are varying degrees of defeminization (female) or masculinization (male). Treatment is by surgery and if necessary, replacement therapy.

Hyperaldosteronism

Hyperaldosteronism is frequently the result of adrenal adenomas. In some cases congenital aldosteronism may be indicated. There is, of course, Na^+ retention with K^+ loss, via the urine, sweat, and saliva. The reninangiotensin system is suppressed. The onset is frequently insidious with hypertension being the only early symptom of the disease. There is generally some muscle weakness, headache, polydipsia, polyuria, and nocturia. Cardiomegaly often results in undiagnosed cases. Treatment involves the removal of the adenoma.

Secondary hyperaldosteronism can also occur due to malignant hypertensin, stenosis of renal arteries, or other renal impairment and hepatic cirrhosis. In the case of congenital hyperplasia, a bilateral adrenalectomy is usually performed. Patients with the later require indefinite replacement therapy.

CONCLUSIONS

This chapter has attempted to present an overview of the adrenal cortex. It by no means is an exhaustive search of the literature. For the serious student of endocrinology there are several excellent textbooks dealing with the adrenal cortex.

ACKNOWLEDGMENTS

The author wishes to thank Bobby James and Ruth York for their clerical assistance, Nick Aston for art work, and Robert Barrenger for photographic prints.

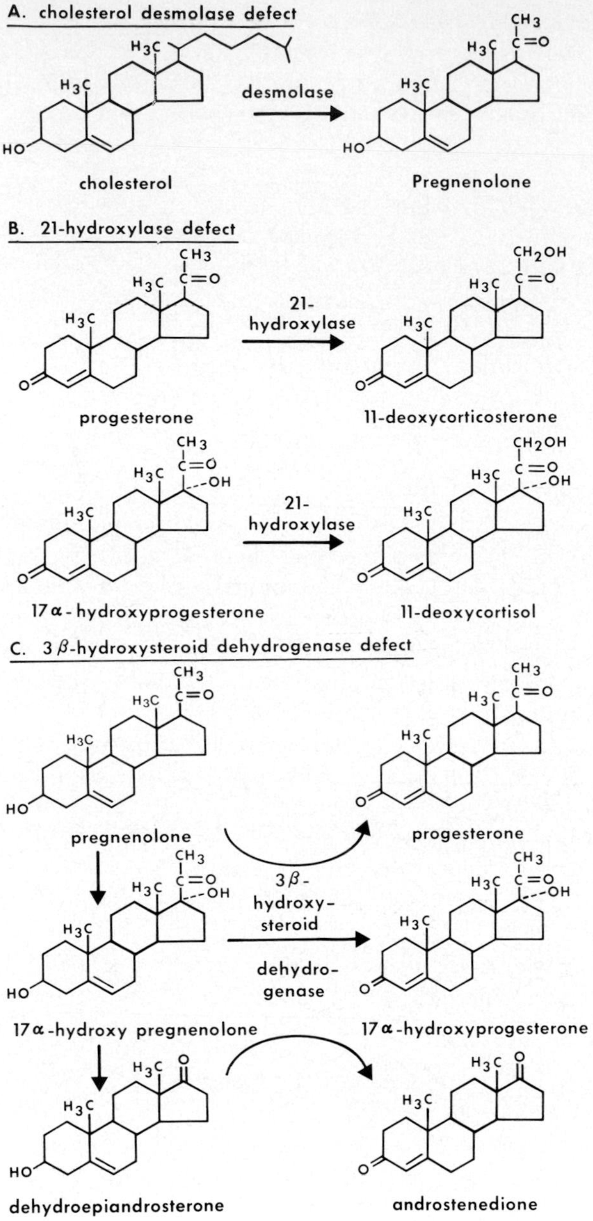

A. cholesterol desmolase defect

cholesterol → (desmolase) → Pregnenolone

B. 21-hydroxylase defect

progesterone → (21-hydroxylase) → 11-deoxycorticosterone

17α-hydroxyprogesterone → (21-hydroxylase) → 11-deoxycortisol

C. 3β-hydroxysteroid dehydrogenase defect

pregnenolone → progesterone

17α-hydroxy pregnenolone → (3β-hydroxysteroid dehydrogenase) → 17α-hydroxyprogesterone

dehydroepiandrosterone → androstenedione

FIGURE 12. Enzymatic defects leading to adrenogenital syndromes. These inborn errors in enzyme production produce effects caused by the absence of specific steroidogenic hormones. (See text).

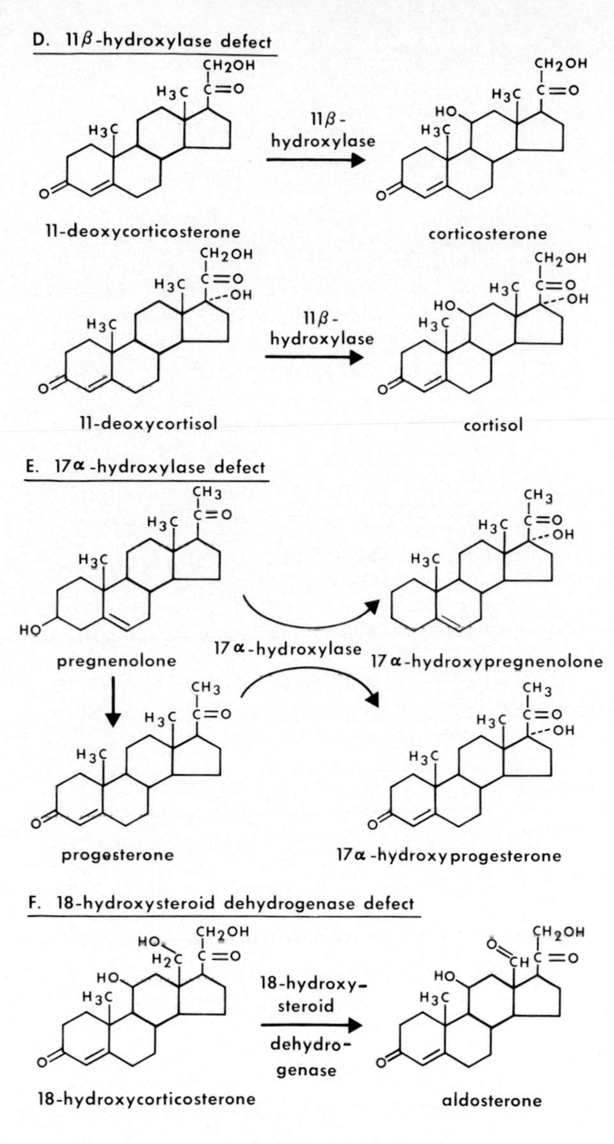

FIGURE 12 (continued).

RECOMMENDED READING

Anderson, D. C., Conway, D. I., and Bu'Lack, D. E., Adrenal Enzyme Defects, in *Adrenal Androgens,* Genazyani, A. R., Thyssen, J. H. H., and Suteri, P. K., Eds., Raven Press, New York, 1980, 115.

Barrington, E. J. W., Hormones and vertebrate evolution, *Experimenta,* 18:201, 1962.

Barrington, E. J. W., in *Introduction to General and Comparative Endocrinology,* Clarendon Press, Oxford, 1975, 197.

Bird, C. E. and Clark, A. F., The Adrenals. in *Systemic Endocrinology,* Ezrin, C., Gadden, J. O., and Valpe, R. Eds., Harper & Row, New York, 1979, 188.

Brownie, A. C. and Skelton, F. R., Adrenocortical function and structure in adrenal-regeneration and methylandrostenediol hypertension, in *Functions of the Adrenal Cortex,* Vol. 2, McKerns, F. W., Ed., Appleton-Century-Crofts, New York, 1968, 691.

Ri Tiore, M. S. H., *Atlas of Human Histology, 4th ed.,* Lea and Febiger, Philadelphia, 1976, 190.

Dunn, J. D., Circadian variation in the adrenocortical and anterior pituitary hormones, in *Biological Rhythms in Neuroendocrine Activity,* Kawakami, M., Ed., Igaku Shoin Ltd., Tokyo, 1974, 119.

Edelman, I. S., Aldosterone and sodium transport, in *Functions of the Adrenal Cortex,* Vol. 1, McKerns, F. W., Ed., Appleton-Century-Crofts, New York, 1968, 79.

Fieser, L. F. and Fieser, M., *Steroids,* Reinhold, New York, 1959, 26.

Fraser, R., The Effect of steroids on the transport of electrolytes through membranes, in *The Biochemistry of Steroid Hormone Action,* Academic Press, New York, 1971, 101.

Frieden, E. H., *Chemical Endocrinology,* Academic Press, New York, 1976, 48.

Gaunt, R., History of the adrenal cortex, in *Handbook of Physiology, Section 7,* Vol. 6, Adrenal Gland, Greep, R. O., Astwood, E. B., Blachko, H., Sayers, G., Smith, A. D., Geiger, S. B., Eds., American Physiology Society, Washington, D.C., 1975, 1.

Gower, D. B., Regulation of steroidogenesis, in *Biochemistry of Steroid Hormones,* Makin, H. L. J., Ed., Blackwell Scientific, Oxford, 1975, 27.

Gower, D. B., Biosynthesis of the Corticosteroids, in *Biochemistry of Steroid Hormones,* Makin, H. L. J., Ed., Blackwell Scientific, Oxford, 1975, 47.

Gray, H. and Goss, C. M., *Anatomy of the Human Body,* 29th ed., Lea and Febiger, Philadelphia, 1973, 1349.

Greep, R. O., The Structure of the adrenal cortex, in *The Adrenal Cortex,* Moon, H. D., Ed., International Academy of Pathology, Paul B. Haeber, New York, 1961, 23.

Gower, D. B., Catabolism and excretion of steroids, in *Biochemistry of Steroid Hormones,* Makin, H. L. J., Ed., Blackwell Scientific, Oxford, 1975, 149.

Hadd, H. and Blickenstaff, R. T., *Conjugates of Steroid Hormones,* Academic Press, New York, 1969.

Ham, A. W. and Comack, D. H., *Histology,* 8th ed., Lippincott, Philadelphia, 1979, 815.

Harrison, R. C., A comparative study of vascularization of the adrenal gland in the rabbit, rat and cat, *J. Anat. (London),* 85, 1951, 12.

Hiroshige, T., Circadian rhythm of corticotropin-releasing activity in the rat hypothalamus: an attempt at physiological validation, in *Biological Rhythms in Neuroendocrine Activity,* Kawaksami, M., Ed., Igaku Shoin Ltd, Tokyo, 1974, 267.

Kent, G. C., *Comparative Anatomy of the Vertebrates,* C. V. Mosby, St. Louis, 1973, 366.

Jubiz, W., The adrenals, in *Endocrinology: A Logical Approach for Clinicians,* McGraw-Hill New York, 1979, 80.

Junqueira, L. C., Carneiro, J., and Contopoulos, A. N., *Basic Histology,* Lang, Los Altos, CA, 1975, 383.

Lee, J. and Laycock, J., *Essential Endocrinology,* Oxford University Press, Oxford, 1978, 43.

Long, J. A., Zonation of the mammalian adrenal cortex, in *Handbook of Physiology, Section 7,* Vol. 6, Greep, R. O., Astwood, E. B., Blachko, H., Sayers, G., Smith, A. D., Geiger, S. B., Eds., American Physiology Society, Washington, D.C., 1975, 13.

Malamed, S., Ultrastructure of the mammalian adrenal cortex in relationship to secretory function, in *Handbook of Physiology, Section 7,* Endocrinology, Vol. 6, Greep, R. O., Astwood, E. B., Blachko, H., Sayers, G., Smith, A. D., Geiger, S. B., Eds., American Physiology Society, Washington, D.C., 1975, 25.

McKelvey, J. F., Charli, J. L., Joseph-Bravo, P., Sherman, T., and Laudes, C., Cellular biochemistry of brain peptides: biosynthesis, degradation, packaging, transport, and release, in *Comprehensive Endocrinology: The Endocrine Function of the Brain,* Motto, M., Ed., Raven Press, 1980, 171.

Monder, C. and Bradlow, H. L., Cortic acids: exploration at the frontier of corticosteroid metabolism, in *Recent Progress in Hormone Research,* Greep, R. O., Ed., Academic Press, New York, 1980, 345.

Maroulis, G. B. and Abrahm, G. E., Concentration of androgens and cortisol in the zones of the adrenal cortex, in *Adrenal Androgens,* Genazyani, A. R., Thyssen, J. H. H., and Suteri, P. K., Ed., Raven Press, New York, 1980, 49.

Netter, F. H., The ciba collection of medical illustration, Forsham, P. H., Ed., CIBA Pharmaceutical, Summit, New Jersey, 1974, 77.

Rimon, D. L. and Schimke, R. N., *Genetic Disorders of the Endocrine Glands,* C. V. Mosby, St. Louis, 1971, 217.

Roberts, S. and Creange, J. E., The role of 3′5′-adenosine phosphate in the subcellular localization of regulatory processes in corticosteroidogenesis, in *Functions of the Adrenal Cortex,* Vol. 1, McKerns, F. W., Ed., Appleton-Century-Crofts, New York, 1968, 339.

Schneeberg, N. G., The adrenal cortex, in *Essentials of Clinical Endocrinology,* C. V. Mosby St. Louis, 1970, 196.

Samuels, L. T. and Nelson, D. H., Biosynthesis of corticosteroids, in *Handbook of Physiology, Section 7,* Vol. 7, Greep, R. O., Astwood, E. B., Blachko, H., Sayers, G., Smith, A. D., and Geiger, S. B., Eds., American Physiology Society, Washington, D.C., 1975, 55.

Sayers, H., Regulation of the secretory activity of the adrenal cortex: cortisol and corticosterone, in *Handbook of Physiology, Section 7,* Vol. 7, Greep, R. O., Astwood, E. B., Blachko, H., Sayers, G., Smith, A. D., and Geiger, S. B., Eds., American Physiology Society, Washington, D.C., 1975, 41.

Schrader, W. T. and O'Malley, B. W., Similarities of structure among steroid receptor proteins, in *Receptors and Human Disease,* Bearn, A. G. and Choppin, P. W., Eds., Josiah Macy, Jr. Foundation, New York, 1979, 183.

Selye, H., Effect of steroids on Resistance, in *Hormones and Resistance,* Springer-Verlag, New York, 1971, 109.

Tchen, T. T., Conversion of cholesterol to pregnenolone in the adrenal cortex: enzymology and regulation, in *Functions of the Adrenal Cortex,* Vol. 1, McKerns, F. W., Ed., Appleton-Century-Crofts, New York, 1968, 3

Villee, D. B., *Human Endocrinology: A Developmental Approach,* W. B. Saunders, Philadelphia, 1975, 58.

REFERENCES

1. **Thorn, G. W.,** The adrenal cortex. I. Historical Aspects, *John Hopkins Med. J.,* 123, 49, 1968.
2. **Addison, T.,** *On the Constitutional and Local Effects of Disease of the Suprarenal Capsules,* S. Higley, London, 1855.
3. **Brown-Sequard, C. E.,** Recherches experimentales sur la physiologie et la pathologie des capsules surrenales, *Compt. Rend.,* 43, 422-425, 1856.
4. **Philipeaux, M.,** Note sur l'exstirpation des capsules surrenales chez les rats albinos, *Compt. Rend.,* 43, 904, 1155, 1856.
5. **Biedl, A.,** *The Internal Secretory Organs. Their Physiology and Pathology,* William Woods, New York, 1913.
6. **Hartman, F. A.,** The general physiology and experimental pathology of the suprarenal glands, in *Endocrinol. Metab., Vol. 2.,* Barker, L. F., Ed., Appleton, New York, 1922, 119.
7. **Houssay, B. A. and Lewis, J. I.,** The relative importance to life of cortex and medulla of the adrenal glands, *Am. J. Physiol.,* 64, 513, 1923.
8. **Wheeler, T. D. and Vincent, S.,** The question as to the relative importance to life of cortex and medulla of the adrenal bodies, *Trans. Roy. Soc. Can.,* 11, 125, 1917.
9. **Swingle, W. W. and Pfiffner, J. J.,** An aqueous extract of the suprarenal cortex which maintains life of bilaterally adrenalectomized cats, *Science,* 71, 321, 1930.
10. **Swingle, W. W. and Pfiffner, J. J.,** Studies on the adrenal cortex. I. The effect of a lipid fraction upon the life span of adrenalectomized cats, *Am. J. Physiol.,* 96, 153, 1931.
11. **Hartman, F. A. and Brownell, K. A.,** The hormone of the adrenal cortex, *Science,* 72, 76, 1930.
12. **Hartman, F. A. and Brownell, K. A.,** A further study of the hormone of the adrenal cortex, *Am. J. Physiol.,* 95, 670, 1930.
13. **Gaunt, R. and Gaunt, H. J.,** Survival of adrenalectomized rats after cortical hormone treatment, *Proc. Soc. Expt. Biol., Med.,* 31, 490, 1934.
14. **Rountree, L. G., Green, C. H., Swingle, W. W., and Pfiffner, J. J.,** The treatment of patients with Addisons disease with the "cortical hormone" of Swingle and Pfiffner, *Science,* 72, 482, 1930.
15. **Kendall, E. C.,** *Cortisone,* Scribners, New York, 1971, 10.
16. **Kendall, E. C.,** A chemical and physiological investigation of the suprarenal cortex, in Cold Spring Harbor Symp. Quant. Biol., Vol. 5, Long Island Biological Association, Ed., Darwin Press, New York, 1937, 299.
17. **Steiger, M. von and Reichstein, T.,** Desoxy-cortico-steron (21-oxyprogesteron) aus Δ^5-3-oxy-atio-cholensaure, *Helv. Chem. Acta,* 20, 1164, 1937.

18. **Marshall, E. K. and Davis, D. M.,** Influences of adrenals on the kidneys, *J. Pharmacol. Exper. Therap.*, 8, 525, 1916.
19. **Marine, D. and Baumann, E. J.,** Duration of life after suprarenalectomy in cats and attempts to prolong it by injections of solutions containing sodium salts, glucose and glycerol, *Am. J. Physiol.*, 81, 86, 1927.
20. **Baumann, E. J. and Kurland, S.,** Changes in the inorganic constituents of blood in suprarenalectomized cats and rabbits, *J. Biol. Chem.*, 71, 281, 1927.
21. **Loeb, R. G.,** Effect of sodium chloride in treatment of a patient with Addison's disease, *Proc. Soc. Exptl. Biol.*, 30, 808, 1933.
22. **Allers, W. D. and Kendall, E. C.,** Maintenance of adrenalectomized dogs without cortin through contact of the mineral constituents of the diet, *Am. J. Physiol.*, 118, 87, 1937.
23. **Britton, S. W. and Silvatte, H.,** The apparent prepotent function of the adrenal glands, *Am. J. Physiol.*, 100, 701, 1932.
24. **Britton, S. W. and Silvatte, H.,** Effects of cortico-adrenal extract on carbohydrate metabolism in normal animals, *Am. J. Physiol.*, 100, 693, 1932.
25. **Long, C. N. H., Katzin, B., and Frey, E. G.,** The adrenal cortex and carbohydrate metabolism, *Endocrinology*, 26, 309, 1940.
26. **Bullock, W. and Sequeira, J.,** On the relationship of the suprarenal capsules to sexual organs, *Trans. Pathol. Soc. (London)*, 56, 189, 1905.
27. **Glynn, E. E.,** The adrenal cortex, its rests and tumors; its relationship to the other ductless glands and especially to sex, *Quant. J. Med. (Oxford)*, 5, 157, 1911.
28. **Rogoff, J. M. and Stewart, G. N.,** Studies on adrenal insufficiency: influence of "heat" on the survival period of dogs after adrenalectomy, *Am. J. Physiol.*, 84, 660, 1928.
29. **Gaunt, R. and Hays, W.,** Role of progesterone and other hormones in survival of pseudopregnant adrenalectomized ferrets, *Am. J. Physiol.*, 124, 767, 1938.
30. **Smith, P. E.,** Hypophysectomy and a replacement therapy in the rat, *Am. J. Anat.*, 45, 205, 1930.
31. **Ingle, D. J. and Kendall, E. C.,** Atrophy of the adrenal cortex of the rat produced by the administration of large amounts of cortin, *Science*, 86, 245, 1937.
32. **Sayers, G.,** The adrenal cortex and homeostatis, *Physiol. Rev.*, 30, 241, 1950.
33. **Kendall, E. C.,** A chemical and physiology investigation of the suprarenal cortex, *Sympos. Quant. Biol.*, 5, 299, 1937.
34. **Grollman, A.,** Physiological and chemical studies on the adrenal cortical hormone, *Sympos. Quant. Biol.*, 5, 313, 1937.
35. **Reichstein, T. J. and Von Eaw, J.,** Uber Bestedteile der Nebennierenrinde: isalierung der Substanzen Q (desoxy-corticosterone) und R sowie Weitere, Staffe. *Helvet. Chim. Acta*, 21, 1197, 1938.
36. **Steiger, M. and Reichstein, T.,** Desoxycorticosterone (21-oxyprogesterone aus 5-3-oxyatio cholensaure), *Helvet. Chim. Acta*, 20, 1164, 1937.
37. **Merklin, R. J.,** Arterial supply of the suprarenal gland, *Anat. Rec.*, 144, 359, 1962.
38. **Gagnon, R.,** The arterial supply of the human adrenal gland, *Rev. Can. Biol.*, 16, 421, 1957.
39. **Flint, J. M.,** The blood vessels, angioesis, organogensis, reticulum and histology of the adrenal, *Johns Hopkins Hosp. Rep.*, 2, 153, 1900.
40. **Minot, C. W.,** On the hitherto unrecognized form of blood circulation without capillaries in the organs of the vertebrata, *Proc. Bos. Soc. Nat. Hist.*, 29, 185, 1900.
41. **Gersh, I. and Grollman, A.,** The vascular pattern of the adrenal gland of the mouse and rat and its physiological responses to changes in glandular activity, *Contrib. Embryol. Carnegie Inst., (Wash.,)* 29, 113, 1941.
42. **Brunn, A. Von,** Ueber das Vorkommen organischer Muskelfasern in den Nebennieren. *Dachr. Ges. Wiss., (Gottengen)*, 421, 1873.
43. **Dahbie, J. W. and Symington, T.,** The human adrenal gland with special reference to vasculature, *Endocrinology*, 34, 479, 1966.
44. **Arnold, J.,** Ein Beitrag za der feinere Struktur und dem Chemismus der Nebennieren, *Arch. Path. Anat. Physiol. Klin. Med.*, 35, 64, 1866.
45. **Cater, D. B. and Lever, J. D.,** The zona intermedia of the adrenal cortex: a correlation of possible functional significance with development, morphology and histochemistry, *J. Anat.*, 88, 437, 1954.
46. **Howard, E. and Migeon, C. J.,** Sex hormone secretion by the adrenal cortex, *Hambuch. Exptl. Pharmakol.*, 14(1), 570, 1962.
47. **Lanman, J. T.,** The fetal zone of the adrenal gland. Its development, cause, comparative anatomy and possible physiological functions, *Medicine*, 32, 389, 1953.
48. **Gottschau, M.,** Struktur und Embryonale entwicklung der Nebennieren bei Saugetieren, *Ark. Anat. Physiol. (Leipzig)*, 1883, 412, 1883.
49. **Swann, H. G.,** The pituitary-adenocortical relationship, *Physiol. Rev.*, 20, 493, 1940.
50. **Tonutti, E.,** Uber die Stukturelle Funktionsanpassung der Nebennierenrinde, *Endokrinologie*, 28, 1, 1951.

51. **Chester Jones, I.,** *The adrenal cortex,* London-Cambridge University Press, London, 1957.
52. **Greep, R. O. and Deane, H. W.,** Histological, cytochemical and physiological observations on the regeneration of the rat's adrenal gland following enucleation, *Endocrinology,* 45, 42, 1949.
53. **Ingle, D. J. and Higgins, G. M.,** Regeneration of the adrenal gland following enucleation. *Am. J. Med. Sci.,* 196, 232, 1938.
54. **Skelton, F. R.,** Adrenal regeneration and adrenal-regeneration hypertension, *Physiol. Rev.,* 39, 162-182, 1959.
55. **Holly, M. P.,** The size of nuclei in the adrenal cortex, *J. Pathol. Bacteriol.,* 90, 289, 1965.
56. **Deane, H. W. and Greep, R. O.,** A morphological and histochemical study of the rat's adrenal cortex after hypophysectomy, with comments on the liver, *Am. J. Anat.,* 79, 117, 1946.
57. **Stark, E., Palkowits, M., Fochet, J., and Hajtmann, B.,** Adrenocortical nuclear volume and adrenocortical function, *Acta Med.* (Hungary), 21, 263, 1965.
58. **Ganong, W. F. and Van Brunt, E. E.,** Control of aldosterone secretion, *Hambuch Expt. Pharmakol.,* 14(3), 4, 1968.
59. **Hartroft, P. M. and Hartroft, W. S.,** Studies on renal juxtaglomerular cells, II. Correlations of the degree of granulation of juxtaglomerular cells and width of the zona glomerulosa of the adrenal cortex, *J. Exper. Med.,* 102, 205, 1955.
60. **Goldman, M. L., Ronzoni, E., and Schroeder, H. A.,** The response of the adrenal cortex of the rat to dietary salt restriction and replacement. *Endocrinology,* 58, 57, 1956.
61. **Marx, A. J. and Deane, H. W.,** Histophysiological changes in the kidneys and adrenal cortex in rats on a low sodium diet, *Endocrinology,* 73, 317, 1963.
62. **Hartroft, P. M. and Eisenstein, A. B.,** Alterations in the adrenal cortex of the rat induced by sodium deficiency: correlation of histologic changes with steroid hormone secretion, *Endocrinology,* 60, 641, 1957.
63. **Koviacs, K. and David, M. A.,** Effect of cortisone on the morphological reactions of the adrenal cortex due to changes in the Na/K intake, *Acta Anat.,* 36, 169, 1959.
64. **Hartroft, P. M.,** Juxtaglomerular cells, *Circ. Res.,* 12, 525, 1963.
65. **Deane, H. W. and Masson, G. M. G.,** Adrenal cortical change in rats with various types of experimental hypertension, *J. Clin. Endocrinol. Metab.,* 11, 193, 1951.
66. **Marx, A. J., Deane, H. W., Mowles, T. F., and Sheppard, H.,** Chronic administration of angiotensin in rats: changes in blood pressure, renal and adrenal histopathology and aldosterone production, *Endocrinology,* 73, 329, 1963.
67. **Giroud, C. J. P., Stachenko, J., and Venning, E. H.,** Secretion of aldosterone by the zona glomerulosa of rat adrenal glands incubated *in vitro, Proc. Soc. Exper. Biol. Med.,* 92, 154, 1956.
68. **Stachenko, J. and Giroud, C. J. P.,** Further observations on the functional zonation of the adrenal cortex, *Can. J. Biochem.,* 42, 1777, 1964.
69. **Brostec, L. R. and Vines, H. W. C.,** *The Adrenal Cortex,* Lewis, London, 1933.
70. **Race, G. J. and Wu, H. M.,** Adrenal cortex functional zonation in the whale (Physter catadom), *Endocrinology,* 68, 156, 1961.
71. **Ofstad, J., Lamirk, J., Stoa, K. F., and Emberland, R.,** Adrenal steroid synthesis in amyloid degeneration localized exclusively to the zona reticularis, *Acta Endocrinology,* 37, 321, 1961.
72. **Griffiths, K. and Cameron, E. H. D.,** Steroid biosynthetic pathways in the human adrenal, *Adv. Ster. Biochem. Pharmacol.,* 2, 223, 1970.
73. **Baird, D. T., Vno, A., and Milby, J. C.,** Adrenal secretion of androgens and oestrogens, *J. Endocrinol.,* 45, 135, 1969.
74. **Fawcett, D. W., Long, J. A., and Jones, A. L.,** The ultrastructure of endocrine glands, *Rec. Progr. Horm. Res.,* 25, 315, 1969.
75. **Sabatini, D. D. and De Robertis, E.,** Ultrastructure zonation of the adrenal cortex in the rat, *J. Biophys. Biochem. Cytol.,* 9, 105, 1961.
76. **Long, J. A. and Jones, A. L.,** Observations on the fine structure of the adrenal cortex of man, *Lab. Invest.,* 17, 355, 1967.
77. **Rhodin, J. A. G.,** The ultrastructure of the adrenal cortex of the rat under normal and experimental conditions, *J. Ultrastruct. Res.,* 34, 23, 1971.
78. **Idelman, E. S.,** Contributions a la cytophysiologic infrastructural de la cortico surrende chez le rat albinos. *Ann. Sci. Nat. Zool. Biol.* An. 8, 205, 1966.
79. **Idelman, S.,** Ultrastructure of the mammalian adrenal cortex, *Intern. Rev. Cytol.,* 27, 181, 1970.
80. **Shelton, J. H. and Jones, L.,** The fine structure of the mouse adrenal cortex and the ultrastructural changes in zona glomerulosa with low and high sodium diets, *Anat. Rec.,* 170, 147, 1971.
81. **Rittenberg, D. and Schoenheimer, R.,** Deuterium as an indicator in the study of intermediate metabolism. XI. Further studies on the biological uptake of deuterium into organic substances, with special references to fat and cholesterol formation, *J. Biol. Chem.,* 121, 235, 1937.
82. **Bloch, K. and Rittenberg, D.,** The biological formation of cholesterol from acetic acid, *J. Biol. Chem.,* 143, 297, 1942.

83. **Bloch, K.**, Biological synthesis of cholesterol, *Rec. Chem. Progr.*, 15, 103, 1953.
84. **Dauben, W. G. and Takemura, K. H.**, A study of the mechanism of the conversion acetate to cholesterol via squalene, *J. Am. Chem. Soc.*, 75, 6302, 1953.
85. **Cornforth, J. W. and Popjak, G.**, The biosynthesis of cholesterol. III. Distribution of ^{14}C in squalene biosynthesized from [Me-^{14}C]-acetate, *Biochem. J.*, 58, 403, 1954.
86. **Cornforth, J. W., Youhatsky-Gore, I., and Popjak, A. J.**, Absolute configuration of cholesterol, *Nature*, 173, 536, 1954.
87. **Dauben, W. G. and Hutton, T. W.**, The biosynthesis of steroids and triterpenes. The origin of carbon 11 and 12 of ergosterol, *J. Am. Chem. Soc.*, 78, 2647, 1956.
88. **Wolf, D. E., Hoffman, C. H., Aldrich, P. E., Skeggs, H. R., Wright, L. D., Falkers, L. D., and Falkers, K.**, β-Hydroxy-β-methyl-γ-valeralactone (divaloric acid): a new biological factor, *J. Am. Chem. Soc.*, 78, 4499, 1956.
89. **Tavoimini, P. A., Gibbs, M. H., and Huff, J. W.**, The utilization of β-hydroxy-β-methyl-γ-valeralactone in cholesterol biosynthesis, *J. Am. Chem. Soc.*, 78, 2647, 1956.
90. **Tavoimini, P. A. and Gibbs, M. H.**, The metabolism of β,γ-dihydroxy-methylvaloric acid by liver homogenates, *J. Am. Chem. Soc.*, 78, 6210, 1956.
91. **Popjak, G.**, Recent advances in the study of sterol biosynthesis. Metab. Physiol. Significance of lipids, *Proc. 6th Inter. Congr. Biochem.*, Cambridge, 1963, 45.
92. **Donniger, C. and Popjak, G.**, The steriochemistry of hydrogen transfer catalyzed by liver alcohol dehydrogenase: IR[1-^{3}H] geronial as a substrate, *Biochem. J.*, 91, 10P, 1964.
93. **Donniger, C. and Ryback, G.**, The steriochemistry of hydrogen transfer catalyzed by mevaldale reductase, *Biochem., J.*, 91, 11P, 1964.
94. **Altman, L. J., Koerski, R. C., and Rilling, H. G.**, Synthesis and conversion of presqualene alcohol to squalene, *J. Am. Chem. Soc.*, 93, 1782, 1971.
95. **Danielsson, H. and Tchen, T. T.**, Steroid metabolism, in *Metabolic Pathways*, Vol. 2, (3rd ed.), Greenburg, D. M., Ed., Academic Press, New York, 1968, 117.
96. **Rilling, H. C., Paulter, C. D., Epstein, W. W., and Larsen, B.**, Studies on the mechanism of squalene biosynthesis. Presqualene pyrophosphate, stereochemistry and a mechanism of its conversion to squalene, *J. Am. Chem. Soc.*, 93, 1783, 1971.
97. **Goodman, D. S., Avigan, J., and Wilson, H.**, The *in vivo* metabolism of desmosterol with adrenal and liver preparations, *J. Clin. Invest.*, 41, 2135, 1962.
98. **Lipsett, M. B. and Hakfelt, B.**, Conversion of 17-alpha-hydroxy-pregnenelone to cortisol. *Experimenta*, 17, 449, 1961.
99. **Whitehouse, B. J. and Vinson, G. P.**, Corticosteroid biosynthesis from pregnenolone and progesterone by human adrenal tissue *in vitro*. A kinetic study, *Steroids*, 11, 245, 1968.
100. **Wieland, R. G., Levy, R. P., Katz, D., and Hirshmann, H.**, Evidence for secretion of 3-beta-hydroxyandrost-5-en-17-one sulfate by measurement in normal human adrenal venous blood, *Biochim. Biophys. Acta*, 78, 566, 1963.
101. **Solomon, S.**, Formation and metabolism of neutral steroids in the human placenta and fetus, *J. Clin. Endocrinol. Metab.*, 26, 762, 1966.
102. **Smith, S. W. and Axelrod, L. R.**, Studies on the metabolism of steroid hormones and their precursors by the human placenta at various stages of gestation of 3-beta-hydroxyandrost-5-en-17-one, *J. Clin. Endocrinol. Metab.*, 29, 1182, 1969.
103. **Hellman, L., Bradlow, H. L., Zumoff, B., and Gallagher, T. F.**, The influence of thyroid hormone on hydrocortisone production and metabolism, *J. Clin. Endocrinol. Metab.*, 21, 1231, 1961.
104. **Kelly, W. G., Lieberman, S. O., and Bandi, L.**, Isolation and characterization of human urinary metabolites of aldosterone. IV. The synthesis and stereochemistry of two bicyclicacetal metabolites, *Biochemistry (Washington)*, 2, 1243, 1963.
105. **Kelly, W. G. and Lieberman, S. O.**, Isolation and characterization of human urinary metabolites of aldosterone, in *Aldosterone, A Symposium*, Baulieu, E. E. and Rabel, P., Eds., Blackwell, Oxford, 1964, 103.
106. **Munck, A. and Brenck-Johnsen, C.**, Specific and non-specific physiochemical interactions of glucocorticoids and related steroids with rat thymus cells *in vitro*, *J. Biol. Chem.*, 243, 5556, 1968.
107. **Pinskey, L. and DiGeorge, A. M.**, Cleft palate in the mouse: a teratogenic index of glucocorticoid potency, *Science*, 147, 402, 1965.
108. **Rowland, J. R. and Hendrick, A. G.**, Triamcinolone acetonide tetratogenesis in Sprague-Dawley rats, *Teratology*, 19, 449, 1979.
109. **Reinisch, J. M., Simon, N. G., Karow, W. G., and Gandelmon, R.**, Prenatal exposure to prednisone in humans and animals retards interuterine growth, *Science*, 202, 436, 1978.
110. **Terrell, T. G.**, Development of the Lymphoid System in the Rhesus Monkey Fetus: a Comparison of Normal Development to Teratogenic Defects Induced by the Corticosteroid Triamcinolone, Doctoral dissertation, University of California, Davis, 1975.
111. **Sydnor, K. L. and Sayers, G.**, Blood and pituitary ACTH in intact and adrenalectomized rats after stress, *Endocrinology*, 55, 621, 1954.

112. **Sayers, G., Beall, R. J., and Sulig, S.,** Modes of action of ACTH, in *MTP International Review of Science,* Vol. 8, Butterworths, London, 1975, chap. 7.
113. **Haynes, R. C.,** Theories on the mode of action of ACTH in stimulating secretory activity of the adrenal cortex, in *Handbook of Physiology, Section 7,* Vol. 6, Greep, R. O., Astwood, E. B., Blachko, H., Sayers, G., Smith, A. D., Geiger, S. B., Eds., American Physiological Society, Washington, D.C., 1975, 69.
114. **Seelig, S. and Sayers, G.,** Isolated adrenal cortex cells: ACTH agonists, partial agonists, antagonists; cyclic AMP and corticosterone productivity, *Arch. Biochem. Biophys.,* 154, 230, 1973.
115. **Fujino, M., Hatanaka, C., and Nisgunyra, A.,** Synthesis of peptides related to corticotropin (ACTH). VI. Synthesis and biological activity of the peptide corresponding to the amino sequences 4-23, 5-23, 6-24, 7-23 in ACTH, *Chem. Pharm. Bull.,* 19, 1066, 1971.
116. **Hofmann, K.,** Preliminary observations relating structure and function in same pituitary hormones, *Brookhaven Symp. Biol.,* 13, 184, 1960.
117. **Ramachandran, J., Chung, D., and Li, C. H.,** Adrenocorticotropins. XXXIV. Aspects of structure-activity relationship of the ACTH molecule. Synthesis heptadecopeptide amide, an octadecapeptide amide and a nanodecapeptide amide possessing high biological activities, *J. Am. Chem. Soc.,* 87:2696-2708, 1965.
118. **Schwyzer, R.,** Chemistry and metabolic action of nonsteroid hormones, *Ann. Rev. Biochem.,* 33, 259, 1964.
119. **Schwyzer, R. and Sieler, P.,** Total synthesis of adrenocorticotropic hormone, *Nature,* 199, 172, 1963.
120. **Sayers, G. and Portanoua, R.,** Regulation of secretory activity of the adrenal cortex: cortisol and corticosterone, in *Handbook of Physiology, Section 7,* Vol. 6, Greep, R. O., Astwood, E. B., Blachko, H., Sayers, G., Smith, A. D., and Geiger, S. B., Eds., American Physiological Society, Washington, D.C., 1975, 41.
121. **Schwyzer, R.,** Chemistry and metabolic action of non-steroid hormones, *Ann. Rev. Biochem.,* 33, 259, 1964.
122. **Seelig, S. and Sayers, G.,** Isolated adrenal cortex cells: ACTH agonist, partial agonists, antagonists; cyclic AMP and corticosterone production, *Arch. Biochem. Biophys.,* 154, 230, 1973.
123. **Hofmann, K., Andreatta, R., Bohn, H., Moroder, H., and Moroder, L.,** Studies on polypepetides. XLV. Structure-function studies in the β-corticotropin series, *Med. Chem.,* 13, 339, 1970.
124. **Ney, R. L., Ogata, E., Shimizu, N., Nicholson, W. E., and Liddle, G. W.,** Structure-function relationships in ACTH and MSH analogues, in *Proceedings of the Second International Congress of Endocrinology,* Taylor, S., Ed., Excerpta Medica Foundation, Amsterdam, 1965, 1184.
125. **Besser, G. M. and Orth, D. N.,** Dissociation of the disappearance of bioactive and radioimmunoreactive ACTH from plasma and man, *J. Clin. Endocr.,* 32, 595, 1971.
126. **Green, J. R., and Harris, G. W.,** Observations of the hypophysial-portal vessels of the living rat, *J. Physiol. (London),* 108, 359, 1949.
127. **Harris, G. W. and Jackson, D.,** Proliferative capacity of the hypophysial portal vessels, *Nature,* 165, 854, 1950.
128. **Jones, M. T. and Hillhouse, E. W.,** Neurotransmitter regulation of corticotropin releasing factor *in vitro, Ann. N.Y. Acad. Sci.,* 297, 536, 1977.
129. **Buckingham, J. C. and Hodges, J. R.,** Production of corticotropin releasing hormone of the isolated hypothalamus of the rat, *J. Physiol. (London),* 272, 469, 1977.
130. **Jones, M. T., Hillhouse, E. W., and Burden, J. L.,** Secretion of corticotropin releasing hormone *in vitro,* in *Frontiers in Neuroendocrinology,* Vol. 5, Martini, L. and Ganong, W. F., Eds., Raven Press, New York, 1976, 194.
131. **Jones, M. T.,** Control of andrenocortical hormone secretion, in *Comprehensive Endocrinology. The Adrenal Gland,* Raven Press, New York, 1979, 93.
132. **Hodges, J. R., Jones, M. T., and Stockman, M. S.,** Effect of emotion on blood corticotrophin and cortisol concentrations in man, *Nature,* 193, 1187, 1962.
133. **Gallagher, T. F., Yoshida, K., Roffwarg, H. D., Fukushima, D. K., Weitzman, E. D., and Hellman, L.,** ACTH and cortisol secretory patterns in man, *J. Clin. Endocrinol.,* 36, 1058, 1973.
134. **Krieger, D. T.,** Regulation of circadian periodicity of plasma ACTH levels, *Ann. N.Y. Acad. Sci.,* 27, 561, 1977.
135. **Scapaznini, U., Moberg, G. P., Van Lakin, G. R., DeGroat, J., Ganong, W. F.,** Relationship between brain 5-HT content to the diurnal variation in plasma corticosterone in the rat, *Neuroendocrinology,* 7, 90, 1971.
136. **Ganong, W. F.,** Evidence for a central nonadrenergic system that inhibits ACTH secretion, in *Brain and Endocrinology Interactions: Median Eminence Structure and Function,* Krigge, H. M., Scott, D. E., and Weindle, A., Eds., S. Karger, Basel, 1977, 254.
137. **Jones, M. T., Hillhouse, E. W., and Burden, D. L.,** Effect of various putative neurotransmitters on the secretion of corticotropin releasing hormone from the rat hypothalamus *in vitro* — a model of the neurotransmitters involved, *J. Endocrinol.,* 69, 1, 1976.

138. **McCann, S. M.,** The ACTH-releasing activity of extracts of the posterior lobe of the pituitary *in vivo, Endocrinology,* 60, 644, 1957.
139. **McCann, S. M. and Brobeck, J. R.,** Evidence for a role of the supraoptico-hypophyseal system in regulation of adrenocorticotrophin secretion, *Proc. Soc. Exptl. Biol. Med.,* 87, 318, 1954.
140. **Royce, P. C. and Sayers, G.,** Purification of hypothalamic corticotrophin releasing factor, *Proc. Soc. Exptl. Biol. Med.,* 103, 447, 1960.
141. **Jones, M. T., Hillhouse, E. W., and Burden, J. L.,** Secretion of corticotrophin releasing hormone *in vitro,* in *Frontiers in Neuroendocrinology,* Vol. 5, Ganong, W. F. and Martini, L., Eds., Raven Press, New York, 1976, 194.
142. **Pollack, J. J. and LaBella, F. S.,** Inhibition by cortisol of ACTH release from the anterior pituitary tissue *in vitro, Can. J. Physiol. Pharmacol.,* 44, 549, 1966.
143. **Arimura, A., Bowers, C. Y., Schally, A. V., Saito, M., and Miller, M. C., III.,** Effect of corticotropin-releasing factor, dexamethasone and actinomycin D on the release of ACTH from rat pituitaries *in vivo* and *in vitro, Endocrinology,* 83, 1232, 1968.
144. **Fleischer, N. and Vale, W.,** Inhibition of vasopressin-induced ACTH release from the pituitary by glucocorticoids *in vitro, Endocrinology,* 83, 1232, 1968.
145. **Vernikos-Danellis, J.,** Effects of stress, adrenalectomy, hypophysectomy and hydrocortisone on the corticotropin-releasing activity of rat median eminence, *Endocrinology,* 76, 122, 1965.
146. **Takebe, K., Kunta, H., Sakakuro, M., Yoskihiko, H., and Mashimo, D.,** Suppressive effect of dexamethasone on the rise of CRF activity in the median eminence induced by stress, *Endocrinology,* 89, 1014, 1971.
147. **Motta, M., Fraschini, F., Peva, F., and Martini, L.,** Hypothalamic and extrahypothalamic mechanism controlling adrenocorticotropin secretion, *Men. Soc. Endocrinol.,* 17, 3, 1967.
148. **Motta, M., Mangili, B., and Martini, L.,** A "short" feedback loop in the control of ACTH secretion, *Endocrinology,* 77, 392, 1965.
149. **Sieden, G. and Brodish, A.,** Physiological evidence for "short-loop" feedback effects of ACTH on hypothalamic CRF, *Neuroendocrinology,* 8, 154, 1971.
150. **Scapagnini, U., Van Loon, G. R., Moberg, G. P., Preziosi, P., and Ganong, W. F.,** Evidence for central norepinephrine-mediated inhibition of ACTH secretion in the rat, *Neuroendocrinology,* 10, 155, 1972.
151. **VanLoon, G. R., Scapagnini, U., Cohen, R., and Ganong, W. F.,** Effect of intraventricular administration of adrenergic drugs on the adrenal venous 17-hydroxycorticosteroid response to surgical stress in the dog, *Neuroendocrinology,* 8, 257, 1971.
152. **Jones, M. T. and Hillhouse, E. W.,** Structure-activity relationship and the mode of action of corticosteroid feedback on corticotrophin-releasing factor (Corticoliberin), *J. Steroid Biochem.,* 7, 1189, 1976.
153. **Lippa, A. S., Antelman, S. M., Fahringer, E. E., and Redgate, E. S.,** Relationship between catecholamines and ACTH-effect of 6-hydroxydopamine, *Nat. New Biol.,* 241, 24, 1973.
154. **Sayers, G. and Sayers, M. A.,** Regulation of pituitary adrenocorticotropic activity during the response of the rat to acute stress, *Endocrinology,* 40, 265, 1947.
155. **Sirett, N. E. and Gibbs, F. P.,** Dexamethasone suppressions of ACTH release: effect of the interval between steroid administration and the application of stimuli known to release ACTH, *Endocrinology,* 85, 355, 1969.
156. **Kendall, J. W., Egans, M. L., Stott, A. K., Kramer, R. M., and Jacobs, J. J.,** The importance of stimulus intensity and duration of steroid administration in supression of stress-induced ACTH secretion, *Endocrinology,* 90, 525, 1972.
157. **Dallman, M. F. and Yates, F. E.,** Dynamic asymmetrics in the corticosteroid feedback pathway and distribution binding and metabolism of elements of the adrenocortical system, *Ann. N.Y. Acad. Sci.,* 156, 696, 1969.
158. **Buckingham, J. C. and Hodges, J. R.,** Corticosteroids on corticotrophin releasing hormone production by the rat hypothalamus *in vivo* and *in vitro, J. Endocrinol.,* 77, 53p, 1978.
159. **Bradbury, M. W. B., Burden, J. L., Hillhouse, E. W., and Jones, M. T.,** Stimulation electrically and by acetylcholine of the rat hypothalamus in vitro, *J. Physiol. (London),* 239, 269, 1974.
160. **Arimura, A., Bowlers, C. V., Schally, A. V., Saito, M., Miller, M. C., and Miller, M.,** Effect on corticotropin releasing factor, dexamethasone and actinomycin D on the release of ACTH from rat pituitaries, *Endocrinology,* 85, 300, 1969.
161. **James, V. H. T., Tunbridge, R. D. G., Wilson, G. A., Hutton, J., Jacobs, H. S., and Rippon, A. E.,** Steroid profiling: a technique for exploring adrenocortical physiology, in *The Endocrine Function of the Human Adrenal Cortex,* James, V. H. T., Serio, M., Giusti, G., Martini, L., Eds., Academic Press, London, 1978, 179.
162. **Birmingham, M. K. and Ward, P. J.,** The identification of the Porter-Silber chromogen secreted by the rat adrenal, *J. Biol. Chem.,* 236, 1661, 1961.

163. **Ward, P. J. and Birmingham, M. K.**, Properties of the ultraviolet-absorbing lipids produced by rat adrenals *in vitro, Biochem. J.*, 76, 269, 1960.
164. **Brodish, A.**, Hypothalamic and extrahypothalamic corticotrophin-releasing factors in peripheral blood, in *Brain-Pituitary-Adrenal Interrelationships*, Brodish, A. and Redgate, E. S., S. Karger, Basel 1973, 128.
165. **Egdall, R. H.**, Adrenal cortical and medullary responses to trauma in dogs with isolated pituitaries, *Endocrinology*, 66, 200, 1960.
166. **Atcheson, J. B. and Taylor, F. H.**, Circadian rhythm: man and animals, in *Handbook of Physiology, Section 7*, Vol. 6, Greep, R. O., Astwood, E. B., Blachko, H., Sayers, G., Smith, A. O., and Geiger, G. R., Eds., American Physiological Society, Washington, D.C. 1975, 127.
167. **Deane, H. W. and Masson, G. M. C.**, Adrenal cortical changes in rats with various types of experimental hypertension, *J. Clin. Endocrinol. Metab.*, 11, 193, 1951.
168. **Hartroft, P. M. and Hartroft, W. S.**, Studies on renal juxtaglomerular cells. I. Variations produced by sodium chloride, and desoxycorticosterone acetate, *J. Exptl. Med.*, 97, 415, 1953.
169. **Hartroft, P. M.**, Juxtaglomerular cells, *Circ. Res.*, 12, 525, 1963.
170. **Dunhue, F. W. and Robertson, W. V. B.**, The effect of desoxycorticosterone acetate and of sodium on the juxtaglomerular apparatus, *Endocrinology*, 61, 293, 1957.
171. **Davis, J. O.**, Discussion remarks, *Rec. Prog. Horm. Res.*, 15, 298, 1959.
172. **Davis, J. O.**, Mechanisms regulating the secretion and metabolism of aldosterone in experimental secondary hyperaldosteronism, *Rec. Prog. Horm. Res.*, 17, 293, 1961.
173. **Davis, J. O.**, Adrenocortical and renal hormonal function in experimental cardiac failure, *Circulation*, 25, 1002, 1962.
174. **Davis, J. O., Anderson, E., Carpenter, C. E., Ayers, C. R., Haymaker, W., and Spence, W. T.**, Aldosterone and corticosterone secretion following midbrain transection, *Am. J. Physiol.*, 200, 437, 1961.
175. **Davis, J. O., Hartroft, P. M., Titus, E. O., Carpenter, C. C. J., Ayers, C. R., and Spiegel, H. E.**, The role of the renin-angiotensin system in the control of aldosterone secretion, *J. Clin. Invest.*, 41, 378, 1962.
176. **Davis, J. O., Carpenter, C. C. J., Ayers, C. R., Holman, J. E., and Bahn, R. C.**, Evidence for secretion of an aldosterone-stimulating hormone by the kidney, *J. Clin. Invest.*, 40, 684, 1961.
177. **Laragh, J. H., Angers, M., Kelley, W. G., and Lieberman, S.**, The effect of epinephrine, norepinephrine, angiotensen II, and others on the secretory rate of aldosterone in man, *J. Am. Med. Assoc.*, 174, 234, 1960.
178. **Genest, J. E., Koiw, E., Nowaczynski, W., and Sandor, T.**, Study of urinary adrenocortical hormones in human arterial hypertension, Proc. Intern. Congr. Endocrinol., 1, Copenhagen, 1960, p. 173.
179. **Ross, E. J.**, *Aldosterone and Aldosteronism*, Lloyd-Luke Ltd., London, 1975, pp. 62, 90.
180. **Davis, J. O.**, Regulation of aldosterone secretion, in *Handbook of Physiology, Section 7*, Vol. 6, Greep, R. O., Astwood, E. B., Blachko, H., Sayers, G., Smith, A. D., and Geiger S. R. Eds., American Physiology Society, Washington, D.C., 1975, 77.
181. **Muller, J.**, *Regulation of Aldosterone Biosynthesis*, Springer-Verlag, Basel, 1971.
182. **Muller, J. and Ziegler, W. H.**, Steriodogenic effects of stimulators of aldosterone biosynthesis upon separate zones of the rat adrenal cortex. Influence of sodium and potassium deficiency, *Eur. J. Clin. Invest.*, 1, 180, 1970.
183. **Davis, J. O. and Friedman, R. H.**, The other angiotensin, *Biochem. Pharmacal.*, 26, 93, 1977.
184. **Servop, C. G., Katic, S., Jay, M. D., and Lowe, R. D.**, The importance of central vasomotor effects in angiostensin induced hypertension, *Br. Med. J.*, 1, 324, 1977.
185. **Simpson, J. B. and Rautenburg, A.**, Subfornical organs: site of drinking illicitations by angiotensin II, *Science*, 181, 1172, 1973.
186. **Lucus, O. J., Dyrenfurth, I., and Venning, E. H.**, Effects of various preparations of pituitary and diencephalon on the *in vitro* secretion of aldosterone and corticosterone by the rat adrenal gland, *Can. J. Biochem. Physiol.*, 39, 901, 1961.
187. **Finkelstein, J. W., Kowarski, A., Spaulding, J. S., and Migeon, C. J.**, Effect of various preparations of human growth hormone on aldosterone secretion rate of hypopituitary dwarfs, *Am. J. Med.*, 38, 517, 1965.
188. **Westphal, U.**, Steroid-protein interactions. XII. Concentrations and binding affinities of cortico steroid-binding globulins in sera of man, monkey, rat, rabbit, and guinea pig, *Arch. Biochem. Biophys.*, 118, 556, 1967.
189. **Westphal, U.**, Binding of corticosteroids by plasma proteins, in *Handbook of Physiology, Section 7*, Vol. 6, Greep, R. O., Astwood, E. B., Blachko, H., Sayers, G., Smith, A. D., and Geiger, S. R., Eds., American Physiological Society, Washington, D.C., 1975, 117.
190. **Gala, R. R. and Westphal, U.**, Corticosteroid-binding globulin in the rat: studies on the sex difference, *Endocrinology*, 77, 841, 1965.

191. **Cake, M. H. and Litwack, G.,** The glucocorticoid receptor, in *Biochemical Actions of Hormones,* Vol. 3, Litwick, G., Ed., Academic Press, New York, 1975, 317.
192. **Henkin, R. I.,** The role of adrenal corticosteroids in sensory processes, in *Handbook of Physiology,* Section 7, Vol. 6, Greep, R. O., Astwood, E. B., Blachko, H., Sayers, G., Smith, A. D., Geiger, S. R., Eds., American Physiology Society, Washington, D.C., 1975, 209.
193. **Spain, D. M.,** Corticosteroids, inflammation, and connective tissue, in *Handbook of Physiology, Section 7,* Vol. 6, Greep, R. O., Astwood, E. B., Blachko, H., Sayers, G., Smith, A. D., and Geiger, S. R., Eds., American Physiological Society, Washington, D.C., 1975, 263.
194. **Handler, J. S., Preston, A. S., and Orloff, J.,** The effect of aldosterone on glycolysis in the urinary bladder of the toad, *J. Biol. Chem.,* 244, 3194, 1969.
195. **Sharp, G. W. G. and Leaf, A.,** Mechanisms of action of aldosterone, *Physiol. Rev.,* 46, 593, 1966.
196. **Kirsten, E., Kirsten, R., Leaf, A., and Sharp, G. W.,** Increased activity of enzymes of the tricarboxylic acid cycle in response to aldosterone in the toad bladder, *Arch. Geo. Physiol.,* 300, 213, 1968.
197. **Wilks, S.,** On disease of the suprarenal capsules: or morbus Addisonii, *Guy's Hosp. Rep.,* 8, 1, 1862.

ADRENAL MEDULLA

George M. Brenner

ANATOMY

The adrenal gland consists of a yellow outer cortex and an inner pearly gray medulla. The medulla constitutes 10% of the gland and is found mainly in the gland's head and body.[1] The demarcation between the cortex and medulla is generally distinct, although islands of cortical cells are occasionally encountered within the medulla.

The component cells of the adrenal medulla are called pheochromocytes (dark-colored cells) or chromaffin cells because they are intensely stained by chrome salts. These cells are derived embryonically from immigrant neuroectodermal cells and are members of the "amine precursor uptake and decarboxylation (APUD) cells" series.[2] According to the APUD concept, these cells arise from a neuroectodermal cell coming from the neural crest and they have the ability to store various amines and produce low molecular weight peptides. Pheochromocytes are ovoid or polygonal cells with vesicular nuclei containing one or more prominent nucleoli.[3] The cytoplasm is basophilic and finely granular. The chromaffin granules are stained golden yellow to brown when the tissue is fixed in chrome salts.

The vascular supply to the adrenal medulla arises from three sources. The main medullary supply is derived from the *arteriae comitantes* which accompany the central vein. In addition, some of the small arteries which arise from the subcapsular arterial plexus pass through the cortex to supply the medulla. A third source consists of effluent blood from the cortex which passes into medullary sinusoids. All medullary blood is eventually collected into the large central vein.

The pheochromocytes are innervated by preganglionic fibers of the sympathetic nervous system. Each sympathetic fiber innervates a group of medullary cells forming a functional unit. Since epinephrine and norepinephrine are stored in different medullary cells, these functional units may provide the basis for different secretory responses to various stimuli.[3]

The primary secretory products of the adrenal medulla are the catecholamines, which are stored in the chromaffin granules. Norepinephrine is the principal hormone in the human medulla during the first year of life. The epinephrine content begins to increase at approximately age 2 years and eventually becomes the dominant hormone, with norepinephrine comprising only 14% of the total catecholamine content.[3]

BIOSYNTHESIS OF CATECHOLAMINES

The pathway for the biosynthesis of catecholamines in the adrenal medulla is shown in Figure 1. The amino acid tyrosine is converted to dihydroxyphenylalanine (DOPA) by a specific cytoplasmic enzyme, tyrosine hydroxylase. Tetrahydropteridine is a cofactor for this enzyme. DOPA is then decarboxylated to form dopamine by a relatively nonspecific cytoplasmic enzyme, L-aromatic amino acid decarboxylase. This enzyme requires pyridoxal phosphate as a cofactor. Dopamine enters the catecholamine storage granule where it is converted to norepinephrine by another relatively nonspecific enzyme, dopamine beta-hydroxylase (DBH). DBH is a copper-containing enzyme requiring ascorbate as a cofactor.

The pathway for conversion of tyrosine to norepinephrine is identical in sympathetic nerves and the adrenal medulla. In the adrenal medulla most of the norepinephrine leaves the granules and is converted to epinephrine by another nonspecific cytoplasmic

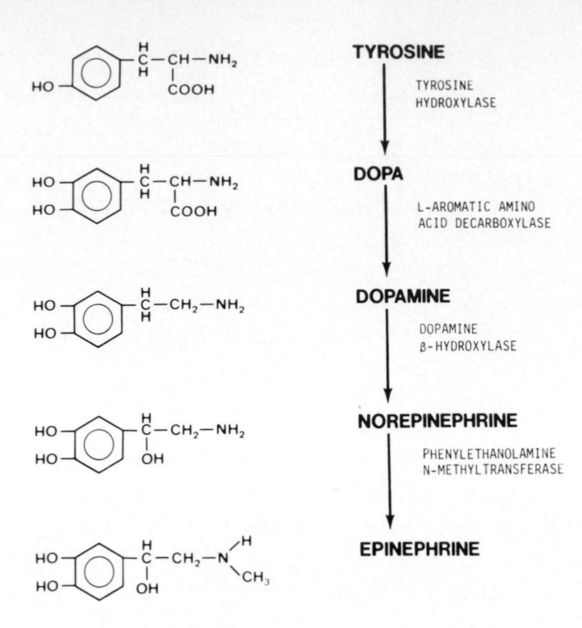

FIGURE 1. The pathway for the biosynthesis of catecholamines.

enzyme, phenylethanolamine N-methyl transferase (PNMT). The methyl group is donated by S-adenosylmethionine which serves as a cofactor in this reaction. PNMT is found in significant quantities only in the adrenal medulla.

The sequence of reactions in the biosynthesis of epinephrine was first proposed by Blaschko.[4] Udenfriend et al.[5] later demonstrated the production of ^{14}C-epinephrine from ^{14}C-tyrosine. The rate-limiting step in this pathway is the conversion of tyrosine to DOPA by tyrosine hydroxylase.[6] Norepinephrine and dopamine inhibit this step and may thereby act to control their own synthesis. PNMT is also inhibited by physiologic concentrations of epinephrine and norepinephrine. The activity of PNMT is dependent on the presence of glucocorticoids which are transported to the adrenal medulla by the portal circulation from the adrenal cortex. Glucocorticoids probably induce the synthesis of PNMT.

Hypophysectomy produces a profound fall in PNMT activity and the epinephrine content of the adrenal medulla.[7] This effect is reversed by glucocorticoid or corticotropin (ACTH) injections. Hypophysectomy also decreases the activity of tyrosine hydroxylase and DBH in the adrenal medulla.[8] Both effects are reversed by ACTH but not by glucocorticoids.

In addition to the regulation of epinephrine biosynthesis by feedback inhibition, ACTH and glucocorticoids, the stimulation of adrenal catecholamine release increases the rate of its own synthesis in the gland. This is probably due to an increased formation of tyrosine hydroxylase, the rate-limiting enzyme in the biosynthesis of epinephrine.[9]

STORAGE AND RELEASE OF ADRENAL CATECHOLAMINES

Adrenal Medullary Granules

Lever[10] first described the electron-dense membrane-bound vesicles which store catecholamines within the adrenal medullary cells. These chromaffin granules were found to contain 6.7% wet wt of catecholamine as well as ATP, protein, calcium, lipid, and mucopolysaccharide.[11] The proteins contained in the granules include a soluble protein fraction which is released upon hypotonic lysis and accounts for about 75% of granule protein. This fraction contains 20 to 50% DBH, depending on the species, as well as other proteins known as chromogranins.

The chromaffin granule catecholamines and ATP occur in a 4:1 *M* ratio which suggests that they form some type of storage complex. Berneis et al.[12,13] using a catecholamine to ATP ration of 3.5:1, found that catecholamine/ATP aggregates could form in concentrated aqueous solutions in vitro. The addition of calcium chloride could produce a separate liquid phase containing 60% wet wt catecholamine and ATP. This phase was most stable at low temperatures. However, such aggregates would not be sufficiently stable at body temperature to account for catecholamine storage in the chromaffin granule. This suggests that other factors such as the granule proteins are involved in catecholamine storage in vivo.

Several populations of chromaffin granules are found in the adrenal medulla. Epinephrine and norepinephrine are stored in different populations of granules within separate cells.[14] There are also subpopulations of granules containing different amounts of DBH and different proportions of ATP in the adenine nucleotide pool.

Uptake of Catecholamines

Isolated chromaffin granules gradually lose their catecholamine content because of the passive permeability of the chromaffin granule membrane to catecholamines. The addition of ATP and magnesium chloride substantially reduces the loss of catecholamines from the granules, and there is now strong evidence that this effect is due to a specific catecholamine uptake mechanism.[15,16] When ATP and magnesium are present, chromaffin granules accumulate catecholamines against a concentration gradient. In addition to the energy requirement, this uptake mechanism is temperature dependent, stereoselective, and saturable and shows substrate competition among catecholamines. As would be expected, dopamine is taken up by this mechanism into the chromaffin granule where it is converted to norepinephrine by DBH. Reserpine inhibits the uptake of catecholamines by the chromaffin granules and prevents the conversion of dopamine to norepinephrine. Continued exposure to reserpine leads to a depletion of adrenal catecholamines. Isolated chromaffin granule membranes can concentrate catecholamines, indicating that the specific energy-dependent uptake process is located in the granule membrane.

Release of Catecholamines

Stimulation of the isolated perfused adrenal gland causes the release of catecholamines, ATP, DBH, and chromogranins into the perfusate. The catecholamines and ATP are released in the same ratio as they occur in isolated chromaffin granules,[17] while DBH and the chromogranins are released in the same relative amounts as are found in the water-soluble fraction of the granule. Enzymes located in the cell cytoplasm or mitochondria are not released by stimulation of the isolated adrenal gland.[18,19] Viveros et al.[20,21] found that the loss of water-soluble DBH from adrenal glands is proportional to the loss of catecholamines, but this relationship is not found for the membrane-bound DBH. They also found that the ratio of total DBH to catecholamine is the same in chromaffin granules isolated from unstimulated glands and in glands partially depleted of catecholamines by insulin administration. This suggests that the granule contents are released in a quantum fashion.

The contents of the chromaffin granules are released by a process known as exocytosis,[22] in which the chromaffin granule membrane fuses with the plasma membrane and the catecholamines are emptied into the extracellular fluid.[14,23] Indirect evidence suggests that calcium may mediate the fusion of the chromaffin granule and plasma membranes. Stimulation of chromaffin cells with carbamylcholine and other secretogogues produces a calcium-dependent increase in the number of invaginations of the chromaffin cell membranes.[24] Calcium binding proteins have been isolated from the adrenal medulla, but their role in catecholamine secretion remains uncertain.

A calcium-binding phosphoprotein has been isolated from the adrenal medulla and later found to increase adenylate cyclase activity in the brain. However, the role of cyclic AMP in catecholamine secretion remains equivocal.[25,26] Kuo and Coffe[27] isolated a calcium-binding troponin-C-like protein from bovine adrenal medulla. This protein may participate in a contractile system involving actin- and myosin-like proteins that transport chromaffin granules to the cell membrane.[28,29] Microtubules may also play a role in catecholamine secretion from the adrenal medulla since drugs inhibiting or promoting microtubule formation also inhibit or increase acetylcholine-induced secretion of catecholamines. Calcium, however, inhibits microtubule formation in the adrenal gland, and the exact role of microtubules in catecholamine secretion remains uncertain.

CONTROL OF MEDULLARY SECRETION

In 1911, Canon and De La Paz[30] showed that adrenal gland secretion can be elicited by emotional excitement, and they defined the role of the adrenal gland in the "fight or flight" reaction. The hypothalamus is a major site of the central nervous system control of adrenal medullary secretion. Stimulation of different areas in the median and anterior hypothalamus produces adrenal gland secretions having different ratios of epinephrine to norepinephrine.[31] The two types of adrenal medullary cells previously described appear to be innervated by different populations of nerves having distinct hypothalamic representations. Adrenal medullary secretion is also affected by a cortical control system, and stimulation of specific cortical areas serves to either increase or decrease medullary secretions. Most of these corticofugal pathways pass through the hypothalamus, but several fibers do not and may influence adrenal secretion by other pathways, yet to be defined.

The secretion of catecholamines from the adrenal medulla can be elicited directly by stimulation of the splanchnic nerves. Acetylcholine is released from the preganglionic sympathetic nerve endings and depolarizes the adrenal medullary cells leading to catecholamine secretion. The acetylcholine-induced depolarization is accompanied by sodium and calcium flux into the medullary cells.[32] The sodium flux is primarily responsible for the depolarization whereas the secretion of catecholamines is directly proportional to the external concentration of calcium.

Calcium is a secretagogue and produces maximal catecholamine secretion when introduced following a period of perfusion of the gland with a calcium-free medium. Calcium ionophores which mediate the transmembrane flux of calcium can increase catecholamine release from adrenal glands and chromaffin cells, whereas secretion is prevented by the calcium uptake inhibitor, verapamil.[33,34]

In addition to emotional excitement, other stimuli which increase adrenal medullary catecholamine secretion include hypoglycemia, hypoxia and hypercapnia. The effect of hypoglycemia can be prevented by denervating the adrenal medulla. Crone[35] demonstrated that the increased medullary secretion induced by hypoglycemia is initiated in an area of the brainstem caudal to the hypothalamus. Himsworth[36] found that application of the local anesthetic lidocaine to the hypothalamus can prevent the catecholamine-releasing effect of hypoglycemia.

Hypoxia induces adrenal medullary secretion in proportion to the fall in P_{O_2}. In the fetal calf, this effect is not prevented by denervation of the adrenal medulla. With fetal development, the direct effect of hypoxia is replaced by a splanchnic nerve-mediated effect which becomes fully developed two to three weeks postpartum.[37] Exposure of individuals to high altitudes has been found to double plasma catecholamine levels, an effect which is not seen in people born and raised above an altitude of 3200 m.[38]

Hypercapnia and acidosis increase adrenal catecholamine secretion by a mechanism that is independent of the P_{O_2}. The effect of hypercapnia is mediated primarily by the direct effect of acidosis on the adrenal glands and is not prevented by denervation.[39] In dogs, the catecholamine secretion is doubled if the pH of the medium perfusion an adrenal gland is reduced to 6.95 to 7.16.[40]

Many other stimuli, including several hormones, autocoids, and drugs increase adrenal medullary secretion of catecholamines. These include glucagon, nicotine, histamine, angiotensin, and others.[41]

CLEARANCE AND METABOLISM OF CIRCULATING CATECHOLAMINES

Metabolic Clearance

Catecholamines released from the adrenal medulla are rapidly removed from the circulation, and they appear to accelerate their own metabolic clearance.[42] Using graded infusions of epinephrine and norepinephrine, it is possible to calculate their metabolic clearance rates at various steady state concentrations.[43,44] The average plasma clearance rate of epinephrine is 52 ± 4 mℓ/kg/min at steady-state plasma epinephrine concentrations of 24 to 74 pg/mℓ (values in the normal basal range). The mean clearance rate is 70% higher (89 ± 6 mℓ/kg/min) at steady-state epinephrine concentrations of 90 to 1020 pg/mℓ.

Norepinephrine clearance also increases as the steady state plasma concentration is increased.

Catecholamines are cleared from the extracellular fluid by two tissue uptake mechanisms. Uptake 1 is an active, high affinity and low-capacity system located in the sympathetic nerves. It is sodium-dependent, saturable and it has a higher affinity for norepinephrine than epinephrine.[45,46] In contrast, uptake 2 is an extraneuronal system found in cardiac and smooth muscle and in the liver. Uptake 2 is a low affinity, high-capacity system with a higher affinity for epinephrine than norepinephrine.[47] Isoproterenol, a synthetic β-adrenergic agonist, can serve as a substrate for uptake 2 but not for uptake 1. Uptake 2 is able to control the access of catecholamines to catabolic enzymes in the tissues.[48] Whitby et al.[49] found that intravenous ^{3}H-epinephrine and norepinephrine are rapidly removed from the circulation and that a large proportion remains unmetabolized, presumably owing to uptake and storage in sympathetic nerves.

Evidence indicates that catecholamines are cleared through mechanisms modulated by β-adrenergic receptors.[50] β-Adrenergic blockade with propranolol reduces the clearance rate of epinephrine by more than 75% whereas α-adrenergic blockade with phentolamine has no effect on epinephrine clearance. β-Adrenergic antagonists inhibit uptake 2,[51] which decreases enzymatic degradation of catecholamines. There is also evidence for β-adrenergic receptor regulation of membrane bound catechol-o-methyltransferase[52] which may be the rate-limiting step in uptake 2.

Metabolic Pathways

Catecholamines are metabolized by two principal enzymes, monoamine oxidase (MAO),[53] and catechol-O-methyltransferase (COMT)[54] (Figure 2). COMT is found in nearly all tissues and is primarily responsible for metabolizing circulating catecholamines. Methylation of epinephrine and norepinephrine produces metanephrine and normetanephrine, respectively. Conjugation with sulfate is another route of catecholamine metabolism. MAO is associated with the mitochondria of sympathetic and central nervous system neurons and adrenal chromaffin cells. In these tissues MAO serves to deaminate cytoplasmic catecholamines. In the liver, the combined effects of MAO

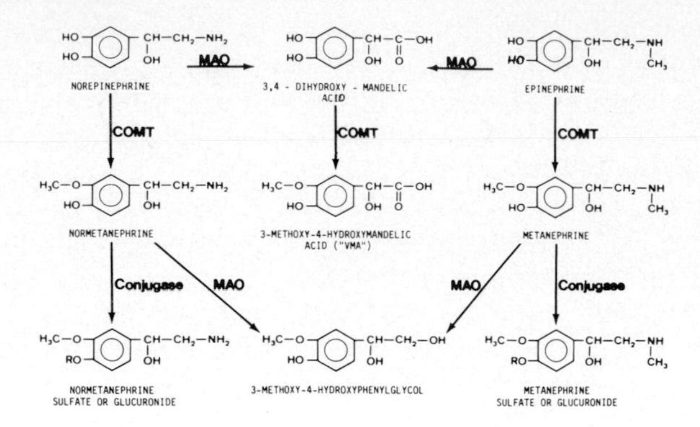

FIGURE 2. Pathways of catecholamine metabolism.

and COMT convert the catecholamines into several end products. These include 3′ methoxy-4′-hydroxy mandelic acid, also known as vanillyl mandelic acid (VMA), which is a major excretory product of catecholamine metabolism.

Considerable species differences have been detected in the metabolism of peripheral catecholamines.[55] In the rabbit and guinea pig, plasma catecholamines are inactivated mainly by MAO deamination. In dog and man, O-methylation and O-sulphation are the preferential pathways for metabolism and excretion.[56] In human plasma, 90% or more of the catecholamines exist as O-methylated or O-sulfurated derivatives.

Measurement of Catecholamines and Their Metabolites

The measurement of catecholamines and their metabolites in plasma and urine provides a useful biochemical index of the level of sympathoadrenal activity. Urine and tissue catecholamines can be quantitated by spectrofluorometry, but these methods are not sufficiently sensitive to measure the much lower levels found in plasma. The recent development of radioenzymatic methods for quantitating catecholamines facilitates the analysis of these compounds and their metabolites in plasma with remarkable sensitivity and specificity.[57,58,59] These methods are based on the use of a partially purified COMT which catalyzes the transfer of a tritium-labeled methyl group from S-adenosyl methionine to the catecholamines, forming the radioactive O-methylated derivatives. The methylated derivatives are extracted into an organic solvent, separated by thin-layer chromatography, and finally eluted, oxidized, and measured by liquid scintillation counting. The technique has a detection limit of 1 pg/mℓ epinephrine and norepinephrine and 5 pg/mℓ dopamine. Modifications of the method permit the measurement of free and conjugated catecholamines including DOPA, dopamine, and epinephrine as well as their methoxylated and deaminated metabolites.[56]

The radioenzymatic methods have permitted the analysis of plasma levels of epinephrine and norepinephrine in humans in various physiologic and pathophysiologic states.[42] Resting levels of free epinephrine are in the range of about 20 to 80 pg/mℓ, and moderate exercise produces levels of about 100 to 140 pg/mℓ. Heavy exercise produces epinephrine levels greater than 400 pg/mℓ. Resting norepinephrine levels are approximately 200 to 250 pg/mℓ and moderate and heavy exercise produces levels of 1000 to 1600 pg/mℓ and 2000 pg/mℓ, respectively.

PHYSIOLOGIC EFFECTS OF EPINEPHRINE

Receptors for Catecholamines

The first indication of the endocrine role of the adrenal medulla was the demonstration that electrical stimulation of the splanchnic nerves decreased the amplitude of intestinal contraction and increased blood pressure.[60] These effects were attributed to inhibitory and excitatory effects of epinephrine. Ahlquist[61] postulated the existence of two types of adrenergic-receptors, α and β, to explain the different potencies of catecholamines in eliciting excitatory and inhibitory effects in various tissues. He observed that α-receptors were much more sensitive to epinephrine and norepinephrine than to isoproterenol whereas β-receptors were more sensitive to isoproterenol than to epinephrine and norepinephrine.

In general, α-receptors mediate effects which are excitatory or motor such as vasoconstriction whereas the effects mediated by β-receptors are predominantly inhibitory such as relaxation of the uterine and bronchial musculature. The notable exception is the β-receptor-mediated excitatory effects of catecholamines on the heart.

β-receptors are subdivided into two classes, β_1- and β_2-receptors, based on distinctions in the order of potency of catecholamines.[62] At β_1-receptors, located in the heart, isoproterenol is more potent than epinephrine which is equipotent with norepinephrine. At β_2-receptors, isoproterenol is equal to or more potent than epinephrine which is much more potent than norepinephrine.[63]

Adrenergic-receptor concentration in tissues is regulated by catecholamines. A sustained decrease in catecholamine levels increases the number of adrenergic-receptors in target cells and increases their responsiveness to catecholamines. A sustained increase in catecholamine levels produces the opposite effects.[64] Tohmek and Cryer[65] found that the intravenous infusion of isoproterenol produces a biphasic change in receptor number and tissue responsiveness to catecholamines. During the first 30 min of isoproterenol infusion, the number of receptors on mononuclear cells increases by nearly twofold, whereas continued infusion produces a 50% decrease after 4 hr. Other studies indicate that the early increase in β-receptor number is associated with an increased phospholipid methylation and membrane fluidity.[66,67]

Metabolic Effects

Epinephrine affects the metabolism of carbohydrates, lipids, and proteins through both direct and indirect effects.[42] Epinephrine produces hyperglycemia by elevating glucose delivery from the liver and by decreasing glucose clearance from the circulation.[68] These effects contribute to the prevention of hypoglycemia during physiologic fluctuations in plasma glucose. With continuous intravenous infusion of epinephrine, glucose delivery returns to the baseline after 60 to 90 min, but the reduced clearance persists. The reduced glucose clearance is apparently responsible for the prolonged hyperglycemia induced by epinephrine.

The direct effects of glucose on glucose delivery and clearance are mediated by β-receptors.[69] Epinephrine also indirectly reduces glucose clearance by inhibiting the secretion of insulin, an effect which is mediated by α-adrenergic-receptors.[70]

The epinephrine-induced increase in glucose output from the liver is due to increased glycogenolysis and increased gluconeogenesis.[71] Epinephrine increases glycogenolysis by activation, via cyclic adenosine monophosphate (cyclic AMP), of hepatic glycogen phosphorylase.[72] This enzyme converts glycogen to glucose-1-phosphate which is the rate-limiting step in the output of glucose from the liver. In addition, cyclic AMP results in an inactivation of glycogen synthetase, the enzyme which catalyzes the transfer of glycosyl units to glycogen.

The stimulation of cyclic AMP production by epinephrine is mediated by adrenergic β-receptors in man.[73] Activation of β-receptors increases the activity of adenylate cyclase which catalyzes the formation of cyclic AMP from adenosine triphosphate (ATP). Epinephrine also activates muscle phosphorylase.[74] Since muscle lacks the enzyme, glucose-6-phosphatase, which is required to deliver glucose into the circulation, the end product of glycogenolysis in muscle is lactate, which arises from the anaerobic metabolism of glucose. The increased blood lactate produced by this process may serve as an energy substrate in other tissues.

Epinephrine is a potent lipolytic agent and it raises the concentration of free fatty acids in blood by activation of triglyceride lipase.[75] This enzyme accelerates the breakdown of triglycerides to form free fatty acids and glycerol. The activation of triglyceride lipase is mediated by cyclic AMP via activation of adrenergic β_1-receptors. As a consequence of increased lipolysis and free fatty acid delivery to the circulation, epinephrine stimulates ketoacid formation. Epinephrine infusions also increase plasma cholesterol and low density lipoproteins. It has been suggested that the increased incidence of atheroslcerosis and coronary artery disease associated with chronic stress may be partly due to the metabolic effects of elevated sympathoadrenal activity.[75]

Other metabolic effects of epinephrine include a calorigenic action which may elevate oxygen consumption by 20 to 30% in man. Epinephrine decreases the plasma levels of certain amino acids after prolonged infusion, an effect mediated by adrenergic β-receptors.[76]

Cardiovascular Effects

Epinephrine is a powerful cardiac stimulant and vasopressor substance.[63,77] It increases heart rate by accelerating the diastolic depolarization of pacemaker cells located in the sinoatrial node. Epinephrine also increases the strength of ventricular contraction and shortens cardiac systole. Cardiac work and oxygen consumption are both increased by epinephrine, but the amount of work performed relative to oxygen consumption (cardiac efficiency) is decreased.

All of the direct cardiac effects of epinephrine are mediated primarily by adrenergic β_1-receptors in the pacemaker cells and myocardium.[78] The increased contractile force induced by epinephrine is probably mediated by cyclic AMP which may increase the Ca^{++} permeability of the plasma membrane. β-Adrenergic stimulation also causes the phosphorylation of a subunit of the contractile protein, troponin. This effect may augment cardiac contraction.[79]

Epinephrine exerts several effects on the cardiac conduction system, some of which are secondary to the increased heart rate.[80] In the Purkinje fibers, epinephrine accelerates diastolic depolarization and facilitates the activation of latent pacemaker cells. Conduction velocity is increased in the bundle of His, Purkinje fibers, and ventricle. Epinephrine speeds atrioventricular (AV) conduction and decreases the degree of AV block occurring as a result of vagal stimulation or disease.

Epinephrine produces vasoconstriction and decreases blood flow in many vascular beds, due to stimulation of adrenergic α-receptors.[81] This effect is exerted primarily on the smaller arterioles and precapillary sphincters, although larger veins and arteries are also affected. The skin, mucosa, and kidney are major sites of vasoconstrictive effect of epinephrine. In other vascular beds, particularly in skeletal muscle, epinephrine produces vasodilatation and increased blood flow due to an action on adrenergic β_2-receptors.[82] These receptors are quite sensitive to epinephrine. Low doses of epinephrine decrease peripheral vascular resistance and blood pressure whereas high doses produce marked vasoconstriction which contributes to the vasopressor effect.

Studies on the effects of graded infusions of epinephrine in human subjects indicate that the threshold plasma level for increasing the heart rate is 50 to 100 pg/mℓ, while the threshold plasma level for a systolic pressor effect is 75 to 125 pg/mℓ.[42]

These levels are achieved during moderate exercise as well as in certain pathophysiologic states.

Other Effects

Epinephrine has effects on smooth muscles which depend on the type of adrenergic receptor present in the given muscle. Epinephrine relaxes gastrointestinal muscle except for the pyloric and ileocecal sphincters. These are relaxed by epinephrine if their tone is already high and contracted if their tone is low.[83] The effect of epinephrine or uterine muscle depends on the phase of the sexual cycle, gestational age, and the dose. During the last month of pregnancy and at parturition, epinephrine causes relaxation of uterine muscle. Epinephrine relaxes the detrusor muscle of the bladder due to activation of β-receptors while contracting the trigone and sphincter muscles through α-receptor stimulation. Epinephrine relaxes bronchial smooth muscle, an effect mediated by β_2-receptors. Because of this effect, epinephrine is employed in the treatment of bronchial asthma.

REFERENCES

1. **Dobie, J. W., Mackay, A. M., and Symington, T.,** The human adrenal gland with special reference to the vasculature, *J. Endocrinol.*, 34, 479, 1966.
2. **Pearse, A. G. E. and Takor, T. T.,** Neuroendocrine embryology and the APUD concept, *Clin. Endocrinol.*, 5, (Suppl.), 229s, 1976.
3. **Neville, A. M.,** The adrenal medulla, in *Functional Pathology of the Human Adrenal Gland,* Symington, T., Ed., Livingstone, Edinburgh, 1969, 219.
4. **Blaschko, H.,** The specific action of L-DOPA decarboxylase, *J. Physiol. (London),* 96, 50, 1939.
5. **Udenfriend, S., Cooper, S. J. R., Clark, C. T., and Baer, J. E.,** The rate of turnover of epinephrine in the adrenal medulla, *Science,* 117, 663, 1953.
6. **Levitt, M., Spector, S., Sjoerdsma, A., and Udenfriend, S.,** Elucidation of the rate-limiting step in norepinephrine biosynthesis in the perfused guinea-pig heart, *J. Pharmacol. Exp. Ther.*, 148, 1, 1965.
7. **Wurtman, R. J. and Axelrod, J.,** Control of enzymatic synthesis of adrenaline in the adrenal medulla by adrenal cortical slices, *J. Biol. Chem.*, 241, 2301, 1966.
8. **Weinshilboum, R. and Axelrod, J.,** Dopamine-β-hydroxylase activity in the rat after hypophysectomy, *Endocrinology,* 87, 894, 1970.
9. **Sedvall, G. C. and Kopin, I. J.,** Acceleration of norepinephrine synthesis in the rat submaxillary gland in vivo during sympathetic nerve stimulation, *Life Sci.*, 6, 45, 1976.
10. **Lever, J. D.,** Electron microscopic observations on the normal and denervated adrenal medulla of the rat, *Endocrinology,* 57, 621, 1955.
11. **Winkler, H.,** The composition of adrenal chromaffin granules: an assessment of controversial results, *Neuroscience,* 1, 65, 1976.
12. **Berneis, K. H., Pletscher, A., and Da Prada, M.,** Metal-dependent aggregation of biogenic amines: a hypothesis for their storage and release, *Nature,* 224, 281, 1969.
13. **Berneis, K. H., Pletscher, A., and Da Prada, M.,** Phase separation in solutions of noradrenaline and adenosine tri-phosphate: influence of bivalent cations and drugs, *Br. J. Pharmacol.*, 39, 382, 1970.
14. **Grynszpan-Winograd, O.,** Ultrastructure of the chromaffin cell, in *Handbook of Physiology, Section 7,* Vol. 6, Blaschko, H., Sayers, G., and Smith, A. D., Eds., American Physiological Society, Washington, D.C., 1975, 295.
15. **Kirshner, N.,** Uptake of catecholamines by a particular fraction of the adrenal medulla, *J. Biol. Chem.*, 237, 2311, 1962.
16. **Taugner, G. and Hasselback, W.,** Über den Mechanismus der Catecholamin-speicherung in den "Chromaffinen Granula" des Nebennierenmarks, *Arch. Pharmakol. Exp. Pathol.*, 255, 266, 1966.
17. **Douglas, W. W. and Poisner, A. M.,** On the relation between ATP splitting and secretion in the adrenal chromaffin cell: extrusion of ATP (unhydrolysed) during release of catecholamines, *J. Physiol. (London),* 183, 249, 1966.
18. **Kirshner, N., Holloway, C., and Kamin, D. L.,** Permeability of catecholamine granules, *Biochim. Biophys. Acta,* 112, 532, 1966.
19. **Kirshner, N., Sage, J. J., and Smith, W. J.,** Mechanism of secretion from the adrenal medulla. II. Release of catecholamines and storage vesicle protein in response to chemical stimulation, *Mol. Pharmacol.*, 3, 251, 1967.
20. **Viveros, O. H., Arqueros, L., and Kirshner, N.,** Mechanism of secretion from the adrenal medulla. V. Retention of storage vesicle membranes following release of adrenaline, *Mol. Pharmacol.*, 5, 342, 1969.

21. **Viveros, O. H., Arqueros, L., and Kirshner, N.,** Mechanism of secretion from the adrenal medulla. VII. Effect of insulin administration on the buoyant density, dopamine-β-hydroxylase and catecholamine content of adrenal storage vesicles, *Mol. Pharmacol.,* 7, 441, 1971.
22. **De Duve, C.,** Footnote, in *Lysosomes,* de Reuck, A. V. S. and Cameron, M. P., Eds., Little, Brown, Boston, 1963, 126.
23. **De Robertis, E. D. P. and Sabatini, D. D.,** Submicroscopic analysis of the secretory process in the adrenal medulla, *Fed. Proc.,* 19, (Suppl.), 70, 1960.
24. **Smith, U., Smith, D. S., Winkler, H., and Ryan, J. W.,** Exocytosis in the adrenal medulla demonstrated by freeze-etching, *Science,* 179, 79, 1973.
25. **Hockman, J. and Perlman, R. L.,** Catecholamine secretion by isolated adrenal cells, *Biochim. Biophys. Acta,* 421, 168, 1976.
26. **Peach, M. J.,** Stimulation of release of adrenal catecholamine by adenosine 3′:5′-cyclic monophosphate and theophylline in the absence of extracellular calcium, *Proc. Natl. Acad. Sci. U.S.A.,* 68, 834, 1972.
27. **Kuo, I. C. Y. and Coffe, C. R.,** Purification and characterization of a troponin-C-like protein from bovine adrenal medulla, *J. Biol. Chem.,* 251, 1603, 1976.
28. **Burridge, K. and Philips, J. H.,** Association of actin and myosin with secretory membranes, *Nature,* 254, 526, 1975.
29. **Frifaró, J. M. and Ulpian, C.,** Actomyosin-like protein isolated from the adrenal medulla, *FEBS Lett.,* 5, 198, 1975.
30. **Cannon, W. B. and De La Paz, D.,** Emotional stimulation of adrenal secretion, *Am. J. Physiol.,* 28, 64, 1911.
31. **Folkow, B. and Von Euler, U. S.,** Selective activation of noradrenaline and adrenaline producing cells in the cat's adrenal gland by hypothalamus stimulation, *Circ. Res.,* 2, 191, 1954.
32. **Douglas, W. W., Kanno, T., and Sampson, S. R.,** Influence of the ionic environment of the membrane potential of adrenal chromaffin cells and in the depolarizing effect of acetylcholine, *J. Physiol. (London),* 191, 107, 1967.
33. **Garcia, A. G., Kirpekar, S. M., and Prat, J. D.,** A calcium ionophore stimulating the secretion of catecholamines from the cat adrenal, *J. Physiol. (London),* 244, 253, 1975.
34. **Chalfie, M., Hoadley, D., Pastan, S., and Perlman, R. L.,** Calcium uptake into rat pheochromocytoma cells, *J. Neurochem.,* 26, 1405, 1976.
35. **Crone, C.,** The secretion of adrenal medullary hormones during hypoglycaemia in intact, decerebrate and spinal sheep, *Acta Physiol. Scand.,* 63, 213, 1965.
36. **Himsworth, R. L.,** Hypothalamic control of adrenaline secretion in response to insufficient glucose, *J. Physiol. (London),* 206, 411, 1970.
37. **Comline, R. S. and Silver, M.,** The development of the adrenal medulla of the foetal and new born calf, *J. Physiol. (London),* 183, 305, 1966.
38. **Moncloa, F., Gómez, M., and Hurtado, A.,** Plasma catecholamines at high altitudes, *J. Appl. Physiol.,* 20, 1329, 1965.
39. **Morris, M. E. and Millar, R. A.,** Blood pH/plasma catecholamine relationships: respiratory acidosis, *Br. J. Anaesth.,* 34, 672, 1962.
40. **Nakas, G. G., Zagury, D., Milhaud, A., Manger, W. M., and Pappas, G. D.,** Acidemia and catecholamine output of the isolated canine adrenal gland, *Am. J. Physiol.,* 213, 1186, 1967.
41. **Lightman, S.,** Adrenal medulla, in *The Adrenal Gland,* James, V. H. T., Ed., Raven Press, New York, 1979, 283.
42. **Cryer, P. E.,** Physiology and pathophysiology of the human sympathoadrenal neuroendocrine system, *N. Engl. J. Med.,* 303, 436, 1980.
43. **Silverberg, A. B., Shah, S. D., Haymond, M. W., and Cryer, P. E.,** Norepinephrine: hormone and neurotransmitter in man, *Am. J. Physiol.,* 234, E252, 1978.
44. **Clutter, W., Bier, D., Shah, S., and Cryer, P.,** Epinephrine plasma metabolic clearance rates and physiologic thresholds for metabolic and hemodynamic actions in man, *J. Clin. Invest.,* 66, 94, 1980.
45. **Iversen, L. L.,** Uptake of noradrenaline in the isolated perfused rat heart, *Br. J. Pharmacol.,* 25, 18, 1963.
46. **Iversen, L. L.,** Uptake processes for biogenic amines, in *Handbook of Psychopharmacology, Section 1,* Vol. 3, Iversen, L. L., Iversen, S. D., and Snyder, S. H., Eds., Plenum Press, New York, 1975, 381.
47. **Lightman, S. L. and Iversen, L. L.,** The role of uptake 2 in the extraneuronal metabolism of catecholamines in the isolated rat heart, *Br. J. Pharmacol.,* 37, 638, 1969.
48. **Lightman, S. L. and Hims, D. A.,** Metabolism of adrenaline in the isolated perfused liver of the rat, *Biochem. Pharmacol.,* 22, 2419, 1973.
49. **Whitby, L. G., Axelrod, J., and Wiel-Malherbe, H.,** The fate of H^3 norepinephrine in animals, *J. Pharmacol. Exp. Ther.,* 132, 195, 1976.

50. **Cryer, P. E., Rizza, R. A., Haymond, M. W., and Gerich, J. E.,** Epinephrine and norepinephrine are cleared through β-adrenergic, but not α-adrenergic, mechanisms in man, *Metabolism,* 29, (11 Suppl. 1), 1114, 1980.
51. **Eisenfeld, A. J., Axelrod, J., and Krakoff, L.,** Inhibition of the extraneuronal accumulation and metabolism of norepinephrine by adrenergic blocking agents, *J. Pharmacol. Exp. Ther.,* 156, 107, 1967.
52. **Wrenn, S., Homcy, C., and Haber, E.,** Evidence for the β-adrenergic receptor regulation of membrane-bound catechol-O-methyltransferase activity in myocardium, *J. Biol. Chem.,* 254, 5708, 1979.
53. **Axelrod, J.,** Methylation reactions in the formation and metabolism of catecholamines and other biogenic amines, *Pharm. Rev.,* 18, 95, 1966.
54. **Gorkin, V. J.,** Monamine oxidases, *Pharm. Rev.,* 18, 115, 1966.
55. **Da Prada, M., Picotti, G. B., Carruba, M. O., and Haefly, W. E.,** in *Catecholamines: Basic and Clinical Frontiers,* Usdin, E., Kopin, I. J. and Barchas, J., Eds., Pergamon Press, New York, 1979, 915.
56. **Da Prada, M.,** Concentration dynamics, and functional meaning of catecholamines in plasma and urine, in *Trends in Pharmacological Sciences,* 1, 157, 1980.
57. **Engleman, K., Portnoy, B., and Lovenbug, W.,** A sensitive and specific double-isotope derivative method for the determination of catecholamines in biological specimens, *Am. J. Med. Sci.,* 255, 259, 1968.
58. **Da Prada, M. and Zurcher, G.,** Simultaneous radio-enzymatic determination of plasma and tissue adrenaline, noradrenaline and dopamine within the fentamole range, *Life Sci.,* 19, 1673, 1976.
59. **Cryer, P. E.,** Isotope-derivative measurements of plasma norepinephrine and epinephrine in man, *Diabetes,* 25, 1071, 1976.
60. **Dreyer, G. P.,** On secretory nerves to the suprarenal capsules, *Am. J. Physiol.,* 2, 203, 1898.
61. **Ahlquist, R. P.,** A study of adrenotropic receptors, *Am. J. Physiol.,* 153, 586, 1948.
62. **Lands, A. M., Arnold, A., McAuliff, J. P., Luduena, F. P., and Brown, T. G.,** Differentiation of receptor systems activated by sympathomimetic amines, *Nature,* 214, 597, 1967.
63. **Weiner, N.,** Norepinephrine, epinephrine and the sympathomimetic amines, in *The Pharmacological Basis of Therapeutics,* 6th ed., Gilman, A. G., Goodman, L. S., and Gilman, A., Eds., Macmillan, New York, 1980, 138.
64. **Lefkowitz, R. J.,** Direct binding studies of adrenergic receptors: biochemical, physiological and clinical implications, *Ann. Intern. Med.,* 91, 450, 1979.
65. **Tohmek, J. F. and Cryer, P. E.,** Biphasic adrenergic modulation of β-adrenergic receptors in man: agonist-induced early increment and late decrement in β-adrenergic receptor number, *J. Clin. Invest.,* 65, 836, 1980.
66. **Hirata, F., Strittmatter, W. J., and Axelrod, J.,** β-Adrenergic receptor agonists increase phospholipid methylation, membrane fluidity, and β-adrenergic receptor-adenylate cyclase coupling, *Proc. Natl. Acad. Sci. U.S.A.,* 76, 368, 1979.
67. **Strittmatter, W. J., Hirata, F., and Axelrod, J.,** Phospholipid methylation unmasks cryptic β-adrenergic receptors in rat reticulocytes, *Science,* 204, 1205, 1979.
68. **Rizza, R., Haymond, M., Cryer, P., and Gerich, J.,** Differential effects of epinephrine on glucose production and disposal in man, *Am. J. Physiol.,* 237, E356, 1979.
69. **Rizza, R. A., Cryer, P. E., Haymond, M. W., and Gerich, J. E.,** Adrenergic mechanisms for the effects of epinephrine on glucose production and clearance in man, *J. Clin. Invest.,* 65, 682, 1980.
70. **Clarke, W. L., Santiago, J. V., Thomas, L., Ben-Galim, E., Haymond, M. W., and Cryer, P. E.,** Adrenergic mechanisms in recovery from hypoglycemia in man: adrenergic blockade, *Am. J. Physiol.,* 236, E147, 1979.
71. **Exton, J. H. and Park, C. R.,** The stimulation of gluconeogenesis from lactate by epinephrine, glucagon, and cyclic 3′-5′-adenylate in the perfused rat liver, *Pharmacol. Rev.,* 18, 181, 1966.
72. **Sutherland, E. W. and Robison, G. A.,** The role of cyclic-3′-5′-AMP in responses to catecholamine and other hormones, *Pharmacol. Rev.,* 18, 145, 1966.
73. **Rall, T. W.,** Role of adenosine 3′-5′-monophosphate (cyclic AMP) in actions of catecholamines, *Pharmacol. Rev.,* 24, 399, 1972.
74. **Krebs, E. G., De Lange, R. J., Kemp, R. G., and Riley, W. D.,** Activation of skeletal muscle phosphorylase, *Pharmacol. Rev.,* 18, 163, 1966.
75. **Himms-Hagen, J.,** Effects of catecholamines on metabolism, in *Handbuch der Experimentellen Pharmakologie, Vol. 33, Catecholamines,* Blaschko, H. and Muscholl, E., Eds., Springer-Verlag, Berlin, 1972, 363.
76. **Shamoon, H., J. R. and Sherwin, R. S.,** Epinephrine-induced hypoaminoacidemia in man: a β-adrenergic effect, *Clin. Res.,* 27, 595A, 1979.
77. **Eckstein, J. W. and Abboud, F. M.,** Circulatory effects of sympathomimetic amines, *Am. Heart J.,* 63, 119, 1962.

78. **Minneman, K. P., Hegstrand, L. R. and Molinoff, P. B.,** Simultaneous determination of β_1- and β_2-adrenergic-receptors in tissues containing both receptor subtypes, *Mol. Pharmacol.,* 15, 286, 1979.
79. **Brunton, L. L., Hayes, J. S., and Mayer, S. E.,** Hormonally-specific phosphorylation of troponin I., *Nature,* 280, 78, 1979.
80. **Bellet, S.,** Mechanism and treatment of A-V heart block and Adams-Stokes syndrome, *Prog. Cardiovasc. Dis.,* 2, 691, 1960.
81. **Aviado, D. M., Jr.,** *Sympathomimetic Drugs,* Charles C Thomas, Springfield, Ill., 1970, 64.
82. **Caldwell, R. W. and Goldberg, L. I.,** An evaluation of the vasodilation produced by mephentermine and certain other sympathomimetic amines, *J. Pharmacol. Exp. Ther.,* 172, 297, 1970.
83. **Furness, J. B. and Burnstock, G.,** Role of circulating catecholamines in the gastrointestinal tract, in *Handbook of Physiology, Section 7,* Vol. 6, Blaschko, H., Sayers, G., and Smith, A. D., Eds., American Physiological Society, Washington, D.C., 1975, 515.

THE THYROID GLAND

Harold M. Kaplan and George H. Gass

ANATOMY

Historical

Galen was first to describe the thyroid gland in his book *De Voce*. In 1543, Vesalius expanded the description. Wharton in 1656 named the organ the thyroid, which means an oblong shield. The term is a misnomer for the shape of the thyroid, referring only to the nearby shield-like thyroid cartilage of the larynx. Stevenson[1] has a more detailed historical account of the gland.

Location and Description

The thyroid gland is in the ventral aspect of the neck, opposite cervical nerves 5, 6, and 7. It is present in all vertebrates, but in varying shapes and locations. In the human adult it weighs at least 20 g, but it is very labile, varying in size with age, diet, reproductive state, and other conditions. It is larger in the female than in the male. Only about 3 g of healthy thyroid tissue are needed to maintain the body in a euthyroid state.

The thyroid gland is covered by two layers of connective tissue. The outer, fibrous sheath is continuous with the cervical fascia; its central layer encloses infrahyoid muscles while its dorsal layer encloses esophagus, trachea, and recurrent laryngeal nerves. The inner, or second layer of connective tissue, is a structure that tightly adheres to the surface of the gland. The existence of two layers in the capsule affords a plane of cleavage which for the surgeon facilitates removal of the gland. As seen from in front, the gland is H- or U-shaped. Two freely movable lobes on either side of the trachea are usually connected by an isthmus which stretches over the ventral aspect of the trachea. The glandular isthmus covers rings 2, 3, and 4 of the trachea.

Each lobe has an apex, base, and three surfaces. The apex lies superoposteriorly, situated between the sternothyroid muscle and the inferior pharyngeal constrictor. The base lies inferomedially. The lateral surface is beneath the omohyoid, sternohyoid, and sternothyroid muscles. The medial surface is related to the cricothyroid muscles, trachea, inferior constrictor of the pharynx, and also the external and recurrent laryngeal nerves. The posterior surface is related to the carotid sheath, prevertebral muscles, parathyroid glands, and sympathetic trunk.

Each anatomic lobe is composed of smaller lobes, each of which in turn consists of many lobules. Each lobule has 20 to 40 follicles, bound into a unit by connective tissue. Each lobule has its own artery.

A pyramidal lobe sometimes occurs, extending superiorly from the isthmus and usually fixed to the hyoid bone by connective tissue or muscle. The presence of colloid for extracellular thyroglobulin storage is unique. In all the other endocrine glands, the storage is intracellular and the holding capacity is limited.

Blood and Lymph Supply

Except for the adrenal glands, more blood supplies the thyroid, relative to its size, than any other bodily organ. The superior thyroid artery comes from the external, or less usually, from the common carotid artery. It has two main branches to the thyroid gland; the larger branch is the principal artery to the central surface and the smaller supplies the dorsal aspect of the gland.

The inferior thyroid artery comes from the thyrocervical trunk of the subclavian.

At the inferior border of the thyroid gland, the inferior thyroid artery divides into two. These divisions supply the postero-inferior aspects of the thyroid and they anastomose with the superior thyroid artery as well as with the corresponding contralateral artery.

An inconstant artery called the arteria thyroidea ima arises from the brachiocephalic trunk, right common carotid, aortic arch, or even elsewhere. It rises to the isthmus where it divides profusely.

The veins form a plexus on the gland surface. The plexus is drained on the right and left by the superior and middle thyroid veins. This blood reaches the internal jugular vein. There is a plexus in front of the trachea formed by the inferior thyroid veins and the plexus drains into the brachiocephalic veins.

The lymphatic vessels run in the interlobular connective tissue. They drain either superiorly to lower deep cervical nodes or inferiorly to paratracheal nodes. Isthmus lymphatics travel superiorly to prelaryngeal nodes or inferiorly to pretracheal nodes.

Nerve Supply

The nerves to the thyroid gland are the parasympathetic vagi and especially the sympathetics. The vagi supply the thyroid through their superior and recurrent laryngeal branches. These nerves accompany the blood vessels into the gland as postganglionics which arise in cervical ganglia. Sympathetic terminals have a close relation to the follicle cells as well as to capillaries and arteriolar walls. This suggests that sympathetic impulses have an influence not only on the blood vessels, but also have a nonvascular or direct secretory effect on the follicle cells.[2] This is a modification of the older view that the nerves are vasomotor and not secretory.

Sympathetic stimulation induces secretion of thyroid hormone, mediated by norepinephrine released at the nerve endings in the gland, the hormone reacting with α-adrenergic receptors. The subsequent action is on thyroid follicle cells. Catecholamines can increase iodination and synthesis of thyroid hormone, as shown for the calf.[2] Catecholamines stimulate adenyl cyclase, increasing the formation of cAMP which then leads to the release of the known hormones of the thyroid.

The neural secretory control is not a major one, but it provides for quick responses of the gland to appropriate stimuli. The mechanisms for maintained regulation will be considered later.

Microscopic Anatomy

Histology-Light Microscope

The units of microscopic structure are spherical or ovate, cyst-like follicles, 0.2 to 0.9 mm in diameter. The small follicles predominate in man. Surrounding each follicle is a very thin basement lamina. A capillary plexus surrounds each follicle, greatly enriching the thyroid in vascular supply. Some histiocytes and lymphocytes are found in these regions. Lymphatic capillaries lie between the capillary nets.

Each follicle has a secretory epithelium consisting of one-layered, cuboidal or squamous cells. The squamous type usually predominates when activity is low and the columnar type usually predominates when the gland is very active.

The central lumen of each follicle contains colloid, which is an optically homogeneous and gelatinous globulin. The colloid is formed from the epithelial cells functioning to store the cellular secretions. The colloid stains markedly with the periodic acid-Schiff reaction since the thyroglobulin stored therein is a glycoprotein, containing hexosamine and also carbohydrates such as galactose, mannose, and others. The colloid thyroglobulin contains iodinated amino acids in peptide linkage, e.g., thyroxine and triiodothyroine, the latter two constituting what may be called the "thyroid hormone" when released into the blood.

There are two populations of cells in the thyroid follicles. The principal cells have been briefly described above. They have cytoplasmic granules of many sizes, the variations depending upon the secretory state. The cell nucleus is spheroidal, centrally placed, with one or more nucleoli. The basal cell membrane is highly folded. The apical cell surface shows prominent microvilli. The cytoplasmic organelles are typical, including thin-rod mitochondria, a supranuclear Golgi apparatus, lipid droplets, granules of many sizes, and ergastoplasm. There are numerous apical vesicles below the microvilli.

There is a second, smaller population of cells, found in the follicular epithelium and in the interfollicular spaces. These are parafollicular cells. They originate from follicular epithelial cells and migrate to their definitive location. They produce the hormone thyrocalcitonin, which counteracts the action of parathyroid hormone, thus being a part of the homeostatic regulation system for plasma calcium ion concentration. The parafollicular cells contain relatively little granular endoplasmic reticulum. They display numerous membrane limited vesicles about 1500 Å in diameter.

Developmental Aspects

The thyroid gland is not a derivative of any branchial arch or pouch, although its primordium appears in the human embryo of about 1.5 mm as a single midventral endodermal evagination from the floor of the pharynx at the level of the first and second branchial pouches. At 2.5 mm (end of 4th week) the outgrowth is a hollow tube, which keeps its connection with the floor of the pharynx by a tubular stalk. The stalk is termed the thyroglossal duct. In later development, this duct temporarily connects the developing thyroid with the tongue which is also forming from the pharyngeal floor. Although the duct atrophies at 6 to 8 weeks, its original place of origin is permanently marked by a pit called the foramen cecum at the base of the tongue. During the 6th week the thyroid loses its lumen and is changed into solid epithelial plates. The structure grows backward and attains its definitive position with a lobe on the right and left sides of the trachea. Connection with the tongue is lost. During the 8th week, discontinuous cavities appear in the solid plates. The cavities become the follicles which acquire colloid. This embryonic formation of follicles ceases at the close of the 4th month, but new follicles arise by budding and cell division of existing follicles. The colloid is not an important component of the follicles until after birth.

The thyroid grows slowly but steadily throughout the prenatal period until at birth its weight is about 0.12% of the total body weight. Although its absolute weight increases after birth, its relative weight declines, being at most 40 g in the normal adult.

The pituitary-thyroid system differentiates to a functional status by the close of the first trimester of pregnancy.[3] Secretion of thyrotropin and thyroid hormones is minimal, however, until midgestation. The thyroxine (T_4) secretion rate near term appears to be relatively high.

The fetal somatic growth is probably not thyroid-dependent. The human placenta is impermeable to thyrotropin and is hardly permeable to thyroid hormones. There is a period of T_4 dependency a few weeks prior to term for bone, brain, and perhaps lung growth and development.

In pathology following 24 hr of neonatal thyrotoxicosis involving marked T_3 increase but much less T_4 increase, thyroid function becomes gradually depressed, probably due to feedback inhibition of thyrotropin release.

Thyroid growth roughly parallels body growth. The gland increases in size from about 1.5 g at birth to 10 to 12 g at age 10 years. There is a significant decrease in both serum T_4 and T_3 concentrations with age. Reverse T_3 (rT_3) is unchanged or increases slightly in childhood and adolescence. Serum thyrotropin concentrations are essentially constant during childhood. There appears to be a decrease in thyroid responsiveness with age. For a detailed description of the embryology of the pituitary-thyroid axis, refer to Werner.[4,5]

In regard to the influence of T_3 and T_4 upon certain vital processes in the embryo, these hormones importantly influence lung maturation and surfactant production in several mammals and they appear to act similarly in man.[6] Fetal serum thyroid hormone levels correlate with the amniotic fluid lecithin to sphingomyelin ratios, and such L/S ratios correlate with lung maturation and surfactant activity. Total and free T_4 are low until 30 weeks of gestation, after which they rise. At birth, free T_4 of serum is at least as high as that of the adult.

Comparative Anatomy (Phylogeny)

Iodine and compounds containing iodine are essential to various plants and animals at all levels of biologic complexity. Some algae contain iodine and so do all marine intertebrates. Certain sponges have high concentrations of diiodotyrosine. Thyroid hormones and their precursor chemicals were observed in organisms before the evolution of a discrete thyroid gland.

There has been a controversy as to whether a hypobranchial groove in the pharyngeal floor of Amphioxus, a protochordate, is a homologue of the thyroid gland. There are no thyroid follicles in protochordates, nor in the invertebrate phyla preceding them in racial history. A structure called the endostyle, seen in the larval lamprey, has developed the capacity to concentrate iodine and synthesize thyroxine. The endostyle, however, can hardly be classified as an endocrine gland.

The adult lamprey has a primitive thyroid gland. The bony fishes have the gland in the form seen in the higher vertebrates. Functionally, however, only warm blooded vertebrates have a gland with all the actions of the thyroid in man, including effects upon metabolism.

It is said to be possible to produce thyroxine without a thyroid gland, as evidenced in some mammals.[7] If so, this suggests that tyrosine synthesis to thyroid hormone is a general biologic property and that the thyroid is a specialized adaptation for hormone synthesis and storage.

NEUROENDOCRINE REGULATION OF THYROID SECRETION

Hypothalamus

Neural impulses to specific hypothalamic centers may stimulate the formation of a thyroid releasing hormone (TRF or TRH). This is produced over a wide area of the hypothalamus and is stored in the median eminence. TRH is a tripeptide pyroglutamyhistidylproline amide. It has been synthesized.

TRH is released into the portal veins running through the stalk from the hypothalamus to the anterior pituitary gland. It activates the release from the pituitary of thyroid stimulating hormone (TSH; thyrotropin). If the hypothalamus is destroyed or the pituitary stalk is severed, the secretion of TSH is markedly reduced, perhaps because TRH reaches the pituitary in less concentrated form from the general circulation. The blood levels of T_3 and T_4 tend to affect the release of TSH by negative feedback possibly on the hypothalamus, but much more likely by action on the pituitary gland, bypassing the hypothalamus.

Anterior Pituitary

TSH is secreted responsively by the basophil cells of the anterior pituitary and in turn controls the activity of the thyroid gland. TSH stimulates iodide trapping, synthesis of T_3 and T_4, breakdown of thyroglobulin, and release of T_3 and T_4 into the plasma. TSH combines with thyroid tissue and is inactivated by it. If TSH is missing, which is possible in hypopituitarism, the thyroid involutes and its own hormone output is greatly reduced.

Increasing levels of thyroid hormones moderate the degree of output of TSH by negative feedback. There is a question as to whether the pituitary produces more than one type of TSH. Abnormal types have been detected in the serum of thyrotoxic persons. T_3 and T_4 in the circulation feed back particularly upon the pituitary. When they are excessive in concentration, less TSH is produced. If T_3 or T_4 become deficient, the secretory centers are stimulated by release of negative feedback and TSH is secreted. It also appears to be possible for T_3 and T_4 to control the thyroid gland directly.

TSH is a glycoprotein with a molecular weight of 28,000. It is composed of two noncovalently linked glycosylated polypeptides called α and β. The α is biologically inactive; it is almost identical to that in luteinizing hormone, follicle stimulating hormone, and chorionic gonadotropin. The β subunit has slight biologic activity; it confers biologic specificity. Production of TSH displays circadian rhythm, probably controlled by TRH.

Environmental Stimuli Affecting Reflex Centers

Warm blooded animals exposed to cold initially increase their thyroid activity. The rapidity of the response suggests a response to cold through afferent neural fibers, the adjustment center being in the hypothalamus. The center(s) respond by release of pituitary thyrotropin and also sympathetic activity.

An intact thyroid is essential for survival during acute exposure to cold, although it may not be necessary when acclimation takes place.[8] Acute exposure stimulates the utilization of T_3 and T_4, mediated by release of norepinephrine from sympathetic nerves. Overall, nonshivering thermogenesis appears to be regulated by the hypothalamus, chiefly due to the calorigenic action of the sympathetic output of norepinephrine. The thyroid hormones allow or potentiate the calorigenic responses. Climatic adaptation does not involve the thyroid significantly over long periods of time.

Thyroid function decreases in response to heat and the metabolic rate is depressed. No firm conclusions can be drawn, however, about the relationships among heat, the basal metabolic rate, and the mechanisms of thyroid response.

Bodily Stimuli Affecting Reflex Centers

Physical stressing agents (trauma, irritating injections) produce lessened release of thyrotropin and they inhibit thyroid secretion. Emotional reactions are usually inhibitory, but the mechanisms may involve the nervous system since thyroxin concentration decreases in the blood; if thyrotropin were involved the feedback effect would increase plasma thyroxine. Note that these stimuli exert effects on thyroid activity opposite to those of cold environments.

BIOCHEMICAL CONTROL OF THYROID SECRETION

cAMP Mediation (“B” Effects)

In all species studied including man, thyrotropin activates adenylate cyclase which enhances cAMP accumulation. It is not certain that cAMP then mediates the known effects of thyrotropin in all species. If so, these are called “B” effects (β-adrenergic). In man, cAMP mediates the action of thyrotropin on iodothyronine release, protein iodination, and glucose oxidation. Most effects are in the B category. The influence of thyrotropin on growth is a B effect, aided by somatotropin, somatomedin, insulin, and/or corticosteroids.

The mechanisms responsible for B effects are relatively well defined. Adenylate cyclase may be activated by thyrotropin by a mechanism similar to that described for cholera toxin, in which some gangliosides are part of the receptor, and the β subunit of thyrotropin binds to specific gangliosides on the plasma membrane. This produces conformational change in thyrotropin which causes the alpha subunit to be translocated within the membrane. The α unit then activates adenylate cyclase. There are other elements of the cAMP system in the thyroid that are similar to those in other tissues. Examples include guanosine 5′-triphosphate-activated adenylate cyclase, three phosphodiesterases, and two cAMP-dependent protein kinases.

"A" effects are analogous to those of the α-adrenergic system. They are not mediated by cAMP.

It is not known whether A and B effects of thyrotropin result from activation of a single receptor by the hormone or if they correspond to binding and activation of several receptors. The mechanism responsible for "A" effects of thyrotropin is unknown.[9,10]

Prostaglandins (PG)

PG, adrenergic agents, HCG and ACh activate thyroid adenylate cyclase in the same manner as thyrotropin does. PG-E_1 and E_2 activate adenylate cyclase probably in the follicular cells. The normal role of this action is unknown.

Adrenergic Agents

Adrenergic compounds bind to thyroid membranes and aid the accumulation of cAMP. The β-adrenergic receptors are not the same as the "B" receptors of thyrotropin. The physiologic role of adrenergic controls is unknown.

Human Chorionic Gonadotropin (HCG)

HCG activates thyroid adenylate cyclase in the same manner as thyrotropin does.

Acetylcholine (ACh)

There are several regulators that control thyroid function by inhibiting the thyrotropin-induced accumulation of cAMP. In the dog, ACh via a muscarinic receptor increases free Ca^{++} levels in cells, which increases the level of cyclic guanosine 3′,5′-monophosphate, decreasing the accumulation of thyrotropin-induced cAMP, directly inhibiting thyroid secretion and activating iodination of protein and PG-E_2 and F-2α, as well as the formation of thromboxane B-2. In man there are cholinergic terminals and ACh increases the level of cyclic guanosine 3′,5′-monophosphate, but it does not inhibit cAMP accumulation caused by thyrotropin.

α-Adrenergic Compounds

These compounds may act by increasing Ca^{++} levels in cells, in turn inhibiting thyrotropin-induced thyroid secretion.

Iodides

Iodides in drug doses decrease thyroid blood flow secretion, iodide trapping, protein iodination, and thyrotropin activity. The effects of iodides may be mediated by an organic form of iodine. Iodide control is adaptive since it lowers thyroid metabolism when iodides are in high supply, gearing the gland toward effective use when iodide is scarce.

Thyroid Hormones

Thyroid hormones inhibit thyrotropin secretion and thus thyroid secretion by a feedback mechanism primarily to the anterior pituitary. These hormones may also be effective at the adenylate cyclase level, although this short loop control is questionable in humans.

THYROID REGULATION IN CERTAIN PATHOLOGY

Immunoglobulins

The essential endocrine disturbance in toxic goiter (Graves disease, von Basedow's disease, and thyrotoxicosis) is excessive secretion of thyroid hormones in response to a nonpituitary stimulus. The output of thyrotropin is low and treatment with even large doses of thyroid hormones does not depress thyroid function. However, the reciprocal relationship between the pituitary and the thyroid is retained. The evidence supports the view that there is a humoral thyroid-stimulating agent.[11] This is termed the long-acting thyroid stimulator (LATS). It has been found in about 80% of persons with this disorder when their serum has been concentrated. The substance is an immunoglobulin, IgG, produced by lymphocytes and behaving as an antibody against the thyroid (whose antigens may be located in the follicular cell membrane). LATS has an action similar to that of thyrotropin (TSH). Both stimulate the production of cAMP. TSH is affected by T_4 and T_3 whereas LATS is unaffected by suppression of T_4 and T_3. LATS is probably not the primary cause of thyrotoxicosis, but rather an indicator of the disease in response to a thyroid abnormality.

PHYSIOLOGIC EFFECTS OF THYROID HORMONES (TH) ON SOME BODILY PROCESSES

Basal Metabolic Rate

In homoiotherms, TH increases energy production and oxygen consumption of most tissues. The brain, retina, spleen, testis, and lungs are exceptions.[12] Large amounts of TH can increase the basal metabolic rate (BMR) even up to 100%. The BMR falls after thyroidectomy and is elevated upon giving TH. In most humans with severe hypothyroidism, the BMR is 40 to 60% elevated. In severe hypothyroidism, the BMR is minus 30 to 45%.

T_3 increases the oxygen consumption far more than T_4 does and has greater therapeutic value in this regard.

In ectotherms, it is difficult to demonstrate any calorigenic effects of thyroid hormones. However, environmental temperature may condition thyroid responses, the specific temperature changing the threshold needed to elicit a response.

In hibernating mammals, the gland is inactive in the winter, but rises to very high activity as the animals leave hibernation in the spring. The reverse is true for seasonal changes in hibernating ectotherms.

Nervous System

Thyroid hormone sensitizes the brain. The BMR correlates with the frequency of α waves. In hypothyroidism, there is increased threshold to light and sound stimuli, decreased α rhythm, and blunted reaction to electric shock. In hyperthyroidism, the BMR is elevated, but brain oxygen consumption stays normal. Increased neural excitability appears to be separable from the metabolic effects of thyroid hormone. Although reaction time is hastened by TH, peripheral nerve activity is not influenced, as evidenced by normal conduction velocity in nerve trunks.

Effect on Muscles

A slight increase in TH secretion increases muscle vigor. A large increase causes protein breakdown and weakens muscle force. A sustained decrease in TH secretion produces sluggishness of muscle contraction.

In pathology, excessive sustained secretion produces fine muscle tremors, due to effects on the ventral horn cell motor neurons. The neuromuscular involvement produces chronic fatigue, although difficulty in sleeping may occur because of increased neuron excitability.

Effect on Respiration

In tissues with elevated BMR there is greater energy output and oxygen demand. Together with elevated carbon dioxide excretion, ventilation increases in rate and depth.

Effect on Digestion

An increase in TH secretion increases the rate of secretion of digestive fluids and enzymes as well as motility. Digested foods are absorbed more readily. Appetite and food intake increase. A decrease in TH secretion is associated with constipation.

Cardiovascular Effects

Blood flow to an area depends upon the status of metabolism therein and the consequent oxygen demand. Hypoxia causes local vasodilation of the tissue beds and increased exchange of nutrients and gases. In high physical activity, these effects are pronounced in the skin vasculature, especially as heat elimination increases. The cardiac output is elevated in response to increased TH secretion.

TH may directly affect cardiac myocardial fiber excitability and contractility, resulting in an increased heart rate and force. In sustained excessive TH secretion, the high rate and force are gradually converted to weaker cardiac output as protein catabolism continues. Cardiac failure can occur in severe thyrotoxicosis. In hypothyroidism, the heart may enlarge, with a decrease in rate and force.

The normal effect of TH on blood volume is one of slight increase, partly a result of vasodilation. An increased cardiac output increases the arterial pressure, although the tendency becomes offset by the cutaneous dilation needed to eliminate heat.

BIOCHEMICAL EFFECTS OF THYROID HORMONES

Carbohydrates

T_3 and T_4 may have little effect on carbohydrate metabolism[11] or they may increase such metabolism if enzyme reactions are accelerated. There is an increase in the rate of glucose absorption into tissue cells. Glyogenolysis, glycolysis, and gluconeogenesis can all be stimulated. Because of this, there may be hyperglycemia attended by glucosuria in hyperthyroidism.

Water and Electrolytes

T_3 and T_4 increase the renal excretion of calcium and phosphorus. In normal persons, T_3 and T_4 administration mobilizes fluid, the urine flow being increased and rich in potassium. The hypothyroid person tends to retain sodium chloride and water.

Protein Metabolism

TH (T_4, T_3) cause an increase in protein metabolism in almost all tissues. The translation process, which involves protein formation by ribosomes, occurs directly after hormone administration. After hours to days, RNA synthesis by genes, which is called transcription, is increased and it results in the synthesis of almost every type of protein.

Increased enzymatic activity caused by TH augments protein anabolism and also catabolism, the processes being essential to growth. If other types of foods are exhausted, TH mobilizes proteins for an energy function. Conversion to sugar, or gluconeogenesis, is accelerated.

Giving TH to hypothyroid persons causes nitrogen retention and a resumption of growth. Liver enlargement and excess plasma globulin are reduced. Although physiologic doses of TH produce protein anabolic changes, large toxic doses of TH do not stimulate growth. TH relieves an excess mucoprotein deposit in tissues of persons with cretinism and myxedema. Thyroid deficiency favors increased nitrogen excretion. Following thyroidectomy, there are marked shifts in protein reserves from organs such as liver and kidney into the plasma.

Bones

Thyroid hormones, by increasing protein formation, favor the growth of bone. However, because epiphyses close rapidly, the rate of growth is first stimulated but then prematurely ended. TH also increases osteoclastic activity, thus causing osteoporosis. Calcium leaves the bone.

Fat Metabolism

Thyroid hormones mobilize lipids from storage deposits, increasing free fatty acid concentration in the blood as well as fat oxidation in tissue cells. Simultaneously, cholesterol, phospholipids, and triglyceride concentrations are decreased in the blood. The reason for cholesterol reduction is an increased excretion in the intestine and conversion to bile acids in the liver. A decreased TH secretion increases these three substances in the blood and excessive fat deposition occurs in the liver.

Vitamins

Thyroid hormones cause an increased need for vitamins, the latter forming essential parts of enzymes in biochemical reactions. Thus, hyperthyroidism may be associated with a greater need for vitamins. T_4 in excess increases the body's need for members of the B complex. In hypothyroidism, carotene accumulates, producing yellowing of the skin, but not the sclera.

Mitochondria

Thyroid hormones cause an increase in size and number of mitochondria in most cells, increasing their membrane surface. This probably stimulates the rate of formation of ATP as a mechanism to meet increased metabolic demands. Very high experimental concentrations of TH cause mitochondrial swelling and uncoupling of oxidative phosphorylation. The effect of increases in T_3 and T_4 is marked on mitochondrial enzymes that are involved in oxidations and electron transport. The increased enzyme concentrations may be associated with increased protein synthesis.

EFFECTS OF THYROID HORMONE ON REPRODUCTIVE PROCESSES

Species and Age Differences

Testes of young animals are more easily impaired than those of adults. Hypothyroidism delays sexual development in the young male. Toxic levels of thyroxine in the young male can impair reproductive functions, although moderate doses may stimulate spermatogenesis.

Effects on Ovaries

Thyroid deficiency or excess can impair ovarian function, causing irregularity or loss of cycles. Thyroidectomized animals can reproduce, but with subnormal fecundity. In rat hypothroidism, litter size is reduced and maternal ability for lactation is suppressed; the ovary becomes susceptible to cyst formation. Infertility in human beings may occur in hypofunction.

Mechanism of Influence over Reproductive Processes

Mechanisms relating the thyroid gland to reproduction are unclear. Some involve protein metabolic disturbances; other involve pituitary malfunction. The anterior pituitary secretes considerable TSH after thyroidectomy. In hypophysectomized rats, thyroxine increases heart rate and rate of consumption, but does not restore body growth or reproductive function. It is possible that the thyroid hormones somehow control pituitary release of somatotropin, corticotropin and gonadotropins.

EFFECTS OF THYROID HORMONE ON DEVELOPMENT IN VARIOUS VERTEBRATES

Growth and Differentiation

Thyroid hormones are essential for mitotic increase in size and for differentiation of form. The thyroid and the anterior pituitary somatotropin act synergistically in skeletal growth. Thyroxine prevents the loss of endochondral ossification observed in hypophysectomized young rats. Thyroxine in the absence of the pituitary does not maintain chondrogenesis. In growing hypothyroid children, growth is markedly retarded. In such children, growth is excessive at first, but the epiphyses close prematurely, shortening eventual height.

Molting

Thyroxine promotes molting, but the influence varies with the species. Thyroid hormones are especially important in urodeles, acting directly upon the skin. Thyroid hormones influence shedding of the outer surface of lizards. In thyroidectomized snakes, skin sloughing increases.

Metamorphosis

Thyroid hormones are essential for the metamorphosis of amphibian larvae.[13] Thyroidless tadpoles grow normally, but remain gigantic larvae. The thyroid action is not essentially dependent upon the capacity to elevate the metabolic rate. The temperature effect on metamorphosis is largely independent of thyroid activity. Metamorphosis in fishes is related to thyroid activity in some species, e.g., salmonids, but not in cyclostomes or most teleosts.

Neotony

Axolotols, which retain the larval form throughout life, can be induced to metamorphose by thyroxine or by inorganic iodine. It is thought that failure to metamorphose is due to the inability of the thyroid to secrete hormone or else to a low sensitivity of the tissues to thyroid hormone. The latter may be true for perennibranchiate salamanders which retain larval characteristics despite thyroid administration.

MECHANISMS OF ACTION OF THYROID HORMONES

Thyroid hormones act on tissues by a variety of mechanisms. Some involve transport of amino acids and electrolytes into cells. Others involve synthesis or activation of cellular enzymes and proteins. The major sites of hormone action include cell membranes, mitochondria, ribosomes, and cell nuclei.

Thyroid hormones may affect the rate of metabolism in cells through action at steps in the TCA cycle. The hormones may alter the membrane permeability of mitochondria or they uncouple oxidative phosphorylation in which oxidative release of energy is coupled to production of ATP. After acting upon cells and processes, T_3 and T_4 are degraded and the released iodine rejoins the iodine pool.

ANTITHYROID SUBSTANCES

Thioureas

Thiocarbamide derivates, e.g., thiourea, thiouracil, and propylthiouracil are very active antithyroid compounds. These drugs produce goiters by blocking iodination of any amino acid residue of proteins, thus causing failure of thyroxine synthesis. In turn, this stimulates thyrotropin, which produces hyperplasia, hypertrophy, and colloid loss in the thyroid.

Propylthiouracil does not prevent the formation of thyroglobulin. However, the lack of T_3 and T_4 in the thyroglobulin produces considerable thyrotropin secretion by feedback upon the anterior pituitary. Thus the compound is goitrogenic.

Goiters due to thioureas are reduced by feeding iodine. The same treatment intensifies the goitrous changes in sulfonamide-induced goiters.

The thiouracils, which represent a class of drugs blocking thyroid peroxidase activity, are distinct from a second class, e.g., perchlorate, which does not inhibit iodination, but blocks the trapping of iodide.

Thiocyanate and Others

Thiocyanate may be chiefly an inhibitor of iodide transport, but it is also a powerful inhibitor of iodination. Aromatic inhibitors of thyroid function are inhibitors of peroxidase-catalyzed iodination.

Cyanides, which inhibit hemoprotein enzymes, inhibit iodination.

REGENERATING CAPACITY OF THYROID TISSUE

Thyroid tissue regenerates rapidly after surgical procedures, if the excision is subtotal and the dietary intake of iodine is moderated. Administration of exogenous thyroid hormone inhibits regeneration of thyroid tissue.

THYROGLOBULIN

Biosynthesis

Thyroglobulin (T_G), which acts as a prohormone, is produced in the thyroid follicle cells and its origin is exclusively the thyroid gland. Its synthesis accounts for more than 50% of the total protein synthesis within the thyroid.

There is little information about the location and transcription of the T_G gene or genes. The nuclear premessenger RNA undergoes polyadenylation and probably capping prior to transportation to the cytoplasm.[14] In the regulation of transcription, continuous stimulation of the thyroid by thyrotropin is necessary to sustain the expression of the thyroglobulin gene.[15]

Messenger RNA with a polyadenylated sequence has been purified from thyroglobulin-synthesizing polyribosomes (from cows).[16,17] Large polyribosomes are found in the thyroids of many mammals and they are engaged in synthesizing thyroglobulin subunits. The messenger RNA from cows can code for a polypeptide with a possible molecular weight of 330,000 daltons. Vassart et al.[16,17] report the translation of bovine 33S messenger RNA into 300,000 dalton polypeptides related to thyroglobulin from the cow. The primary translation products correspond to 12.5 half-thyroglobulin molecules that form 195 dimers of thyroglobulin. The view that thyroglobulin is synthesized only through translation of 33S thyroglobulin messenger RNA has been challenged.[18] In regulation at the level of translation, it may be that thyrotropin stimulates T_G synthesis by promoting the translation of a pool of inactive T_G messenger RNA. This process is mediated by cAMP.

The polypeptide chains are synthesized on the polyribosomes which are found on the rough endoplasmic reticulum (RER) of the follicle cells. The first carbohydrates, which are N-acetylglucosamine and mannose, are attached before the compound leaves the RER. All other polysaccharide chains are attached as the protein migrates from the rough to the smooth endoplasmic reticulum and thence to the Golgi apparatus. In that apparatus, glycolysation of T_G takes place. This process involves synthesis of a core carbohydrate chain attached to the membrane as a dolichol derivative.[19] The carbohydrate transfers to the T_G chain where it produces the three kinds of carbohydrate units found in the complete T_G. Sialic acid is added to some chains, explaining the presence of 23 sialic acid residues per 19S molecule of human T_G. Following sialic acid residues attachment, T_G is released into the colloid space by means of small apical vesicles.

In moving thyroglobulin from the endoplasmic reticulum to colloid storage, thyrotropin controls the process. The mechanism of secretion into the colloidal area is by fusion of exocytotic residues within the apical membrane of the cell.[20]

The last stage in biosynthesis involves iodination and hormone synthesis. These processes continue in the T_G stored within the follicular colloid. Although most of the iodine incorporation occurs after completion of the carbohydrate units, iodination can also occur in incomplete T_G molecules.

Chemical Properties

Thyroglobulin is a large glycoprotein whose molecular weight is about 660,000. The sedimentation coefficient is 19S. The isoelectric point of pH about 4.58 has been estimated by extrapolation of electrophoretic mobility data. The isolated molecule is ovoid in shape, about 300 × 150 Å. The molecule is composed of two symmetric halves, probably representing two 12S subunits. The term thyroglobulin refers most strictly to the 19S protein, but the 12S half-molecules and 27S dimers can be isolated. The 27S molecules contain more iodine and are richer in thyroxine content than is the 19S T_G. The 27S is produced by union of two molecules of 19S as a product of iodination.

It has been difficult to determine the number of peptide chains in T_G since the 19S molecule has different amounts of monoidotyrosine, diiodityrosine, T_3 and T_4. The molecule also contains iodinated histidyl residues, iodotyrosyl derivatives, oxidation products of other residues, and the oxidative coupling of iodotyrosyl to iodothyronyl residues. The fundamental polypeptide chain synthesized by the thyroid cell is probably 12S, and all other species represent products resulting from the action of iodine or proteolysis. T_G is stable between pH 5 and 11. Stability is enhanced with increasing iodine content.

The amino acids of T_G are similar among vertebrates. The composition of T_G in diseased thyroid tissue shows no differences from that of the normal. The 19S molecule contains about 2% of tyrosine and about 100 disulfide bonds. The data on amino acid sequence are very limited.

The function of the carbohydrate chains in T_G is unknown. They probably limit the rate of T_G synthesis and are essential to T_G secretion from the follicle cells. T_G contains about 10% carbohydrate. There are two main types of oligosaccharide chains, attached to aspariginyl residues. One, called unit A, contains N-acetylglucosamine and mannose. A second, called unit B, has branched chains ending in fucose or in N-acetylneuraminic acid (sialic acid). A third chain, isolated in the human, contains mostly B-acetylgalactosamine and sialic acid.

Assay Techniques

Hjort[21] and Assem[22] demonstrated thyroglobulin in the circulation by hemagglutination inhibition or by electrophoretic immunoretention technique. Early clinical assays were reported in 1973 and 1975 by Van Herle et al.,[23,24] followed by others,[25] all based on the double-antibody technique.

Sensitive and specific radioimmunoassay for humans was reviewed in 1979 by Van Herle et al.[9,10] They listed a normal mean serum value of 5.1 ng/mℓ, with a range of about 1.6 to 20.7. Day to day variations rarely exceed the normal range of the assay. There are no age-related variations in the human male, but women have higher values than men. In the rat, the mean thyroglobulin level is high (101.5 ng/mℓ) and the range of normals is wide (12.0 to 258 ng/mℓ). Thyroglobulin was long undetected in the human circulation because it was considered that the compound served only to provide the body with active thyroid hormones.

Control of Thyroglobulin Secretion from the Thyroid

Thyroglobulin is a normal secretory product of the thyroid gland and the process is regulated by thyrotropin. Administration of thyroxine in rats and man reduces serum thyroglobulin levels. Thus, T_4 (and also T_3) suppress serum thyroglobulin levels. If thyroglobulin is to be classified as a secretory product, a dose-response relation should exist between an amount of thyroid-stimulating hormone injected and the amount of thyroglobulin released. This relation has been proved.[26] Various thyroid stimulators can induce the release of thyroglobulin into the circulation.[24]

Mechanism of Release of T_G from the Gland

The mechanism of secretion (release) is unknown. It is possibly released by endocytosis of primary colloid droplets or secondary lysosomes or by escaping via relaxation of junctions.[9,10] The secretion rate for the hormonal iodine components of T_G is 60 μg/day. This constitutes a 30 day supply of iodine. The secretion rate for iodine in the form of iodotyrosines represents a 20 day supply of iodine.[27]

Circulating Thyroglobulin

Thyroglobulin gets into the circulation via thyroidal lymphatics. Its role in the general circulation is still unproved. It is also uncertain whether circulating thyroglobulin is involved in thyroid autoregulation. The compound is not an antigen since it occurs in the circulation of almost all normal persons.

Metabolism and Fate

The half-life of thyroglobulin may be about 24 hr.[10] It is known that the ready uptake of asialoglycoproteins by liver explains the rapid removal of glycoproteins from blood. This can explain the rapid removal of asialothyroglobulin since thyroglobulin has carbohydrate moieties. The half-life of thyroglobulin varies with the size of the molecule, small molecules clearing faster than native 19S thyroglobulin. Tissues other than the liver can bind the intact or desialylated form of thyroglobulin.

The metabolic activity of thyroglobulin in the microenvironment of the tissues is not known. Studies are lacking on the metabolism of thyroglobulin following its release from the thyroid gland.

Functions of T_G in Hormone Production

T_G is part of a mechanism for the efficient synthesis of diodotyrosines and for their coupling to form thyroid hormones. Additionally, T_G provides for the storage of the thyroid hormones T_3 and T_4, adaptively releasing these hormones into the plasma.

T_G contains 0.2 to 1% iodine, incorporated into monoiodotyrosine (MIT), diodotyrosine (DIT), T_3 and T_4. Of considerable importance in the economy of iodine utilization is the fact that the concentration of MIT is as low as 5% and this will not exceed 10% of the entire tyrosyl residues.

The relative amounts of T_3 and T_4 within T_G are determined by the amounts of MIT and DIT present. The iodoamino acid composition is determined by the iodine content of T_G. Most T_G is stored in colloid and very little is stored in the secretory cells. This extracellular storage is unique to the thyroid gland.

With an adequate supply of dietary iodine, the T_G of the colloid contains 5 to 7 mg of iodine, 1/3 present as T_3 and T_4, 2/3 as iodotyrosines. These are retained in the poorly diffusible T_G form until the thyroid cells utilize them by proteolysis in lysosomes.

THYROXINE (T_4)

Cell Source and Description of Biosynthesis

In 1915, Edward Kendall at the Mayo Clinic isolated a biologically active compound from the thyroid gland and named it thyroxin. A corrected spelling to thyroxine occurred later, when it was found to be an amine.

Thyroxine (T_4) (and triiodothyronine, T_3) are iodinated amino acids produced outside of the cells of the thyroid follicle or at the outside of the apical membrane. Inside the follicle they are incorporated within the protein prohormone thyroglobulin. This is stored in the colloid. T_4 is the principal circulating thyroid hormone, although T_3 is the most biologically active one. To release the two hormones, the iodinated thyroglobulin is transported from colloid to follicular epithelial cell and digested.

To synthesize T_4 (and T_3), iodine and tyrosine are needed in adequate amounts. Iodine, whose source is food and water, is ingested mainly as inorganic iodide. It is released as reduced iodide (I^-) in the intestine and it is absorbed into the plasma. The reduced iodide is trapped by the follicle cells, entering against an electrochemical gradient, thus requiring ATP energy expediture. About 50% of all the iodide in the body becomes stored in the thyroid gland. Other tissues in mammals can trap iodide, but cannot synthesize it to a hormone. The regulation of iodide trapping involves a response to anterior pituitary thyrotropin and may even involve self regulation.

Inside the follicle cell, reduced iodide (I^-) is oxidized to iodine (I_2) which then becomes capable of iodinating tyrosine residues already incorporated within the thyroglobulin molecule. This process is called organification. The reactions involve an enzyme called thyroid peroxidase (molecular weight about 64,000). The process of iodination occurs at the cell-colloid interface close to the apical membranes. Tyrosine within the thyroglobulin molecule is iodinated to monoiodotyrosine (MIT) and then to diiodotyrosine (DIT). Excess iodide inhibits the process of iodination of thyroglobulin.

Organification subsequently involves coupling or condensing of the two iodotyrosines formed within the thyroglobulin molecules and this activity produces the iodothyronines. To produce T_4, two molecules of DIT oxidatively couple with the loss of one alanine side chain. This intramolecular coupling is catalyzed by thyroid peroxidase. The synthetic process for T_4 (and T_3) is outlined in Table 1. Prior to thyroglobulin being iodinated (as described), the T_G molecule is synthesized by epithelial cells of the follicle and then secreted as colloid into the lumen of the follicle.

T_G is not unique in its ability to form T_4 since the latter is produced in several proteins iodinated in a peroxidase system, but T_G is the most efficient of the proteins tested experimentally. This efficiency is relative in the light of the fact that the 660,000 mol wt T_G secretes only three or four T_4 molecules into the plasma.

T_4 (and T_3) are freed into the plasma by proteolytic hydrolysis of thyroglobulin. In this process, thyroglobulin is taken from the colloid and trapped in lysosomes in the cytoplasm of the follicular cells. Enzymatic activity in the lysosomes splits thyroglobulin such that T_3 and T_4 are released. Simultaneously, remaining iodotyrosines (MIT and DIT) are deiodinated by deiodinase to iodide and they become available again for synthesis.

T_3 and T_4 can escape from the follicle. MIT and DIT ordinarily do not escape because they are effectively deiodinated. Thyroglobulin was once thought incapable of entering the plasma, but there are claims that it is a normal component of blood.[9,10] T_3 appears in the plasma in relatively small amounts, but it is about seven times as active as T_4 (which constitutes 60 to 90% of the circulating organically bound iodine).

Normal Role of Iodine in T_4 Synthesis

Thyroid hormone formation depends initially upon the trapping of iodide from the circulation and the iodination of tyrosine. This process, noted previously, demands

Table 1
CHEMICAL STRUCTURE AND SCHEMA SHOWING PATHWAY OF BIOSYNTHESIS OF T_3 AND T_4

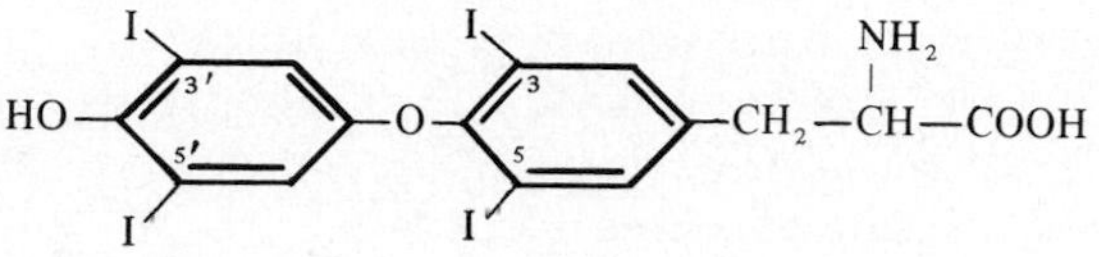

Thyroxine

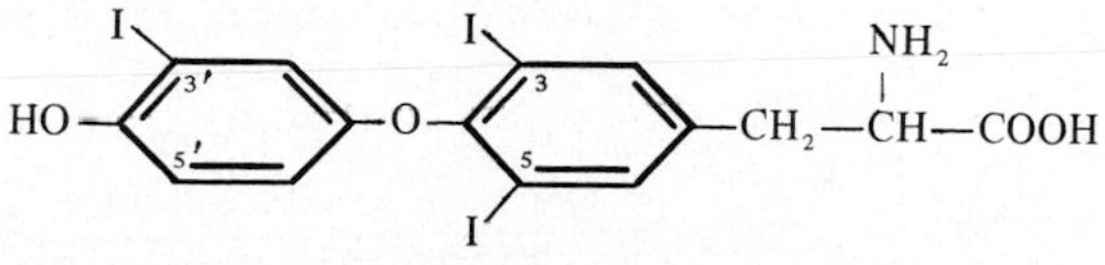

Triiodothyronine

The structures of thyroxine (T_4) and triiodothyronine (T_3).

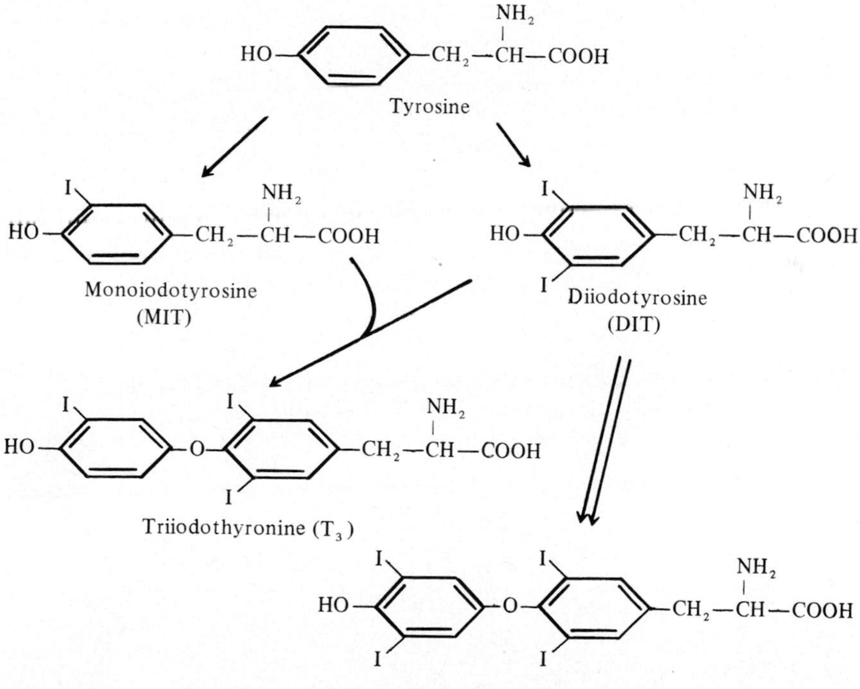

Tyrosine

Monoiodotyrosine
(MIT)

Diiodotyrosine
(DIT)

Triiodothyronine (T_3)

Throxine (Tetraiodothyronine, T_4)

Synthesis of the iodotyrosines (MIT, DIT) and the iodothyronines (T_3, T_4) from tyrosine.

the oxidation of inorganic iodide to iodine, I_2, in the presence of thyroid peroxidase. Normally, all the iodide is taken up by the gland, oxidized quickly, and bound to thyroglobulin. The high storage capacity of thyroglobulin for iodine and of the colloid lumen for thyroglobulin permits the thyroid to maintain a steady secretion of the iodothyronines long after any pathologic block of synthesis. The site of iodide transport in thyroid epithelial cells is most likely via the basal membrane, by active transport.

To form T_4, 100 to 150 μg of ingested iodine are required per day. The need increases in puberty, pregnancy, or stress of any kind including cold climates. Several forms of iodine may be ingested. Following reduction chiefly to iodide prior to intestinal absorption, the plasma concentration stays low since thyroid follicle cells trap (concentrate) iodide from blood by an iodide pump, at about 2 μg/hr. In maximal activity, the iodide can be concentrated to about 350 times the iodide concentration in the blood.[12] The ability to trap iodides is not unique to the thyroid. The substance is in high concentration in saliva, gastric juice, and the milk of nursing women, although none of these tissues uses the iodide to form T_4 (or T_3).

Thyrotropin is the most important factor affecting iodide transport in the thyroid and cAMP is the mediator of most thyrotropin effects on the thyroid including transport. Iodide transport is also subject to an autoregulatory mechanism which involves the total organic iodine concentration within the thyroid.

Forms of Iodine in Plasma

The iodine content within the plasma exists in several discrete fractions. The total amount in a normal adult is about 6 μg/100 mℓ or even more.[28] Of this, 90% represents organic iodine and the rest is "free" (inorganic). Almost all of the organic iodine is bound to protein and this is termed protein bound iodine (PBI). Diagnostically, the normal range of PBI is defined as 4 to 8 μg/100 mℓ serum. Excessive values occur in hyperthyroidism and low values in hypothyroidism. The major source of plasma iodide is dietary and the major route of any loss from the plasma is renal excretion.

Conservation of Iodine

Thyroglobulin contains T_3, T_4, and uncoupled mono and deiodityrosines. Upon thyroglobulin digestion these iodotyrosines are liberated and deiodinated by the enzyme deiodinase. The products are recirculated and used again to form thyroglobulin. There are thus two iodide pools (although they may not be distinctly separated).

Chemical Properties of T_4

The naturally occurring hormone is levorotatory. Synthetic thyroxine is a mixture of D- and L-isomers (racemic) and is considerably less active than the natural hormone.

Assay Techniques for T_4

Thyroxine is normally present in peripheral blood, accounting for 85 to 90% of organic iodine - containing compounds in the circulation. The plasma concentration of T_4 is 5 to 12 μg/100 mℓ. Radioimmunoassay (RIA) methods for T_4 (and T_3) came into use late in that field because the overall size of T_4 and T_3 convinced workers that they were not suitable antigens.

The methods for RIA of T_4 (and T_3) use variations of three basic steps (1) preparation of specific anti-T_4 (or anti-T_3) antibodies; (2) addition of isotopically labeled T_4 (or T_3) standards or serum to be tested and reaction with anti-T_4 (or T_3) antibody; and (3) separation of antibody-bound and free T_4 (or T_3). For a detailed discussion with references, the paper by Prasad and Hollander[29] is recommended.

Physiologic Actions and Mechanisms of Thyroxine

The actions have been described for T_4 (and T_3). Most of the actions can be explained on the basis of translation of specific RNA messages for synthesis of proteins and protein enzymes. Because of the diversity of actions, receptors must be very widespread in the body.

Transport of T_4 in the Blood

T_4 is secreted into the blood with great constancy, from 80 to 90 μg/day.[30] Upon release from the thyroid, T_4 (and T_3) are quickly bound to plasma proteins and very little remains free. T_4 (and T_3) are bound to proteins in the following decreasing order of affinity; thyroxine-binding globulin (TBG), thyroxine-binding prealbumin (TBPA), and albumin. These three carriers account for 60%, 30%, and 10%, respectively, of the T_4 binding capacity of serum. In regard to T_3, its affinity for TBG is two to six times less than that of T_4. There is more T_3 bound to albumin than to TBPA. The binding process is not a vital function, but it moderates losses of free hormones in passage through the liver and kidney. It also serves to adaptively regulate the rates of passage of the hormones to cells where metabolism and degradation occur.

The presence of more than a single protein binder has a purpose, e.g., TBG serves as a relatively inert hormonal reservoir whereas TBPA produces a labile, quickly available supply of hormones in response to demand.

Alterations of protein binding occur in several diseases, thyroid and extrathyroid, but the alterations do not upset the thyroid status because a feedback mechanism provides an adequacy in free hormone levels.

In the tissue areas, T_4 (and T_3) are freed from the binding proteins and pass through the capillaries to enter the tissue cells. It is thought that thyroid hormones can be bound to tissue proteins.

Metabolism and Fate of Thyroxine

T_4 (and T_3) can be processed in the liver and sent via the bile to the intestine. About 10% of T_4 is excreted daily by this route, mainly as free T_4, but to some extent conjugated as the beta glucuronide. In an alternate pathway, T_4 (and T_3) are oxidatively deaminated in the liver to pyruvic acid derivatives. Some T_4 is deiodinated in the periphery and the released iodide is recycled by the thyroid or excreted in the urine. The kidney is importantly involved in regulating T_4 (and T_3) plasma concentrations by excreting free and conjugated forms of T_4 (and T_3). Some of the metabolites passed into the intestine are resorbed and utilized again. Very little iodide is lost in the urine. T_4 metabolism also involves muscle where there are deiodination, oxidative deamination, and conjugation. T_4 may convert to T_3 in the tissues, perhaps 1/3 of the T_4 metabolized daily being deiodinated to T_3. The specific mechanisms are speculative.[31] The stepwise degrading of T_4 can give rise not only to T_3 but also to reverse T_3 (3,3,5-triiodothyronine). Reverse T_3 is a metabolically inactive hormone.

The deiodination of T_4 to T_3 in tissues is an important aspect of iodothyronine metabolism. It shows that T_3 within cells can have an extra thyroidal source. This explains the fact that there is much more T_3 turned over in the body than can be accomplished solely by thyroid secretion. T_3 can be produced from T_4 in the liver, kidneys, striated muscle, and elsewhere.

Relation of T_4 to Reverse T_3

Reverse T_3 (rT_3), or 3,3′,5′-triiodothyronine, which is physiologically inactive, occurs in human plasma. Its origin is the monodeiodination of the inner ring of T_4. This contrasts with T_3 which arises from monodeiodination of the outer ring of T_4.

There is current interest in rT_3 because its concentration is measurable in human serum by RIA and because its concentration is diagnostic in some pathologic conditions. The normal concentration in serum is about 40 ng/100 mℓ for a human adult, increasing in hyperthyroidism and decreasing in hypothyroidism.

The rT_3 in serum is mostly bound to proteins, about 0.3% remaining free. The secretion of about 90 ng of T_4 per day is accompanied by a secretion of about 1.2 μg of rT_3. Almost all rT_3 comes from peripheral deiodination of T_4.

TRIIODOTHYRONINE

Cell Source and Biosynthesis

Triiodothyronine (T_3) was described in 1952 and 1953 as a substance in the thyroid gland, by Gross and Pitt-Rivers.[32,33]

The cell source and the biosynthesis of T_3 from the amino acid tyrosine have been touched upon in the section discussing thyroxine. T_3 may be formed within the thyroid gland by coupling one molecule of DIT and one molecule of MIT. Within tissue cells T_3 may be formed by deiodination of T_4. This extrathyroid increment contrasts with T_4 which normally is derived only from thyroid activity, making T_4 the primary secretory product of the gland.

Iodide availability is important in regulating the formation of T_3 relative to T_4. A progressive increase in DIT/MIT with increasing degree of iodination favors T_4 over T_3 formation. Thus T_3 is enhanced in an iodine deficiency where MIT is greatly increased relative to DIT.

Chemical Structure

Refer to previous section on thyroxine.

Chemical Properties

Refer to previous section on thyroxine.

Assay Techniques

The techniques of RIA are discussed for T_3 by Prasad and Hollander.[26] The normal T_3 concentration in plasma is 100 to 160 ng/100 mℓ. This decreases in hypothyroidism and increases in hyperthyroidism. The RIA allows delineation of several clinical situations in which T_3 has a marked role, the outstanding situation being T_3 toxicosis. The current RIA methods for T_3 are suitable for routine clinical use.

Release of T_3 from Thyroglobulin (T_G)

The proteolysis of T_G releases its peptide-linked amino acids, T_3 (and T_4), into the circulation as free amino acids. The T_G digestion is brought about by an active proteolytic system of enzymes in the gland that have a lysosomal origin. The iodotyrosines do not escape into the plasma, but are deiodinated within the thyroid by a deiodinase which is active for iodotyrosines but not for iodothyronines.

Release of T_3 and T_4 into the circulation can be inhibited by many agents, including iodide, lithium, colchicine and others. Iodide in high doses is especially inhibitory.

The secretion (release) of thyroid hormones T_3 and T_4 is regulated by thyrotropin. Unlike the mechanism of secretion of insulin and pituitary hormones, where there is expulsion of contents to the cell exterior, T_3 and T_4 do not utilize an exocytotic process. Microtubules may be involved in thyroid hormone release.

Transport of T_3 in the Blood

Refer to the section on thyroxine. T_3, like T_4, is almost at once, and almost completely bound to serum proteins. Both T_3 and T_4 are predominantly bound to an inter-*d*-globulin called thyronine-binding globulin. Both T_3 and T_4 are bound to a lesser degree to albumin. T_3, unlike T_4, is hardly bound to a prealbumin. The proteins prolong the availability of the hormones and modulate the effects of any changes in their concentrations. They also serve as a reservoir for extrathyroid storage. The extrathyroid T_3 pool is about 5% of that for T_4.[30] Because of weaker binding, T_3 and T_4 tend to diffuse from blood to interstitial fluid as free hormones.

In distribution from blood to tissues, T_3 is found chiefly within cells in slowly equilibrating tissues whereas T_4 is found chiefly in plasma, interstitial fluid, and rapidly equilibrating tissues.

Metabolism and Fate of T_3

In the disposal of T_3 (and T_4), little or none of the glucuronide and sulfate conjugates sent from liver to bile is reabsorbed from the intestine. There is no enterohepatic cycle for T_3 and T_4. The conjugates are split in the intestine, thus explaining the presence of unconjugated residues in the feces.

T_3 is also disposed of by deiodination, without intermediate metabolite formation. Contrary to this, T_4 uses pathways involving the appearance of intermediary metabolites, including reverse T_3 and tetraiodothyroacetic acid, the former being biologically inactive and the latter active.

CALCITONIN

Cell Source of Calcitonin

Copp et al.[34,35] in 1961 and 1962, reported the presence of a hormone in blood, now called calcitonin (CT), which lowers plasma calcium and inorganic phosphorus. The origin of CA was said to be in the parathyroid gland. Foster et al.[36] established the fact that CA is secreted by the thyroid gland and they suggested that CA in the dog thyroid is formed in the parafollicular (C) cells. It is now known that the C cells are the major source of CA in the thyroid gland of man. The C cells in the human thyroid are the prime source of the 32 amino acid calcitonin monomer.

C cells in man comprise less than 0.1% of the epithelial cell mass of the thyroid. These cells are located in both parafollicular and intrafollicular regions, the former predominating. C cells tend to be isolated and are densest in the middle third of the lateral lobes, deep inside the parenchyma. Since CT in man is also present in the parathyroids and thymus,[31] the term calcitonin is preferable to the earlier term thyrocalcitonin. Also, in lower vertebrates, e.g., the chicken, a structure called the ultimobranchial bodies (UB) contains a large amount of CT whereas the thyroid gland has no detectable amount.

In vertebrate embryology there are relationships among the parafollicular cells, the UB, and the neural crest. Unlike the thyroid follicular cells, the parafollicular cells are derived from the neural crest and migrate to the region of the last branchial pouch. The UB also arise from the neural crest. The UB are paired glands originating at the level of the fourth and fifth pairs of gill pouches. They migrate near the caudal border of the thyroid gland. The C cells, originating in the neural crest, enter the thyroid with the UB component of the caudal pharyngeal pouches. Being of neural crest origin, in part or completely, C cells are related to the argentaffin cells of the adrenal medulla. This can explain why malignant degeneration of C cells, as in medullary thyroid carcinoma, may be associated with adrenal medullary tumors (pheochromocytoma).

Chemical Structure

All known chemical species of calcitonins consist of a single sequence, 32 amino acid polypeptide chain. The chain contains a 1 to 7 disulfide bridge at the NH_2-end and prolinamide at the carboxy-terminal amino acid residue. CTs from various animal species differ in specific residues within the chain, producing marked variations in immunologic activity.

The major C-cell secretory product, calcitonin monomer, has a molecular weight of about 3500 daltons. Rat CT most closely resembles the hormone in man, differing by only two amino acids. Salmon CT, which differs from human CT in 16 amino acids, is the only form available therapeutically in the U.S. The salmon form is immunogenic. Salmon CT is the most potent one to lower serum calcium.

An outline of the amino acid sequence of human CT is shown in Table 2. The entire sequence of 32 amino acids has been thought to be essential to its biologic activity, but modifications with bioactivity are under experimentation.[37]

Table 2
OUTLINE OF AMINO ACID SEQUENCE OF HUMAN CALCITONIN

H_2N-	Cys-	Gly-	Asn-	Lev-	Ser-	Thr-	Cys-	Met-	Leu-	Gly-		
	1	2	3	4	5	6	7	8	9	10		
-	Thr-	Tyr-	Thr-	Gln-	Asp-	Phe-	Asn-	Lys-	Phe-	His-	Thr-	
	11	12	13	14	15	16	17	18	19	20	21	
-	Phe-	Pro-	Gln-	Thr-	Ala-	Ile-	Gly-	Val-	Gly-	Ala-	Pro[a]-	C = 0
	22	23	24	25	26	27	28	29	30	31	32	NH_2

[a] Pro is prolinamide.

Bioassays

Procedures which measure CT in serum are amply discussed elsewhere.[37,38] Early CA measurements were based on the hypocalcemic effect resulting from CT injection into young rats, but this method is insufficiently sensitive for normal human plasma.

Several RIA procedures easily measure CT in normal human blood. The value of plasma immunoreactive CT during fasting is less than 100 pg/mℓ,[37] although some investigators report up to 600 pg/mℓ. The major biologically active species in blood appears to be the CT monomer.

Assays with less sensitivity than the RIA include radioreceptor and adenylate cyclase assays.[37]

Chemical Properties of Calcitonin

Although the complete 32 amino acid peptide is essential for full biologic activity, the integrity of the first nine amino acids appears to be of primary importance.

Regulation of Secretion

There is uncertainty about the chief physiologic regulator of CT secretion. High calcium concentrations in extracellular fluids stimulate CT release whereas low calcium concentrations inhibit it. The major stimulus may be hypercalcemia. Magnesium increase is also implicated, but the importance of magnesium is unclear.

Among the gut hormones, gastrin is a potent secretagogue for CT, but in pharmacologic doses only.

The autonomic nervous system may be involved. β-adrenergic agonists are experimentally found to increase CT secretion.

Overall, a large number of substances stimulate or inhibit CT secretion. No firm conclusions can yet be drawn about the mechanisms involved.

Physiologic Actions of Calcitonin

CT, like parathyroid hormone, is involved in actions upon bone, kidney, and gut. It is a part of the mechanism for calcium homeostasis, acting with the parathyroid to maintain blood level calcium constancy. In lower vertebrates it is part of the fluid and electrolyte control mechanisms.

CT protects bone by inhibiting osteoclastic bone resorption, permitting the ingress of calcium and phosphate, bu preventing their egress. CT regulates the rate of skeletal remodeling. It is thought that CT plays a role in prenatal as well as postnatal bone development. In the fetus, CT is much higher in umbilical arterial blood than it is in venous blood at term, indicating a fetal rather than a placental origin.[39]

Pharmacologic administration of CT in man decreases renal tubular resorption of calcium and phosphate and also of sodium, potassium, and magnesium.[37] A deficiency of CT, however, is not known to disturb renal processing of calcium, phosphate, or sodium, thus suggesting that physiologic levels of CT do not affect the kidney.

Pharmacologic doses of CT decrease gastrin and gastric acid secretion and they increase small-bowel secretion of sodium, potassium, chloride, and water. CT does not appear to affect intestinal absorption of calcium.[37]

Mechanism and Site of Action of Calcitonin

CT binds to membrane receptors in target cells and stimulates cAMP production. Whether cAMP is the second messenger is inconclusive.

The primary site of action of CT is the skeleton where it blocks bone resorption caused by parathyroid hormone. The mechanism of action of CT within the cells is uncertain. In bone cells it lowers calcium concentration in the cytosol. This may be brought about by enhancing calcium loss from the cells and increasing calcium uptake by the mitochondria. The decrease in cell calcium activates adenylate cyclase and leads to increased cAMP. Bone resorption is inhibited because calcium lowering in the cytosol inactivates some phosphoprotein products of the protein kinases which are cAMP dependent.

Metabolism and Fate of Calcitonin

CT occurs in human blood at less than 100 pg/mℓ. The CT monomer when injected leaves the plasma with a half-life of about 10 min.[37] Metabolism takes place chiefly in the kidney. The monomer is processed therein by filtration and resorption. Subsequent degradation may occur in human plasma partly by a heat-labile factor. Other, unknown mechanisms for degradation must exist.

Calcitonin in Disease

There are no definite syndromes associated with a deficiency of CT. However, CT elevation is the serum is seen in human thyroid medullary carcinomas, which are tumors of the C cells. These persons have no known abnormality of mineral or skeletal metabolism. The plasma phosphorus and magnesium levels may not be affected. In all other clinical disorders associated with increased CT in the blood there are also no consistent mineral or skeletal abnormalities attributable specifically to the calcitonin excess.

Despite the uncertainty about CT effects, the hormone has therapeutic value in man primarily in the treatment of Paget's disease of bone. It decreases the number of osteoclasts and lowers alkaline phosphatase and also the urinary excretion of hydroxyproline. The parenteral administration of CT can often restore the calcium balance.

THE HYPOTHALAMIC-PITUITARY-THYROID AXIS IN RELATION TO THYROID DEVELOPMENT IN THE HUMAN FETUS AND NEONATE

This brief discussion is an amplification of that considered in a previous section on anatomy. The reader is referred to a review by Fisher and Klein[40] for an excellent, detailed account, from part of which the present data have been abstracted.

Embryology

The human placenta does not allow passage of T_3, T_4, rT_3, and TSH, so that the thyroid control system of the fetus is not maternally regulated. The fetal system can be influenced by pharmacologic, but not physiologic concentrations of TRH.

By at most the 12th week of gestation, the histologic structures of the thyroid and pituitary are generally well developed and the ability exists to produce pituitary TSH, resulting in measurable amounts of T_4 in the serum. By the 35th week at most, the hypothalamus and its portal blood system have matured, TRH being detectable at 10 to 12 weeks in the serum.

At 18 to 20 weeks, thyroid activity is increasing, with corresponding increases in serum T_4. At the same period, TSH levels have increased, peaking in the serum by the early third trimester of gestation.

The concentration of serum T_3 continues to increase from an unmeasurable amount at 30 weeks to about 50 ng/dℓ at term, with an additional sixfold increase in the first neonatal day.

The serum rT_3 levels keep decreasing from 250 ng/dℓ in the early third trimester to term and the levels drop further in the first 10 or so neonatal days.

Negative Feedback Regulation

As T_4 levels rise, they exert an inhibitory effect upon TSH output. It is probable that T_4 is first monodeiodinated to T_3 which in turn feeds back upon the pituitary. This control system is present at term and is not identifiable in the preterm fetus. An increased enzyme protein synthesis and/or activation of existing enzyme protein may produce the conversion of T_4 to T_3, in the liver.

Thyroid Regulation by TSH

TSH levels are fairly constant from the early 3rd trimester to term whereas the T_4 levels are rising in the same period. It appears that the responsiveness of the thyroid to TSH is continually increasing in late pregnancy.

Whereas the fetal thyroid is controllable by T_4/T_3 interactions with pituitary TSH output, the thyroid gland in the adult can autoregulate iodine uptake and transfer even without regard to TSH variations.

Maturation of Responsive Processes in Target Organs

How and when the end-organs in tissues develop responsiveness to thyroid secretions is virtually unknown. It is found in the rat that hepatic nuclear T_3-receptors mature the 1st few weeks after birth. There is even earlier maturation of the T_3-receptors in the rat brain and it is suggested that nerve growth factor is the mediator of thyroid effects on brain maturation.

The Neonate

TSH rises abruptly in the serum at birth, peaking in about ½ hr, and then decreasing quickly to the end of the first day, followed by a slower decrease for the succeeding 48 hr.

Serum T_3 and free T_3 levels increase up to sixfold in the first few hours after birth. Most of the increase is attributable to a conversion of T_4 to T_3. There is a delayed, second T_3 peak from 24 to 36 postnatal hr, again because of high T_4 levels which are quickly converted to T_3.

Serum T_4 and free T_4 levels are highest at about 24 hr, decreasing gradually for several weeks.

The quick release of the thyroid hormones into the circulation is a result of the stress of the cool neonatal environment upon the pituitary, which then activates the thyroid by TSH release.

REFERENCES

1. **Stevenson, G. F.,** The early history of the thyroid gland, in *Evaluation of Thyroid and Parathyroid Functions,* Sunderman, F. W., and Sunderman, F. W., Jr., Eds., J. P. Lippincott, Philadelphia, 1963, 3.
2. **Melander, A.,** Sympathetic nervous-adrenal medullary system, in *The Thyroid,* 4th ed., Werner, S. C. and Ingbar, S. H., Eds., Harper & Row, New York, 1978, 216.
3. **Fisher, D. A.,** Thyroid physiology and function tests in infancy and childhood, in *The Thyroid,* 4th ed., Werner, S. C. and Ingbar, S. H., Eds., Harper & Row, New York, 1978, 375.
4. **Werner, S. C. and Ingbar, S. H.,** *The Thyroid,* 4th ed., Harper & Row, New York, 1978.
5. **Werner, S. C.,** Embryology: normal and anomalous development and clinical aspects, in *The Thyroid,* 4th ed., Werner, S. C. and Ingbar, S. H., Eds., Harper & Row, New York, 1978, 397.
6. **Chopra, I. S.,** Thyroid hormones and respiratory distress syndrome of the newborn, *N. Eng. J. Med.,* 295, 335, 1976.
7. **Turner, C. D. and Bagnara, J. T.,** *General Endocrinology,* 6th ed., W. B. Saunders, Philadelphia, 1976.
8. **Carlson, L. D.,** Nonshivering thermogenesis and its endocrine control, *Fed. Proc.,* 19, (Suppl. 5), 25, 1960.
9. **Van Herle, A. J., Vassart, G., and Dumont, J. E.,** Control of thyroglobulin synthesis and secretion, *N. Eng. J. Med.,* 301, 239, 1979.
10. **Van Herle, A. J., Vassart, G., and Dumont, J. E.,** Control of thyroglobulin synthesis and secretion, *N. Eng. J. Med.,* 301, 307, 1979.
11. **Montgomery, D. A. D. and Welbourn, R. B.,** *Medical and Surgical Endocrinology,* Williams & Wilkins, Baltimore, 1975.
12. **Guyton, A. C.,** *Textbook of Medical Physiology,* 5th ed., W. B. Saunders, Philadelphia, 1976.
13. **Gudernatsch, J. F.,** Feeding experiments on tadpoles, *Arch. Entwicklungsmechanik. Organismen,* 35, 457, 1912.
14. **Furuichi, Y., Muthukrishnan, S., Thomasz, J., and Shatkin, A. J.,** Mechanism of formation of reovirus mRNA 5 -terminal blocked and methylated sequence, m^7GpppG^mpC, *J. Biol. Chem.,* 251, 5043, 1976.
15. **Pavlovic-Hournac, M., Rappaport, L., and Nunez, J.,** Incorporation of labelled amino acid into protein by thyroid glands from hypophysectomized rats. I. *In vitro* studies, *Endocrinology,* 89, 1477, 1971.
16. **Vassart, G., Brocas, H., Lecocq, R., and Dumont, J. E.,** Thyroglobulin messenger RNA: translation of 33-S mRNA into a peptide immunologically related to thyroglobulin, *Eur. J. Biochem.,* 55, 15, 1975.
17. **Vassart, G., Refetoff, S., Brocas, H., Dinsart, C., and Dumont, J. E.,** Translation of thyroglobulin 33-S messenger RNA as a means of determining thyroglobulin quarternary structure, *Proc. Natl. Acad. Sci. U.S.A.,* 72, 3839, 1975.
18. **De Nayer, P., Caucheteux, D., and Luypaert, B.,** Identification of RNA species with messenger activity in the thyroid gland, *FEBS Lett.,* 76, 316, 1977.
19. **Waechter, C. J. and Lennarz, W. J.,** The role of polyprenol-linked sugars in glycoprotein synthesis, *Ann. Rev. Biochem.,* 45, 95, 1976.
20. **Ekhohm, R., Engstrom, G., Ericson, L. E., and Melander, A.,** Exocytosis of protein into the thyroid follicle lumen: an early effect of TSH, *Endocrinology,* 97, 337, 1975.
21. **Hjort, T.,** Determination of serum-thyroglobulin by a haemagglutination-inhibition test, *Lancet,* 1, 1262, 1961.
22. **Assem, E. S. K.,** Thyroglobulin in the serum of parturient women and newborn infants, *Lancet,* 1, 139, 1964.
23. **Van Herle, A. J., Uller, R. P., Matthews, N. L., and Brown, J.,** Radioimmuneassay for measurement of thyroglobulin in human serum, *J. Clin. Invest.,* 52, 1320, 1973.
24. **Van Herle, A. J., Klandorf, H., and Uller, R. P.,** A radioimmuneassay for serum rat thyroglobulin: physiologic and pharmacological studies, *J. Clin. Invest.,* 56, 1073, 1975.
25. **Bodlaender, P., Arjonilla, J. R., Sweat, R., and Twomey, S. L.,** A practical immunoassay of thyroglobulin, *Clin. Chem.,* 24, 267, 1978.
26. **Uller, R. P., Van Herle, A. J., and Chopra, I. J.,** Thyroidal response to graded dose of bovine thyrotropin, *J. Clin. Endocrinol. Metab.,* 45, 312, 1977.
27. **Edelhoch, H. and Robbins, J.,** Thyroglobulin: chemistry and biosynthesis, in *The Thyroid,* 4th ed., Werner, S. C. and Ingbar, S. H., Eds., Harper & Row, New York, 1978, 62.
28. **Brobeck, J. R.,** Ed., *Best & Taylor's Physiological Basis of Medical Practice,* 10th ed., Williams & Wilkins, Baltimore, 7, 37, 1977.

29. **Prasad, J. A. and Hollander, C. S.,** Thyroxine and triiodothyronine, in *Methods of Hormone Radioimmuneassay,* Jaffe, B. M. and Behrman, H. R., Eds., Academic Press, New York, 1979, 375.
30. **Nicoloff, J. T.,** Thyroid hormone transport and metabolism: pathophysiologic implications, in *The Thyroid,* 4th ed., Werner, S. C. and Ingbar, S. H., Eds., Harper & Row, New York, 1978, 88.
31. **Hall, R., Anderson, J., Smart, G. A., and Besser, M.,** *Fundamentals of Clinical Endocrinology,* 2nd ed., Pitman, New York, 1974, 73.
32. **Gross, J. and Pitt-Rivers, R.,** The identification of 3:5:3′-1-triiodothyronine in human plasma, *Lancet,* 262, 439, 1953.
33. **Gross, J. and Pitt-Rivers, R.,** 3:5:3′ triidothyronine - isolation from thyroid gland and synthesis, *Biochem. J.,* 53, 645, 1953.
34. **Copp, D. H., Davidson, A. G. F., and Cheney, B. A.,** Evidence for a new parathyroid hormone which lowers blood calcium, *Proc. Canad. Fed. Biol. Soc.,* 4, 17, 1961.
35. **Copp, D. H., Cheney, B. A., Davidson, A. G. F., and Dube, W. J.,** Hypercalcemia after parathyroidectomy. The homeostatic role of calcitonin, *Fed. Proc.,* 21(2), 206, 1962.
36. **Foster, G. F., MacIntyre, I., and Pearse, A. G. E.,** Calcitonin production and the mitochondrion-rich cells of the dog thyroid, *Nature (London),* 203, 1029, 1964.
37. **Austin, L. A., and Heath, H.,** Calcitonin, physiology and pathophysiology, *N. Eng. J. Med.,* 304, 269, 1981.
38. **Tashjian, A. and Voelkel, E. F.,** Human calcitonin: application of affinity chromatography, in *Methods of Hormone Radioimmuneassay,* Jaffe, B. M. and Behrman, H. R., Eds., Academic Press, New York, 1979, 355.
39. **Samaan, N. A., Anderson, G. D., and Adam-Mayne, M. E.,** Immunoreactive calcitonin in the mother, neonate, child and adult, *Am. J. Obst. Gynecol.,* 121, 622, 1975.
40. **Fisher, D. A. and Klein, A. H.,** Thyroid development and disorders of thyroid function in the newborn, *N. Eng. J. Med.,* 304, 702, 1981.

THE PARATHYROID GLAND

Jerry G. Hurst

ANATOMY OF THE PARATHYROID GLAND (PTG)

Embryologic Origin

Most mammals have two pairs of PTG. The superior PTGs originate from the fourth pharyngeal pouch and the inferior ones from the third one, although there is some evidence that they originate as placodes of neuroectoderm. They are often found in association with the thyroid and/or thymus.

Number and Location

The location of the PTGs in the adult animal varies considerably among species and between individuals within a species. Table 1 gives the number and general location of the PTG of some mammalian species. It is not unusual, however, to find ectopic PTG tissue. This plus the fact that a PTG may be small, accounts for the difficulty often encountered in attempts to remove PTG adenomas.

Histology

The PTG is encased in a delicate connective tissue capsule which dips down into the gland at irregular places, forming incomplete and odd-sized segments. These septa carry blood vessels and autonomic nerve fibers into the gland. The parenchyma of the PTG consists of chief cells (which synthesize and secrete PTH) and, in some species beyond a certain age, oxyphilic cells (whose functions remain unknown). Many species do not have oxyphilic cells, but humans and ruminants do. The infant and young human PTG has no oxyphilic cells, but commencing at about age 7 years they first appear and increase in number thereafter. The PTG of older individuals also contain fat cells.

Chief Cells

The chief cells are the most numerous and, in most mammals, the only parenchymal cells in the PTG. They are 4 to 8 μm in diameter and are arranged more or less into cords or clumps. The small size means that the nuclei, when seen through the light microscope, appear close together. The cytoplasm is never very darkly staining, but it is darker in some cells than others. These are called "dark chief cells" or simply "dark cells" to distinguish them from the light cells whose cytoplasm is less darkly staining. The cytoplasm of some chief cells stains so poorly that they are called clear cells. The lighter ones contain more glycogen than darker ones and are considered to be inactive cells. The chief cells are slightly acidophilic, contain membrane bound secretory granules (200 to 400 nm in diameter) which have a denser center than periphery, have a well developed Golgi complex and show a rough endoplasmic reticulum.

A chief cell undergoes cyclic change going from a resting to a synthesizing to a packaging to a secreting cell and then back to a resting stage. The ratio of resting to active chief cells is about 4 to 1 during normocalcemia and 10 to 1 during chronic hypercalcemia.

Oxyphilic Cells

The oxyphilic cells, present in postjuvenile humans and ruminants are 6 to 10 μm in diameter. They have cytoplasmic granules which stain brightly with eosin stain and they are rich in mitochondria and oxidative enzymes. Their functions, if any, are unknown. Since they appear after the chief cells, they may be derived from them.

Table 1
NUMBERS AND LOCATIONS OF PTGs IN SOME MAMMALS[204]

Species	Number of PTGs	
Human	4	Two superior and two inferior glands located on the posterior quadrants of the thyroid gland. They are themselves encapsulated and, although often enclosed by the fascia encompassing the thyroid, they are usually outside the thyroid capsule.
Bovine Sheep Goat	4	Two large superior (often called external) glands lie several centimeters anterior to the anterior borders of the thyroid near the common carotid and often associated with the thymus. Two much smaller inferior (internal) glands, usually attached to the posterior (inferior) poles of the thyroid.
Dog Cat	4	Two superior glands near the anterior border of the thyroid gland. 2 inferior glands on the medial surface of thyroid glands. The superior glands are somewhat larger than inferior ones.
Horse	4	Two superior glands anterior to the upper poles of the thyroid gland. Two inferior glands many centimeters below the thyroid near the bifurcation of the bicarotid trunk near the 1st rib.
Pig	2	They would correspond to superior PTGs of other animals. They are in the thymus and near the bifurcation of the common carotid.
Rat	2	They are located close to the thyroid gland.

Fat Cells

There are few fat cells in the young human PTG but they increase with age and may constitute over 50% of the PTG weight in old age.

CHEMISTRY AND BIOSYNTHESIS OF PARATHYROID HORMONE (PTH)

Extraction and Purification of PTH

In 1925 Collip was the first to successfully extract a factor from bovine parathyroid tissue which would elevate the plasma Ca when injected into a dog.[1] He used hot HCl to extract this factor, a rather harsh extraction procedure which extracts many other components. Later, phenol and other solvents were used to extract this active factor which could be removed from the solution by salt fractionation or by precipitation with organic solvents or trichloroacetic acid.[2] The precipitate may be further purified by gel filtration followed with ion exchange chromatography on carboxymethylcellulose in a urea buffer.[3] Such treatment results in an active factor (PTH) of sufficiently high purity for analysis. Basically, this procedure has been used to purify bovine, porcine and human PTH.

Structure of PTH

Primary and Secondary Structure

Amino acid analysis of the highly purified PTH has shown PTH to be a single chain polypeptide of 84 amino acids for the three species in which its amino acid sequence has been determined. It has no cysteine residues and consequently no disulfide bridges. The primary structure of PTH is shown in Table 2[4-6,8] with the amino terminal residue being number 1 and the carboxyl terminal residue being number 84. Since bovine PTH

Table 2
THE PRIMARY STRUCTURE OF bPTH, pPTH AND hPTH

Residue Number	Amino Acid in This Position			Residue Number	Amino Acid in This Position		
	bPTH[4]	pPTH[5]	hPTH[6,8]		bPTH	pPTH	hPTH
1	NH_2-Ala	Ser	Ser	46	Gly		Ala
2	Val			47	Ser		Gly
3	Ser			48	Ser		
4	Glu			49	Gln		
5	Ile			50	Arg		
6	Gln			51	Pro		
7	Phe		Leu	52	Arg		
8	Met			53	Lys		
9	His			54	Lys		
10	Asn			55	Glu		
11	Leu			56	Asp		
12	Gly			57	Asn		
13	Lys			58	Val		
14	His			59	Leu		
15	Leu			60	Val		
16	Ser		Asn	61	Glu		
17	Ser			62	Ser		
18	Met	Leu		63	His		
19	Glu			64	Gln		Glu
20	Arg			65	Lys		
21	Val			66	Ser		
22	Glu		Glu? Gln?	67	Leu		
23	Trp			68	Gly		
24	Leu			69	Glu		
25	Arg			70	Ala		
26	Lys			71	Asp		
27	Lys			72	Lys		
28	Leu		Leu? Lys?	73	Ala		
29	Gln			74	Aps	Ala	
30	Asp		Asp? Leu?	75	Val		
31	Val			76	Asp		
32	His			77	Val		
33	Asn			78	Leu		
34	Phe			79	Ile		Thr
35	Val			80	Lys		
36	Ala			81	Ala		
37	Leu			82	Lys		
38	Gly			83	Pro		Ser
39	Ala			84	Gln-COOH		
40	Ser		Pro				
41	Ile		Leu				
42	Ala	Val					
43	Tyr	His	Pro				
44	Arg						
45	Asp						

Note: See any standard biochemistry textbook for meaning of the symbols for the various amino acids.

(bPTH) was the first to be isolated and sequenced, it is given in full. In the other columns of Table 2 the amino acids of human (hPTH) and porcine PTH (pPTH) are given where they differ from bPTH. The preponderance of basic amino acid residues (arginine and lysine) impart an overall positive electrical charge to the molecule.[7] The molecule appears to have some secondary structure with α-helixes in the ends and random coil in the middle.

There is close homology between the PTH molecules of the three species (Table 2). This has permitted the measurement by radioimmunoassay of PTH (iPTH) in several species using the more readily available bPTH as a tracer hormone and for inducing the formation of antisera which are used in the assay.

Minimum Primary Structure Required for Biologic Activity

Utilizing the in vivo chick hypercalcemic or the in vitro renal adenylate cyclase responses, the amino-terminal 1-34 (amino acid) fragment of bPTH retains full biologic activity when compared on an equimolar basis. Removal of the amino-terminal residue (alanine) of bPTH 1-34 results in a marked decrease in biologic activity and removal of the first and second residues (alanine and valine, see Table 2) completely abolishes biologic activity. Shortening of the bPTH 1-34 fragment at the carboxyl end results in diminished activity with minimal activity still retained by bPTH 1-27. Further shortening results in complete loss of activity.[9]

bPTH is considerably more potent than hPTH or pPTH in some in vitro assays and the same is true for the 1-34 fragments of bPTH. This is probably due to the amino-terminal serine of hPTH 1-34. When replaced by alanine the activity of hPTH 1-34 approaches that of bPTH 1-34. In some in vivo assays, the potency of bPTH 1-34 and hPTH 1-34 are comparable.[7]

Analogues of PTH

Various modifications of the synthetic PTH 1-34 molecule have been made in attempts to either increase the potency of the hormone or to develop biologically inactive analogues which will act as competitive inhibitors with the native hormone to be used to block the action of endogenous PTH in the treatment of hyperparathyroidism. A few such blocking hormones have been synthesized. Clinical usefulness of such analogues awaits the development of forms which have a high affinity for the PTH receptors of target tissues.

Biosynthesis of PTH

Several reviews on the biosynthesis of PTH have been published.[10-13]

Precursors of PTH

Proparathyroid Hormone (ProPTH)

Until about 1970 it was thought that PTH was synthesized as an 84 amino acid peptide. In 1971 Cohn et al.[14] reported the presence of a non-PTH calcemic factor in bPTG tissue and a year later their group[15] as well as Kempter et al.[16] reported it to be a precursor to PTH. It is called proparathyroid hormone (ProPTH) and contains (in all species thus far studied) six additional amino acid residues as a straight chain hexapeptide attached to the amino-terminal end of the PTH 1-84 molecule. These six have been numbered -1 through -6, starting with the one attached to the N terminal amino acid residue of PTH 1-84. Thus, ProPTH consist of 90 amino acids, -6 through 84 (Table 3). Dilute trypsin or PTG extracts can convert ProPTH to PTH.

Preproparathyroid Hormone (PreProPTH)

After the discovery of ProPTH, Kemper et al.[17] discovered that RNA from parathyroid tissue could synthesize, in a cell-free system, a molecule which was immunologically and chemically related to both PTH and ProPTH, except that it was larger by 25 amino acid residues than ProPTH. They named this product preproparathyroid hormone (PreProPTH) and offered evidence that it was a precursor to ProPTH. The additional amino acid residues of PreProPTH are attached to the amino-terminal end of ProPTH and are numbered -7 through -31. Thus, PreProPTH has 115 amino acid residues which, from the amino-terminal to carboxyl-terminal end, are numbered -31 through 84 (Table 3).

Table 3
THE AMINO ACID SEQUENCE OF BOVINE PREPROPARATHYROID HORMONE (bPreProPTH) AND BOVINE PROPARATHYROID HORMONE (bProPTH) AND HOW THEY RELATE TO bPTH

Name of molecule	Amino acid residue number	Amino acid in this position
PreProPTH (−31 to 84)	−31	NH_2 — Met
	−30	Met
	−29	Ser
	−28	Ala
	−27	Lys
	−26	Asp
	−25	Met
	−24	Val
	−23	Lys
	−22	Val
	−21	Met
	−20	Ile
	−19	Val
	−18	Met
	−17	Leu
	−16	Ala
	−15	Ile
	−14	Cys
	−13	Phe
	−12	Leu
	−11	Ala
	−10	Arg
	−9	Ser
	−8	Asp
	−7	Gly
ProPTH (−6 to 84)	−6	Lys
	−5	Ser
	−4	Val
	−3	Lys
	−2	Lys
	−1	Arg
PTH (1 to 84)	1	Ala
	2	Val
	3	Ser
	See Table 2 for the 4—83 Sequence	
	84	Gln-COOH

Biosynthesis of PreProPTH and ProPTH

Messenger RNA (mRNA) extracted from PTG tissue codes for the synthesis of PreProPTH. It is not known whether this mRNA is a direct transcription of nuclear DNA or if it has been changed after it is transcribed. Evidence[10-13] from in vitro experiments supports a general outline of PreProPTH synthesis:

Transcription Phase	Nuclear DNA	—Triphosphoribonucleotides / RNA Polymerase→	mRNA	Post Transcriptional Modifications?
			↓	"Excision"?
Transitional Phase	PrePro PTH	←tRNA-Amino Acid / Polyribosomes (on rough endoplasmic reticulum)—	mRNA	"Clipping"? "Rejoining"? "Capping"?

Translation of mRNA occurs on polyribosomes of the endoplasmic reticulum (ER) of the PTG chief cells utilizing amino-acid bearing (transfer RNA) molecules. When the growing polypeptide chain is 20 to 30 amino acid residues long (i.e., when it extends from -31 to -10 or so amino acid residues), it emerges from the polyribosome and the amino terminal methionine(s) is(are) removed. This leaves exposed the -29 to -10 or so end which is hydrophobic and which attaches to the wall of the ER and directs the growing polypeptide chain into the cisternal lumen of the ER. Soon after or even before the number 84 residue (the 115th amino acid) of PreProPTH is released from the ribosome, the presequence (-29 through -7), also known as the leader sequence or signal segment/sequence, of PreProPTH is cleaved.[19] This results in the formation of ProPTH in the lumen of the ER. Translation of the 115 amino acid PreProPTH takes about 1 min. The function of the presequence (leader, signal sequence) of PreProPTH is probably to get the molecule into the lumen of the ER so it can be transported into the Golgi Apparatus for packaging into secretory granules.

A leader sequence may be a general property of most or even all polypeptides which are destined to be secreted (e.g., insulin, placental lactogenic hormone, pancreatic enzymes, immunoglobulins, growth hormone, prolactin, and serum albumin). In all cases, the leader sequence is located on the amino-terminal end of the molecule.

There may be a minimal length requirement for mRNA to span the polyribosome. Since the minimal length appears to be about 50 codons (50 amino acids) and since PTH has 84 amino acids, it would appear that PTH exceeds this minimal length and does not require the leader sequence for this function.

Biosynthesis of PTH

The result of the transcription, translation, and peptide cleavage of PreProPTH results in the presence of ProPTH in the lumina of the endoplasmic reticulum (ER). From there, ProPTH is transported to the Golgi apparatus where the pro-portion of the molecule (-6 through -1 amino acid residues) is cleaved, yielding the native PTH 1-84. It takes 15 min from the time radioactive amino acids are added to the incubation medium of PTH tissue until both rdioactive ProPTH and radioactive PTH are found in the Golgi apparatus.[22]

The function of ProPTH is unknown and although it is tempting to ascribe to it a role in intracellular transport or packaging of PTH, there is no direct evidence that it functions thus.

The cleavage of ProPTH occurs at basic amino acid sites (lysine-arginine-alanine site, -2, -1, and 1 residue) between arginine and alanine and is catalyzed by an endopeptidase with trypsin-like activity.[23,24] Cohn's group has named the enzyme, which is found mainly in the microsomal fraction of PTG homogenates, convertase[10] and has shown that it is like but not identical to trypsin.[24] The result of this cleavage in vitro is PTH 1-84 and a hexapeptide (-6 through -1, see Table 3). The hexapeptide is attacked by exopeptidases and converted into a mixture of penta- and tetrapeptides. In vivo experiments have failed to show the presence of any of these peptides in intact PTG.[10] Whether the hexapeptide or any of its metabolites has a physiologic function is unknown.

Packaging, Secretion, and Intracellular Degradation of PTH

In the Golgi apparatus newly formed PTH is packaged into membrane bound vesicles known as secretory granules. The PTH can be (1) immediately secreted to the cell surface by exocytosis; (2) immediately degraded; or (3) stored within the gland for future secretion or degradation.[10] As currently understood from in vitro experiments, the PTG does all three. Within 30 to 45 min after adding radiolabeled amino acids to the incubation medium, radiolabeled PTH is detectable in the medium. Since it takes

15 min for PTH to appear in the Golgi apparatus, an additional 15 to 30 min are required for packaging of PTH, transport to the cell surface membrane and exocytosis to occur. Not much newly synthesized hormone is added to the intracellular store of hormone after the addition of radiolabelled amino acids. Most of it is secreted or undergoes intracellular degradation.

There appear to be two types of PTH-containing secretory granules in the PTG cells. One type is more electron dense than the other. The denser ones are known as mature granules and the others are called immature granules. Not much is known about the preferential release of one over the other, but some evidence has been presented which indicates that secretion of the immature granules may occur independently of secretion of the more mature ones.[25] Most of the iPTH in the chief cells is located in these secretory granules and essentially none is found in the nucleus or mitochondria.[26,27,30,31] The relative proportion of intracellular PTH located in the two kinds of granules probably varies with age and/or physiologic state of the gland.[31]

Some PTH and/or ProPTH undergoes intracellular degradation within the chief cells and the degradation is directly related to the concentration of Calcium in the incubation medium.[28,29] ECF Ca concentration is the main regulator of PTH secretion rate. A high Ca concentration inhibits and a low Ca concentration "stimulates" PTH secretion rate. Thus, intracellular degradation of PTH (or ProPTH) may play a major role in regulating PTH secretion rate from the PTG cells.[10]

PARATHYROID SECRETORY PROTEIN

It has been recognized since 1970 that the PTG secretes, in vitro, newly synthesized proteins which are different from PTH or its fragments.[32,33] Among these non-PTH proteins a major one is parathyroid secretory protein (PSP).[34] It is a dimere made up of two identical subunits (monomeres) with molecular weights of about 70,000 each. The secretion of PSP is inhibited by calcium as is the secretion of PTH. The secretion ratio of PTH to PSP is about 6 to 1.[34] PSP is a glycoprotein[35] and is found in the same cells and organelles as is PTH.[36] Its function remains unknown, but it is tempting to ascribe to it a role in the intracellular transport of PTH.[35]

SECRETION OF FRAGMENTS OF PTH BY PTG

There is a calcium-independent, nonsuppressible component of parathyroid secretion.[37] Even at very high plasma calcium concentrations there are still significant quantities of immunoreactive PTH (iPTH) secreted. In vivo work from our laboratory utilizing the calf has shown that this material is predominantly carboxyl fragment(s) of the PTH molecule which are biologically inactive.[37,38] The proportion of carboxyl fragments to intact hormone varies with the plasma calcium concentration ([Ca]p). Thus when [Ca]p is high, the secretion of intact PTH is low and nearly all of the iPTH occurs as carboxyl fragment(s). As the [Ca]p is lowered, the PTH secretion rate increases and the ratio of intact hormone to carboxyl fragment increases.[38] If intracellular degradation of PTH plays a major role in the regulation of PTH secretion rate, and if an increase in [Ca]p increases that intracellular degradation of PTH, it is not surprising that the major, nonsuppressible PTH secretory product of the PTG during hypercalcemia is a biologically inactive PTH fragment.

We were unable to demonstrate the secretion of a biologically active, amino-terminal fragment of PTH by the PTG of normal calves, but a small amount of this fragment has been detected in the venous effluent from hyperfunctioning parathyroid glands of man.[39]

REGULATION OF THE SECRETION OF PTH

Although our understanding of the mechanism for the control of PTH secretion is limited,[10,12] much is known about changes which produce alterations in the secretion rate of PTH.

Calcium and Parathyroid Secretion

Plasma Calcium

Calcium is the major regulator of PTH secretion. The plasma calcium concentration ([Ca]p) for man and most domestic animals is near 10 ± 1 mg/dℓ of plasma. (The horse and laying hen are notable exceptions, with [Ca]p of about 13 and 30 mg/dℓ, respectively.) About 46% of the calcium is bound to plasma proteins, mainly albumin, but also some globulins. About 48% is ionized and about 6% is complexed with other substances such as citrates and phosphates. These different varieties are in equilibrium with each other. The protein-bound calcium is pH-dependent, with a lowering of the pH favoring dissociation. It is the ionized calcium which affects the PTH secretory rate. Because of past difficulty of determining ionized calcium, investigators reported total calcium most often in terms of mg/100 mℓ (mg/dℓ) of plasma (or serum). This should be reported as 2.5 m*M*/1 or 5mEq/1.

Effects of PTG on Plasma Calcium

When the PTGs of an animal are removed, the plasma calcium concentration falls, often to a level incompatible with life. The organism is hypocalcemic. Different species display different responses to hypocalcemia. Ruminants develop paresis whereas monogastric animals develop tetany. Birds have discrete ultimobranchial bodies (UB) whereas in mammals this tissue has been incorporated into the thyroid gland in "C" cells. In either case this tissue secretes calcitonin which lowers blood calcium. In our laboratory, when the parathyroids are removed in chickens, the birds are found to develop transient hypocalcemia with a return to normocalcemia in 48 hr. If the PTGs and UBs are both removed, the birds develop severe hypocalcemia and die within 2 to 4 days. This indicates that the UB in birds has the ability to secrete PTH.[40]

Injection of PTH into animals leads to an elevation in plasma calcium concentration, hypercalcemia. PTH secreting tumors also lead to hypercalcemia.

Effect of Plasma Calcium on PTG

When plasma calcium concentration ($[Ca]_p$) falls, the PTGs secrete more PTH. The relationship between $[Ca]_p$ and PTH secretion rate is sigmoidal. This was first shown by the radioimmunoassay of peripheral plasma PTH concentrations in hypocalcemia cows before and during treatment with Ca.[41] It was later shown by radioimmunoassay for PTH of parathyroid venous plasma in calves during alterations of plasma Ca which were induced by the intravenous infusion of EDTA (which chelates Ca) or $CaCl_2$ (which raises plasma Ca).[42]

It was found in our laboratory that

1. Above a $[Ca]_p$ of 11 mg/dℓ the PTH secretion rate is at a minimum of 0.3 ng/kg body wt/min and further increases in $[Ca]_p$ result in no further decrease in PTH
2. In the normocalcemic range of 9 to 11 mg/dℓ slight increases in PTH secretion rate accompany small decreases in $[Ca]_p$
3. In the moderately hypocalcemic range of 7.5 to 9 mg/dℓ small changes in plasma Ca result in large changes in PTH secretion rate
4. Maximal PTH secretion rate (5.5 ng/kg body wt/min) occurs when $[Ca]_p$ drops to 7.5 mg/dℓ

Additional drop in Ca does not produce a further increase in PTH secretion rate.[42] PTG appears to behave appropriately. Its secretion rate change is small in response to small changes in plasma Ca in the normocalcemic range, but it responds much more vigorously when the Ca decreases to mild hypocalcemic levels and it reaches its greatest secretory capacity before the plasma Ca has fallen to lethal levels.[42]

Speed of PTH Secretory Response to Calcium

The response of the PTG to changes in ECF Ca is rapid. Blum et al.[43] estimated that the PTG responds to hypocalcemia by secreting PTH within 20 sec.

Phosphate and Parathyroid Secretion

That elevated blood phosphate levels stimulate the PTG directly has been shown to be incorrect.[44] Phosphate has an indirect effect on the PTG via its effect on plasma calcium. High plasma phosphate lowers plasma ionic calcium,[44] presumably by increasing the deposition of calcium and phosphate into bone, and it is the low plasma calcium which stimulates PTH secretion. This becomes a problem in some renal patients where the clearance of phosphate from blood is reduced. This results in an elevated blood phosphate, which leads to decreased calcium, which in turn stimulates excessive PTH release secondary renal hyperparathyroidism.

Magnesium and Parathyroid Secretion

Magnesium affects the secretion of PTH in the same direction as does Ca; an increase in plasma Mg concentration inhibits and a decrease stimulates PTH secretion rate.[45,46] However, on a molar basis the potency of Mg in this respect is only 1/3 to 1/2 that of Ca.[45,46] It appears unlikely that in the normal range Mg plays a significant role in regulating PTH secretion rate.

Exceptionally low plasma Mg concentrations, due to chronic deficiency in dietary Mg or Mg absorption from the gut, results in hypocalcemia and inappropriately low blood levels of PTH (hypoparathyroidism). The hypocalcemia often causes low Ca tetany. The intravenous administration of Mg salts alone corrects not only the hypomagnesemia but also the hypoparathyroidism and consequently also the hypocalcemia.[47] Such a rapid response indicates that some minimal level of Mg is required for the release of PTH.

Severe hypomagnesemia is produced in calves by feeding them a low magnesium diet. After about one month the magnesium level in the blood decreases to as low as 0.6 mg/dℓ. The calves do not develop hypocalcemia or hypoparathyroidism during the treatment. Infusion of $MgCl_2$ into the calves does not significantly enhance the PTH secretory response. The discrepancy between these data and the human data may be due to the more chronic nature of the human hypomagnesemia or the difference in the degree of hypomagnesemia.

Epinephrine and Parathyroid Secretion

Infusion of catecholamines increases peripheral blood levels of iPTH in cows[48] and man.[49] It must be assumed that epinephrine has a direct effect on the PTG because when it is added to PTG slices in vitro it stimulates the release of PTH into the incubation medium.[50] Measurement of iPTH secretion rate in calves has shown that the intravenous infusion of epinephrine causes a dramatic increase in PTH secretion rate.[51] The doses of epinephrine utilized have been within the physiologic range.

The basal level of peripheral iPTH decreases following the administration of propranolol, a β-adrenergic blocking agent.[49] These observations support the idea that endogenous epinephrine may play a physiologic role in the regulation of PTH secretion.[51] The effectiveness of epinephrine in stimulating PTH has been shown in the rat to persist for up to five weeks.[52]

Effect of Cyclic AMP on PTH Secretion

There is a close correlation between the amount of cAMP and the amount of iPTH released into the incubation medium by PTG slices.[53] The release of both is increased by decreasing the concentration of calcium in the medium and decreased by increasing the calcium. Also, substances known to increase intracellular cAMP (e.g., thiophylline and dibutyrl cyclic adenosine monophosphate, dcAMP) cause an in vitro increase in PTH release from PTG. The intracellular cAMP concentration of dispersed bPTH cells increases as the PTH release increases in response to a wide range of substances known to stimulate PTH secretion.[54] The release of PTH is linear in relation to the intracellular log concentration of cAMP regardless of what secretagogue is used to stimulate the PTG.[54] These observations indicate that cAMP is the second messenger for a variety of stimulators of the PTG. That is, the interaction between the stimulator of the PTG and its receptors on the PTG results in the formation of intracellular cAMP which then mediates the effects of the secretagogue on the PTG. Conversly, inhibitors of the PTG decrease intracellular cAMP as well as PTH release.

The level of ECF calcium seems to modify the effect of intracellular cAMP on PTH release. At high ECF calcium levels, the PTH released in response to a particular level of intracellular cAMP is less than that released at the same intracellular level of cAMP when the ECF calcium is low.

Effect of Vitamin D Metabolites on PTH Secretion

Vitamin D must be converted into a more polar compound to be effective. Vitamin D_3 is a hormone which is synthesized in the skin. The D_3 is hydroxylated in the 25 position by the liver and then in either the 1 or 24 position by the kidney and becomes 1,25-DHCC, a very potent hypercalcemic hormone, or 24,25-DHCC. Because of the tropic action of PTH on 1,25-DHCC formation it has been tempting to speculate that 1,25-DHCC acts in a negative feedback manner on the PTG and inhibits PTH secretion. Many investigators have probed this theory and the results have often been conflicting.[68-71,205,206] It seems unsafe at present to ascribe to any of the metabolites of vitamin D a definite, direct effect on the PTG. 1,25-DHCC does inhibit the PTG indirectly via its hypercalcemic action. The chick PTG can concentrate 1,25-DHCC.

Effects of Other Substances on PTH Secretion

The effects of other substances on PTH secretion rate have been tested. In most instances the physiologic significance of their effects is nebulous.

Gastrin

PTH, when administered directly into the antrum circulation of the stomach of pigs, stimulates the secretion of gastrin even when it has no detectable effects on plasma calcium.[55] Since PTH stimulates gastrin secretion it seems appropriate to ask if gastrin affects, in a negative feedback manner, the secretion of PTH. Experiments to test this have been performed, and apparently gastrin has no effects on PTH secretion rate by isolated bovine PTG cells in vitro[56] or by the intact PTG of calves in vivo.

Secretin

Secretin, at 10^{-8} molar concentration, increases cAMP and PTH release from dispersed bovine parathyroid cells.[56]

Ethanol

Ingestion of ethanol at the rate of 0.8 g/kg body wt over a 1 hr period by human subjects, results in an increase in plasma iPTH concentration to 132% above its concentration before ethanol was drunk. Bovine PTG slices in vitro are also stimulated in a dose-related manner by ethanol. It seems that the effect is a direct one on the PTG.[57]

Growth Hormone (GH or STH)

Because acromegalic patients often have elevated plasma calcium concentrations, the possibility exists that GH stimulates PTH secretion or 1,25-DHCC synthesis, which is responsible for the hypercalcemia. Prolonged administration of bovine GH (1 mg/da) or rat GH (0.2 mg/da) to rats for 4 weeks results in an elevation of plasma calcium and iPTH concentrations. This indicates that the hypercalcemic effect of GH is due to the PTG because if GH produces hypercalcemia by some other route (e.g., increasing directly 1,25-DHCC release), there would be decreased plasma PTH.[59] The administration of GH to 9 GH-deficient children (9 to 18 years of age) fails to produce any change in the circulating level of iPTH or vitamin D metabolites.[60] The GH-induced changes in calcium and phosphate are said not to be mediated by changes in PTH or vitamin D status.[60] The effect of GH on PTH secretion may be a way of enhancing bone growth and/or mineralization during body growth.

Somatostatin

Somatostatin is an inhibitory hormone first isolated from the hypothalamus and named for its action in inhibiting the release of GH (somatotropic hormone, somatotropin) from the anterior pituitary. It also inhibits the secretion of other peptide hormones (e.g., glucagon, insulin, and gastrin). The possibility exists that somatostatin may inhibit yet another peptide hormone, PTH, directly or indirectly by inhibiting GH which, as shown above, may be a stimulating hormone to the PTG. Consequently, experiments were undertaken to determine if somatostatin affects the blood levels of PTH. It was found that it decreases blood concentrations of PTH in rats and monkeys and that the addition of somatostatin antisera to bovine PTG slices causes an increase in PTH. This suggests that endogenous somatostatin is inhibiting the PTG and that this inhibition is removed when the somatostatin reacts with its antisera.[61] Some workers have found no effect of somatostatin on PTH secretion.[62] The physiologic significance of the somatostatin effect may be the same as that for GH.

Prostaglandins

Prostaglandins may play an essential role in mediating the action of some hormones.[63] Prostaglandin E_2 (PGE_2) causes half-maximal stimulation of PTH release and intracellular cAMP accumulation in dispersed PTG cells at about 10^{-7} and 10^{-6} *M*, respectively.[64] The effects are evident within 15 min. PGE_2 also causes release of PTH from rat PTG slices in vitro. $PGF_{2\alpha}$ inhibits PTH release from and cAMP accumulation in isolated PTG cells.[65] The physiologic significance of prostaglandins is unknown.

Vitamin A

Vitamin A has been reported to stimulate PTH release from bovine PTG tissue and to increase the plasma iPTH concentration in vivo.[72]

Calcitonin

Calcitonin is a hormone of the ultimobranchial bodies in birds and fishes and the "C" cells of the thyroid glands in mammals. It lowers plasma calcium and consequently would be expected to stimulate PTH secretion in vivo. That it may have a direct stimulatory effect on the PTG has been shown in PTG cultures in vitro.[207]

Cortisol

Cortisol stimulates the release of PTH from rat PTG tissue cultures.[208] It can raise the blood levels of PTH in man and the effect is not attributable to changes in plasma calcium.[209]

RATE OF PTH SECRETION, STORAGE OF PTH, AND PLASMA TRANSPORT OF PTH

PTH Secretion Rate

It is difficult to directly measure PTH secretion rate. Indirect estimates based upon changes in peripheral plasma concentrations of PTH are difficult to quantitate because PTH exists in the blood in different forms (intact hormone and fragments) with different biologic half-lives. From PTH infusion studies it has been learned that large changes in PTH infusion rates product small changes in plasma iPTH concentrations and small changes in PTH infusion rates produce indiscernible changes in plasma iPTH concentrations.

Our laboratory has determined the PTH secretion rate in the calf.[42] This is made possible because in this species the superior parathyroids are anatomically well separated from the thyroid, are rather large, and have a venous drainage which permits one to collect the blood draining a single PTG. Our technique involves collection of the venous effluent of a single superior PTG in an anesthetized 3-to-6-week-old calf. Simultaneously, we also collect blood from a peripheral artery. The PTH concentration of parathyroid venous and peripheral arterial plasma is determined using two antisera, one which is specific to the amino-terminal end and another which is specific to the carboxyl-terminal end of the PTH molecule. By collecting timed samples of parathyroid venous blood, the blood flow rate can be calculated and from this and the hematocrit we can calculate the plasma flow rate. From the plasma flow rate and the concentration of PTH in the plasma, we can calculate the amount of PTH emanating from the single superior PTG per unit of time. Since the arterial blood entering the PTG contains PTH, the PTH concentration of peripheral arterial plasma is used to correct for this. The total PTH secretion rate can be calculated by adjusting the secretion rate for the single gland, which represents about 42% of the total PTG tissue in the calf, to the total amount of PTG tissue. This can be expressed meaningfully on the basis of body weight and we usually give our results in terms of ng of PTH/kg of body wt/min.

The PTH secretion rate curve in relation to plasma Ca concentration is sigmoid. During normocalcemia the PTH secretion rate is about 1 ng/kg/min. It is maximally stimulated by a plasma Ca concentration of about 7.5 mg/dℓ; at this plasma Ca concentration and lower ones, the PTG secretion rate is 5 ng/kg/min. At 10.5 mg/dℓ plasma Ca concentration, the PTG is maximally inhibited and the PTH secretion rate is 0.3 ng/kg/min. It is not further suppressed even when the plasma Ca concentration is raised to 15 mg/dℓ.

In the normocalcemic range of 9.5 to 10.5 mg/dℓ, small changes in plasma Ca result in small changes in PTH secretion rate. In the moderate to moderately severe plasma Ca concentration range (7.5 to 9.5 mg/dℓ), small changes in plasma Ca result in large changes in PTH secretion rate.

Why there should be nonsuppressible PTH secretion rate during hypercalcemia is not clear. The animal does not need PTH to elicit bone resorption and to elevate plasma Ca during hypercalcemia. Almost all of the PTH released during hypercalcemia is inactive carboxyl fragments(s)[38] which do not contribute to the hypercalcemia. But, why should the PTG secrete any form of PTH during hypercalcemia? A possible explanation is that the PTG keeps its PTH synthesizing machinery operative to respond rapidly to a hypocalcemic challenge and that this machinery is synthesizing new PTH which, because of the high Ca, is being degraded into biologically inactive carboxyl fragments.

Another way to establish the PTH secretion rate is to determine the infusion rate of exogenous PTH which is required to maintain plasma Ca at a constant level in parathyroidectomized animals. This approach has been used in the dog where it is found that a continuous infusion rate of 0.1 μ/kg/hr is required to maintain plasma Ca.[73] Since the most highly purified PTH preparations have a potency of about 3000 μ/mg, 0.1 μ/kg/hr $\simeq$ 30 ng/kg/hr or 0.5 ng/kg/min. This is in excellent agreement with the endogenous secretion rate of 1 ng/kg/min which we find in calves during normocalcemia.

Storage of PTH in the PTG

A mg of bovine PTG tissue contains 0.2 μg of extractable PTH.[73] Our calves, which have about 75 mg of PTG tissue, have about 15 μg of PTH in their parathyroids. During normocalcemia when the secretion rate is 1 ng/kg/min, a 50-kg calf has enough stored hormone to last for about 5 hr. Even during severe hypocalcemia there is enough stored hormone to last about 1 hr.[42]

Transport of PTH in the Blood

PTH and its carboxyl fragments appear to be transported in the blood in their free form rather than complexed with carrier protein.

PERIPHERAL METABOLISM OF PTH[77]

Circulating Forms of PTH

The PTH found in the peripheral circulation of man and cattle consists of both intact PTH and carboxyl-terminal fragments. This raises some questions (1) do these fragments come from the PTG; or (2) do they arise peripherally; and if so, (3) which organ or organs are responsible for the cleavage of the intact hormone and the generation of these fragments? We have shown in our laboratory, as have others, that the PTG does indeed secrete carboxyl-fragments, especially during hypercalcemia.[38] There is no doubt that the PTG contributes to the heterogeneity of circulating PTH. That the intact PTH molecule is also cleaved peripherally has been well documented.[75,76] Following the injection of purified PTH into rats and dogs, PTH undergoes rapid and specific cleavage between the 33 to 34 and 36 to 37 amino acid residues, yielding an amino-terminal fragment which is biologically active and a carboxyl-terminal fragment which may be biologically inactive.[75] The same results hold for man and cattle.

Biologic Half-Life ($T_{1/2}$) of PTH

Numerous studies are available on the biologic half-life ($T_{1/2}$) of injected or infused exogenous PTH, as determined by radioimmunoassay (RIA). Since PTH in peripheral plasma is heterogeneous (i.e., intact hormone plus fragments), it is important that the recognition sites on the PTH molecule of the antisera used in the RIA be known because the $T_{1/2}$ of PTH, as opposed to its carboxyl-fragment, is short, on the order of 15 min at most. The $T_{1/2}$ of the carboxyl-fragment of PTH is about 1 hr.[75,78]

Where is PTH Cleaved and/or Cleared?

The disappearance of bPTH is slow in nephrectomized rats, dogs, and man and in partially hepatectomized rats. Singer et al.[78] measured the arteriovenous (A-V) difference in plasma PTH concentration across specific organs or regions of the body of dogs. They infused purified PTH into the right atrium of dogs. When a steady state (i.e., when a constant arterial blood level of bPTH) was reached, they measured the bPTH in plasma collected concurrently from the aorta, renal vein, the hepatic vein, femoral vein, pulmonary artery, and the left atrium (to stimulate pulmonary venous blood). They found the A-V difference of iPTH across various structures to be as follows: liver, 23%; kidney, 19%; hind leg, 0%; and lungs, 0%. They also found that only about 0.1% of the total bPTH which had been infused appeared in the urine. Since these experiments were conducted using a radioimmunoassay which employed an antisera with recognition sites in both the amino- and carboxyl-terminal portions of PTH, they were measuring both intact PTH and its fragments. In human studies using antisera with primarily amino-terminal recognition sites (i.e., probably measuring intact hormone almost exclusively), this same group showed that the A-V differences of endogenous PTH across the liver of hyperparathyroid patients is 44%, across the kidney it is 34%, and across the leg (muscle and/or bone) it is 16%.[79] The liver and kidneys, but also muscle/bone, clear intact, exogenous, (and presumably endogenous) PTH from the circulation at a rather rapid rate.

Role of the Kidney in the Catabolism of PTH

The kidney clears the renal arterial blood of about 30% of its intact PTH.[79] It does this through both glomerular filtration (with subsequent reabsorption of most of the filtered load of PTH since very little is found in the urine) and by uptake of the hormone at the peri-tubular side of the renal tubular cells.[80] (In this connection it may be noted that when purified bPTH is incubated with urine, only about 40% is recoverable.)[78] The kidney also apparently takes up the biologically inactive carboxyl-terminal fragments, but only by glomerular filtration and subsequent reabsorption. The importance of the kidney in clearance of both intact PTH and fragments has been demonstrated in human patients with chronic renal failure. These patients have a high iPTH concentration in their blood. After they receive a renal transplant from a living, near-relative donor (which results in immediate renal function), the plasma iPTH concentration decreases rapidly and reaches 20% of the pretransplantation value with 24 hr.[81] This marked fall in iPTH is due primarily to a fall in the carboxyl-terminal fragments.[77]

The kidney is probably a source of the PTH fragments found in the general circulation because the perfusion of the isolated dog kidney with intact PTH results in the appearance of both amino- and carboxyl-terminal fragments in its venous effluent.[82] The perfusate calcium concentration affects the rate at which the kidney degrades PTH. When it is low the degradation of PTH is accelerated and when it is high degradation is retarded.[82]

Role of the Liver in the Catabolism of PTH

The arteriovenous (A-V) difference for intact PTH of the liver is about 45%.[79] This indicates that the liver extracts intact PTH from the blood. That the liver cleaves intact PTH into two products or two groups of similar products has been shown by analysis of the hepatic venous effluent from isolated rat livers which are perfused with fluid containing bPTH. One of these products (or group of products) has carboxyl-terminal immunoreactivity, a mol wt of about 7000, and is biologically inactive. The other has amino-terminal immunoreactivity, a mol wt of about 3500, and is biologically active. The presence of a low calcium concentration in the perfusion fluid speeds up this fragment formation and a high calcium concentration slows it.[83] This is similar to the kidney studies.[82]

The liver apparently does not selectively take up amino- or carboxyl-terminal fragments.[77] This has been shown in anesthetized dogs where the liver fails to take up ^{125}iodinated PTH 1-34 or PTH 43-84 fragments even though it takes up over 30% of intact PTH over a wide range of plasma PTH concentration. On a molar basis it also takes up about the same amount of the ^{125}iodinated PTH 28-48 fragment as it does PTH 1-84. The hepatic receptor for PTH recognizes some essential binding site which resides on the PTH molecule in its 28-48 position and which is absent or partly absent from the two terminal fragments tested. This would account for the liver's selective uptake of PTH 1-84 and 28-48, but not PTH 1-34 or 43-84.

Since the liver selectively takes up intact PTH[88] and generates an active fragment,[83] (especially when the blood Ca concentration is low), it is tempting to speculate that the liver is required to activate PTH (i.e., produce an amino-terminal fragment) before it can act on its target organs (mainly kidney and bone).

Role of Bone in the Peripheral Metabolism of PTH

It was reported in 1967 that when 25 USP units of PTH/kg of body wt is added to blood perfusing the isolated tibia of a cat, there is no increase in the mobilization of calcium from the bone. However, when the PTH is injected into a cat whose isolated tibia is being perfused by arterial blood from the cat itself, there is (within 20 min) an increase (20% above baseline) in calcium mobilization from the bone.[84] This observation suggested that PTH must undergo some systemic change before it can be effective on bone or else give rise to some other substance which then acts on bone.

Considering the generation of fragments of PTH by the liver and kidney, it is logical to assess the effects of the active, amino-terminal PTH 1-34 fragment on bone. In 1978 Martin et al.[85] reported that isolated, perfused bone extracts 36% of the synthetic PTH 1-34 which has been added to the perfusion fluid, but it does not extract oxidized (biologically inactive) PTH 1-34 and only insignificant amounts of intact bPTH 1-84. They also reported that the biologically active bPTH 1-34 significantly increases the amount of cAMP released from the bone whereas the oxidized bPTH 1-34 does not and that PTH 1-84 stimulates only minimal increases in cAMP release.[85]

These experiments suggest that intact PTH has either no effect or at best a marginal effect on bone and, since the amino-terminal fragment is effective, raise the possibility that PTH must undergo peripheral cleavage before it can act on bone. In vitro studies prevent us from accepting this theory without further work because when isolated fetal or neonatal bone cells or minced fetal or neonatal calvaria are incubated with PTH 1-84, they quickly degrade PTH 1-84, but not oxidized (biologically inactive) PTH 1-84.[86] The degradation is not due to the medium because it occurs only when bone cells or minced calvaria are present.

Carboxyl-terminal fragments and intact PTH, but no amino-terminal fragments, were found in the medium in this study.[86] That the bone was being affected by PTH and not merely degrading it was shown by the increased production of cAMP by both the isolated cells and minced calvaria.

In another attempt to answer the question of whether PTH must be cleaved to exert its effect on bone, Goltzman[87] incubated PTH 1-84 with rabbit calvaria and got cAMP production. Analysis of the incubation medium, however, by very sensitive techniques fails to show even traces of PTH fragment. Goltzman concluded that PTH 1-84 is effective on bone and does not require cleavage.[87] Thus it is not presently known whether peripheral cleavage of PTH is required for it to have an in vivo effect on bone or whether bone can cleave PTH and contribute to the pool of fragments in the general circulation.

PHYSIOLOGIC ACTIONS OF PTH[89]

The principal actions of PTH are

1. PTH increases bone resorption (catabolism of bone)
2. PTH increases bone formation (anabolism of bone)
3. PTH increases phosphate excretion by the kidney
4. PTH decreases renal calcium excretion
5. PTH increases (indirectly via vitamin D metabolism) the absorption of dietary calcium by the gut

Effects of PTH on Bone

Catabolic Effects of PTH on Bone

One of the most observable effects of PTH is its destruction of bone (osteolysis). This was discovered in osteitis fibrosa to be due to PTG adenomas. This destruction is mimicked by chronic injection of parathyroid extract (PTE). PTH can also stimulate bone formation.

Bone resorption due to PTE (the active component of which is PTH) may require "supraphysiologic" doses, like those due to PTH injection or PTG adenoma. Even in normal subjects PTH concentration may become great enough to stimulate bone resorption when blood calcium is low, such as after an overnight fast or during times when there is a deficiency of calcium in the diet. In the person with normal calcium absorption and a normal calcium diet, the low levels of PTH in the blood are probably more anabolic than catabolic.[89-91]

Histologic Evidence

Evidence that bone resorption (catabolic effect) is a direct response to PTH is found when PTGs are implanted next to bone. These cause an increase in the number of osteoclasts and an erosion of bone near the transplant whereas other tissues transplanted to similar sites are without such effects.[97] Also, single large doses of PTH or PTE depress osteoblastic and enhance osteoclastic activity.[90]

PTH appears to act on osteoprogenitor cells, stimulating them to undergo mitosis and to differentiate into osteoclasts. The formation of osteoclasts is probably due to coalescence of osteoprogenitor cells because after treatment with PTH at least 12 hr must elapse before one finds an increase in DNA synthesis, but only 2 hr before one finds an increase in the number of osteoclasts.[98]

PTH stimulates osteocytes to reabsorb bone. PTH given to rats causes an increase in the amount of Golgi apparatus, in the amount of rough endoplasmic reticulum, and in the number of lysosomes in osteocytes. It also causes the cell surface opposite the eccentrically placed nucleus to assume a ruffled-like appearance. Under this ruffled-like border the lacunar space is widened and in this space many free ends of demineralized collagen fibers can be seen sticking out from the bone. Many large vesicles are also seen in the cytoplasm near the ruffled-like border. Thus, PTH produces numerous changes in the osteocytes which show intense metabolic activity which is consistent with the hypothesis that the PTH-stimulated osteocytes are busy synthesizing enzymes and resorbing bone.[99] This is in keeping with the observation that PTH causes such a marked and rapid calcium mobilization from bone that it is impossible to conceive of all of it being due to preexisting osteoclasts.

Biochemical Evidence

Biochemical evidence also indicates that PTH increases bone catabolism. Collagen makes up around 20% of the dry weight of bone. Consequently, measurements of the breakdown products of collagen which appear in the urine, blood or culture medium, if distinguishable from products from other tissues, are useful indicators of the rate of bone organic matrix catabolism.

Collagen contains two unique amino acids, hydroxyproline and hydroxylysine. Injection of PTH increases the plasma level and urinary excretion of these two hydroxylated amino acids. Thus, changes in concentration of small molecules containing hydroxyproline and hydroxylysine in the plasma reflect changes in collagen breakdown and consequently, bone organic matrix breakdown. These results can be misinterpreted if there is simultaneously skin collagen breakdown. However, more specific analyses can differentiate between hydroxylysine derived from skin and from bone, because the former is in plasma mainly as a diglycoside and the latter as a monoglycoside. PTH also increases the amount of calcium and phosphate in the blood and the amount of increase is too great to have come from any source other than bone.

Surfaces of bone, whether endosteal, periosteal, or the Haversian canal appear to be covered with a functional cellular layer (the osteoprogenitor cells, which are also known as surface osteocytes) which maintain the ionic composition of the bone fluid compartment (BFC) different from the systemic extracellular fluid compartment. This layer concentrates K in and decreases Ca, Mg, and Na in the bone fluid compartment.[104] This probably requires a Ca pump to move calcium out of the BFC. One of the early actions of PTH on bone is thought to cause a net efflux of Ca across this functional cellular layer from BFC to ECF compartment. This movement of Ca is not accompanied by phosphate and strongly suggests that this early effect of PTH is on the rapidly exchangeable bone Ca and not on mineralized bone because the latter will result in mobilization of both Ca and iP, not just Ca.[105,106] This early effect of PTH occurs within a few hours whereas the bone resorbing action of PTH requires a day or more, in tissue culture studies.[105]

Although we usually think of the action of PTH on bone mobilization as being leisurely, several experiments have shown a rapid action.[84,107,108]

Summary of Catabolic Effect of PTH on Bone

PTH mobilizes Ca from bone. It has early effects of increasing the exit of Ca from bone unaccompanied by phosphate, of causing osteocytic osteolysis, and of inhibiting osteoblasts and hence inhibiting bone formation. It has a more delayed effect on Ca resorption by activation and recruitment of osteoclasts. This delayed effect appears to require "supraphysiologic" amounts of PTH.

Anabolic Actions of PTH on Bone

The catabolic action of PTH on bone has been considered its dominant action for a half-century. However, more recent studies have emphasized the anabolic action of PTH on bone. See reviews by Parsons[91] and Parfitt.[90]

Parsons et al.[109] pointed out that the response to PTH is different at different dose levels. Based upon the infusion rate of PTH required to maintain a normal plasma calcium concentration in acutely parathyroidectomized animals[73] the PTH plasma concentration is estimated to be $10^{-11} M$ (0.1 ng/mℓ). However, the bone Ca resorption effects of PTH require concentrations of the hormone of about $10^{-8} M$, a 1000-fold greater than is required to produce its renal phosphaturic and calcemic effect. The rat renal membrane adenylate cyclase system, in vitro, requires an even higher level (10^{-6} to 10^{-5} M) of PTH in the medium. Thus, of the hypercalcemic actions of PTH, only the ones on the kidney and indirectly on the gut have been shown at apparently physiologic dose levels.

In bone remodeling, bone formation is strongly coupled with bone resorption. Whether bone turnover is normal, subnormal, or supranormal, there seems to be a high positive correlation between bone resorption and bone formation.[110] Thus, when searching for an anabolic action of PTH on bone, one is confronted with the question of whether increased bone formation after PTH treatment is a direct action of PTH on bone formation or secondary to the PTH induced bone resorption.

Early workers[96,111] presented histologic evidence that large daily injections of parathyroid extract into rats causes an increase in blood calcium, osteoblasts, and osteoclasts. The increases reach a peak in 4 days. By 12 days of continued PTE treatment, plasma calcium and osteoblast count returned to normal, but the number of osteoblasts remained elevated. When the PTE treatment is reduced to ¼ of the daily dose and given every other day, there is an increase in osteoblasts without a prior increase in osteoclasts. Hermann-Erlee et al.[103] have found that relatively low doses of PTH 1-34 ($5 \times 10^{-9} M$) causes, after 48 hr, an increase in osteoblast count in embryonic mouse radii in tissue culture. Treatment of embryonic chick bones in vitro with 10^{-12} M PTH over a 12 day period shows that for up to 16 hr of incubation, collagen synthesis (as assessed by uptake of ^{3}H Proline) is depressed, but then stimulated for the remainder of the time, even though PTH is included in the medium only for the initial 24 hr.[108] Hydroxyproline release is enhanced from the 4th hr through the 12th day of the incubation.[108]

In summary, small physiologic doses of PTH given chronically have mainly an anabolic effect on bone whereas larger doses produce mainly a catabolic effect. At least one small clinical trial has been conducted on three postmenopausal osteoporotic patients with 100 μg/da of hPTH 1-34 over a 6 month period. A marked positive calcium balance was seen in all three patients.[112]

Other Actions of PTH on Bone

Bone Cell Receptors for PTH

Plasma membranes of osteoblasts and osteoprogenitor cells of the parietal bone selectively bind rat PTH.[113]

Adenylate Cyclase System of Bone

PTH activates the adenylate cyclase enzyme system in bone cells and results in the production of cAMP by these cells.[114,115] According to this concept, PTH binds to specific receptors on bone cells and this activates adenylate cyclase. This produces cAMP, which in turn acts intracellularly to produce the various effects of PTH on bone cells. Caution in assigning cAMP the role of second messenger is urged.[115]

The effect of PTH in producing cAMP is rapid. Its concentration reaches a peak in 15 min and declines by 60 min. In isolated bone cells the PTH-induced cAMP production can be detected within 30 sec in response to physiologic levels of PTH.[116]

Several observations point to cAMP as a mediator of the PTH response:

1. PTH usually produces a substantial increase in cAMP when acting upon bone

2. Dibutyryl cAMP (dcAMP), an analogue of cAMP, which results in an accumulation of intracellular cAMP by blocking cAMP breakdown, can induce bone resorption in vitro

3. dcAMP can increase lactate production by bone cells

4. It can increase the release of lysosomal enzymes.[118]

Calcium Entry into Bone Cells

PTH increases the entry of Ca into isolated bone cells. The Ca-entry effect can be seen within five min, may precede the production of cAMP and may be the second messenger, cAMP being a third messenger.[117]

Cohn's group[118] isolated bone cells and segregated them into osteoclastic-like and osteoblastic-like cells. Using these two cell populations, they showed that increasing the Ca concentration of the incubation medium over a range of 1.8 to 5.3 m*M* mimics, in time and magnitude of response, the action of PTH on the production of hyaluronate by the osteoclastic-like cells and on the inhibition of citrate decarboxylation by the osteoblastic-like cells.[118] When Ca is absent from the medium, PTH is ineffective in producing these biochemical responses, but it is effective in increasing bone cell cAMP. Ca by itself does not increase cAMP, but it produces the other two biochemical responses. Thus, Ca does not mimic PTH by activating the adenylate cyclase system.

The results indicate that Ca plays a role in mediating the action of PTH. They are consistent with the hypothesis that PTH stimulates the adenylate cyclase system, which increases cAMP production, which then increases intracellular Ca, which in turn brings about the biochemical changes in hyaluronate and citrate decarboxylation. When the Ca of the medium is raised, and presumably also the intracellular Ca, the cAMP step in the above hypothesis is possibly bypassed. These data are consistent with the idea that cAMP can be the second messenger and Ca the third messenger.

Lactic Acid Production

Bone cells make lactic acid, and acid production is increased within two min by PTH. Its production probably represents an overall change in bone cell metabolism due to PTH.[90]

Citric Acid Production

Bone cells make citrate. The citrate concentration of osteoclasts has been reported to be 100 times higher than that of nonbone cells. PTH increases citrate of bone cells by inhibiting its decarboxylation. There is usually a good correlation between PTH-induced citrate accumulation and bone resorption, in tissue culture experiments.[121] The exact role of citrate in bone resorption is still not clear.

Carbonic Acid Production

Osteoclasts contain abundant carbonic anhydrase whereas other bone cells contain but little. Inhibitors of carbonic anhydrase as well as decreases in CO_2 decrease the effectiveness of PTH in producing hypercalcemia.[122]

Lysosomal Enzymes and Collagenase Release from Bone Cells

Bone resorption occurs under the ruffled borders of osteoclasts (and under similar structures in osteocytes). The clear area around the ruffled border probably seals this structure to the underlying bone and produces a microenvironment between cell and bone where products from the bone resorbing cell can degrade bone. The ruffled border is characterized by having long cytoplasmic projections and many vacuoles, all in close association with lysosomes. There is evidence of much endocytotic and exocytotic activity occurring in the ruffled borders and evidence that mineral and organic constituents of bone are broken down under the ruffled border. Several lysosomal enzymes are released by the osteoclasts and, in tissue culture, several of these escape into the culture medium and can be assayed. The production and/or release of some of these lysosomal enzymes are increased by PTH. Collagen fibers are apparently completely solubilized outside the cytoplasm because they are never seen intracellularly.

Acid phosphatase is found in most of the vacuoles of the osteoclasts as well as in the resorptive space under the ruffled borders. PTH increases the amount of acid phosphatase in the osteoclasts.

The production and release of the following lysosomal enzymes are increased by PTH and are correlated with bone resorption in tissue culture[123,124] (1) β-glucuronidase; (2) N-acetyl-β-glucosaminidase; (3) β-galactosidase; (4) acid protease, cathepsin D; and (5) deoxyribonuclease.

The release of two nonlysosomal enzymes, alkaline phosphatase and catalase, decreases during the resorption process. It appears that PTH stimulates the osteoclasts to empth their lysosomes. What the lysosomal enzymes are doing for bone resorption is not known.

Substances which increase the rate of bone resorption, including prostaglandin E_2, dibutyryl cAMP, isobutylmethylxanthine, and the Ca ionophore, A23187, increase lysosomal enzyme release from fetal rat bone in tissue culture at concentrations which also increase ^{45}Ca release from bones.[124] The possibility that the increase in lysosomal enzyme release is the result of cell destruction has been ruled out. Conversely, inhibitors of bone resorption, calcitonin, cortisol, and colchicine, block both lysosomal enzyme and ^{45}Ca release. It is safe to say that PTH stimulates the release of lysosomal enzymes and the release can be correlated with bone resorption. However, the exact role of these released enzymes in bone resorption is still not clear. In some studies,[124] the changes in the release of the lysosomal enzyme, β-glucuronidase, subsequent to PTH treatment precede the change in ^{45}Ca release. This suggests that the release of the enzymes may be responsible for the resorption of mineral from bone.

Collagenase (or procollagenase) is released from bone which is grown in tissue culture. Studies by Vaes and others[123,124] fail to show a correlation between the PTH-induced resorption of bone and the release of collagenase. This does not mean that collagenase is not involved in matrix removal or that its synthesis and release are not increased by PTH. It may be that it is bound or prevented from appearing in greater quantities during increased bone resorption. It may be bound to solubilized collagen and taken up by endocytosis.

Effects of PTH on the Kidney

Effects of PTH on Renal Phosphate Excretion

When pains are taken to maintain a constant glomerular filtration rate (GFR), renal blood flow and filtered load, PTH still shows a marked depressant effect on the reabsorption by the proximal convoluted tubule (PCT) of all ions so far tested. Thus, the reabsorption of phosphate, Ca, Na, and HCO_3 ions as well as tubular water by the PCT is depressed by fairly large doses of PTH.[128,129] Since PTH produces an increase in urinary phosphate excretion, a decrease in Ca excretion, a variable but usually increase in HCO_3 excretion, and usually no or only minimal increases in Na excretion, it is apparent that the more distal nephron is further modifying the tubular fluid.

In vivo evidence from micropuncture techniques in the rat[130] and dog[129] indicates that most phosphate reabsorption occurs in the proximal convoluted tubule (PCT) and that the phosphate which is not absorbed there is not reabsorbed, but is excreted in the urine. Large doses of PTH inhibit this proximal phosphate reabsorption. Thus, by decreasing the Tmax of phosphate in the PCT, large doses of PTH result in an increased excretion of phosphate and a greater clearance of phosphate from the blood.

The distal nephron also has the capability to reabsorb phosphate, but this capacity is suppressed by physiologic levels of endogenous PTH. Following parathyroidectomy, this characteristic of the distal tubule becomes manifested.[131,134] Also, physiologic levels of PTH have no consistent effect on the reabsorption of phosphate by the PCT.[132] It may be that the main action of low levels of PTH on phosphate clearance is exerted via its depression of phosphate reabsorption by the distal nephron. Higher levels depress phosphate reabsorption in the PCT. Thus the effect of PTH is to increase phosphate excretion by depressing phosphate reabsorption in both the PCT and DCT.

Effects of PTH on Renal Calcium Excretion

Relatively large doses of PTH inhibit Ca reabsorption by the PCT, but unlike phosphate the amount of Ca excreted in the urine decreases.[129] This indicates that PTH acts in the distal nephron (which includes the distal convoluted tubule and collecting duct) to increase the reabsorption of Ca. Small, physiologic doses of PTH do not inhibit reabsorption of Ca by the PCT, but result in a decreased urinary Ca excretion.[126] Thus, it may be that at physiologic levels, PTH is affecting both Ca and phosphate reabsorption in the distal nephron where it inhibits the reabsorption of phosphate (i.e., it decreases $TmPO_4$) and stimulates the reabsorption of Ca. At higher levels, the effects of PTH on $TmPO_4$ in the distal nephron are already maximal, so its only additional effect on phosphate is to inhibit its Tmax in the PCT. The higher doses of PTH appear to further enhance the distal tubular reabsorption of Ca while paradoxically inhibiting its reabsorption by the PCT. The effects on the distal tubule apparently dominate because the amount of Ca in the urine is decreased by the larger doses of PTH.[129]

According to Puschett,[126] the reabsorption of Ca in the nephron closely parallels that of sodium and is as follows: 50 to 65% in PCT, 20 to 30% in the outer medullary portion of tbe ascending limb of the loop of Henle, 5 to 8% in the cortical portion of the ascending limb of Henle's loop, 2 to 3% in the DCT and perhaps another 1 to 2% in the collecting ducts. The exact place(s) in the distal nephron where PTH enhances Ca reabsorption is not known.[126]

In some cases, PTH will cause an increase in urinary Ca excretion. This is despite the fact that it has increased the renal reabsorption of Ca and is due to the fact that PTH produces hypercalcemia which increases the filtered load of Ca.

Effects of PTH on Bicarbonate Excretion

Large doses of PTH impair bicarbonate resorption by the PCT. Whether or not it increases bicarbonate in the urine depends upon whether or not the distal tubule reabsorbs this extra bicarbonate which is delivered to it.[126]

Effects of PTH on Magnesium Excretion

The effects of PTH on the handling of Mg by the kidney is less clear than for Ca and PO_4. PTH enhances the reabsorption of Mg, decreases the clearance of Mg from the blood, and decreases urinary Mg.[141]

Other Effects of PTH on the Kidney

cAMP

Administration of PTH to parathyroidectomized rats produces large increases in the excretion of cAMP in the urine. The response is rapid and precedes the appearance of phosphaturia.[133] The administration of dibutyryl cAMP (but not 5' AMP) to the dog nearly mimics the effect of PTH in inhibiting the proximal renal tubular reabsorption of phosphate, sodium, calcium, and water and in producing a marked phosphaturia.[128,129] Thus, cAMP may be acting as the second messenger for the action of PTH in the kidney as it may also be doing in bone.

In vitro studies show that PTH stimulates the adenylate cyclase system in the kidney but there are species variation as to which parts of the kidney are responsive to the hormone.[135]

Guanine Triphosphate

Synthetic analogues of GTP may potentiate the effects of PTH on the renal adenylate cyclase system.[136] This means that naturally occurring guanyl nucleotides may play a role in the activation of adenylate cyclase by PTH.

Uptake of Calcium by Renal Microsomes

Homogenates of renal cortical and papillary microsomes, devoid of mitochondria, from cat kidneys which have been perfused with PTH-containing perfusate, enhance Ca uptake. The uptake is about 95% dependent upon the presence of ATP in the suspension medium.[137]

Renal Receptors for PTH

PTH initiates its action in the kidney by binding with PTH-specific receptors on the surface of cell membranes of certain renal tubular cells.[138] The renal PTH-receptor has been studied by Nissenson and Arnaud.[142] They state that there is a single type of binding site, which has a high affinity for bPTH 1-34 (Kd = 7-10 n*M*) and which is high in number (4-6 *M*/mg of protein).

Injection of ^{3}H-labeled PTH into thyroparathyroidectomized rats 10 min before they are killed shows, by thaw-mount autoradiography, that the label is concentrated mainly in the apical (next to the tubular lumen) regions of the cells of the PCT and that the uptake of the PTH diminishes toward the distal end of the PCT. The epithelium of the DCT, collecting ducts, and glomeruli are not labeled.[139] This may be a means for removal of PTH from the blood for catabolism rather than a means whereby PTH exerts its physiologic action.[141] The perfused rat kidney removes about 70% of the plasma PTH via a process of glomerular filtration followed by renal tubular reabsorption of 95% of the filtered load of PTH. The resorbed PTH is subsequently catabolized.[140]

Effects of PTH on Formation of Vitamin D Metabolites

PTH stimulates the kidney to hydroxylate 25-(OH)D_3 on the number 1 carbon to form 1,25$(OH)_2D_3$, a potent vitamin D metabolite which acts on the gut to stimulate calcium and phosphate absorption.

Effects of PTH on the Gut

PTH stimulates the gut to absorb calcium and phosphate, but this action is indirect. It depends upon the action of PTH on the renal production of vitamin D metabolites which then act on the gut.

ASSAYS FOR PTH

For many years only biologic assays (bioassays) were available for measuring PTH. These assays depend upon some biologic response, historically an elevation in plasma calcium concentration, in test animals. They are relatively insensitive. There is no bioassay sensitive enough to enable one to determine the amount of PTH in unconcentrated body fluids or where its concentration is in the order of 10^{-12} to 10^{-11} mol/ℓ.

There are both in vitro and in vivo bioassays and they continue to be essential for determining the potency of PTH preparations and for validating the more recently employed protein binding assays. The latter are many times more sensitive than the bioassays, but are limited because they often do not distinguish between biologically active and inactive PTH. This deficiency of the protein binding assay is reduced by the use of multiple assays employing more specific binding proteins.

Bioassays

Units of PTH

Since highly purified PTH and essentially pure PTH 1-34 were not originally available, impure preparations of PTH were used. The preparations were obtained by extracting PTH from parathyroid glands and yielded parathyroid extract (PTE). Because much of the extracted material is not PTH, expressing PTH by weight of the material is not correct. Instead, the amount of PTH in the extract is expressed on the basis of the biologic potency of the extract, in units. By definition, 100 USP units is that amount of PTH required to increase the plasma calcium concentration of a 10 to 12 kg dog by 1 mg/100 mℓ of plasma, 16 hr after injection of the extract. The most highly purified bPTH has a potency of 2500 to 3500 USP units/mg.

In Vivo Bioassay

The hypercalcemic response of the dog to the injection of PTH solutions has been used to assay PTH and to establish a unit of PTH. This assay is insensitive. The most common in vivo bioassay is probably the chick hypercalcemic response, which utilizes 10-day-old chicks given hormone preparations intravenously. The working range of this assay is 1 to 10 USP units or about 300 to 3000 ng of PTH.[101] Since normal concentrations of PTH in peripheral plasma are about 0.5 ng/mℓ, one would have to inject about 600 mℓ of plasma into a 50-g chick to see a response. Thus, this assay is not suitable for measuring peripheral plasma PTH, but it may be useful for measuring PTH in plasma from the parathyroid vein or for measuring PTH in parathyroid extracts of homogenates.

In Vitro Bioassays

These assays measure biologic responses by a cultured organ or tissue to PTH. For example, the release of calcium from mouse calvaria in tissue culture has been used as an assay for PTH with a working range of 0.06 to 1.2 units/2 mℓ of incubation medium.[211] A similar assay and one probably more widely utilized is the rat kidney adenylate cyclase assay which measures the production of 3-,5-cAMP by rat renal membranes in vitro after the addition of PTH. This assay has a working range of 0.2 to 1.0 USP units.[102,103]

A cytochemical bioassay for PTH has been reported to have a detection limit as low as 0.1 fg/mℓ (10^{-16} g/mℓ).[58] The usefulness of this assay will have to await further trials.

Binding Assays

Protein-Binding Assays

The theory of protein-binding assays is to use a protein which binds specifically with PTH, mix the sample containing an unknown amount of PTH (cold PTH) with this protein and add some PTH which has been labeled with a radioisotope (hot PTH). Let the components interact and then separate the hot PTH into a fraction which has been bound to the binding-protein and a fraction which is free. Express the two values as a ratio. Compare this number with a series of standards which were prepared the same way except that in place of unknown amounts of cold PTH, add known amounts of cold PTH to the mixture of binding-protein and hot PTH. The more cold PTH added, the less the hot hormone can bind to the binding-protein, and consequently more of the hot hormone will remain free. This is an extremely sensitive, highly specific assay which can detect the circulating levels of PTH in blood.

Radioimmunoassays

The most commonly employed protein-binding assays for PTH are the radioimmunoassays (RIA). Antibodies (Abs) are used as the binding protein. The Abs are produced by injecting animals with multiple doses of relatively pure heterologous PTH or PTH fragment. After the animal has developed a high titer of antibodies against PTH, it is bled and the serum separated from the cells. The serum containing the antibodies is referred to as antiserum. It is diluted to give a suitable concentration for binding with the amount of PTH in the samples to be assayed.

We use two antisera. One is produced by a guinea pig into which we inject bPTH 1-84. This antiserum is diluted so that the final dilution in the incubation test tubes is 1 to 100,000. It has at least two recognition sites for PTH, one in the 53-84 amino acid region of bPTH and another in the 35-52 region of tbe molecule. However, it does not have a recognition site in the 1-34 biologically active region of the molecule. Thus, this antiserum recognizes intact bPTH and inactive carboxyl fragments of PTH, but not amino-terminal fragments up to 34 amino acid residues long.

Our other antiserum is raised in a rabbit against synthetic bPTH 1-34. It has its recognition site(s) in the 1-34 region of PTH and thus recognizes intact PTH and amino-terminal fragments but not carboxyl-terminal fragments. Thus, our antisera are region specific and they have proven useful in determining the relative proportion of intact hormone and fragment secreted by the PTG of our test animal.[212-214]

REFERENCES

1. **Collip, J. B.,** Extraction of a parathyroid hormone which will prevent or control parathyroid tetany and which regulates the level of blood calcium, *J. Biol. Chem.*, 63, 395, 1925.
2. **Aurbach, G. D.,** Isolation of parathyroid hormone after extraction with phenol, *J. Biol. Chem.*, 234, 3179, 1959.
3. **Keutmann, H. T., Aurbach, G. D., Dawson, B. F., Niall, H. D., Deftos, L. J., and Potts, J. T. Jr.,** Isolation and characterization of the bovine parathyroid isohormones, *Biochemistry*, 10, 2779, 1971.
4. **Brewer, H. B., Jr. and Ranan, R.,** Bovine parathyroid hormone: amino acid sequence, *Proc. Natl. Acad. Sci. U.S.A.*, 67, 1862, 1970.
5. **Saver, R. T., Niall, H. D., Hogan, M. L., Keutmann, H. T., O'Riordan, J. L. H., and Potts, J. T., Jr.,** The amino acid sequence of porcine parathyroid hormone, *Biochemistry*, 13, 1994, 1974.
6. **Keutmann, H. T., Saver, M. M., Hendy, G. M., O'Riordan, J. L. H., and Potts, J. T., Jr.,** The complete amino acid sequence of human parathyroid hormone, *Biochemistry*, 17, 5723, 1978.
7. **Keutmann, H. T.,** Chemistry of parathyroid hormone, in *Endocrinology, Vol. 2,* DeGroot, L. J., Cahill, G. F., Jr., Martini, L., Nelson, D. H., Odell, W. D., Potts, J. T., Jr., Steinberger, E., and Winegard, A. I., Eds., Grune & Stratton, San Francisco, 1979, 593.
8. **Niall, H. D., Saver, R. T., Jacobs, J. W., Keutmann, H. T., Segre, G. V., O'Riordan, J. L. H., Aurbach, G. D., and Potts, J. T., Jr.,** The amino acid sequence of the amino-terminal 37 residues of human parathyroid hormone, *Proc. Natl. Acad. Sci. U.S.A.*, 71, 384, 1974.
9. **Tregear, G. W., Van Rietschoten, J., Green, E., Keutmann, H. T., Niall, H. D., Reit, B., Parsons, J. A., Potts, J. T., Jr.,** Bovine parathyroid hormone: minimum chain length of synthetic peptide required for biological activity, *Endocrinology*, 93, 1349, 1973.
10. **MacGregor, R. R. and Cohn, D. V.,** The intracellular pathway for parathormone biosynthesis and secretion, *Clin. Orthop. Rel. Res.*, 137, 244, 1978.
11. **Habener, J. R. and Kronenberg, H. M.,** Parathyroid hormone biosynthesis: structure and function of biosynthetic precursors, *Fed. Proc.*, 37, 2561, 1978.
12. **Habener, J. F. and Potts, J. T., Jr.,** Biosynthesis of parathyroid hormone, *N. Eng. J. Med.*, 299, 580 and 635, 1978.
13. **Habener, J. F., Kemper, B. W., Rich, A. and Potts, J. T., Jr.,** Biosynthesis of parathyroid hormone, *Rec. Prog. Horm. Res*, 33, 249, 1977.
14. **Hamilton, J. W., MacGregor, R. R., Chu, L. L. H., and Cohn, D. V.,** The isolation and partial purification of non-parathyroid calcemic fraction from bovine parathyroid glands, *Endocrinology*, 89, 1440, 1971.
15. **Cohn, D. V., MacGregor, R. R., Chu, L. L. H., Kimmel, J. R., and Hamilton, J. W.,** Calcemic fraction-A: biosynthetic peptide precursor of parathyroid hormone, *Proc. Natl. Acad. Sci. U.S.A.*, 69, 1521, 1972.
16. **Kemper, B., Habener, J. F., Potts, J. T., Jr., and Rich, A.,** Proparathyroid hormone: identification of a biosynthetic precursor to parathyroid hormone, *Proc. Natl. Acad. Sci. U.S.A.*, 69, 643, 1972.
17. **Kemper, B., Habener, J. F., Mulligan, R. C., Potts, J. T., Jr., and Rich, A.,** Preproparathyroid hormone: a direct translation product of parathyroid messenger RNA, Proc. Natl. Acad. Sci. U.S.A., 71, 3731, 1974.
18. **Blobel, G. and Dobberstein, B.,** Transfer of proteins across membranes: presence of proteolytically processed and unprocessed nascent immunoglobulin light chains on membrane-bound ribosomes of murine myeloma, *J. Cell. Biol.*, 67, 835, 1975.
19. **Habener, J. F., Potts, J. T., Jr., and Rich, A.,** Preproparathyroid hormone: evidence for an early biosynthetic precursor of proparathyroid hormone, *J. Biol. Chem.*, 251, 3893, 1976.
20. **Habener, J. F., Amherdt, M., and Orci, L.,** Subcellular organelles involved in the conversion of biosynthetic precursors of parathyroid hormone, *Trans. Assoc. Am. Physicians*, 90, 366, 1977.
21. **Chu, L. L. H., MacGregor, R. R., and Cohn, D. V.,** Energy-dependent intracellular translocation of proparathormone, hormone to parathyroid hormone: the use of amides as specific inhibitors, *Endocrinology*, 95, 1431, 1974.
22. **Chu, L. L. H., MacGregor, R. R., Hamilton, J. W., and Cohn, D. V.,** Conversion of proparathyroid hormone to parathyroid hormone: the use of amides as specific inhibitors, *Endocrinology*, 95, 1431, 1974.
23. **Goltzman, D., Callahan, E. N., Tregear, G. W., and Potts, J. T., Jr.,** Conversion of proparathyroid hormone to parathyroid hormone: studies *in vitro* with trypsin, *Biochemistry*, 15, 5076, 1976.
24. **MacGregor, R. R., Chu, L. L. H., and Cohn, D. V.,** Conversion of proparathyroid hormone to parathyroid hormone by a particulate enzyme of the parathyroid gland, *J. Biol. Chem.*, 251, 6711, 1976.
25. **MacGregor, R. R., Hamilton, J. W., and Cohn, D. V.,** The by-pass of tissue hormone stores during the secretion of newly synthesized parathyroid hormone, *Endocrinology*, 97, 178, 1975.

26. **Limacher, W., Wild, P., Manser, E., and Lutz, H.**, Identification of immunoreactive sites in bovine parathyroid cells to antibodies raised against the NH_2-terminal sequence of parathyroid hormone, *J. Histochem. Cytochem.*, 27, 1209, 1979.
27. **Futrell, J. M., Su, S. P., Roth, S. I., Habener, J. F., Segre, G. V., and Potts, J. T., Jr.**, Localization of parathyroid hormone in bovine and human parathyroid glands using a peroxidase-labelled antibody, in *Endocrinology of Calcium Metabolism*, Copp, D. H. and Talmage, R. V., Eds., Excerpta Medica, Amsterdam, 1978, 353.
28. **Chu, L. L., MacGregor, R. R., Anast, C. S., Hamilton, J. W., and Cohn, D. V.**, Studies on the biosynthesis of rat parathyroid hormone and proparathyroid hormone: adaptation of the parathyroid gland to dietary restriction of calcium, *Endocrinology*, 93, 915, 1973.
29. **Habener, J. F., Kemper, B., and Potts, J. T., Jr.**, Calcium-dependent intracellular degradation of parathyroid hormone: a possible mechanism for the regulation of hormone stores, *Endocrinology*, 97, 431, 1975.
30. **MacGregor, R. R., Chu, L. L. H., Hamilton, J. W., and Cohn, D. V.**, Studies on the subcellular localization of proparathyroid hormone and parathyroid hormone in the bovine parathyroid gland: separation of newly synthesized from mature forms, *Endocrinology*, 93, 1387, 1973.
31. **Habener, J. F. and Potts, J. T., Jr.**, Subcellular distribution of parathyroid hormone, hormonal precursors, and parathyroid secretory protein, *Endocrinology*, 104, 265, 1979.
32. **Au, W. Y. W., Poland, A. P., Stern, P. H. and Raisz, L. G.**, Hormone synthesis and secretion by rat parathyroid gland in tissue culture, *J. Clin. Invest.*, 49, 1639, 1970.
33. **Sherwood, L. M., Rodman, J. S., and Lundberg, W. B.**, Evidence for a precursor to circulating parathyroid hormone, *Proc. Natl. Acad. Sci. U.S.A.*, 67, 1631, 1970.
34. **Kemper, B., Habener, J. F., Rich, A. and Potts, J. T., Jr.**, Parathyroid secretion: discovery of a major calcium-dependent protein, *Science*, 184, 167, 1974.
35. **Morrissey, J. J., Hamilton, J. W., and Cohn, D. V.**, The secretion of parathormone and glycosylated proteins by parathyroid cells in culture, *Biochem. Biophys. Res. Commun.*, 82, 1279, 1978.
36. **Ravazzola, M., Orci, L., Habener, J. F., and Potts, J. T., Jr.**, Parathyroid secretory protein: immunochemical localization within cells that contain parathyroid hormone, *Lancet*, 12, 371, 1978.
37. **Mayer, G. P., Habener, J. F., and Potts, J. T., Jr.**, Parathyroid hormone secretion *in vivo* : demonstration of a calcium-independent, nonsuppressible component of secretion, *J. Clin. Invest.*, 57, 678, 1976.
38. **Mayer, G. P., Keaton, J. A., Hurst, J. G., and Habener, J. F.**, Effects of plasma calcium concentration on the relative proportion of hormone and carboxyl fragments in parathyroid venous blood, *Endocrinology*, 104, 1778, 1979.
39. **Flueck, J. A., DiBella, F. P., Edis, A. J., Kehrwald, J. M., and Arnaud, C. D.**, Immunoheterogeneity of parathyroid hormone in venous effluent serum from hyperfunctioning parathyroid glands, *J. Clin. Invest.*, 60, 1367, 1977.
40. **Hurst, J. G. and Newcomer, W. S.**, Functional parathyroid tissue in ultimobronchial bodies of chickens, *Proc. Soc. Exptl. Biol. Med.*, 132, 55, 1969.
41. **Blum, J. W., Mayer, G. P., and Potts, J. T., Jr.**, Parathyroid hormone response during spontaneous hypocalcemia and induced hypercalcemia in cows, *Endocrinology*, 95, 84, 1974.
42. **Mayer, G. P. and Hurst, J. G.**, Sigmoidal relationship between parathyroid hormone secretion rate and plasma calcium concentration in calves, *Endocrinology*, 102, 1036, 1978.
43. **Blum, J. W., Fischer, J. A., Schwoerer, D., Hunziker, W., and Binswanger, U.**, Acute parathyroid hormone response: sensitivity, relationship to hypocalcemia, and rapidity, *Endocrinology*, 95, 753, 1974.
44. **Sherwood, L. M., Mayer, G. P., Ramberg, C. F., Jr., Kronfeld, D. S., Aurbach, G. D., and Potts, J. T., Jr.**, Regulation of parathyroid hormone secretion: proportional control by calcium, lack of effect of phosphate, *Endocrinology*, 83, 1043, 1968.
45. **Mayer, G. P. and Hurst, J. G.**, Comparison of the effects of calcium and magnesium on parathyroid hormone secretion rate in calves, *Endocrinology*, 102, 1803, 1978.
46. **Habener, J. F. and Potts, J. T., Jr.**, Relative effectiveness of magnesium and calcium on the secretion and biosynthesis of parathyroid hormone *in vitro*, *Endocrinology*, 98, 197, 1976.
47. **Anast, C. S., Winnacker, J. L., Forte, L. R., and Burns, T. W.**, Impaired release of parathyroid hormone in magnesium deficiency, *J. Clin. Endocrinol. Metab.*, 42, 707, 1976.
48. **Fischer, J. A., Blum, J. W., and Binswanger, U.**, Acute parathyroid hormone response to epinephrine *in vivo*, *J. Clin. Invest.*, 52, 2434, 1973.
49. **Kukreja, S. C., Hargis, G. K., Bowser, E. M., Henderson, W. J., Fisherman, E. W., and Williams, G. A.**, Role of adrenergic stimuli in parathyroid hormone secretion in man, *J. Clin. Endocrinol. Metab.*, 40, 478, 1975.
50. **Williams, G. A., Hargis, G. K., Bowser, E. N., Henderson, W. J., and Martinez, N. J.**, Evidence for a role of adenosine 3′5′-monophosphate in parathyroid hormone release, *Endocrinology*, 92, 687, 1973.

51. **Mayer, G. P., Hurst, J. G., Barto, J. A., Keaton, J. A., and Moore, M. P.,** Effects of epinephrine on parathyroid hormone secretion in calves, *Endocrinology,* 104, 1181, 1979.
52. **Harney, A. M., Kukreja, S. C., Hargis, G. K., Johnson, P. A., Bowser, E. N. and Williams, G. A.,** Effect of long-term administration of epinephrine and propranolol on serum calcium, parathyroid hormone and calcitonin in the rat, *Proc. Soc. Exptl. Biol. Med.,* 159, 266, 1978.
53. **Abe, M. and Sherwood, L. M.,** Regulation of parathyroid hormone secretion by adenyl cyclase, *Biochem. Biophys. Res. Commun.,* 48, 396, 1972.
54. **Brown, E. M., Gardner, D. G., Windeck, R. A., and Aurbach, G. D.,** Relationship of intracellular 3′5′-adenosine monophosphate accumulation to parathyroid hormone release from dispersed bovine parathyroid cells, *Endocrinology,* 103, 2323, 1978.
55. **Bolman, R. M., III, Cooper, C. W., Garner, S. C., Munson, P. L., and Wells, S. A., Jr.,** Stimulation of gastrin secretion in the pig by parathyroid hormone and its inhibition by thyrocalcitonin, *Endocrinology,* 100, 1014, 1977.
56. **Windeck, R., Brown, E. M., Gardner, D. G., and Aurbach, G. D.,** Effect of gastrointestinal hormones on isolated bovine parathyroid cells, *Endocrinology,* 103, 2020, 1978.
57. **Williams, G. A., Bowser, E. N., Hargis, G. K., Kukreja, S. C., Shah, J. H., Vora, N. M., and Henderson, W. J.,** Effect of ethanol on parathyroid hormone and calcitonin secretion in man, *Proc. Soc. Exptl. Biol. Med.,* 159, 187, 1978.
58. **Chambers, D. J., Dunham, J., Zanelli, J. M., Parsons, J. A., Bitensky, L. and Chayen, J.,** A sensitive bioassay of parathyroid hormone in plasma, *Clin. Endocrinol.,* 9, 373, 1978.
59. **Lancer, S. R., Bowser, E. N., Hargis, G. K., and Williams, G. A.,** The effect of growth hormone on parathyroid function in rats, *Endocrinology,* 98, 1289, 1976.
60. **Gertner, J. M., Horst, R. L., Broadus, A. E., Rasmussen, H., and Genel, M.,** Parathyroid function and vitamin D metabolism during human growth hormone replacement, *J. Clin. Endocrinol. Metab.,* 49, 185, 1979.
61. **Williams, G. A., Hargis, G. K., Ensinck, J. W., Kukreja, S. C., Bowser, E. N., Chertow, B. S., and Henderson, W. J.,** Role of endogenous somatostatin in the secretion of parathyroid hormone and calcitonin, *Metabolism,* 28, 950, 1979.
62. **Deftos, L. J., Lorenz, M., and Bohanon, M.,** Somatostatin does not suppress plasma parathyroid hormone, *J. Clin. Endocrinol. Metab.,* 43, 205, 1976.
63. **Sato, S., Szabo, M., Kowalski, K., and Burke, G.,** Role of prostaglandin in thyrotropin action on thyroid, *Endocrinology,* 90, 343, 1972.
64. **Gardner, D. G., Brown, E. M., Windeck, R., and Aurbach, G. D.,** Prostaglandin E_2 stimulation of adenosin 3′5′-monophosphate accumulation and parathyroid hormone release in dispersed bovine parathyroid cells, *Endocrinology,* 103, 577, 1978.
65. **Gardner, D. G., Brown, E. M., Windeck, and Aurbach, G. D.,** Prostaglandin $F_{2\alpha}$ inhibits 3′5′-adenosine monophosphate accumulation and parathyroid hormone release from dispersed bovine parathyroid cells, *Endocrinology,* 104, 1, 1979.
66. **Deluca, H. F.,** Recent advances in our understanding of the vitamin D endocrine system, *Steroid Biochem.,* 11, 35, 1979.
67. **Haussler, M. R. and McCain, T. A.,** Basic and clinical concepts related to vitamin D metabolism and action, *N. Eng. J. Med.,* 297, 974 and 1041, 1977.
68. **Golden, P., Mazey, R., Greenwalt, A., Martin, K., and Slatopolsky, E.,** Vitamin D: a direct effect on the parathyroid gland?, *Miner. Electrolyte Metab.,* 2, 1, 1979.
69. **Tanaka, Y., DeLuca, H. F., Ghayarian, J. G., Hargis, G. K., and Williams, G. A.,** Effects of vitamin D and its metabolites on serum parathyroid hormone levels in the rat, *Miner. Electrolyte Metab.,* 2, 20, 1979.
70. **Oldham, S. B., Smith, R., Hartenbower, D. L., Henry, H. L., Norman, A. W., and Coburn, J. W.,** The acute effects of 1,25-dihydroxycholecalciferol on serum immuno-reactive parathyroid hormone in the dog, *Endocrinology,* 104, 248, 1979.
71. **Dietel, M., Dorn, G., Monty, R., and Altenahr, E.,** Influence of vitamin D_3,1,25-dihydroxyvitamin D_3 and 24,25-dihydroxy vitamin D_3 on parathyroid hormone secretion, adenosine 3′5′-monophosphate release, and ultrastructure of parathyroid glands in organ culture, *Endocrinology,* 105, 237, 1979.
72. **Chertow, B. S., Williams, G. A., Norris, R. M., Baker, G. R., and Hargis, G. K.,** Vitamin A stimulation of parathyroid hormone: interactions with calcium, hydrocortisone, and vitamin E in bovine parathyroid tissues and effects of vitamin A in man, *Eur. J. Clin. Invest.,* 7, 307, 1977.
73. **Copp, D. H., Moghadam, H., Mensen, E. D., and McPherson, G. D.,** The parathyroids and calcium homeostasis, in: *The Parathyroids,* Greep, R. O. and Talmage, R. V., Eds., Charles C Thomas, Springfield, Ill., 1961, 203.
74. **Hamilton, J. W., Spierto, F. W., MacGregor, R. R., and Cohn, D. V.,** Studies on the biosynthesis *in vitro* of parathyroid hormone. II. The effects of calcium and magnesium on synthesis of parathyroid hormone isolated from bovine parathyroid tissues and incubation medium, *J. Biol. Chem.,* 246, 3224, 1971.

75. **Segre, G. V., D'Amour, P., and Potts, J. T., Jr.**, Metabolism of radioiodinated bovine parathyroid hormone in the rat, *Endocrinology*, 99, 1645, 1976.
76. **Habener, J. F., Mayer, G. P., Dee, P. C., and Potts, J. T., Jr.**, Metabolism of amino and carboxyl sequence immunoreactive parathyroid hormone in the bovine: evidence for peripheral cleavage of hormone, *Metabolism*, 25, 385, 1976.
77. **Martin, K. J., Kruska, K. A., Freitag, J. J., Klahr, S., and Slatopolsky, E.**, The peripheral metabolism of parathyroid hormone, *N. Eng. J. Med.*, 301, 1092, 1979.
78. **Singer, F. R., Segre, G. V., Habener, J. F., and Potts, J. T., Jr.**, Peripheral metabolism of bovine parathyroid hormone in the dog, *Metabolism*, 24, 139, 1975.
79. **Oldham, S. B., Finck, E. J., and Singer, F. R.**, Parathyroid clearance in man, *Metabolism*, 27, 993, 1978.
80. **Martin, K. J., Hruska, K. A., Lewis, J., Anderson, C., and Slatopolsky, E.**, The renal handling of parathyroid hormone: role of peritubular uptake and glomerular filtration, *J. Clin. Invest.*, 60, 808, 1977.
81. **Freitag, J. J., Martin, K. J., Kruska, K., Anderson, C., Ladenson, J., and Slatopolsky, E.**, Impaired parathyroid hormone metabolism in patients with chronic renal failure, *N. Eng. J. Med.*, 298, 29, 1978.
82. **Kruska, K., Martin, K., Mennes, P., Greenwalt, A., Anderson, C., Klahr, S., and Slatopolsky, E.**, Degradation of parathyroid hormone and fragment production by the isolated perfused dog kidney: the effect of glomerular filtration rate and perfusate Ca^{++} concentrations, *J. Clin. Invest.*, 60, 501, 1977.
83. **Canterbury, J. M., Bricker, L. A., Levey, G. S., Kozlouskis, P. L., Ruiz, E., Zull, J. E., and Reiss, E.**, Metabolism of parathyroid hormone: immunological and biological characteristics of fragments generated by liver perfusion, *J. Clin. Invest.*, 55, 1245, 1975.
84. **Parsons, J. A. and Robinson, C. J.**, A rapid indirect hypercalcemic action of parathyroid hormone demonstrated in isolated blood-perfused bone, in *Parathyroid Hormone and Thyrocalcitonin (Calcitonin)*, Talmage, R. V. and Belanger, L. F., Eds., Excerpta Medica, Amsterdam, 1968, 329.
85. **Martin, K. J., Freitag, J. J., Conrades, M. B., Kruska, K., Klahr, S., and Slatopolsky, E.**, Selective uptake of the synthetic amino terminal fragment of bovine parathyroid hormone by isolated perfused bone, *J. Clin. Invest.*, 62, 256, 1978.
86. **Freitag, J. J., Martin, K. J., Conrades, M. B., and Slatopolsky, E.**, Metabolism of parathyroid hormone by fetal rat calvaria, *Endocrinology*, 104, 510, 1979.
87. **Galtzman, D.**, Examination of the requirement for metabolism of parathyroid hormone in skeletal tissue before biological action, *Endocrinology*, 102, 1555, 1978.
88. **D'Amour, P., Huet, P. M., Segre, G. V., and Rosenblatt, M.**, Structural requirements for uptake and cleavage of iodinated bovine parathyroid hormone by the dog liver *in vivo, Prog. Abstr. 61st Ann. Meet. Endocr. Soc., Anaheim, Calif.*, (Abstr. No. 172) p. 115, 1979.
89. **Parsons, J. A.**, Physiology of parathyroid hormone, in *Endocrinology, Vol. 2,* DeGroot, L. J, Cahill, G. F., Jr., Martini, L., Nelson, D. H., Odell, W. D., Potts, J. T., Jr., Steinberger, E., and Winegard, A. I., Eds., Grune & Stratton, New York, 1979, 621.
90. **Parfitt, A. M.**, The action of parathyroid hormone on bone: relation to bone remodelling and turnover, calcium homeostasis and metabolic bone disease (a four part report), *Metabolism*, 25, 809, 1976.
91. **Parsons, J. A.**, Parathyroid physiology and the skeleton, in *The Biochemistry and Physiology of Bone*, Vol. 4, Bourne, G. H., Ed., Academic Press, New York, 1976, 159.
92. **Jaworski, Z. F. and Lok, E.**, The rate of osteoclastic bone erosion in Haversian remodelling sites of adult dogs rib, *Calcif. Tiss. Res.*, 10, 103, 1972.
93. **Rowland, R. E.**, Exchangeable bone calcium, *Clin. Orthop.*, 49, 233, 1966.
94. **Riggs, B. L., Bassingthwaite, J. B., Jowsey, J., and Pequegnat, E. P.**, Autoradiographic methods for quantitation of deposition and distribution of radiocalcium in bone, *J. Lab. Clin. Med.*, 75, 520, 1970.
95. **Groer, P. G. and Marshall, J. H.**, Mechanism of calcium exchange at bone surfaces, *Calcif. Tiss. Res.*, 12, 175, 1973.
96. **Selye, H.**, On the stimulation of new bone formation with parathyroid extract and irradiated ergosterol, *Endocrinology*, 16, 547, 1932.
97. **Barnicot, N. A.**, The local action of the parathyroid and other tissues on bone in intracerebral graft, *J. Anat. (London)*, 82, 233, 1948.
98. **Tatevossian, A.**, Effect of parathyroid extract on blood calcium and osteoclast count in mice, *Calicif. Tiss. Res.*, 11, 251, 1973.
99. **Krempien, B. and Ritz, E.**, Effects of parathyroid hormone on osteocytes. Ultrastructural evidence for anisotropic osteolysis and involvement of the cytoskeleton, *Metab. Bone Dis. Rel. Res.* 1, 55, 1978.

100. **Raisz, L. G., Trummel, C. T., and Simmons, H.,** Induction of bone resorption in tissue culture: prolonged response after brief exposure to parathyroid hormone or 25-hydroxycholecalciferol, *Endocrinology,* 90, 744, 1972.
101. **Parsons, J. A., Reit, B., and Robinson, C.J.,** A rapid and sensitive hypercalcemic assay for parathyroid hormone using the chicken, *Endocrinology,* 92, 454, 1973.
102. **Marcus, R. and Aurbach, G. D.,** Bioassay of parathyroid hormone, *in vitro* with a stable preparation of adenyl cyclase from rat kidney, *Endocrinology,* 85, 801, 1969.
103. **Herrmann-Erlee, M. P. M., Heersche, J. N. M., Hekkelman, J. W., Gaillard, P. J., Tregear, G. W., Parsons, J. A., and Potts, J. T., Jr.,** Effects on bone, *in vitro* of bovine parathyroid hormone and synthetic fragments representing residues 1-34, 2-34, 3-34, *Endocrine Res. Commun.,* 3, 21, 1976.
104. **Neuman, W. F.,** The *milieu interieur* of bone: Claude Bernard revisited, *Fed. Proc.,* 28, 1846, 1969.
105. **Ramp, W. K. and McNeil, R. W.,** Selective stimulation of net calcium efflux from chick embryo tibiae by parathyroid hormone *in vitro, Calcif. Tiss. Res.,* 25, 227, 1978.
106. **Talmage, R. V.** Calcium homeostasis — calcium transport — parathyroid action. The effect of parathyroid hormone on the movement of calcium between bone and fluid, *Clin. Orthop.,* 67, 210, 1969.
107. **Aurbach, G. D.,** Parathyroid hormone: mechanism of actions and cyclic AMP, *Fed. Proc.,* 29, 1179, 1970.
108. **Howard, G. A., Battemiller, B. L., and Baylink, D. J.,** Evidence for the coupling of bone formation to bone resorption *in vitro, Metab. Bone. Dis. Rel. Res,* 2, 131, 1980.
109. **Parsons, J. A., Rafferty, B., and Gray, D. et al.,** Pharmacology of parathyroid hormone and some of its fragments and analogues, in *Calcium-Regulating Hormones,* Talmage, R. V., Owen, M., and Parsons, J. A., Eds. Excerpta Medica, Amsterdam, 1975, 33.
110. **Harris, W.H. and Heaney, R. P.,** Skeletal renewal and metabolic bone disease, *New Engl. J. Med.,* 280, 253, 1969.
111. **Pugsley, L. I. and Selye, H.,** The histological changes in the bone responsible for the action of parathyroid hormone on the calcium metabolism of the rat, *J. Physiol. (London),* 79, 113, 1933.
112. **Reeve, J., Tregear, G. W.,and Parsons, J. A.,** Preliminary trial of low doses of human parathyroid hormone 1-34 peptide in treatment of osteoporosis, *Calcif. Tiss. Res.,* (Suppl. 21), 469, 1976.
113. **O'Grady, R. L. and Cameron, D. A.,** Demonstration of binding sites of PTH in bone cells, in *Endocrinology (London),* Taylor, S. and Heinemann, W., Eds., 1972, 374.
114. **Peck, W. A., Carpenter, J., Messinger, K., and Debra, D.,** Cyclic 3′5′ adenosine monophosphate in isolated bone cells: response to low concentrations of parathyroid hormone, *Endocrinology,* 92, 692, 1973.
115. **Peck, W.,** Cyclic AMP as a second messenger in the skeletal actions of parathyroid hormone: a decade-old hypothesis, *Calcif. Tiss. Int.,* 29, 1, 1979.
116. **Rodan, S. B. and Rodan, G. A.,** The effect of parathyroid hormone and thyrocalcitonin on the accumulation of cyclic adenosine 3′5′-monophosphate in freshly isolated bone cells, *J. Biol. Chem.,* 249, 3068, 1974.
117. **Oziak, R. and Stern, P. H.,** Calcium transport in isolated bone cells. III. Effects of parathyroid hormone and cyclic 3′5′-AMP, *Endocrinology,* 97, 1281, 1975.
118. **Wong, G. L., Kent, G. N., Ku, K. Y., and Cohn, D. V.,** The interaction of parathormone and calcium on the hormone-regulated synthesis of hyaluronic acid and citrate decarboxylation in isolated bone cells, *Endocrinology,* 103, 2274, 1978.
119. **Neuman, W. F., Mulryan, B. J., and Martin, G. R.,** A chemical view of osteoclasis based on studies with yttrium, *Clin. Orthop.,* 17, 124, 1960.
120. **Firschein, H. E. and Alcock, N. W.,** Rate of removal of collagen and mineral from bone and cartilage, *Metabolism,* 18, 115, 1969.
121. **Nisbet, J. A., Hellwell, S., and Nordin, B. E. C.,** Relation of lactic and citric acid metabolism to bone resorption in tissue culture, *Clin. Orthop.,* 70, 220, 1970.
122. **Waite, L. C.,** Carbonic anhydrase inhibitors, parathyroid hormone and calcium metabolism, *Endocrinology,* 91, 1160, 1972.
123. **Vaes, G.,** Collagenase, lysosomes and osteoclastic bone resorption, in *Collagenase in Normal and Pathological Connective Tissue,* Wolley, D. E. and Evanson, J. M., Eds., John Wiley & Sons, New York, 1980, 185.
124. **Eilon, G. and Raisz, L. G.,** Comparison of the effects of stimulators and inhibitors of resorption on the release of lysosomal enzymes and radioactive calcium from fetal bone in organ culture, *Endocrinology,* 103, 1969, 1978.
125. **McPartlin, J., Skrabanek, P., and Powell, D.,** Early effects of parathyroid hormone on rat calvarian bone alkaline phosphatase, *Endocrinology,* 103, 1573, 1978.
126. **Puschett, J. B.,** Renal tubular effects of parathyroid hormone: an update, *Clin. Orthop.,* 135, 249, 1978.
127. **Pang, P. K., Tenner, T. E., Jr., Yee, J. A., Yang, M., and Janssen, H. F.,** Hypotensive action of parathyroid hormone preparations on rats and dogs, *Proc. Natl. Acad. Sci. U.S.A.,* 77, 675, 1980.

128. **Agus, Z. S., Puschett, J. B., Senesky, D., and Goldberg, M.**, Mode of action of parathyroid hormone and cyclic adenosine 3′,5′-monophosphate on renal tubular phosphate reabsorption in the dog, *J. Clin. Invest.*, 50, 617, 1971.
129. **Augus, Z. S., Gardner, L. B., Beck, L. H., and Goldberg, M.**, Effects of parathyroid hormone on renal tubular reabsorption of calcium, sodium and phosphate, *Am. J. Physiol.*, 224, 1143, 1973.
130. **Strickler, J. C., Thompson, D. D., Klose, R. M., and Giebisch, G.**, Micropuncture study of inorganic phosphate excretion in the rat, *J. Clin. Invest.*, 43, 1596, 1964.
131. **Beck, L. H. and Goldberg, M.**, Effects of acetazolamide and parathyroidectomy on renal transport of sodium, calcium and phosphate, *Am. J. Physiol.*, 224, 1136, 1973.
132. **Dennis, V. W., Bello-Reuss, E., and Robinson, R. R.**, Response of phosphate transport to parathyroid hormone in segments of rabbit nephron, *Am. J. Physiol.*, 233, F29, 1977.
133. **Chase, L. R. and Aurbach, G. D.**, Parathyroid function and the renal excretion of 3′,5′-adenylic acid, *Proc. Natl. Acad. Sci., U.S.A.*, 58, 518, 1967.
134. **Pastoriza-Munoz, E., Colindres, R. E., Lassiter, W. E., and Lechene, C.**, Effect of parathyroid hormone on phosphate reabsorption in rat distal convolution, *Am. J. Physiol.*, 235, F321, 1978.
135. **Jackson, B. A., Hui, Y. S. F., Northrup, T. E., and Dousa, T. P.**, Differential responsiveness of adenylate cyclase from rat, dog and rabbit kidney to parathyroid hormone, vasopressin and calcitonin, *Mineral Electrolyte Metab.*, 3, 136, 1980.
136. **Goltzman, D., Callahan, E. N., Tregear, G. W., and Potts, J. T., Jr.**, Influence of guanyl nucleotides on parathyroid hormone — stimulated adenylyl cyclase activity in renal cortical membranes, *Endocrinology*, 103, 1352, 1978.
137. **Harada, E., Laychock, S. G., and Rubin, R. P.**, Parathyroid hormone induced stimulation of calcium uptake by renal microsomes, *Biochem. Biophys. Res. Commun.*, 84, 396, 1978.
138. **Dibella, F. P., Dousa, T. P., Miller, S., Dousa, T. P., Miller, S. S., and Arnaud, C. D.**, Parathyroid hormone receptors of renal cortex: specific binding of biologically active ^{125}I-labelled hormone and relationship to adenylate cyclase activation, *Proc. Natl. Acad. Sci. U.S.A.*, 71, 723, 1974.
139. **Stumpf, W. E., Sar, M., Narbaitz, R., Reid, F. A., DeLuca, H. F., and Tanaka, Y.**, Cellular and subcellular localization of 1,25-$(OH)_2$-Vitamin D_3 in rat kidney: comparison with localization of parathyroid hormone and estradiol, *Proc. Natl. Acad. Sci. U.S.A.*, 77, 1149, 1980.
140. **Kau, S. T. and Maack, T.**, Transport and catabolism of parathyroid hormone in isolated rat kidney, *Am. J. Physiol.*, 233, F445, 1977.
141. **Massry, S. G., Coburn, J. W., Friedler, R. M., Kurokawa, K., and Singer, F. R.**, Relationship between the kidney and parathyroid hormone, *Nephron*, 15, 197, 1975.
142. **Haussler, M. R. and McCain, T. A.**, Basic and clinical concepts related to vitamin D metabolism and action, *New Eng. J. Med.*, 297, 974, and 1041, 1977.
143. **Norman, A. W. and Henry, H. L.**, Vitamin D to 1,25-dihydroxycholecalciferol: evolution of a steroid hormone, *Trends Biochem. Sci.*, 4, 14, 1979.
144. **Fraser, D. R.**, The metabolism and function of vitamin D, *World Rev. Nutr. Diet*, 31, 168, 1978.
145. **Arnaud, C. D.** Calcium homeostasis: regulatory elements and their integration, *Fed. Proc.*, 37, 2557, 1978.
146. **Hay, A.**, Complexities of vitamin D metabolism still increasing, *Nature*, 278, 510, 1979.
147. **Deluca, H. F.**, Recent advances in our understanding of the vitamin D endocrine system, *J. Steroid Biochem*, 11, 35, 1979.
148. **Drezner, M. K. and Harrelson, J. M.**, Newer knowledge of vitamin D and its metabolites in health and disease, *Clin. Orthop.*, 139, 206, 1979.
149. **Coburn, J. W., Hartenbower, D. L., and Norman, A. W.**, Metabolism and action of the hormone Vitamin D. Its relation to diseases of calcium homeostatis, *West. J. Med.*, 121, 22, 1974.
150. **Thompson, M. L.**, Relative efficiency of pigment and horny later thickness in protecting the skin of Europeans and Africans against solar ultraviolet radiation, *J. Physiol. (London)*, 127, 236, 1955.
151. **Tucker, G., Gragnon, R., and Haussler, M.**, Vitamin D_3-25-hydroxylase: tissue occurrence and apparent lack of regulation, *Arch. Biochem. Biophys.*, 155, 47, 1973.
152. **Fraser, D. R. and Kodicek, E.**, Unique biosynthesis by kidney of a biologically active vitamin D metabolite, *Nature*, 228, 764, 1970.
153. **Haussler, M. R., Myrtle, J. F., and Norman, A. W.**, The association of a metabolite of vitamin D_3 with intestinal mucosa chromatin, *in vivo*, *J. Biol. Chem.*, 243, 4055, 1968.
154. **Tanaka, Y., Halloran, B., Schnoes, H. K., and DeLuca, H. F.**, *In vitro* production of 1,25-dihydroxyvitamin D_3 by rat placental tissue, *Proc. Natl. Acad. Sci. U.S.A.*, 76, 5033, 1979.
155. **Sunaga, S., Horiuchi, N., Takahashi, N., Okuyama, K., and Suda, T.**, The site of 1α,25-Dihydroxyvitamin D_3 production in pregnancy, *Biochem. Biophys. Res. Commun.*, 90, 948, 1979.
156. **Boyle, I. T., Gray, R. W., and DeLuca, H. F.**, Regulation by calcium of *in vivo* synthesis of 1,25-dihydroxycholecalciferol and 21,25-dihydroxycholecalciferol, *Proc. Natl. Acad. Sci. U.S.A.*, 68, 2131, 1971.
157. **Tanaka, Y. and DeLuca, H. F.**, The control of 25-hydroxyvitamin D metabolism by inorganic phosphorus, *Arch. Biochem. Biophys.*, 154, 566, 1973.

158. **Madhok, T. C. and DeLuca, H. F.**, Characteristics of the rat liver microsomal enzyme system converting cholecalciferol into 25-hydroxycholecalciferol, *Biochem. J.*, 184, 491, 1979.
159. **Henry, H. L.**, Response of chick kidney cell cultures to 1,25-Dihydroxyvitamin D_3, *Prog. Abstr. 61st Ann. Meet. Endocr. Soc.*, Anaheim, Calif., (Abstr. No. 755), p. 261, 1979.
160. **Spanos, E., Pike, J. W., Haussler, M. R., Colston, K. W., Evans, I. M. A., Goldner, A. M., McCain, T. A., and MacIntyre, I.**, Circulating 1 α,25-dihydroxyvitamin D in the chicken: enhancement by injection of prolactin and during egg laying, *Life Sci.*, 19, 1751, 1976.
161. **Boass, A., Toverud, S. U., and McCain, T. A., Pike, J. W., and Haussler, M. R.**, Elevated serum levels of 1α,25-dihydroxycholecalciferol in lactating rats, *Nature*, 267, 630, 1977.
162. **Brown, D. J., Spanos, E., and MacIntyre, I.**, Hormonal control of plasma 1,25-dihydroxyvitamin D_3 in man, *J. Endocrinol.* 83, 54P, 1979.
163. **Halloran, B. P., Barthell, E. N., and DeLuca, H. F.**, Vitamin D metabolism during pregnancy and lactation in the rat, *Proc. Natl. Acad. Sci. U.S.A.*, 76, 5549, 1979.
164. **Baksi, S. N. and Kenny, A. D.**, Vitamin D_3 metabolism in immature Japanese Quail: Effects of ovarian hormones, *Endocrinology*, 101, 1216, 1977.
165. **Pike, J. W., Spanos, E., Colston, K. W., MacIntyre, I., and Haussler, M. R.**, Influence of estrogen on renal vitamin D hydroxylases and serum 1α,25-$(OH)_2D_3$ in chicks, *Am. J. Physiol.*, 235, E338, 1978.
166. **Eisman, J. A., Hamstra, A. J., Kram, B. E., and DeLuca, H. F.**, A sensitive, precise and convenient method for determination of 1,25-dihydroxyvitamin D in human plasma, *Arch. Biochem. Biophysic.*, 176, 235, 1976.
167. **Lund, B. and Sorensen, O. H.**, Measurement of 25-hydroxyvitamin D in serum and its relation to sunshine, age, and vitamin D intake in the Danish population, *Scand. J. Clin. Lab. Invest.*, 39, 23, 1979.
168. **Bikle, D. D., Morrissey, R. L., and Zolock, D. T.**, The mechanism of action of vitamin D in the intestine, *Am. J. Clin. Nutr.*, 32, 2322, 1979.
169. **Wasserman, R. H., Kallfelz, F. A., and Comar, C. L.**, Active transport of calcium by rat duodenum *in vivo, Sciences*, 133, 883, 1961.
170. **Schachter, D. and Rosen, S. M.**, Active transport of Ca^{45} by the small intestine and its dependence on vitamin D, *Am. J. Physiol.*, 196, 357, 1959.
171. **Harrison, H. E. and Harrison, H. C.**, Intestinal transport of phosphate: Action of vitamin D, calcium and potassium, *Am. J. Physiol.*, 201, 1007, 1961.
172. **Wasserman, R. H. and Taytor, A. N.**, Intestinal absorption of phosphate in the chick: effect of Vitamin D_3 and other parameters, *J. Nutr.*, 103, 586, 1973.
173. **Walling, M. W.**, Intestinal Ca and phosphate transport differential responses to vitamin D_3 metabolites, *Am. J. Physiol.*, 233, E488, 1977.
174. **Charles, A., Martial, J., Zolock, D., Morrissey, R., Bickle, D., and Baxter, J.**, Regulation of the messenger RNA for calcium binding protein by 1,25-dihydroxycholecalciferol, in *Vitamin D Biochemical, Chemical and Clinical Aspects Related to Calcium Metabolism*, Norman, A. W., Schaefer, K., Coburn, J. W., DeLuca, H. F., Fraser, D., Grigoleit, H. G., and Herrath, D. V., Eds., Walter de Gruyter, New York, 1977, 227.
175. **Corradino, R. A.**, Cyclic AMP regulation of the 1α25-$(OH)_2D_3$ - mediated intestinal calcium absorptive mechanism, in *Vitamin D Biochemical, Chemical and Clinical Aspects Related to Calcium Metabolism*, Norman, A. W., Schaefer, K., Coburn, J. W., DeLuca, H. F., Fraser, D., Grigoleit, H. G., and Herrath, D. V., Eds., Walter de Gruyter, New York, 1977, 231.
176. **Tsai, H. C. and Norman, A. W.**, Studies on the mode of action of calciferol. VI. Effect of 1,25-dihydroxyvitamin D_3 on RNA synthesis in the intestinal mucosa, *Biochem. Biophys. Res. Commun.*, 54, 622, 1973.
177. **Zerwekh, J. E., Haussler, M. R., and Lindell, T. J.**, Rapid enhancement of chick intestinal DNA-dependent RNA polymerase II activity by 1α,25-dihydroxyvitamin D_3, *in vivo, Proc. Natl. Acad. Sci. U.S.A.*, 71, 2337, 1974.
178. **Haussler, M. R., Nagode, L. A., and Rasmussen, H.**, Induction of intestinal brush border alkaline phosphatase by vitamin D and identity with Ca ATPase, *Nature*, 228, 1199, 1970.
179. **Wasserman, R. H., Corradino, R. A., Fullmer, C. S., and Taylor, A. N.**, Some aspects of vitamin D action: calcium absorption and vitamin D-dependent calcium-binding protein, *Vitam. Horm.*, 32, 299, 1974.
180. **Corradino, R. A.**, 1,25-dihydroxycholecalciferol: inhibition of action in organ-cultured intestine by actinomycin D and α-amanitin, *Nature*, 243, 41, 1973.
181. **Bikle, D. D., Zolock, D. T., Morrissey, R. L., and Herman, R. H.**, Independence of 1,25-Dihydroxyvitamin D_3-mediated calcium transport from *de novo* RNA and protein synthesis, *J. Biol. Chem.*, 253, 484, 1978.
182. **Queille, M. L., Miravet, L., Bordier, P., and Redel, J.**, The action of vitamin D metabolites (25 $(OH)D_3$-12, 5 $(OH)_2D_3$ - 25,26$(OH)_2$ D_3) on vitamin D deficient rats, *Biomedicine*, 28, 237, 1978.

183. **Carlsson, A.**, Tracer experiments on the effect of vitamin D on the skeletal metabolism of calcium and phosphorus, *Acta Physiol. Scand.*, 26, 212, 1952.
184. **Rasmussen, H., DeLuca, H., Arnaud, C., Hawker, C., and von Stedingk, M.**, The relationship between vitamin D and parathyroid hormone, *J. Clin. Invest.*, 42, 1940, 1963.
185. **Reynolds, J. J., Holick, M. F., and DeLuca, H. F.**, The role of vitamin D metabolites in bone resorption, *Calicif. Tiss. Res.*, 12, 295, 1973.
186. **Tanaka, Y. and DeLuca, H. F.**, Bone mineral mobilization activity of 1,25-dihydroxycholecalciferol, a metabolite of vitamin D, *Arch. Biochem. Biophys.*, 146, 574, 1971.
187. **Boris, A., Hurley, J. F., and Trimal, T.**, *In vivo* studies in chicks and rats of bone calcium mobilization by 1α,25-dihydroxycholecalciferol (calcitriol) and its congeners, *J. Nutri.*, 109, 1772, 1979.
188. **Raisz, L. G., Maina, D. M., Gworek, S. C., Dietrich, J. W., and Canalis, E. M.**, Hormonal control of bone collagen synthesis *in vitro*: inhibitory effects of 1-hydroxylated vitamin D metabolites, *Endocrinology*, 102, 731, 1978.
189. **Dickson, I. R. and Kodicek, E.**, Effect of vitamin D deficiency on bone formation in the chick, *Biochem. J.*, 182, 429, 1979.
190. **Malluche, H. H., Henry, H., Meyer-Sabellek, W., Sherman, D., Massry, S. G., and Norman, A. W.**, Effects and interation of 24R,25 $(OH)_2D_3$ and 1,25 $(OH)_2D_3$ on bone, *Am. J. Physiol.*, 238, E494, 1980.
191. **Lindgren, J. U. and Lindholm, T. S.**, Effect of 1-alpha-hydroxyvitamin D_3 on osteoporosis in rats induced by oophorectomy, *Calcif. Tiss. Intl.*, 27, 161, 1979.
192. **Boris, A., Hurley, J. F., and Trmal, T.**, Biological activity evaluation of chemically synthesized vitamin D metabolites and analogs, in *Vitamin D Biochemical, Chemical and Clinical Aspects Related to Calcium Metabolism*, Norman, A. W., Schaefer, K., Coburn, J. W., DeLuca, H. F., Fraser, Grigoleit, H. G., and Herrath, D. V., Eds., Walter de Gruyter, New York, 1977, 553.
193. **Deiss, W. P. Jr. and Hern, D. L.**, Bone matrix studies: influences of parathyroid extract, calcitonin, and cholecalciferol and of rickets and its treatment, *Biochem. Biophys. Acta.*, 284, 311, 1979.
194. **Corvol, M. T. and Dumontier, M. F., Garabedian, M. and Rappaport, R.**, Vitamin D and cartilage. II. Biological activity of 25-hydroxycholecalciferol and 24,25- and 1,25- dihydroxycholecalciferols on cultured growth plate chondrocytes, *Endocrinology*, 102, 1269, 1978.
195. **Puschett, J. B., Beck, W. S. Jr., and Jelonek, A.**, Parathyroid hormone and 25-hydroxyvitamin D_3: synergistic and antagonistic effects on renal phosphate transport, *Science*, 190, 473, 1975.
196. **Puschett, J. B., Moranz, J., and Kurnick, W.**, Evidence for a direct action of cholecalciferol and 25-hydroxycholecalciferol on renal transport of phosphate, sodium and calcium, *J. Clin. Invest.*, 51, 373, 1972.
197. **Popoutzer, M. M., Robinette, J. B., DeLuca, H. F., and Holick, M. F.**, The acute effect of 25-hydroxycholecalciferol on renal handling of phosphorus, *J. Clin. Invest.*, 53, 913, 1974.
198. **Puschett, J. B. and Kuhrman, M. S.** Renal tubular effects of 1,25-dihydroxyvitamin D_3: interactions with vasopressin and parathyroid hormone in the vitamin D-depleted rat, *J. Lab. Clin. Med.*, 92, 895, 1978.
199. **DeLuca, H. F. and Holick, M. F.**, Vitamin D: biosynthesis, metabolism and mode of action, in *Endocrinology, Vol. 2*, DeGroot, L. J., Cahill, G. F. Jr., Martini, L., Nelson, D. H., Odell, W. D., Potts, J. T., Jr., Steinberger, E., and Winegard, A. I., Grune & Stratton, New York, 1979, 653.
200. **Hadad, J. G.**, Transport of vitamin D metabolites, *Clin. Ortho. Rel. Res.*, 142, 249, 1979.
201. **Eisman, J. A., Hamstra, A. J., Kream, B. E., and DeLuca, H. F.**, 1,25-dihydroxyvitamin D in biological fluids: a simplified and sensitive assay, *Science*, 193, 1021, 1976.
202. **Bringhurst, F. R. and Potts, J. T. Jr.**, Calcium and phosphate distribution, turnover, and metabolic actions, in *Endocrinology*, Vol. 2, L. J. DeGroot, Cahill, F. G., Jr., Martini, L., Nelson, D. H., Odell, W. D., Potts, J. T., Jr., Steinberger, E., and Winegard, A. I., Eds., Grune & Stratton, New York, 1979, 551.
203. **Urist, M.**, Biochemistry of calcification, in *The Biochemistry and Physiology of Bone*, Vol. 4, G. H. Bourne, Ed., Academic Press, New York, 1976, 1.
204. **McDonald, L. E.**, *Veterinary Endocrinology and Reproduction*, Lea & Febiger, Philadelphia, 1975, 63.
205. **Chertow, B. S., Baker, G. R., Henry, H. L., and Norman, A. W.**, Effects of vitamin D metabolites on bovine parathyroid hormone release *in vitro*, *Am. J. Physiol.*, 238, E384, 1980.
206. **Fischer, J. A. and Blum, J. W.**, Noncalcium control of parathyroid hormone secretion, *Miner. Electrolyte Metab.*, 3, 158, 1980.
207. **Fischer, J. A., Oldham, S. B., Sizemore, G. W. and Arnaud, C. D.**, Calcitonin stimulation of parathyroid hormone secretion *in vitro*, *Horm. Metab. Res.*, 3, 223, 1971.
208. **Au, W. Y. W.** Cortisol stimulation of parathyroid hormone secretion by rat parathyroid glands in organ culture, *Science*, 193, 1015, 1976.
209. **Fucik, R. F., Kukreja, S. C., Hargis, G. K., Bowser, E. N., Henderson, W. J., and Williams, G. A.**, Effect of glucocorticoids on function of the parathyroid glands in man, *J. Clin. Endocrinol., Metab.*, 40, 152, 1975.

210. **Tam, C. S. and Anderson, W.**, Tetracycline labeling of bone *in vivo*, *Calcif. Tiss. Int.*, 30, 121, 1980.
211. **Webster, L. A., Atkins, D., and Peacock, M.**, A bioassay for parathyroid hormone using whole mouse calvaria in tissue culture, *J. Endocrinol.*, 62, 631, 1974.
212. **Mayer, G. P., Keaton, J. A., Hurst, J. G., and Habener, J. F.**, Effects of plasma calcium concentration on the relative proportion of hormone and carboxyl fragments in parathyroid venous blood, *Endocrinology*, 104, 1778, 1979.
213. **Berson, S. A., Yalow, R. S., Aurbach, G. D., and Potts, J. D., Jr.**, Immunoassay of bovine and human parathyroid hormone, *Proc. Natl. Acad. Sci. U.S.A.*, 49, 613, 1963.
214. **Mayer, G. P. and Hurst, J. G.**, Sigmoidal relationship between parathyroid hormone secretion rate and plasma calcium concentration in calves, *Endocrinology*, 102, 1036, 1978.
215. **Saeki, T. and Hurst, J. G.**, Unpublished data, 1981.
216. **Hurst, J. G.**, Unpublished observations, 1981.

VITAMIN D

Jerry G. Hurst

INTRODUCTION

One of the interesting concepts to arise in the field of endocrinology has been the realization that vitamin D is a hormone rather than a dietary constituent required for normal bodily function. Physiologically speaking, vitamin D is not a vitamin; it is only when an animal or person is deprived of a natural environment (sunlight) that vitamin D becomes a dietary requirement.

Because of the role of vitamin D in the regulation of calcium and phosphate, these substances are considered in the course of the chapter.

Several recent review articles on vitamin D are available.[141-148]

CALCIUM (Ca)

Role of Calcium

Calcium plays an important, although not completely understood, role in many processes within the body. Calcium constitutes a major portion of the skeleton. It is involved in muscle contraction, blood coagulation, the activity of many enzymes, hormone release, and in cell adhesiveness, membrane stability, proliferation, and permeability.

Distribution and Turnover of Calcium

The lean adult body contains about 20g of Ca and 10g of phosphate (iP)/kg body wt. This is equivalent to 2% Ca and 1% PO_4.

The plasma Ca concentration in most adult mammals is about 10 mg/dℓ (5 mEq/L, or 2.5×10^{-3}M). It is about 12 mg/dℓ in the horse and even higher in the laying hen. The iP concentration is more variable, but averages, in man, about 3.5 mg/dℓ.

About 99% of the Ca and 85% of the iP is in the skeleton, giving rigidity to the organic matrix. The plasma Ca is in three forms. About 48% is ionized, 46% is protein bound (chiefly albumin), and about 6% complexed to citrate, phophate, or even other compounds. It is the ionized form that influences physiologic processes. Many workers cite the total plasma Ca. Until recently, it was easier to measure total Ca than Ca^{++}. The plasma PO_4 is only about 12% (protein) bound.

Intracellular Ca is hard to measure, but has a concentration of about 10^{-6}*M*. Since this is about three orders of magnitude less than extracellular fluid (ECF) calcium, a Ca pump is probably required to move Ca out of cells.

Approximately 1% of the Ca in bone is freely exchangeable with the Ca of the ECF and it is referred to as labile bone Ca. The Ca in the ECF and the intracellular Ca make up the miscible Ca pool. The remaining bone Ca is in the form of amorphous as well as crystalline calcium phosphate salts. Surprisingly, after a century of effort, the exact chemical structures(s) of bone mineral salts still is not known.[202] The Ca and iP stored in bone may be resorbed and added to the miscible pool when dietary Ca and iP are insufficient to maintain plasma Ca and iP.

Absorption of Ca and iP

The source of Ca and iP is the diet. The intake of both ions varies greatly depending upon the diet. Of the Ca ingested, 25 to 75% is absorbed. The amount absorbed is regulated by PTH (indirectly) via a metabolite of vitamin D. Ca absorption is adaptive and a greater percent is absorbed when the diet is low in Ca. The converse holds. Ca absorption is decreased in old age, and it is inhibited by glucocorticoids, unusually high amounts of iP in the diet, chronic ethanol ingestion, and by anticonvulsants used in treating epilepsy.

Ca is absorbed along the entire small intestine, but the degree of absorption is greatest in the duodenum. Because of the transit time of the chyme in the intestine, probably the greater bulk of Ca is absorbed in the lower small intestine.

iP absorption shows adaptation. It is stimulated by a vitamin D metabolite, it is maximal in the jejunum, and it is inhibited by high Ca content in the diet. About 70% of ingested iP is absorbed.

Excretion of Calcium

The kidney is the major route by which excess calcium is eliminated from the body, although small amounts are lost via sweat and by secretion across the intestine from serosal to mucosal sides. These latter two apparently do not play a significant role in regulating ECF calcium, but the kidney does. The excretion of Ca by the kidney is regulated by PTH (and possibly a vitamin D metabolite). Fifty % of the filtered Ca is resorbed in the proximal convoluted tubule (PCT). The distal convoluted tubule has a transport maximum (Tmax) for Ca and, if the filtered load of calcium exceeds these limites, it is excreted in the urine. PTH increases the Tmax for Ca and hence conserves this cation. On the other hand, the excretion of iP by the kidney is enhanced by PTH because PTH decreases the Tmax for iP.

Regulation of Calcium

Three agents play a central role in regulating the concentration of calcium in the extracellular fluids of the body. They are parathyroid hormone (from the parathyroid glands), a vitamin D metabolite (from hepatic and renal conversion of a prohormone produced in the skin), and calcitonin (from special cells in the thyroid of mammals and the ultimobranchial body of most other higher vertebrates).

VITAMIN D

Historical

Prior to 1920, many children in temperate zones developed rickets, a defective mineralization of their bones. There was considerable controversy up to that time about the cause of this disease; some argued that it was due to a lack of sunshine and others that it was a dietary deficiency. During the ensuing decade it was shown that in essence both schools of thought were correct and that exposure of an animal or person to sunlight (or, as it turned out, to ultraviolet light of wave lengths of about 280 to 320 nm),[146,149] or supplementing the diet with cod liver oil prevented or cured rickets. In the mid 1920s it was also discovered that irradiation of food is effective in preventing rickets.

The structure of the antirachitic substance (vitamin D) was determined. The naturally occurring vitamin D in the irradiated animal is cholecalciferol, which is called vitamin D_3. The form arising from irradiating the diet is ergocalciferol, which is called vitamin D_2. The former is derived by photolysis of 7-dehydrocholesterol in the skin of animals. The latter is derived from photolysis of ergosterol in plants.

The structure of the major vitamin D compounds are shown in Figure 1. It is seen that the D compounds are sterols. It is of interest that D_2 and D_3 are chemically similar and in mammals their actions are also similar. Birds are remarkably insensitive to D_2.

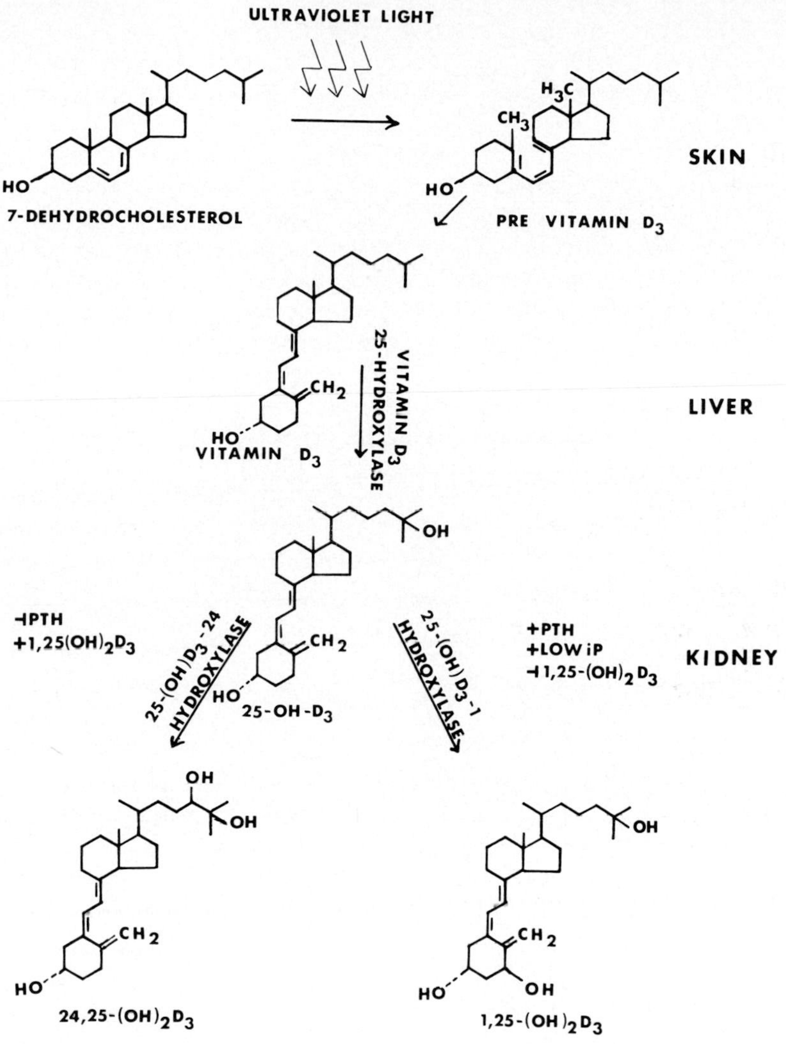

FIGURE 1. The structure of formation of vitamin D_3 and its major metabolites.

Biosynthesis of Vitamin D and Its Metabolites

Vitamin D plays an important role in bone mineralization by providing a proper plasma calcium and phosphorous milieu.[147] However, it is not vitamin D (cholecalciferol or calciferol) itself, but another metabolite which is responsible for this action. To date, the most potent naturally occurring metabolite of vitamin D_3 is 1,25-DHCC, (1,25-dihydroxycholecalciferol, 1,25-$(OH)_2$ D_3) which acts as a hormone.

Figure 1 illustrates the synthesis of vitamin D_3 and its three major metabolites. Ultraviolet light falling on the skin presumably acts on 7-dehydrocholesterol (see Figure 2), which is maximally concentrated in the Malpighian layer of human skin, and cleaves the bond between carbons 9 and 10 located in the B ring of the cyclopentanoperhydrophenanthrine nucleus to yield cholecalciferol (also known as vitamin D_3). This is probably a two step process, with an intermediate compound called previtamin D_3.[215]

The cholecalciferol is carried in the blood by a vitamin D transport protein, called transcalciferin, to the liver. The liver contains a microsomal, cytochrome P-450-dependent vitamin D_3-25-hydroxylase which hydroxylates vitamin D_3 (cholecalciferol) on the carbon 25, yielding 25-hydroxyvitamin D_3 (25-hydroxycholecalciferol, 25(OH)

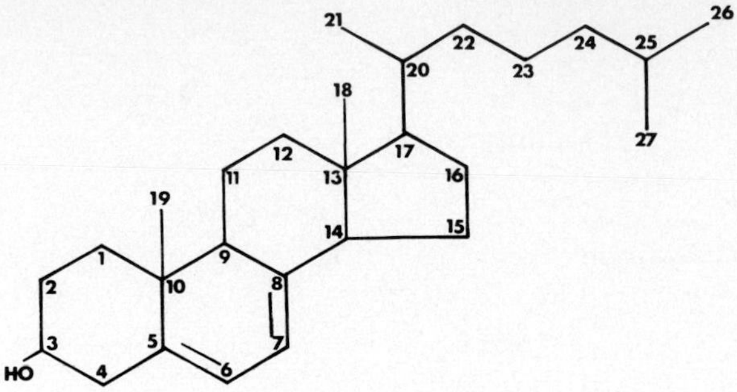

7-DEHYDROCHOLESTEROL

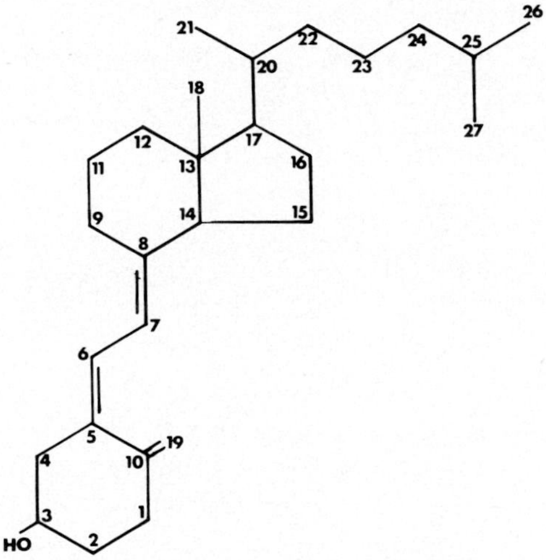

VITAMIN D_3

FIGURE 2. The numbering system for the carbon atoms of vitamin D_3 and its precursor, 7-dihydrocholesterol.

vitamin D_3, 25(OH)D_3, 25-HCC). This compound is picked up by the blood and is bound to the transport protein transcalciferin. 25-Hydroxyvitamin D is the most abundant form of vitamin D found in the circulation.

The hepatic 25-hydroxylation step is not regulated very tightly so that over a wide range either an increase in vitamin D intake or an increase in exposure to sunlight results in an increase in the amount of 25(OH)D_3 in the circulation.[150] The increase in 25(OH)D_3 is not proportionate to the increase in vitamin D_3 so there may be some regulation, presumably via some sort of end-product inhibition by 25(OH)D_3 on its own synthesis.[146] Other organs (intestine, kidney) can apparently 25-hydroxylate vitamin D, but the liver is the major site for this reaction.[146]

Since vitamin D metabolites act (along with PTH) to regulate calcium and phosphate metabolism, something must regulate these metabolites. The mitochondria of the kidney contain a 25-hydroxyvitamin D-1α-hydroxylase[151] which hydroxylates 25-OH-D in the 1 position to yield 1,25-dihydroxyvitamin D (1,25-dihydroxycholecalciferol; 1,25-DHCC; 1,25-$(OH)_2D$). This compound was originally detected in the intestinal mucosa of chicks and was proposed to be the active metabolite of vitamin D_3.[152] It seems certain that the kidney is the sole site of the 1α-hydroxylation of 25-OH-D, except that in the gravid animal the placenta may also produce 1,25-$(OH)_2$-D_3.[153] 1,25-$(OH)_2$-D is the most potent and rapidly acting of the various forms of vitamin D. In bone resorption it is reportedly 100 times more active than 25-OH-D_3.

The process is as follows: under natural conditions ultraviolet light from the sun converts 7-dehydrocholesterol in the skin to vitamin D_3 by cleavage of the B ring. The vitamin D_3 is transported in association with transcalciferin by the blood to the liver where it is 25-hydroxylated to form 25-OH-D_3. The 25-OH-D_3 is then transported by the blood, again in association with transcalciferin to the kidney, where it is 1α-hydroxylated yielding 1,25-$(OH)_2$-D_3. This is the active form of vitamin D_3 and it is transported by the blood throughout the body. The 1,25-$(OH)_2$-D_3 is able to exert its effects wherever it encounters receptors on target cells. Investigators are not sure as to whether or not 1,25-$(OH)_2$-D_3 undergoes further metabolism before it exerts its biologic actions on target tissues.[146]

A renal, mitochondrial enzyme, 25-hydroxyvitamin D_3-24-hydroxylase, is capable of hydroxylating 25-OH-D_3 in the 24 position, yielding 24,25-$(OH)_2D_3$. No clear physiologic role for this product has yet been established, although it has been implicated in bone anabolism and as a way of ridding the body of 25-OH-D_3.[141] Its production is inversely related to that of 1,25-$(OH)_2$-D_3 and it may have some yet undiscovered function.

For the biochemistry of the various vitamin D enzymes, the reader is referred to reviews by DeLuca[146] and Norman and Henry.[142] These enzymes are cytochrome p-450-containing, mixed function monoxygenases; depend upon the generation of NADPH; and incorporate oxygen into the vitamin D molecule.

Regulation of Vitamin D Metabolism

The transformation of 7-dehydrocholesterol in the skin is probably not controlled and the hepatic 25-hydroxylation is not very tightly controlled.[150] However, the renal enzymatic conversion of 25-OH-D to the 1,25- or 24,25-$(OH)_2D$ is regulated and it seems that PTH, extracellular phosphate concentration, and possibly 1,25-$(OH)_2D$ itself, are involved in this regulation. In vitamin D intoxication, when excessive pharmaceutical preparations of vitamin D are taken, the circulating levels of 25-OH-D may be elevated 30-fold and yet the level of 1,25-$(OH)_2D$ shows no increase.[141]

Role of PTH in Regulating Vitamin D Metabolism

DeLuca et al.[146] showed that the production of 1,25-$(OH)_2D_3$ in rats is markedly increased by feeding them a diet low enough in Ca to produce hypocalcemia. Conversely, they found that a high Ca diet decreases 1,25-$(OH)_2D_3$ production. These experiments implicated plasma calcium in the regulation of 1,25-$(OH)D_3$ synthesis. However, DeLuca's group subsequently showed that this response to hypocalcemia was dependent upon the PTG. That is, when the rats are made hypocalcemic by feeding a low Ca diet, the production of 1,25-$(OH)_2D_3$ rises and 24, 25-$(OH)_2D_3$ falls, but when they are then parathyroidectomized, the production of 1,25-$(OH)_2D_3$ falls and 24,25-$(OH)_2D_3$ rises.[146] It appears that the hypocalcemia is activating the renal 25-hydroxy-1α-hydroxylase indirectly by first stimulating the PTG to produce PTH which then activates the 1α-hydroxylase. Additional experiments utilizing various ways of manipulating plasma PTH levels have confirmed that PTH stimulates, in an unknown way, the 25-hydroxyvitamin D_3-1α-hydroxylase and inhibits the 25-hydroxyvitamin D_3-24-hydroxylase enzymes.[141,147]

Role of Phosphate in Regulating Vitamin D Metabolism

Low levels of plasma phosphate (produced by feeding a low phosphate diet) in rats results in an elevated production of 1,25-$(OH)_2D_3$ even in the absence of the PTG.[156] Conversely, hyperphosphatemia produces a decrease in 1,25-$(OH)_2D_3$ and an increase in 24,25-$(OH)_2D_3$ production. Thus, phosphate has an action on 1,25-$(OH)_2D_3$ production independent of the PTG, but how it produces this effect is not known. It is not known whether this effect is a direct or indirect one.[147]

Role of 1,25-$(OH)_2D_3$ in Regulating Its Own Synthesis

In vivo studies suggest that 1,25-$(OH)_2D_3$ inhibits its own formation and stimulates the formation of 24,25-$(OH)_2D_3$. However, these studies are clouded by the fact that PTH modulates the renal production of these two vitamin D metabolites. Since the injection of 1,25-$(OH)_2D_3$ alters plasma Ca and, since this will in turn decrease PTH secretion, the changes in endogenous 1,25-$(OH)_2D_3$ subsequent to its exogenous administration may be accounted for on the basis of changes in PTH. In vitro experiments, using primary cultures of chick kidney cells, have shown that the addition of 1,25-$(OH)_2D_3$ to the incubation medium decreases the synthesis of 1,25-$(OH)_2D_3$ within one hr (maximal inhibition is seen at 20 hr) and increases the synthesis of 24,25-$(OH)_2D_3$ within four hr. (The increase in 24,25-$(OH)_2D_3$ continues linearly for an additional 16 hr). The increased synthesis of 24,25-$(OH)_2D_3$ subsequent to the administration of 1,25-$(OH)_2D_3$ is blocked by substances which inhibit nuclear transcription.[158]

Other Substances Which Regulate Vitamin D Metabolism

Several physiologic states, all of which increase the need of the animal for calcium absorption from the gut or reabsorption from bone, such as growth, pregnancy and lactation, are associated with an increase in circulating levels of 1,25-$(OH)_2D_3$.[141] Lactating rats have elevated levels of 1,25-$(OH)_2D_3$.[160] During the 33 to 34 weeks of pregnancy, the level of this vitamin D metabolite is some three-fold higher than in non-pregnant women (88 vs 29 pg/mℓ of plasma).[161] In the human study the prolactin, placental lactogen, and estrogen (but apparently not PTH) blood levels are elevated and any one of them may be responsible for the elevated plasma 1,25-$(OH)_2D_3$.

The plasma level of 1,25-$(OH)_2D_3$ is elevated three-fold in rats during late pregnancy and sixfold (to 158 pg/mℓ) during lactation.[162] These observations suggest that prolactin is a 1α-hydroxylase stimulator. At the same time plasma levels of 24,25-$(OH)_2D_3$ fall.[162] In these rat experiments the plasma Ca concentration falls and this may account for the changes in plasma 1,25-$(OH)_2D_3$ via the effects of the mild hypocalcemia upon the PTG. Injection of prolactin into chicks stimulates the activity of 1α-hydroxylase and increases the circulating level of 1,25-$(OH)_2D_3$.[159] Thus, prolactin may be a stimulus, directly or indirectly to the 1α-hydroxylase system.

Kidney homogenates of estradiol treated birds increase the conversion of 25-(OH)-D_3 into 1,25-$(OH)_2D_3$.[162] Treatment of chicks with diethylstilestrol is followed by a seven fold decrease in 24-hydroxylase activity and an increase in circulating levels of 1,25-$(OH)_2D_3$.[164] DeLuca's group found that a single estrogen administration to mature male birds produces a marked elevation in 1-hydroxylation and suppression of 24-hydroxylation within 24 hr and that these changes are followed by a dramatic (four-fold) increase in plasma calcium which is sustained for over 1 week. The response is not obtained in immature or castrate birds, but when estradiol plus testosterone or progesterone is injected into the castrate, the response is obtained.[146] Since these experiments with estrogenic compounds involve treatment of the whole animal and not homogenates, they do not rule out the possibility that the estrogenic effect is secondary. It appears reasonably sure that estrogens, either directly or indirectly and, perhaps by acting synergistically with other sex hormones, stimulate the production of 1,25-$(OH)_2D_3$. The latter then increases the availability of Ca for eggshell formation in the bird and possibly for fetal bone formation and for milk formation in the mammal.

Plasma levels of 1,25-$(OH)_2D_3$ are reported in human acromegalic patients to be significantly elevated, but no correlation can be found between these levels and the levels of growth hormone.[161]

It is too early to assign to GH, estrogens or prolactin a direct role in 1α-hydroxylase stimulation. It is still to be demonstrated that these agents have a direct action on this enzyme in organ or tissue culture.

Action of Vitamin D or Its Metabolites

A role for vitamin D in calcium and phosphate metabolism has been recognized for about 60 years, but there is only sketchy information about the mechanisms by which it works. Vitamin D appears to function by being metabolized into more polar metabolites. It acts on the gut, bone, and possibly the kidney, muscle, and the PTG. The target organ which has received the most attention is the gut.

Action of Vitamin D on the Gut

Physiologic Action

In the early 1960s it was shown that vitamin D administration stimulates the small intestine of animals to actively absorb calcium.[168,169] Vitamin D also stimulates the gut to absorb phosphate and this action is independent of calcium absorption.[170,171] It is most likely that the 1,25-DHCC metabolite of vitamin D is the stimulating factor. On a M/cm^2 of gut surface/unit of time basis, 1,25-DHCC-stimulated Ca absorption is greatest in the upper small intestine.[172] Because of the different lengths of the various parts of the small intestine and the time the chyme is in each, the jejunum may be where most Ca is absorbed. 24R,25-DHCC, when given to intact animals, has simlar effects on calcium (and phosphate) absorption, but this metabolite is much less potent. Furthermore, since 24R,25-DHCC is ineffective in stimulating Ca or PO_4 absorption by the gut in nephrectomized animals, its action is probably due to its conversion to 1,24R,25-$(OH)_3D$.[172]

Biochemical Actions

The biochemical mechanisms by which 1,25-$(OH)_2D_3$ exerts its effect on the gut are not known in full, but evidence[141] supports the concept that 1,25-$(OH)_2D_3$ is bound to a cytosolic receptor which is highly specific for 1,25-dihydroxylated secosterols.[146,216] This receptor binds 1,25-$(OH)_2D$ 500 times more strongly than it does 25-(OH)D, 800 times more strongly than 24,25-$(OH)_2D$, and three times more than 1,24R,25-$(OH)_3D$.

After binding, the hormone-receptor complex translocates to the nucleus of intestinal mucosal cells, where it binds with nonhistone, nuclear proteins, and enhances the synthesis of mRNA. The mRNA codes for various proteins, including the 24,000-mol wt calcium-binding protein (CaBP), in birds.[178]

That 1,25-$(OH)_2D_3$ is translocated to and sequestered in the nucleus has been shown by autoradiographic techniques, using tritiated 1,25-$(OH)_2D_3$ of high specific activity. Four hr after injection of this tracer, it is found almost entirely in the nuclear component of intestinal mucosal cells of chicks, with very little in the cytoplasm. The nuclear localization occurs as early as ½ hr post-injection and before intestinal Ca transport or protein synthesis is seen.[217] Thus, it appears that 1,25-$(OH)_2D_3$ acts like other steroid hormones by binding with cytosolic receptors, producing a hormone-receptor complex which goes to the nucleus and initiates gene activation. This results in mRNA synthesis and new protein synthesis. In addition to CaBP, at least three other intestinal, mucosal proteins increase (or appear) in response to 1,25-$(OH)_2D_3$. Their roles, as well as the role of CaBP in calcium and phosphate absorption, are not yet certain.

CaBP may play a role in intestinal calcium absorption. In the intestinal mucosa the amount of CaBP closely parallels changes in Ca absorption by the gut following 1,25-

$(OH)_2D$ administration. However, after the peak of the response, the decrease in Ca absorption is faster than the decrease in CaBP. The appearance of CaBP and the increase in Ca absorption following 1,25-$(OH)_2D$ treatment are inhibited by treatment of the animal with actinomycin D, an inhibitor of nuclear m-RNA synthesis.[179] It is speculated that its role is to accept Ca which enters on the luminal side of the mucosal cells and make it available for active transport out of these cells on their serosal sides.[167] Consistent with this hypothesis is the observation that 1,25-$(OH)_2D_3$ increases the permeability of the mucosal cells to Ca even in the absence of new protein synthesis and thus increases the intracellular Ca of these cells. However, concomitant with an increase in protein synthesis, there is a decrease in intracellular calcium, indicating that the newly synthesized proteins are involved in removal of Ca from the cells.[167]

Bickle et al.,[180] using a gut sac technique in chicks, were able to dissociate the effects of 1,25-$(OH)_2D_3$ on protein synthesis and Ca absorption by the gut and concluded that 1,25-$(OH)D_3$-induced Ca transport is not dependent upon the induction of the synthesis of CaBP, total protein (as measured by leucine incorporation into protein) or alkaline phosphatase. Also, on a time scale, they found that Ca uptake and transport are increased by 1,25-$(OH)_2D_3$ prior to any detectable change in RNA-polymerase, CaBP or alkaline phosphatase.[167]

An effect of 1,25-$(OH)_2D_3$ on intestinal mucosal cells in organ culture is to increase cAMP. The increase precedes the increase in CaBP and ^{47}Ca uptake. The cAMP returns to baseline by two hours and then it gradually rises in parallel with the increase in CaBP and calcium uptake.[174] The role of cAMP in mediating the effects of 1,25-$(OH)D_3$ on the intestine is unknown.

The 1,25-$(OH)_2D_3$ stimulates the production or activity of the following in intestinal mucosal cells (1) nuclear RNA synthesis, an effect seen within 2 or 3 hr; (2) nuclear RNA polymerase II activity, in 2 or 3 hr;[176] and (3) an alkaline phosphatase.[177] This enzyme, known as calcium-ATPase, appears after enhanced Ca absorption has occurred and hence probably plays no role in Ca absorption. It may be involved in phosphate absorption.[141]

The action of 1,25-$(OH)_2D_3$ on the intestine is slow. Except for cAMP production, which increases within 30 min after 1,25-$(OH)_2D_3$ treatment, most other biochemical changes in the gut are found only after two or three hr.

Action of Vitamin D on Bone

Vitamin D, endogenous or exogenous, is required for mineralization of bone. Very little is known concerning the mechanism.

Vitamin D has dual effects on bone. It causes increased mineralization and increased resorption of bone. It may be that 25-(OH)D has the former and 1,25-$(OH)_2D$ the latter effect.[147,181] Vitamin D metabolites, by increasing calcium and phosphate absorption from the gut (and possibly reabsorption by the renal tubules) plays an important (and possibly the only) role in providing mineral for bone. Of the two effects of vitamin D on bone, reabsorption is the easier one to demonstrate, and has been more extensively studied. The direct action (as opposed to its indirect effect by increasing mineral absorption from the gut) of vitamin D on bone mineralization is not clear.

Effect of Vitamin D on Bone Resorption

Physiologic doses of vitamin D increase the mobilization of radioactive Ca from previously radiolabeled bone.[182] Vitamin D deficient animals on a calcium-free diet develop severe hypocalcemia. When they are subsequently given vitamin D but kept on the Ca-free diet, their serum calcium rises and the only pool in their bodies great enough to supply calcium is bone.[183] This shows that vitamin D (or its metabolites) stimulates bone Ca resorption directly or indirectly. This in vivo vitamin D-stimulated bone mineral resorption requires the presence of PTH and therefore may simply be potentiating the action of PTH on bone.

That $1,25\text{-}(OH)_2D_3$ is most effective in mobilizing Ca from bone has been shown by in vitro, embryonic bone culture experiments where concentrations of this hormone as low as 10^{-14} molar causes bone calcium mobilization, 1000 times this amount of 25-$(OH)D_3$ is required to produce the same effect, and vitamin D_3 is without effect.[184] For unknown reasons organ culture systems do not need PTH to show an increased mobilization of Ca subsequent to $1,25\text{-}(OH)_2D_3$ treatment. Just how $1,25\text{-}(OH)_2D_3$ mobilizes Ca from bone is now known. The action is blocked in vivo by actinomycin D.[185]

Based upon daily doses of the various forms of vitamin D required to raise the plasma Ca concentration by 1 mg/dℓ in vitamin D deficient rats, Boris et al.[186] showed that the intestinal absorption of Ca is about 1000 times more sensitive to $1,25\text{-}(OH)_2D_3$, 60 times more sensitive to $25\text{-}(OH)D_3$, and 40 times more sensitive to vitamin D, than is bone mineral mobilization. This assessment was made by measuring the increase in plasma Ca after administration of the vitamin D compound in vitamin D-deficient rats with and without Ca in their diets. The increase in plasma Ca in the animals without Ca in their diet is an assessment of bone calcium mobilization and the increase in plasma Ca in the animals with Ca in their diet is an assessment of intestinal Ca absorption.

Boris et al.[186] found no increase in release of ^{45}Ca from bones of vitamin D-deficient chicks (which had been labeled 2 weeks earlier with ^{45}Ca) at any of the times studied (4 to 30 hr) after the subcutaneous injection of 1 μg of $1,25\text{-}(OH)_2D_3$. However, Ca absorption from the gut is increased three times within 6 hr and is still significantly elevated at 4 and 30 hr. These studies suggest that the major physiologic action of $1,25\text{-}(OH)_2D_3$ in maintaining plasma Ca concentration is via its action on mineral absorption by the gut, not from the bone.

Raisz et al.[187] reported that $1,25\text{-}(OH)_2D_3$ inhibits collagen synthesis in fetal rat calvaria cultured for 24 hr in a chemically defined medium containing 5% serum from vitamin D deficient rats. The vitamin D metabolite is effective over the dose range of 10^{-11} to 10^{-7} *M*, but not at 10^{-12} or 10^{-13} *M*. Also the $1,24R,25\text{-}(OH)_3D_3$ metabolite is effective, but it requires a higher dose of 10^{-9} to 10^{-7}. The non-1-hydroxylated metabolites ($25\text{-}(OH)D_3$ and $24R,25\text{-}(OH)_2D_3$) are not effective at doses up to 10^{-7} *M*. The effective doses of $1,25\text{-}(OH)_2D_3$ are near the normal circulation levels of this hormone in humans and these in vitro studies suggest that $1,25\text{-}(OH)_2D_3$ inhibits bone collagen synthesis at physiologic doses. However, the free $1,25\text{-}(OH)_2D_3$ in the culture media may be much greater at 10^{-11} *M* than in blood at the same molar concentration, due to the presence of vitamin D binding protein in the blood.

Effect of Vitamin D on Bone Mineralization

Vitamin D in some form is required for bone mineralization since vitamin D deficient rickets results in decreased bone mineralization and the bone defect is readily treated by vitamin D.

Does vitamin D have a direct action on bone in increasing mineralization and/or osteoid formation or are its effects indirect by providing a proper extracellular fluid mineral (calcium and phosphate) composition in which mineralization can proceed normally or both? There is little doubt that vitamin D provides the proper composition of extracellular fluid for mineralization, but its direct action on the mineralization process is dubious.

Evidence from in vivo experiments mainly on vitamin D deficient chicks and rats shows that vitamin D and its metabolites improve mineralization of bone. The effects are as follows:

1. Increase in osteoid calcification[188]
2. Acceleration of the conversion of low density to high density bone[188]
3. Decrease in the amount of unmineralized osteoid relative to total dry weight of bone[188,189]

4. ($1,25\text{-}(OH)_2D_3$) maintaining the volume of bone[189]
5. ($1,25$-and $24,25\text{-}(OH)_2D_3$ and $25\text{-}OHD_3$) increasing bone Ca content[181]
6. (Various metabolites) increasing bone ash[190,191]
7. (D_3, $25\text{-}(OH)D_3$, $1,25\text{-}(OH)_2D_3$, and $24,25\text{-}(OH)_2D_3$ decreasing eiphyseal plate width[191]

Based upon increases in tibial ash weight in chicks, vitamin D compounds are ranked in potency[191] as follows: $1,25\text{-}(OH)_2D_3$, $25\text{-}(OH)D_3$, vitamin D, $1,24R,25\text{-}(OH)_3D_3$, $24R, 24\text{-}(OH)_2D_3$.

In most of the in vivo studies, the plasma calcium and/or phosphate is altered by vitamin D treatment. It is possible that the changes in plasma mineral concentrations improves bone mineralization rather than a direct action of vitamin D on bone.

Rats on a vitamin D and phosphate deficient diet develop signs of decreased bone mineralization. These changes are reversed by supplementing the diet with phosphate alone as well as with phosphate plus vitamin D. The reversal is no better with vitamin D plus phosphate than with phosphate alone.[192] These data support the hypothesis that the action of vitamin D on bone mineralization is secondary to improved extracellular mineral composition.[192]

One in vitro study utilizing chondrocytes from the proliferative zone of the growth plate cartilage of young rabbits show that when these cells are grown in tissue culture, the incorporation of $^{35}SO_4$ into proteoglycans or other macromolecules is enhanced by $24\text{-}25\text{-}(OH)_2D_3$ at 2.4×10^{-13} and $2.4 \times 10^{-10} M$, by $1,25\text{-}(OH)_2D_3$ at 2.4×10^{-11} and $2.4 \times 10^{-10} M$, and by $25\text{-}(OH)D_3$ at $2.5 \times 10^{-8} M$. Vitamin D_3 itself is not effective in concentrations as high as $10^{-7} M$. After addition to the medium of $25\text{-}(OH)D_3$, a polar form of vitamin D, one indistinguishable from $24\ 25\text{-}(OH)_2D_3$, is extractable and it possibly accounts for the effectiveness of $25\text{-}(OH)D_3$ in this system.[193]

Overall, a direct action of vitamin D or its metabolites on bone mineralization and/or organic matrix formation can be neither confirmed nor denied.

Action of Vitamin D on the Kidney[147]

It appears that $25\text{-}(OH)D_3$ or $1,25\text{-}(OH)_2D_3$ increases renal reabsorption of phosphate and hence decreases phosphate excretion by the kidney.[194-197] This action may require PTH (or antidiuretic hormone, ADH, VP) since in physiologic amounts $1,25\text{-}(OH)_2D_3$ is ineffective unless small amounts of PTH (which by itself is also ineffective) are simultaneously infused, in thyroparathyroidectomized rats on a vitamin D deficient diet.[197] This combination of ineffective doses of $1,25\text{-}(OH)_2D_3$ and PTH produces a 52% fall in urinary phosphate excretion, a 20% fall in Na excretion and a 22% fall in urinary cAMP. The excretion of Ca rises. This may result from an increased Ca filtered load since this combination increases serum Ca significantly without changing the glomerular filtration rate.[197]

There is some evidence that vitamin D metabolites increase renal resportion of Ca.[195]

Other Effects of Vitamin D

Body Weight Gain

Body weight gain is decreased profoundly by vitamin D deficiency.[197,198] Whether this is a direct effect of vitamin D on growth or secondary to changes in mineral metabolism is not known.

Muscle Strength

Muscle strength, as judged from clinical observation, is improved in rachitic children following vitamin D therapy.[198]

Transport of Vitamin D [200]

Vitamin D sterols are poorly water soluble. When transported in the blood, they are bound to large plasma proteins yielding a water soluble complex. In a large number of mammals, bony fishes and reptiles, the vitamin D binding protein (DBP) is an α globulin. Birds bind vitamin D and 25-(OH)D_3 to β globulins. Amphibians and cartilaginous fishes bind vitamin D to serum lipoproteins.

In humans, DBP appears to be a single polypeptide chain of approximately 55,000 mol wt. It has a greater affinity for 25-(OH)D_3 and 24,25-$(OH)_2D_3$ than for vitamin D_3 or 1,25-$(OH)_2D_3$. This may explain the fact that the latter two are cleared more rapidly from blood than the former two. DBP has a binding capacity of approximately 1 mol of ligand/mol of carrier protein. Based upon radioimmunoassay, human blood has a DBP concentration of approximately 500 mg/ℓ, or 8×10^{-6} M/ℓ. At normal plasma concentrations of vitamin D and its metabolites, DBP is only about 3% saturated. The large excess of DBP binding capacity may protect against vitamin D intoxication. DBP is probably synthesized by the liver. Estrogen therapy, including the oral contraceptives, and pregnancy increase plasma DBP concentrations.

DBP probably functions (1) to solubilize vitamin D sterols; (2) to protect these compounds from rapid degradation and renal clearance; (3) as a storage reservoir for vitamin D compounds, especially 25-(OH)D_3 (the blood is considered to be the major storage organ for 25-(OH)D_3); and (4) in regulating the delivery of these sterols to the tissues.

The great excess of DBP may function to store up D compounds during abundant sunlight (summer), to be used during sunlight deprivation (winter).

Assays for Vitamin D

Bioassays

Bioassays have been devised which depend upon some biologic action of vitamin D (or more likely its biologically active metabolites). For example, vitamin D may be given to a rachitic animal and 24 to 40 hr later a dose of radioactive Ca is given. One hr thereafter the amount of radioactive Ca in the plasma is determined. Such bioassays are relatively insensitive and incapable of distinguishing between the various forms of vitamin D and its metabolites. They were important historically and are still employed in establishing the biologic potency of vitamin D preparations and as standards against which to evaluate nonbiologic assays for vitamin D.

Another type of bioassay involves a biologic response to vitamin D under in vitro conditions. For example, 1,25-$(OH)_2D_3$ is a potent stimulator of bone resorption by osteoclasts. This property has been developed into a very sensitive bioassay which is capable of measuring 1 pg of 1,25-$(OH)_2D_3$.[219]

Protein Binding Assays

Protein binding assays[200] are widely used to assay vitamin D and its metabolites. They are basically like radioimmunoassays (RIA), except that a naturally occurring cytosolic receptor, often obtained from intestinal mucosa of rachitic chicks, is used in lieu of the antibody used in RIA. These assays are very sensitive and can easily quantitate D metabolites in normal blood plasma (around 10 pg/mℓ). Like the bioassays, these assays cannot distinguish between the various vitamin D metabolites. Consequently, plasma samples must be fractionated by various chromatographic means into its various D_3 metabolites before they are quantitated by protein binding assay.

REFERENCES

1. **Collip, J. B.,** Extraction of a parathyroid hormone which will prevent or control parathyroid tetany and which regulates the level of blood calcium, *J. Biol. Chem.*, 63, 395, 1925.
2. **Aurbach, G. D.** Isolation of parathyroid hormone after extraction with phenol, *J. Biol. Chem.*, 234, 3179, 1959.
3. **Keutmann, H. T., Aurbach, G. D., Dawson, B. F., Niall, H. D., Deftos, L. J., and Potts, J. T. Jr.,** Isolation and characterization of the bovine parathyroid isohormones, *Biochemistry*, 10, 2779, 1971.
4. **Brewer, H. B., Jr. and Ranan, R.,** Bovine parathyroid hormone: amino acid sequence, *Proc. Natl. Acad. Sci. U.S.A.*, 67, 1862, 1970.
5. **Saver, R. T., Niall, H. D., Hogan, M. L., Keutmann, H. T., O'Riordan, J. L. H., and Potts, J. T., Jr.,** The amino acid sequence of porcine parathyroid hormone, *Biochemistry*, 13, 1994, 1974.
6. **Keutmann, H. T., Saver, M. M., Hendy, G. M., O'Riordan, J. L. H., and Potts, J. T., Jr.,** The complete amino acid sequence of human parathyroid hormone, *Biochemistry*, 17, 5723, 1978.
7. **Keutmann, H. T.** Chemistry of parathyroid hormine, in *Endocrinology, Vol. 2,* DeGroot, L. J., Cahill, G. F., Jr., Martini, L., Nelson, D. H., Odell, W. D., Potts, J. T., Jr., Steinberger, E., and Winegard, A. I., Eds., Grune & Stratton, San Francisco, 1979, 593.
8. **Niall, H. D., Saver, R. T., Jacobs, J. W., Keutmann, H. T., Segre, G. V., O'Riordan, J. L. H., Aurbach, G. D., and Potts, J. T., Jr.,** The amino acid sequence of the amino-terminal 37 residues of human parathyroid hormone, *Proc. Natl. Acad. Sci. U.S.A.*, 71, 384, 1974.
9. **Tregear, G. W., Van Reitschoten, J., Green, E., Keutmann, H. T., Niall, H. D., Reit, B., Parsons, J. A., and Potts, J. T., Jr.,** Bovine parathyroid hormone: minimum chain length of synthetic peptide required for biological activity, *Endocrinology*, 93, 1349, 1973.
10. **MacGregor, R. R. and Cohn, D. V.** The intracellular pathway for parathormone biosynthesis and secretion, *Clin. Orthop. Rel. Res.*, 137, 244, 1978.
11. **Habener, J. R. and Kronenberg, H. M.,** Parathyroid hormone biosynthesis: structure and function of biosynthetic precursors, *Fed. Proc.*, 37, 2561, 1978.
12. **Habener, J. F. and Potts, J. T., Jr.,** Biosynthesis of parathyroid hormone, *N. Eng. J. Med.*, 299, 580, 1978.
13. **Habener, J. F., Kemper, B. W., Rich, A. and Potts, J. T., Jr.,** Biosynthesis of parathyroid hormone, *Rec. Prog. Horm. Res.*, 33, 249, 1977.
14. **Hamilton, J. W., MacGregor, R. R., Chu, L. L. H., and Cohn, D. V.,** The isolation and partial purification of non-parathyroid calcemic fraction from bovine parathyroid glands, *Endocrinology*, 89, 1440, 1971.
15. **Conn, D. V., MacGregor, R. R., Chu, L. L. H., Kimmel, J. R., and Hamilton, J. W.,** Calcemic fraction-A; biosynthetic peptide precursor of parathyroid hormone, *Proc. Natl. Acad Sci. U.S.A.*, 69, 1521, 1972.
16. **Kemper, B., Habener, J. F., Potts, J. T., Jr., and Rich, A.,** Proparathyroid hormone: identification of a biosynthetic precursor to parathyroid hormone, *Proc. Natl. Acad. Sci. U.S.A.*, 69, 643, 1972.
17. **Kemper, B., Habener, J. F., Mulligan, R. C., Potts, J. T., Jr., and Rich, A.,** Preproparathyroid hormone: a direct translation product of parathyroid messenger RNA, *Proc. Natl. Acad. Sci. U.S.A.*, 71, 3731, 1974.
18. **Blobel, G. and Dobberstein, B.,** Transfer of proteins across membranes: presence of proteolytically processed and unprocessed nascent immunoglobulin light chains on membrane-bound ribosomes of murine myeloma, *J. Cell Biol.*, 67, 835, 1975.
19. **Habener, J. F., Potts, J. T., Jr., and Rich, A.,** Preproparathyroid hormone: evidence for an early biosynthetic precursor of proparathyroid hormone, *J. Biol. Chem.*, 251, 3893, 1976.
20. **Habener, J. F., Amherdt, M., and Orci, L.,** Subcellular organelles involved in the conversion of biosynthetic precursors of parathyroid hormone, *Trans. Assoc. Am. Physicians*, 90, 366, 1977.
21. **Chu, L. L. H., MacGregor, R. R., and Cohn, D. V.,** Energy-dependent intracellular translocation of proparathormone, hormone to parathyroid hormone: the use of amides as specific inhibitors, *Endocrinology*, 95, 1431, 1974.
22. **Chu, L. L. H., MacGregor, R. R., Hamilton, J. W., and Cohn, D. V.,** Conversion of proparathyroid hormone to parathyroid hormone: the use of amides as specific inhibitors, *Endocrinology*, 95, 1431, 1974.
23. **Goltzman, D., Callahan, E. N., Tregear, G. W., and Potts, J. T., Jr.,** Conversion of proparathyroid hormone to parathyroid hormone: studies *in vitro* with tyrpsin, *Biochemistry*, 15, 5076, 1976.
24. **MacGregor, R. R., Chu, L. L. H., and Cohn, D. V.** Conversion of proparathyroid hormone to parathyroid hormone by a particulate enzyme of the parathyroid gland, *J. Biol. Chem.*, 251, 6711, 1976.
25. **MacGregor, R. R., Hamilton, J. W., and Cohn, D. V.,** The by-pass of tissue hormone stores during the secretion of newly synthesized parathyroid hormone, *Endocrinology*, 97, 178, 1975.

26. **Limacher, W., Wild, P., Manser, E., and Lutz, H.,** Identification of immunoreactive sites in bovine parathyroid cells to antibodies raised against the NH_2-terminal sequence of parathyroid hormone, *J. Histochem. Cytochem.*, 27, 1209, 1979.
27. **Futrell, J. M., Su, S. P., Roth, S. I., Habener, J. F., Segre, G. V., and Potts, J. T., Jr.,** Localization of parathyroid hormone in bovine and human parathyroid glands using a peroxidase-labelled antibody, in *Endocrinology of Calcium Metabolism*, Copp, D. H. and Talmage, R. V., Eds., Excerpta Medica, Amsterdam, 1978, 353.
28. **Chu, L. L., MacGregor, R. R., Anast, C. S., Hamilton, J. W., and Cohn, D. V.,** Studies on the biosynthesis of rat parathyroid hormone and proparathyroid hormone: adaptation of the parathyroid gland to dietary restriction of calcium, *Endocrinology*, 93, 915, 1973.
29. **Habener, J. F., Kemper, B., and Potts, J. T., Jr.,** Calcium-dependent intracellular degradation of parathyroid hormone: a possible mechanism for the regulation of hormone stores, *Endocrinology*, 97, 431, 1975.
30. **MacGregor, R. R., Chu, L. L. H., Hamilton, J. W., and Cohn, D. V.,** Studies on the subcellular localization of proparathyroid hormone and parathyroid hormone in the bovine parathyroid gland: separation of newly synthesized from mature forms, *Endocrinology*, 93, 1387, 1973.
31. **Habener, J. F. and Potts, J. T., Jr.,** Subcellular distribution of parathyroid hormone, hormonal precursors, and parathyroid secretory protein, *Endocrinology*, 104, 265, 1979.
32. **Au, W. Y. W., Poland, A. P., Stern, P. H., and Raisz, L. G.,** Hormone synthesis and secretion by rat parathyroid gland in tissue culture, *J. Clin. Invest.*, 49, 1639, 1970.
33. **Sherwood, L. M., Rodman, J. S., and Lundberg, W. B.,** Evidence for a precursor to circulating parathyroid hormone, *Proc. Natl. Acad. Sci. U.S.A.*, 67, 1631, 1970.
34. **Kemper, B., Habener, J. F., Rich, A., and Potts, J. T., Jr.,** Parathyroid secretion: discovery of a major calcium-dependent protein, *Science*, 184, 167, 1974.
35. **Morrissey, J. J., Hamilton, J. W., and Cohn, D. V.,** The secretion of parathormone and glycosylated proteins by parathyroid cells in culture, *Biochem. Biophys. Res. Commun.*, 82, 1279, 1978.
36. **Ravazzola, M., Orci, L., Habener, J. F., and Potts, J. T., Jr.,** Parathyroid secretory protein: immunochemical localization within cells that contain parathyroid hormone, *Lancet*, 12, 371, 1978.
37. **Mayer, G. P., Habener, J. F., and Potts, J. T., Jr.,** Parathyroid hormone secretion *in vivo:* demonstration of a calcium-independent, nonsuppressible component of secretion, *J. Clin. Invest.*, 57, 678, 1976.
38. **Mayer, G. P., Keaton, J. A., Hurst, J. G.,and Habener, J. F.,** Effects of plasma calcium concentration on the relative proportion of hormone and carboxyl fragments in parathyroid venous blood, *Endocrinology*, 104, 1778, 1979.
39. **Flueck, J. A., DiBella, F. P., Edis, A. J., Kehrwald, J. M., and Arnaud, C. D.,** Immunoheterogeneity of parathyroid hormone in venous effluent serum from hyperfunctioning parathyroid glands, *J. Clin. Invest.*, 60, 1397, 1977.
40. **Hurst, J. G. and Newcomer, W. S.,** Functional parathyroid tissue in ultimobronchial bodies of chickens, *Proc. Soc. Exptl. Biol. Med.*, 132, 55, 1969.
41. **Blum, J. W., Mayer, G. P., and Potts, J. T., Jr.,** Parathyroid hormone response during spontaneous hypocalcemia and induced hypercalcemia in cows, *Endocrinology*, 95, 84, 1974.
42. **Mayer, G. P. and Hurst, J. G.,** Sigmoidal relationship between parathyroid hormone secretion rate and plasma calcium concentration in calves, *Endocrinology*, 102, 1036, 1978.
43. **Blum, J. W., Fischer, J. A., Schwoerer, D., Hunziker, W., and Binswanger, U.,** Acute parathyroid hormone response: sensitivity, relationship to hypocalcemia, and rapidity, *Endocrinology*, 95, 753, 1974.
44. **Sherwood, L. M., Mayer, G. P., Ramberg, C. F., Jr., Kronfeld, D. S., Aurbach, G. D., and Potts, J. T., Jr.,** Regulation of parathyroid hormone secretion: proportional control by calcium, lack of effect of phosphate, *Endocrinology*, 83, 1043, 1968.
45. **Mayer, G. P. and Hurst, J. G.,** Comparison of the effects of calcium and magnesium on parathyroid hormone secretion rate in calves, *Endocrinology*, 102, 1803, 1978.
46. **Habener, J. F. and Potts, J. T., Jr.,** Relative effectiveness of magnesium and calcium on the secretion and biosynthesis of parathyroid hormone *in vitro*, *Endocrinology*, 98, 197, 1976.
47. **Anast, C. S., Winnacker, J. L., Forte, L. R., and Burns, T. W.,** Impaired release of parathyroid hormone in magnesium deficiency, *J. Clin. Endocrinol. Metab.*, 42, 707, 1976.
48. **Fischer, J. A., Blum, J. W., and Binswanger, U.,** Acute parathyroid hormone response to epinephrine *in vivo*, *J. Clin. Invest.*, 52, 2434, 1973.
49. **Kukreja, S. C., Hargis, G. K., Bowser, E. M., Henderson, W. J., Fisherman, E. W., and Williams, G. A.,** Role of adrenergic stimuli in parathyroid hormone secretion in man, *J. Clin. Endocrinol. Metab.*, 40, 478, 1975.
50. **Williams, G. A., Hargis, G. K., Bowser, E. N., Henderson, W. J., and Martinez, N. J.,** Evidence for a role of adenosine 3′5′-monophosphate in parathyroid hormone release, *Endocrinology*, 92, 687, 1973.

51. **Mayer, G. P., Hurst, J. G., Barto, J. A., Keaton, J. A., and Moore, M. P.,** Effects of epinephrine on parathyroid hormone secretion in calves, *Endocrinology,* 104, 1181, 1979.
52. **Harney, A. M., Kukreja, S. C., Hargis, G. K., Johnson, P. A., Bowser, E. N., and Williams, G. A.,** Effect of long-term administration of epinephrine and propranolol on serum calcium, parathyroid hormone and calcitonin in the rat, *Proc. Soc. Exptl. Biol. Med.,* 159, 266, 1978.
53. **Abe, M. and Sherwood, L. M.,** Regulation of parathyroid hormone secretion by adenyl cyclase, *Biochem. Biophys. Res. Commun.,* 48, 396,1972.
54. **Brown, E. M., Gardner, D. G., Windeck, R. A., and Aurbach, G. D.,** Relationship of intracellular 3′5′-adenosine monophosphate accumulation to parathyroid hormone release from dispersed bovine parathyroid cells, *Endocrinology,* 103, 2323, 1978.
55. **Bolman, R. M., III, Cooper, C. W., Garner, S. C., Munson, P. L., and Wells, S. A., Jr.,** Stimulation of gastrin secretion in the pig by parathyroid hormone and its inhibition by thyrocalcitonin, *Endocrinology,* 100, 1014, 1977.
56. **Windeck, R., Brown, E. M., Gardner, D. G., and Aurbach, G. D.,** Effect of gastrointestinal hormones on isolated bovine parathyroid cells, *Endocrinology,* 103, 2020, 1978.
57. **Williams, G. A., Bowser, E. N., Hargis, G. K., Kukreja, S. C., Shah, J. H., Vora, N. M., and Henderson, W. J.,** Effect of ethanol on parathyroid hormone and calcitonin secretion in man, *Proc. Soc. Exptl. Biol. Med.,* 159, 187, 1978.
58. **Lancer, S. R., Bowser, E. N., Hargis, G. K., and Williams, G. A.,** The effect of growth hormone on parathyroid function in rats, *Endocrinology,* 98, 1289, 1976.

58a. **Chambers, D. J., Dunham, J., Zanelli, J. M., Parsons, J. A., Bitensky, L., and Chayen, J.,** A sensitive bioassay of parathyroid hormone in plasma, *Clin. Endocrinol.,* 9, 373, 1978.

59. **Gertner, J. M., Horst, R. L., Broadus, A. E., Rasmussen, H., and Genel, M.,** Parathyroid function and vitamin D metabolism during human growth hormone replacement, *J. Clin. Endocrinol. Metab.,* 49, 185, 1979.
60. **Williams, G. A., Hargis, G. K., Ensinck, J. W., Kukreja, S. C., Bowser, E. N., Chertow, B. S., and Henderson, W.J.,** Role of endogenous somatostatin in the secretion of parathyroid hormone and calcitonin, *Metabolism,* 28, 950, 1979.
61. **Deftos, L. J., Lorenz, M., and Bohanon, M.,** Somatostatin does not suppress plasma parathyroid hormone, *J. Clin. Endocrinol. Metab.,* 43, 205, 1976.
62. **Sato, S., Szabo, M., Kowalski, K., and Burke, G.,** Role of prostaglandin in thyrotropin action on thyroid, *Endocrinology,* 90, 343, 1972.
63. **Gardener, D. G., Brown, E. M., Windeck, R., and Aurbach,** Prostaglandin E_2 stimulation of adenosin 3′5′-monophosphate accumulation and parathyroid hormone release in dispersed bovine parathyroid cells, *Endocrinology,* 103, 577, 1978.
64. **Gardner, D. G., Brown, E. M., Windeck, and Aurbach, G. D.,** Prostaglandin $F_{2\alpha}$ inhibits 3′5′ = adenosine monophosphate accumulation and parathyroid hormone release from dispersed bovine parathyroid cells, *Endocrinology,* 104, 1, 1979.
65. **Deluca, H. F.,** Recent advances in our understanding of the vitamin D endocrine system, *Steroid Biochem.,* 11, 35, 1979.
66. **Haussler, M. R. and McCain, T. A.,** Basic and clinical concepts related to vitamin D metabolism and action, *N. Engl. J. Med.,* 297, 974 and 1041, 1977.
67. **Golden, P., Mazey, R., Greenwalt, A., Martin, K., and Slatopolsky, E.,** Vitamin D: a direct effect on the parathyroid gland?, *Miner. Electrolyte Metab.,* 2, 1, 1979.
68. **Tanaka, Y., DeLuca, H. F., Ghayarian, J. G., Hargis, G. K., and Williams, G. A.,** Effects of vitamin D and its metabolites on serum parathyroid hormone levels in the rat, *Miner. Electrolyte Metab.,* 2, 20, 1979.
69. **Oldham, S. B., Smith, R., Hartenbower, D. L., Henry, H. L., Norman, A. W., and Coburn, J. W.,** The acute effects of 1,25-dihydroxycholecalciferol on serum immuno-reactive parathyroid hormone in the dog, *Endocrinology,* 104, 248, 1979.
70. **Dietel, M., Dorn, G., Monty, R.,and Altenahr, E.,** Influence of vitamin D_3 1,25-dihydroxyvitamin D_3 and 24,25-dihydroxy vitamin D_3 on parathyroid hormone secretion, adenosine 3′5′-monophosphate release, and ultrastructure of parathyroid glands in organ culture, *Endocrinology,* 105, 237, 1979.
71. **Chertow, B. S., Williams, G. A., Norris, R. M., Baker, G. R., and Hargis, G. K.,** Vitamin A. stimulation of parathyroid hormone: interactions with calcium, hydrocortisone, and vitamin E ain bovine parathyroid tissues and effects of vitamin A in man, *Eur. J. Clin. Invest.,* 7, 307, 1977.
72. **Copp, D. H., Moghadam, H., Mensen, E. D., and McPherson, G. D.,** The parathyroids and calcium homeostasis, in *Parathyroids,* Greep, R. O. and Talmage, R. V., Eds., Charles C Thomas, Springfield, Ill., 1961, 203.
73. **Hamilton, J. W., Spierto, F. W., MacGregor, R. R., and Cohn, D. V.,** Studies on the biosynthesis *in vitro* of parathyroid hormone. II. The effects of calcium and magnesium on synthesis of parathyroid hormone isolated from bovine parathyroid tissues and incubation medium, *J. Biol. Chem.,* 246, 3224, 1971.

74. **Segre, G. V., D'Amour, P., and Potts, J. T., Jr.,** Metabolism of radioiodinated bovine parathyroid hormone in the rat, *Endocrinology,* 99, 1645, 1976.
75. **Habener, J. F., Mayer, G. P., Dee, P. C., and Potts, J. T., Jr.,** Metabolism of amino and carboxyl sequence immunoreactive parathyroid hormone in the bovine: evidence for peripheral cleavage of hormone, *Metabolism,* 25, 385, 1976.
76. **Martin, K. J., Hruska, K. A., Freitag, J. J., Klahr, S., and Slatopolsky, E.,** The peripheral metabolism of parathyroid hormone, *N. Eng. J. Med.,* 301, 1092, 1979.
77. **Singer, F. R., Segre, G. V., Habener, J. F., and Potts, J. T., Jr.,** Peripheral metabolism of bovine parathyroid hormone in the dog, *Metabolism,* 24, 139, 1975.
78. **Oldham, S. B., Finck, E. J., and Singer, F. R.,** Parathyroid clearance in man, *Metabolism,* 27, 993, 1978.
79. **Martin, K. J., Hruska, K. A., Lewis, J., Anderson, C., and Slatopolsky, E.,** The renal handling of parathyroid hormone: role of peritubular uptake and glomerular filtration, *J. Clin. Invest.,* 60, 808, 1977.
80. **Freitag, J. J., Martin, K. J., Hruska, K., Anderson, C., Ladenson, J., and Slatopolsky, E.,** Impaired parathyroid hormone metabolism in patients with chronic renal failure, *N. Engl. J. Med.,* 298, 29, 1978.
81. **Hruska, K., Martin, K., Mennes, P., Greenwalt, A., Anderson, C., Klahr, S., and Slatopolsky, E.,** Degradation of parathyroid hormone and fragment production by the isolated perfused dog kidney: the effect of glomerular filtration rate and perfusate Ca^{++} concentrations, *J. Clin. Invest.,* 60, 501, 1977.
82. **Canterbury, J. M., Bricker, L. A., Levey, G. S., Kozlouskis, P. L., Ruiz, E., Zull, J. E., and Reiss, E.,** Metabolism of parathyroid hormone: immunological and biological characteristics of fragments generated by liver perfusion, *J. Clin. Invest.,* 55, 1245, 1975.
83. **Parsons, J. A. and Robinson, C. J,.** A rapid indirect hypercalcemic action of parathyroid hormone demonstrated in isolated blood-perfused bone, in *Parathyroid Hormone and Thyrocalcitonin (Calcitonin),* Talmage, R. V. and Belanger, L. F., Eds., Excerpta Medica, Amsterdam, 1968, 329.
84. **Martin, K. J., Freitag, J. J., Conrades, M. B., Hruska, K., Klahr, S., and Slatopolsky, E.,** Selective uptake of the synthetic amino terminal fragment of bovine parathyroid hormone by isolated perfused bone, *J. Clin. Invest.,* 62, 256, 1978.
85. **Freitag, J. J., Martin, K. J., Conrades, M. B., and Slatopolsky, E.,** Metabolism of parathyroid hormone by fetal rat calvaria, *Endocrinology,* 104, 510, 1979.
86. **Galtzman, D.,** Examination of the requirement for metabolism of parathyroid hormone in skeletal tissue before biological action, *Endocrinology,* 102, 1555, 1978.
87. **D'Amour, P., Huet, P. M., Segre, G.V., and Rosenblatt, M.,** Structural requirements for uptake and cleavage of iodinated bovine parathyroid hormone by the dog liver *in vivo, Prog. Abstr. 61st Ann. Meet. Endocr. Soc.* Anaheim, Calif. (Abstr. No. 172) p. 115, 1979.
88. **Parsons, J. A.,** Physiology of parathyroid hormone, in *Endocrinology, Vol. 2,* DeGroot, L. J., Cahill, G. F., Jr., Martini, L., Nelson, D. H., Odell, W. D., Potts, J. T., Jr., Steinberger, E., and Winegard, A. I., Eds., Grune & Stratton, New York, 1979, 621.
89. **Parfitt, A. M.,** The action of parathyroid hormone on bone: relation to bone remodelling and turnover, calcium homeostasis and metabolic bone disease (a four part report), *Metabolism,* 25, 809, 909, 1033, and 1157, 1976.
90. **Parsons, J. A.,** Parathyroid physiology and the skeleton, in *The Biochemistry and Physiology of Bone,* Vol. 4, Bourne, G. H., Ed., Academic Press, New York, 1976, 159.
91. **Jaworski, F. and Lok, E.,** The rate of osteoclastic bone erosion in Haversian remodeling sites of adult dogs rib, *Calcif. Tissue Res.,* 10, 103, 1972.
92. **Rowland, R. E.,** Exchangeable bone calcium, *Clin. Orthop.,* 49, 233, 1966.
93. **Riggs, B. L., Bassingthwaite, J. B., Jowsey, J., and Pequegnat, E. P.,** Autoradiographic methods for quantitation of deposition and distribution of radiocalcium in bone, *J. Lab. Clin. Med.,* 75, 520, 1970.
94. **Groer, P. G.and Marshall, J. H.,** Mechanism of calcium exchange at bone surfaces, *Calcif. Tissue Res.,* 12, 175, 1973.
95. **Selye, H.,** On the stimulation of new bone formation with parathyroid extract and irradiated ergosterol, *Endocrinology,* 16, 547, 1932.
96. **Barnicot, N. A.,** The local action of the parathyroid and other tissues on bone in intracerebral graft, *J. Anat. (London),* 82(4), 233, 1948.
97. **Tatevossian, A.,** Effect of parathyroid extract on blood calcium and osteoclast count in mice, *Calcif. Tissue Res.,* 11, 251, 1973.
98. **Krempien, B. and Ritz, E.,** Effects of parathyroid hormone on osteocytes: ultrastructural evidence for anistotropic osteolysis and involvement of the cytoskeleton, *Metab. Bone Dis. Rel. Res.,* 1, 55, 1978.

99. **Raisz, L. G., Trummel, C. T., and Simmons, H.**, Induction of bone resorption in tissue culture: prolonged response after brief exposure to parathyroid hormone or 25-hydroxycholecalciferol, *Endocrinology*, 90, 744, 1972.
100. **Parsons, J. A., Reit, E., and Robinson, C. J.**, A rapid and sensitive hypercalcemic assay for parathyroid hormone using the chicken, *Endocrinology*, 92, 454, 1973.
101. **Marcus, R. and Aurbach, G.D.**, Bioassay of parathyroid hormone *in vitro* with a stable preparation of adenyl cyclase from rat kidney, *Endocrinology*, 85, 801, 1969.
102. **Herrmann-Erlee, M. P. M., Heersche, J. N. M., Hekkelman, J. W., Gaillard, P. J., Tregear, G. W., Parsons, J. A., and Potts, J. T., Jr.**, Effects on bone *in vitro* of bovine parathyroid hormone and synthetic fragments representing residues 1-34, 2-34, 3-34, *Endocrine Res. Commun.*, 3, 21, 1976.
103. **Neuman, W. F.**, *The milieu interieur* of bone: Claude Bernard revisited, *Fed. Proc.*, 28, 1846, 1969.
104. **Ramp, W. K. and McNeil, R.W.**, Selective stimulation of net calcium efflux from chick embryo tibiae by parathyroid hormone *in vitro*, *Calcif. Tissue Res.*, 25, 227, 1978.
105. **Talmage, R. V.** Calcium homeostasis — calcium transport — parathyroid action: the effect of parathyroid hormone on the movement of calcium between bone and fluid, *Clin. Orthop.*, 67, 210, 1969.
106. **Aurbach, G. D.**, Parathyroid hormone: mechanism of actions and cyclic AMP, *Fed. Proc.*, 29, 1179, 1970.
107. **Howard, G. A., Battemiller, B. L., and Baylink, D. J.**, Evidence for the coupling of bone formation to bone resorption *in vitro*, *Metab. Bone. Dis. Rel. Res.*, 2, 131, 1980.
108. **Parsons, J. A., Rafferty, B., Gray, D. et al.**, Pharmacology of parathyroid hormone and some of its fragments and analogues, in *Calcium-Regulating Hormones*, Talmage, R. V., Owen, M., and Parsons, J. A., Eds., Excerpta Medica, Amsterdam, 1975, 33.
109. **Harris, W.H. and Heaney, R. P.**, Skeletal renewal and metabolic bone disease, *N. Engl. J. Med.*, 280, 253, 1969.
110. **Pugsley, L. I. and Selye, H.**, The histological changes in the bone responsible for the action of parathyroid hormone on the calcium metabolism of the rat, *J. Physiol. (London)*, 79, 113, 1933.
111. **Reeve, J., Tregear, G. W., and Parsons, J. A.**, Preliminary trial of low doses of human parathyroid hormone 1-34 peptide in treatment of osteoporosis, *Calcif. Tissue Res.*, (Suppl. 21), 469, 1976.
112. **O'Grady, R. L. and Cameron, D. A.**, Demonstration of binding sites for PTH in bone cells, in *Endocrinology, (London)*, Taylor, S. and Heinemann, W., Eds., 1972.
113. **Peck, W. A., Carpenter, J., Messinger, K., and Debra, D.**, Cyclic 3′5′ adenosine monophosphate in isolated bone cells: response to low concentrations of parathyroid hormone, *Endocrinology*, 92, 692, 1973.
114. **Peck, W.**, Cyclic AMP as a second messenger in the skeletal actions of parathyroid hormone: a decade-old hypothesis, *Calcif. Tissue Int.*, 29, 1, 1979.
115. **Rodan, S.B. and Rodan, G. A.**, The effect of parathyroid hormone and thyrocalcitonin on the accumulation of cyclic adenosine 3′5′-monophosphate in freshly isolated bone cells, *J. Biol. Chem.*, 249, 3068, 1974.
116. **Oziak, R. and Stern, P. H.**, Calcium transport in isolated bone cells. III. Effects of parathyroid hormone and cyclic 3′5′-AMP, *Endocrinology*, 97, 1281, 1975.
117. **Wong, G. L., Kent, G. N., Ku, K. Y., and Cohn, D. V.**, The interaction of parathormone and calcium on the hormone-regulated synthesis of hyaluronic acid and citrate decarboxylation in isolated bone cells, *Endocrinology*, 103, 2274, 1978.
118. **Neuman, W. F., Mulryan, B. J., and Martin, G. R.**, A chemical view of osteoclasis based on studies with yttrium, *Clin. Orthrop.*, 17, 124, 1960.
119. **Firschein, H. E. and Alcock, N. W.**, Rate or removal of collagen and mineral from bone and cartilage, *Metabolism*, 18, 115, 1969.
120. **Nisbet, J. A., Hellwell, S., and Nordin, B. E. C.**, Relation of lactic and citric acid metabolism to bone resorption in tissue culture, *Clin. Orthop.*, 70, 220, 1970.
121. **Waite, L. C.**, Carbonic anhydrase inhibitors, parathyroid hormone and calcium metabolism, *Endocrinology*, 91, 1160, 1972.
122. **Vaes, G.**, Collagenase, lysosomes and osteoclastic bone resorption, in *Collagenase in Normal and Pathological Connective Tissue*, Wolley, D. E., and Evanson, J. M., Eds., John Wiley & Sons, New York, 1980, 185.
123. **Eilon, G. and Raisz, L. G.**, Comparison of the effects of stimulators and inhibitors of resorption on the release of lysosomal enzymes and radioactive calcium from fetal bone in organ culture, *Endocrinology*, 103, 1969, 1978.
124. **McPartlin, J., Skrabanek, P., and Powell, D.**, Early effects of parathyroid hormone on rat calvarian bone alkaline phosphatase. *Endocrinology*, 103, 1573, 1978.
125. **Puschett, J. B.**, Renal tubular effects of parathyroid hormone: an update, *Clin. Orthop.*, 135, 249, 1978.

126. **Pang, P. K., Tenner, T. E., Jr., Yee, J. A., Yang, M., and Janssen, H. F.**, Hypotensive action of parathyroid hormone preparations on rats and dogs, *Proc. Natl. Acad. Sci. U.S.A.*, 77, 675, 1980.
127. **Agus, Z. S., Puschett, J. B., Senesky, D., and Goldberg, M.**, Mode of action of parathyroid hormone and cyclic adenosine 3′,5′-monophosphate on renal tubular phosphate reabsorption in the dog, *J. Clin. Invest.*, 50, 617, 1971.
128. **Agus, Z. S., Gardner, L. B., Beck, L. H., and Goldberg, M.**, Effects of parathyroid hormone on renal tubular reabsorption of calcium, sodium and phosphate, *Am. J. Physiol.*, 224, 1143, 1973.
129. **Strickler, J. C., Thompson, D. D., Klose, R. M., and Giebisch, G.**, Micropuncture study of inorganic phosphate excretion in the rat, *J. Clin. Invest.*, 43, 1596, 1964.
130. **Beck, L. H. and Goldberg, M.**, Effects of acetazolamide and parathyroidectomy on renal transport of sodium, calcium and phosphate, *Am. J. Physiol.*, 224, 1136, 1973.
131. **Dennis, V. W., Bello-Reuss, E., and Robinson, R. R.**, Response of phosphate transport to parathyroid hormone in segments of rabbit nephron, *Am. J. Physiol.*, 233, F29, 1977.
132. **Chase, L. R.and Aurbach, G. D.**, Parathyroid function and the renal excretion of 3′,5′-adenylic acid, *Proc. Natl. Acad. Sci., U.S.A.*, 58, 518, 1967.
133. **Pastoriza-Munoz, E., Colindres, R. E., Lassiter, W. E., and Lechene, C.**, Effect of parathyroid hormone on phosphate reabsorption in rat distal convolution *Am. J. Physiol.*, 235, F321, 1978.
134. **Jackson, B. A., Hui, Y. S. F., Northrup, T. E., and Dousa, T. P.**, Differential responsiveness of adenylate cyclase from rat, dog and rabbit kidney to parathyroid hormone, vasopressin and calcitonin, *Miner. Electrolyte Metab.*, 3, 136, 1980.
135. **Goltzman, D., Callahan, E. N., Tregear, G. W., and Potts, J. T., Jr.**, Influence of guanyl nucleotides on parathyroid hormone — stimulated adenylyl cyclase activity in renal cortical membranes, *Endocrinology*, 103, 1352, 1978.
136. **Harada, E., Laychock, S. G.,and Rubin, R. P.**, Parathyroid hormone induced stimulation of calcium uptake by renal microsomes, *Biochem. Biophys. Res. Commun.*, 84, 396, 1978.
137. **Dibella, F. P., Dousa, T. P., Miller, S., Dousa, T. P., Miller, S.S., and Arnaud, C. D.**, Parathyroid hormone receptors of renal cortex: specific binding of biologically active ^{125}I-labelled hormone and relationship to adenylate cyclase activation, *Proc. Natl. Acad. Sci. U.S.A.*, 71, 723, 1974.
138. **Stumpf, W. E., Sar, M., Narbaitz, R., Reid, F. A., DeLuca, H. F., and Tanaka, Y.**, Cellular and subcellular localization of 1,25-$(OH)_2$-Vitamin D_3 in rat kidney: comparison with localization of parathyroid hormone and estradiol, *Proc. Natl. Acad. Sci. U.S.A.*, 77, 1149, 1980.
139. **Kau, S. T. and Maack, T.**, Transport and catabolism of parathyroid hormone in isolated rat kidney, *Am. J. Physiol.*, 233, F445, 1977.
140. **Massry, S. G., Coburn, J. W., Friedler, R. M., Kurokawa, K., and Singer, F. R.**, Relationship between the kidney and parathyroid hormone, *Nephron*, 15, 197, 1975.
141. **Haussler, M. R. and McCain, T. A.**, Basic and clinical concepts related to vitamin D metabolism and action, *N. Eng. J. Med.*, 297, 974, and 1041, 1977.
142. **Norman, A. W. and Henry, H. L.**, Vitamin D to 1,25-dihydroxycholecalciferol: evolution of a steroid hormone, *Trends Biochem. Sci.*, 4, 14, 1979.
143. **Fraser, D. R.**, The metabolism and function of vitamin D, *World Rev. Nutr. Diet.*, 31, 168, 1978.
144. **Arnaud, C. D.**, Calcium homeostasis: regulatory elements and their integration, *Fed. Proc.*, 37, 2557, 1978.
145. **Hay, A.**, Complexities of vitamin D metabolism still increasing, *Nature*, 278, 510, 1979.
146. **Deluca, H. F.**, Recent advances in our understanding of the vitamin D endocrine system, *J. Steroid Biochem.*, 11, 35, 1979.
147. **Drezner, M. K. and Harrelson, J. M.**, Newer knowledge of vitamin D and its metabolites in health and disease, *Clin. Orthop.*, 139, 206, 1979.
148. **Coburn, J. W., Hartenbower, D. L.,and Norman, A. W.**, Metabolism and action of the hormone Vitamin D: its relation to diseases of calcium homeostasis, *West. J. Med.*, 121, 22, 1974.
149. **Thompson, M. L.**, Relative efficiency of pigment and horny layer thickenss in protecting the skin of Europeans and Africans against solar ultraviolet radiation, *J. Physiol. (London)*, 127, 236, 1955.
150. **Tucker, G., Gragnon, R., and Haussler, M.**, Vitamin D_3-25-hydroxylase: tissue occurrence and apparent lack of regulation, *Arch. Biochem. Biophys.*, 155, 47, 1973.
151. **Fraser, D. R. and Kodicek, E.**, Unique biosynthesis by kidney of a biologically active vitamin d metabolite, *Nature*, 228, 764, 1970.
152. **Haussler, M. R., Myrtle, J. F., and Norman, A. W.**, The association of a metabolite of vitamin D_3 with intestinal mucosa chromatin, *in vivo*, *J. Biol. Chem.*, 243, 4055, 1968.
153. **Tanaka, Y., Halloran, B., Schnoes, H. K., and DeLuca, H. F.**, *In vitro* production of 1,25-dihydroxyvitamin D_3 by rat placental tissue, *Proc. Natl. Acad. Sci. U.S.A.*, 76, 5033, 1979.
154. **Sunaga S., Horiuchi, N., Takahashi, N., Okuyama, K., and Suda, T.**, The site of 1α,25-Dihydroxyvitamin D_3 production in pregnancy, *Biochem. Biophys. Res. Comm.*, 90, 948, 1979.

155. **Boyle, I. T., Gray, R. W., and DeLuca, H. F.,** Regulation by calcium of *in vivo* synthesis of 1,25-dihydroxycholecalciferol and 21,25-dihydroxycholecalciferol., *Proc. Natl. Acad. Sci. U.S.A.*, 68, 2131, 1971.
156. **Tanaka, Y. and DeLuca, H. F.,** The control of 25-hydroxyvitamin D metabolism by inorganic phosphorus, *Arch. Biochem. Biphys.*, 154, 566, 1973.
157. **Madhok, T. C. and DeLuca, H. F.,** Characteristics of the rat liver microsomal enzyme system converting cholecalciferol into 25-hydroxycholecalciferol., *Biochem. J.*, 184, 491, 1979.
158. **Henry, H. L.,** Response of chick kidney cell cultures to 1,25-Dihydroxyvitamin D_3, *Prog. Abstr. 61st Ann. Meet. Endocr. Soc.* Anaheim, Calif., (Abstr. No. 755), p. 261, 1979.
159. **Spanos, E., Pike, J. W., Haussler, M. R., Colston, K. W., Evans, I. M. A., Goldner, A. M., McCain, T. A., and MacIntyre, I.,** Circulating 1 α,25-dihydroxyvitamin D in the chicken: enhancement by injection of prolactin and during egg laying, *Life Sci.*, 19, 1751, 1976.
160. **Boass, A., Toverud, S. U., and McCain, T. A., Pike, J. W., and Haussler, M. R.,** Elevated serum levels of 1α,25-dihydroxycholecaliciferol in lactating rats, *Nature*, 267, 630, 1977.
161. **Brown, D. J., Spanos, E., and MacIntyre, I.,** Hormonal control of plasma 1,25-dihydroxyvitamin D_3 in man, *J. Endocrinol*, 83, 54P, 1979 (abstract).
162. **Halloran, B. P., Barthell, E. N., and DeLuca, H. F.,** Vitamin D metabolism during pregnancy and lactation in the rat, *Proc. Natl. Acad. Sci. U.S.A.*, 76, 5549, 1979.
163. **Baksi, S. N. and Kenny, A. D.,** Vitamin D_3 metabolism in immature Japanese quail: effects of ovarian hormones, *Endocrinology*, 101, 1216, 1977.
164. **Pike, J. W., Spanos, E., Colston, K. W., MacIntyre, I., and Haussler, M. R.,** Influence of estrogen on renal vitamin D hydroxylases and serum 1α,25-$(OH)_2D_3$ in chicks, *Am. J. Physiol.*, 235, E338, 1978.
165. **Eisman, J. A., Hamstra, A. J., Kream, B. E.,and DeLuca, H. F.,** A sensitive, precise and convenient method for determination of 1,25-dihydroxyvitamin D in human plasma, *Arch. Biochem. Biophysic.*, 176, 235, 1976.
166. **Lund, B. and Sorensen, O. H.,** Measurement of 25-hydroxyvitamin D in serum and its relation to sunshine, age and vitamin D intake in the Danish population, *Scand. J. Clin. Lab. Invest.*, 39, 23, 1979.
167. **Bikle, D. D., Morrissey, R. L., and Zolock, D. T.,** The mechanism of action of vitamin D in the intestine, *Am. J. Clin. Nutr.*, 32, 2322, 1979.
168. **Wasserman, R.H., Kallfelz, F. A., and Comar, C. L.,** Active transport of calcium by rat duodenum *in vivo*, *Science*, 133, 883, 1961.
169. **Schachter, D. and Rosen, S. M.,** Active transport of Ca^{45} by the small intestine and its dependence on vitamin D, *Am. J. Physiol.*, 196, 357, 1959.
170. **Harrison, H. E. and Harrison, H. C.,** Intestinal transport of phosphate: action of vitamin D, calcium and potassium, *Am. J. Physiol.*, 201, 1007, 1961.
171. **Wasserman, R.H. and Taytor, A. N.,** Intestinal absorption of phosphate in the chick: effect of Vitamin D_3 and other parameters, *J. Nutr.*, 103, 586, 1973.
172. **Walling, M. W.,** Intestinal Ca and phosphate transport differential responses to vitamin D_3 metabolites, *Am. J. Physiol.*, 233, E488, 1977.
173. **Charles, A., Martial, J., Zolock, D., Morrissey, R., Bickle, D., and Baxter, J.,** Regulation of the messenger RNA for calcium binding protein by 1,25-dihydroxycholecalciferol, in *Vitamin D Biochemical, Chemical and Clinical Aspects Related to Calcium Metabolism*, Norman, A. W., Schaefer, K., Coburn, J. W., DeLuca, H. F., Fraser, D., Grigoleit, H. G., and Herrath, D. V., Eds., Walter de Gruyter, New York, 1977, 227.
174. **Corradino, R. A.,** Cyclic AMP regulation of the 1α25-$(OH)_2D_3$ - mediated intestinal calcium absorptive mechanism, in *Vitamin D Biochemical, Chemical and Clinical Aspects Related to Calcium Metabolism*, Norman, A. W., Schaefer, K., Coburn, J. W., DeLuca, H. F., Fraser, D., Grigoleit, H. G., and Herrath, D. V., Eds., Walter de Gruyter, New York, 1977, 231.
175. **Tsai, H. C. and Norman, A. W.,** Studies on the mode of action of calciferol. VI: Effect of 1,25-dihydroxyvitamin D_3 and RNA synthesis in the intestinal mucosa, *Biochem. Biophys. Res. Commun.*, 54, 622, 1973.
176. **Zerwekh, J. E., Haussler, M. R., and Lindell, T. J.,** Rapid enhancement of chick intestinal DNA-dependent RNA polymerase II activity by 1α,25-dihydroxyvitamin D_3, *in vivo, Proc. Natl. Acad. Sci. U.S.A.*, 71, 2337, 1974.
177. **Haussler, M. R., Nagode, L. A., and Rasmussen, H.,** Induction of intestinal brush border alkaline phosphatase by vitamin D and identity with Ca ATPase, *Nature*, 228, 1199, 1970.
178. **Wasserman, R. H., Corradino, R. A., Fullmer, C. S., and Taylor, A. N.,** Some aspects of vitamin D action: calcium absorption and vitamin D-dependent calcium-binding protein, *Vitam. Horm.*, 32, 299, 1974.
179. **Corradino, R. A.,** 1,25-dihydroxycholecalciferol: inhibition of action in organ-cultured intestine by actinomycin D and α-amanitin, *Nature*, 243, 41, 1973.

180. **Bickle, D. D., Zolock, D. T., Morrissey, R. L., and Herman, R. H.,** Independence of 1,25-Dihydroxyvitamin D_3-mediated calcium transport from *de novo* RNA and protein synthesis, *J. Biol. Chem.*, 253, 484, 1978.
181. **Queille, M. L., Miravet, L., Bordier, P., and Radel, J.,** The action of vitamin D metabolites (25 $(OH)D_3$-12,5$(OH)_2D_3$-25,26$(OH)_2D_3$) on vitamin D deficient rats, *Biomedicine*, 28, 237, 1978.
182. **Carlsson, A.,** Tracer Experiments on the effect of vitamin D on the skeletal metabolism of calcium and phosphorus, *Acta Physiol. Scand.*, 26, 212, 1952.
183. **Rasmussen, H., DeLuca, H., Arnaud, C., Hawker, C., and von Stedingk, M.,** The relationship between vitamin D and parathyroid hormone, *J. Clin. Invest.*, 42, 1940, 1963.
184. **Reynolds, J. J., Holick, M. F., and DeLuca, H. F.,** The role of vitamin D metabolites in bone resorption, *Calcif. Tissue Res.*, 12, 295, 1973.
185. **Tanaka, Y. and DeLuca, H. F.,** Bone mineral mobilization activity of 1,25-dihydroxycholecalciferol, a metabolite of vitamin D, *Arch. Biochem. Biophys.*, 146, 574, 1971.
186. **Boris, A., Hurley, J. F.,and Trimal, T.,** *In vivo* studies in chicks and rats of bone calcium mobilization by 1α,25-dihydroxycholecalciferol (calcitriol) and its congeners, *J. Nutr.*, 109, 1772, 1979.
187. **Raisz, L. G., Maina, D. M., Gworek, S. C., Dietrich, J. W., and Canalis, E. M.,** Hormonal control of bone collagen synthesis *in vitro:* inhibitory effects of 1-hydroxylated vitamin D metabolites, *Endocrinology*, 102, 731, 1978.
188. **Dickson, I. R. and Kodicek, E.,** Effect of vitamin D deficiency on bone formation in the chick, *Biochem. J.*, 182, 429, 1979.
189. **Malluche, H. H., Henry, H., Meyer-Sabellek, W., Sherman, D., Massry, S. G., and Norman, A. W.,** Effects and interaction of 24R,25 $(OH)_2D_3$ and 1,25 $(OH)_2D_3$ on bone, *Am. J. Physiol.*, 238, E494, 1980.
190. **Lindgren, J. U. and Lindholm, T. S.,** Effect of 1-alpha-hydroxyvitamin D_3 on osteoporosis in rats induced by oophorectomy, *Calcif. Tissue Intl.*, 27, 161, 1979.
191. **Boris, A., Hurley, J. F., and Trmal, T.,** Biological activity evaluation of chemically synthesized vitamin D metabolites and analogs, in *Vitamin D Biochemical, Chemical and Clinical Aspects Related to Calcium Metabolism*, Norman, A. W., Schaefer, K., Coburn, J. W., DeLuca, H. F., Fraser, Grigoleit, H. G., and Herrath, D. V., Eds., Walter de Gruyter, New York, 1977, 553.
192. **Deiss, W. P., Jr. and Hern, D. L.,** Bone matrix studies: influences of parathyroid extract, calcitonin, and cholecalciferol and of rickets and its treatment, *Biochim. Biophys. Acta*, 284, 311, 1979.
193. **Corvol, M. T. and Dumontier, M. F., Garabedian, M. and Rappaport, R.,** Vitamin D and cartilage. II. Biological activity of 25-hydroxycholecalciferol and 24,25- and 1,25- dihydroxycholecalciferols on cultured growth plate chondrocytes, *Endocrinology*, 102, 1269, 1978.
194. **Puschett, J. B., Beck, W. S. Jr., and Jelonek, A.,** Parathyroid hormone and 25-hydroxyvitamin D_3: synergistic and antagonistic effects on renal phosphate transport, *Science*, 190, 473, 1975.
195. **Puschett, J. B., Moranz, J., and Kurnick, W.,** Evidence for a direct action of cholecalciferol and 25-hydroxycholecalciferol on renal transport of phosphate, sodium and calcium, *J. Clin. Invest.*, 51, 373, 1972.
196. **Popoutzer, M. M., Robinette, J. B., DeLuca, H. F., and Holick, M. F.,** The acute effect of 25-hydroxycholecalciferol on renal handling of phosphorus, *J. Clin. Invest.*, 53, 913, 1974.
197. **Puschett, J. B. and Kuhrman, M. S.,** Renal tubular effects of 1,25-Dihydroxyvitamin D_3: interactions with vasopressin and parathyroid hormone in the vitamin D-depleted rat, *J. Lab. Clin. Med.*, 92, 895, 1978.
198. **DeLuca, H. F. and Holick, M. F.,** Vitamin D: biosynthesis, metabolism and mode of action, in *Endocrinology, Vol. 2*, DeGroot, L. J., Cahill, G. F. Jr., Martini, L., Nelson, D. H., Odell, W. D., Potts, J. T., Jr., Steinberger, E., and Winegard, A. I., Grune & Stratton, New York, 1979, 653.
199. **Hadad, J. G.,** Transport of vitamin D metabolites, *Clin. Ortho. Rel. Res.*, 142, 249, 1979.
200. **Eisman, J. A., Hamstra, A. J., Kream, B. E., and DeLuca, H. F.,** 1,25-dihydroxyvitamin D in biological fluids: a simplified and sensitive assay, *Science*, 193, 1021, 1976.
201. **Bringhurst, F. R. and Potts, J. T. Jr.,** Calcium and phosphate distribution, turnover, and metabolic actions, in *Endocrinology, Vol. 2* DeGroot, L. J., Cahill, G. F., Jr., Martini, L., Nelson, D. H., Odell, W. D., Potts, J. T., Jr., Steinberger, E., and Winegard, A. I., Eds., Grune & Stratton, San Francisco, 1979, 551.
202. **Urist, M.,** Biochemistry of calcification, in *The Biochemistry and Physiology of Bone, Vol. 4*, G. H. Bourne, Ed., Academic Press, San Francisco, 1976, 1.
203. **McDonald, L. E.,** *Veterinary Endocrinology and Reproduction*, Lea & Febiger, Philadelphia, 1975, 63.
204. **Chertow, B. S., Baker, G. R., Henry, H. L., and Norman, A. W.,** Effects of vitamin D metabolites on bovine parathyroid hormone release *in vitro*, *Am. J. Physiol.*, 238, E384, 1980.
205. **Fischer, J. A. and Blum, J. W.,** Noncalcium control of parathyroid hormone secretion, *Miner. Electrolyte Metab.*, 3, 158, 1980.

206. **Fischer, J. A., Oldham, S. B., Sizemore, G. W., and Arnaud, C. D.**, Calcitonin stimulation of parathyroid hormone secretion *in vitro, Hormone Metab. Res.*, 3, 223, 1971.
207. **Au, W. Y. W.**, Cortisol stimulation of parathyroid hormone secretion by rat parathyroid glands in organ culture, *Science*, 193, 1015, 1976.
208. **Fucik, R. F., Kukreja, S. C., Hargis, G. K., Bowser, E. N., Henderson, W. J., and Williams, G. A.**, Effect of glucocorticoids on function of the parathyroid glands in man, *J. Clin. Endocrinol. Metab.*, 40, 152, 1975.
209. **Tam, C. S. and Anderson, W.**, Tetracycline labeling of bone *in vivo, Calcif. Tissue Int.*, 30, 121, 1980.
210. **Webster, L. A., Atkins, D., and Peacock, M.**, A bioassay for parathyroid horone using whole mouse calvaria in tissue culture, *J. Endocrinol.*, 62, 631, 1974.
211. **Mayer, G. P., Keaton, J. A., Hurst, J. G., and Habener, J. F.**, Effects of plasma calcium concentration on the relative proportion of hormone and carboxyl fragments in parathyroid venous blood, *Endocrinology*, 104, 1778, 1979.
212. **Berson, S. A., Yalow, R. S., Aurbach, G. D., and Potts, J. D., Jr.**, Immunoassay of bovine and human parathyroid hormone, *Proc. Natl. Acad. Sci. U.S.A.*, 49, 613, 1963.
213. **Mayer, G. P. and Hurst, J. G.**, Sigmoidal relationship between parathyroid hormone secretion rate and plasma calcium concentration in calves, *Endocrinology*, 102, 1036, 1978.
214. **Saeki, T. and Hayashi, M,.** Radioimmunoassay of bovine parathyroid hormone, *Natl. Inst. Anim. Health Q. (Japan)*, 15, 151, 1975.
215. **Holick, M. F., Frommer, J. E., McNeill, S. C., Richtand, N. M., Henley, J. W., and Potts, J. T., Jr.**, Photometabolism of 7-dehydrocholesterol to previtamin D_3 in skin, *Biochem. Biophys. Res. Commun.*, 76, 107, 1977.
216. **Brumbaugh, P. F.and Haussler, M. R.**, 1 alpha, 25-dihydroxyvitamin D_3 receptor: competitive binding of vitamin D analogs, *Life Sci.*, 13, 1737, 1973.
217. **Zile, M., Bunge, E. C., Barsness, L., Yamada, S., Schnoes, H. K., and DeLuca, H. F.**, Localization of 1,25-dihydroxyvitamin D_3 in intestinal nuclei *in vivo, Arch. Biochem. Biophys.*, 186, 15, 1978.
218. **Schnoes, H. K. and DeLuca, H. F.**, Recent progress in vitamin D metabolism and the chemistry of vitamin D metabolites, *Fed. Proc.*, 39, 2723, 1980.
219. **Stern, P. H., Hamstra, A. J., DeLuca, H. F., and Bell, N. H.**, A bioassay capable of measuring 1 picrogram of 1,25-dihydroxyvitamin D_3, *J. Clin. Endoc. Metab.*, 46, 891, 1978.
220. **Garabedian, M., Holick, M. F., DeLuca, H. F., and Boyle, I. T.**, Control of 25-hydroxycholecalciferol metabolism by parathyroid glands, *Proc. Natl. Acad. Sci. U.S.A.*, 69, 1673, 1972.
221. **Golden, P., Greenwalt, A., Martin, K., Bellorunfont, E., Mazey, R., Klahr, S., and Slatopolsky, E.**, Lack of a direct effect of 1,25-Dihydroxycholecalciferol on parathyroid hormone secretion by normal bovine parathyroid glands, *Endocrinology*, 107, 602, 1980.
222. **Walker, D. G.**, Bone resorption restored in osteopetrotic mice by transplants of normal bone marrow and spleen cells, *Science*, 190, 784, 1975.
223. **Mundy, G. R., Altman, A. J., Gonder, M. D., and Bandelin, J. G.**, Direct resorption of bone by human monocytes, *Science*, 196, 1109, 1977.
224. **Lieberherr, M., Garabedian, M., Guillozo, H., Thil, C. L., and Balson, S.**, *In vitro* effects of Vitamin D_3 metabolites on rat calvaria cAMP content, *Calcif. Tissue Int.*, 30, 209, 1980.
225. **Galus, K., Szymendera, J., Zaleski, A., and Schreyer, K.**, Effects of 1 alpha-hydroxyvitamin D_3 and 24R, 25-dihydroxyvitamin D_3 on bone remodeling, *Calicif. Tissue Int.*, 31, 209, 1980.

GASTROINTESTINAL HORMONES

William M. Yau

INTRODUCTION

During the past two decades a truly remarkable series of advances in our understanding of gastrointestinal physiology has taken place. This is particularly apparent because of the increasing number of gastrointestinal peptides which display interesting diversified pharmacologic properties but whose physiologic significance has yet to be determined. It has been demonstrated that many of these peptides possess significant hormonal effects in digestive processes, therefore the concept of the gut as an endocrine organ is now well accepted.

In the digestive system, the regulatory signals may originate from within the lumen and/or from the nervous pathways innervating the various regions. Mechanical distention as a result of the presence of a bolus, and/or the chemical constituents derived from food or its digestion, along with secretion from digestive glands, can be used as signals to trigger the release of peptides from the overlapping endocrine segments.

The array of hormonal messengers released by the intraluminal signals possess a wide spectrum of actions. Stimulation may be superseded by inhibition, depending on the peptide hormones present and their prevailing concentrations. The recognition of hormones by specific receptor sites at the target tissues initiates a sequence of biologic activities which are subjected to modification by the neural signals. Neural mechanisms are also activated by mechanical and chemical stimuli. The amplitude of the signal, whether hormonal or neural, depends on the balance between the intensity of stimulation and the capacity of the body to dispose of the stimulation. Both the affinity of a peptide for a receptor site and the efficacy of a peptide-receptor combination can be modified by other peptides or by neurotransmitters acting on the same or neighboring sites. There may be, however, a greater dependence of one system over the other from one area of the gut to another.

As our ability to quantitatively and qualitatively measure these peptides within the system increases with the availability of pure peptides for development of sensitive radioimmunoassay and for specific localization of the site of origin by immunocytochemical techniques, several important observations have led us to believe that the peptides are not evenly distributed throughout the digestive tract. One region may have an abundance of one type whereas a neighboring region may have an abundance of another type with a dissimilar or opposite biologic action. Many peptides are known to be located both within endocrine cells and nervous tissues, centrally and peripherally. The distribution within the nervous system is also uneven.

The target tissues of the peptides are not limited to digestive glands and muscle cells, but involve neurons and endocrine cells elsewhere, and thereby may assume regulatory functions resulting in release of additional hormones or neurotransmitters. At present many peptides are being considered as both putative neurotransmitters and candidate hormones regulating the activity of the gut. Gut endocrinology has been the subject of many excellent reviews in recent years.[1-20]

The primary aim of this chapter is to briefly update this knowledge of gastrointestinal hormones with only minimal attention to their discovery, isolation, and chemical characterization. A firm separation of the hormonal actions from the paracrine or neurocrine actions of the same peptide is not possible currently. The large number of morphologically distinguishable types of peptide-containing cells compounded by the dispersed nature of peptides distributed both in neural and digestive tissues have made

Table 1
MOLECULAR FORMS OF GASTRIN

Tetrapeptide[a]	(G—4, Component V)	597 (Mol wt.)
Minigastrin	(G—14, Component IV)	1833[b]
		1913[c]
Little gastrin	(G—17, Component III)	2098[b]
		2178[c]
Big gastrin	(G—34, Component II)	3839[b]
		3919[c]
Component I	(between G—34 and Big big gastrin)	
Big big gastrin[d]		20,000
NH_2-terminus tridecapeptide	(NT—13, NT-G-17)	1581[c]

[a] Minimum fragment for gastrin activity
[b] Molecular weight for gastrin-I.
[c] Molecular weight for gastrin-II.
[d] Artifact in assay system.

the gut one of the most complex organ systems in the body. The status of many of these peptides, either as a hormone or as a neurotransmitter, is controversial and remains to be settled.

GASTRIN[21-26]

Gastrin is a hormone, secreted in the antral mucosa of the stomach, that stimulates secretion of hydrochloric acid by the parietal cells of the gastric glands. Of the multiple molecular forms of gastrin (Table 1) that have been isolated and characterized, the most abundant one is G-17 from the antral mucosa. This form accounts for more than 90% of all gastrin immunoreactivity in the body. The G-34 form is the one that is most readily released into the blood upon stimulation and appears to be the second most abundant form. In terms of distribution, G-17 is the tissue hormone while G-34 is the major form present in the circulation. Besides the usual sulfated and unsulfated pair that exists in each molecular form, six forms of component 1 and G-34 and four forms of G-17 and G-14 are known to be present in the blood. The degree of gastrin heterogeneity is complex and our primary limitation is the ability to separate them with modern biochemical techniques.

The significance of the heterogenous molecular forms of gastrin is far from clear. Presumably, component 1 is the preprogastrin and G-34 is the progastrin. The primary active form is the G-17. G-14 is a degradation product still carrying gastrin activity.

The principal form of gastrin in most species examined has long been recognized to be G-17. A recent study, however, indicates that G-4, which is localized in TG cells both in the antral and upper intestinal mucosa, is present in a concentration far higher than that of G-17. Whether TG cells are different from the G cells in which most of the gastrin is secreted, remains to be determined.

Release of Gastrin (Table 2)

The natural stimuli causing gastrin release are the presence of food and the mechanical distention resulting from the presence of food, in the stomach. (See Table 2) Neural signals, vagal in particular, stimulate gastrin release through a direct action on the G cells in the antrum. Partially digested proteins and some amino acids enhance gastrin release by buffering the gastric acidity, thus eliminating the feedback inhibition from low luminal pH on the G cell output of gastrin. At the same time, proteins and amino acids affect gastrin release by a direct stimulation of G cells. Facilitation of

AMINO TERMINAL — CARBOXYL TERMINAL

CCK-V: 39 Tyr-Ile-Gln-Gln-Ala-Arg-33 Lys-Ala-Pro-Ser-Gly-Arg-Val-Ser-Met-Ile-Lys-Asn-Leu-Gln-Ser-Leu-Asp-Pro-Ser-His-Arg-Ile-Ser-Asp-Arg-Asp-Tyr(SO_3H)-Met-Gly-Trp-Met-Asp-Phe-NH_2

G-34-II*: 34 Glp-Leu-Gly-Pro-Gln-Gly-His-Pro-Ser-Leu-Val-Ala-Asp-Pro-Ser-Lys-Lys-17 Gln-Gly-Pro-Trp-Leu-Glu-Glu-Glu-Glu-Glu-Ala-Tyr(SO_3H)-Gly-Trp-Met-Asp-Phe-NH_2

G-17-II*: Glp-Gly-Pro-Trp-Leu-Glu-Glu-Glu-Glu-Glu-Ala-Tyr(SO_3H)-Gly-Trp-Met-Asp-Phe-NH_2

G-14-II*: Trp-Leu-Glu-Glu-Glu-Glu-Glu-Ala-Tyr-Gly-Trp-Met-Asp-Phe-NH_2

G-4: Trp-Met-Asp-Phe-NH_2

FIGURE 1. The Gastrin Family — *No SO_3H for I. Distribution is 2:1 ratio in favor of unsulfated forms.

gastrin release can also result from hypoglycemia and hypercalcemia. Bombesin, a tetradecapeptide first isolated from amphibian (*Bombina bombina*) skin is by far the most potent stimulant of gastrin release in man. Gastrin release by bombesin is unaffected by the presence of high acidity in the antrum, which suggests a possible role bombesin may play in the postprandial phase of gastric acid secretion. Peptides of the secretin family (Figure 1) inhibit gastrin release from G cells and, with the action of gastrin on parietal cell secretion.

Fate of Gastrin in Metabolism

The half-life of circulating G-17 and G-34 is 6 and 40 to 50 min., respectively. The kidney and small intestine are the organs responsible for the degradation and breakdown of gastrin. Neither G-17 nor G-34 is removed by the liver; however, small fragments of them (less than ten amino acids) can be cleared in that organ. The involvement of kidney and intestine is substantiated by the development of hypergastrinemia in patients with renal failure or extensive bowel resection.

Biologic Actions

The carboxyl-terminus tetrapeptide, Trp-Met-Asp-Phe-NH_2, is the smallest fragment that exhibits full biologic activity, but with a far lesser molar potency than the longer G-17. All molecular forms tested, including both sulfated and nonsulfated variants, achieve the same maximal effect in inducing acid secretion. While G-17 and G-14 possess equal potency, G-34 has only 1/6 the potency of G-17 or G-14 on a molar basis. It is therefore important in the calculation of effective concentration to consider both the half-life as well as the relative molar potency of the molecular species in question.

An amino terminal fragment (NT-13), presumably cleaved off from G-17, has been described in the fasting serum of gastrinoma patients. It is a tridecapeptide, which is released in response to intravenously administered secretin. No biologic activities have been demonstrated for NT-13. The biologic actions of gastrin are listed in Table 3.

Pathophysiology

Abnormal gastrin secretion leads to disorders intimately related to gastric secretion. Little is known of any motor disorder associated with abnormal gastrin secretion. Hy-

Table 2
STIMULANTS FOR GASTRIN RELEASE

Peptides
Amino Acids (tryptophan and phenylalanine)
Hypoglycemia
Neural stimulation (vagal or distention-initiated reflex)
Bombesin
Calcium

Table 3
BIOLOGIC ACTIONS OF GASTRIN

Trophic action
- Stomach
- Small intestine
- Pancreas

Water and electrolyte secretion
- Stomach
- Small intestine
- Pancreas
- Liver

Enzyme secretion
- Stomach
- Small intestine
- Pancreas

Stimulation of smooth muscle
- Lower esophageal sphincter
- Stomach
- Small and large intestine
- Gallbladder

Inhibition of smooth muscle
- Pyloric sphincter
- Sphincter of Oddi
- Ileocecal sphincter

Inhibition of water, electrolyte, and glucose absorption
- Small intestine

Release of hormones
- Calcitonin
- Insulin

Increase in blood flow
- Stomach
- Small intestine
- Pancreas

pergastrinemia can be a result of a gastrinoma, which most commonly occurs in the pancreas as in the Zollinger-Ellison syndrome, or less commonly in the duodenum or the antrum. Hypersecretion of acid by the stomach is brought about by hypergastrinemia; however, hypergastrinemia does not always result in hyperchlorhydria. With gastric ulcer, patients have low rates of acid secretion accompanied by hypergastrinemia.

There is evidence to indicate that the molecular species of gastrin in the serum of gastric ulcer patients may be predominantly the less potent G-34. Unfortunately, in the present conventional gastrin radioimmunoassay system, G-17 is likely to cross react with G-34.

Hypergastrinemia is also commonly seen in atrophic gastritis patients. This is mainly the result of a diminished feedback inhibition on gastrin release in the presence of achlorhydria. In this condition, the primary defect is a deficient acid secretory capacity

	AMINO TERMINAL
	1 7 14
VIP	His-Ser-Asp-Ala-Val-Phe-Thr-Asp-Asn-Tyr-Thr-Arg-Leu-Arg-
SECRETIN	His-Ser-Asp-Gly-Thr-Phe-Thr-Ser-Glu-Leu-Ser-Arg-Leu-Arg-
GLUCAGON	His-Ser-Gln-Gly-Thr-Phe-Thr-Ser-Asp-Tyr-Ser-Lys-Tyr-Leu-
GIP*	Tyr-Ala-Glu-Gly-Thr-Phe-Ile-Ser-Asp-Tyr-Ser-Ile-Ala-Met-
	21 28
VIP	Lys-Gln-Met-Ala-Val-Lys-Lys-Tyr-Leu-Asn-Ser-Ile-Leu-Asn-NH_2
SECRETIN	Asp-Ser-Ala-Arg-Leu-Gln-Arg-Leu-Leu-Gln-Gly-Leu-Val-NH_2
GLUCAGON	Asp-Ser-Arg-Arg-Ala-Gln-Asp-Phe-Val-Gln-Trp-Leu-Met-Asp-Thr
GIP	Asp-Lys-Ile-Arg-Gln-Gln-Asp-Phe-Val-Asn-Trp-Leu-Leu-Ala-Gln-Gln-

FIGURE 2. The Secretin Family — *Partial sequence is presented here. Molecular weight: VIP (3326); Secretin (3055); Glucagon (3483); GIP (5104).

in the midst of ample gastrin. Hypergastrinemia in the Zollinger-Ellison disease is caused by the extragastric population of G cells from pancreas. This hypergastrinemia is responsive to challenge by calcium infusion, but not by food.

In view of the many different molecular forms of gastrin that are known to exist both in the circulation and in tissues, attempted correlation of gastrin activity with disease states is of little value with the conventional radioimmunoassay system. Only until molecularly specific antibodies capable of recognizing each individual form within the same family without any cross reactivity are developed, can the pathologic basis begin to be unraveled. Of promise in this area is the successful development of antiserum with almost absolute specificity for G-17.

CHOLECYSTOKININ (CCK)[27-32]

Cholecystokinin, secreted by the I cells of the upper small intestine, is a peptide of 33 amino acids with the carboxyl-terminal pentapeptide identical to that of the corresponding gastrin molecule. In considering homology, this hormone is to be classified as a member of the gastrin family (Figure 2). A CCK-variant (CCK-V), made up of 39 amino acids (six additional amino acids at the amino-terminus portion), has recently been discovered.

Release of CCK

Table 4 shows a list of substances capable of releasing CCK into the circulation. The amino acids which are effective releasers, arranged in decreasing order of potency, are phenylalanine, tryptophan, valine, leucine, and methionine. Neural involvement, if any, in the release of CCK is uncertain. Little is known of the inhibitors of CCK release from the small intestine; however, neurotensin has been shown to inhibit CCK release in response to oleic acid introduced into the duodenum.

Table 4
STIMULANTS FOR CHOLECYSTOKININ RELEASE

Peptides and amino acids
Fat and fatty acids (>10 C)
Bombesin
Calcium
Magnesium

Table 5
BIOLOGIC ACTIONS OF CHOLECYSTOKININ

Trophic action
  Pancreas
Enzyme secretion
  Pancreas
Water and electrolyte secretion
  Pancreas[a]
Stimulation of smooth muscle
  Stomach
  Small intestine
  Gallbladder
Inhibition of smooth muscle
  Lower esophageal sphincter
  Gastric emptying
  Sphincter of Oddi
Inhibition of water and electrolyte absorption
  Small intestine

[a] Primarily potentiate the effect of secretin.

Metabolic Fate of CCK

The biologic half-life of CCK in the circulation is in the order of three minutes. It is uncertain if the liver plays any role in the degradation of the full molecule. Partial inactivation of small fragments by the liver is known to occur.

Biologic Actions

A fragment of this hormone (octapeptide-CCK) is more biologically potent than the entire molecule. Sulfation on the tyrosyl residue is essential for full activity. The non-sulfated counterpart is 100 times less potent in eliciting CCK actions. Carboxyl-terminal fragments smaller than the heptapeptide, even with sulfation on the tyrosine, fail to exhibit full biologic activity.

CCK has the same qualitative spectrum of actions as gastrin. It is a strong stimulant of gallbladder contraction and pancreatic enzyme secretion, but a weaker gastric acid stimulant. In the stomach it behaves as a partial agonist and may competitively inhibit gastrin-stimulated secretion of acid. On the other hand, gastrin is a partial agonist for gallbladder contraction and pancreatic enzyme secretion. In general, the structure-activity relationship holds true for both CCK and gastrin, the only difference being in the relative degree of potency for each. A list of the biologic actions of CCK is shown in Table 5.

Pathophysiology

Disorders associated with either an excessive or deficient level of CCK are not well documented. An elevated basal level of CCK in celiac disease patients has been reported. A lack of reliable radioimmunoassay technique for CCK is partly responsible for the poor understanding in this area.

Table 6
GUT ENDOCRINE CELLS

Peptide	Location	Cell type
Bombesin[a]	Stomach[b]	P
CCK[a]	Small intestine[c]	I
Enteroglucagon	Intestine[d]	L
Gastrin[a]	Antrum and upper small intestine	G
GIP	Small intestine[c]	K
Motilin	Upper small intestine	EC_2
Neurotensin[a]	Lower small intestine	N
PP	Stomach[b], pancreas, and small intestine[c]	PP
Secretin	Small intestine[c]	S
Somatostatin[a]	Pancreas, stomach[b], and upper small intestine	D
Substance p[a]	Stomach[b] and upper small intestine	EC_1
VIP[a]	Pancreas, stomach[b], and intestine[d]	D_1

[a] Also present in neural tissues.
[b] Stomach — present in both body and antrum.
[c] Small intestine — present in both upper and lower small intestine.
[d] Intestine — present in both small and large intestine.

SECRETIN[33-38]

It was the discovery of secretin that led to the formulation of the basic concepts of endocrinology. A number of gut peptides share, to varying degree, a structural resemblance to that of the secretin molecule, although they are secreted from different cell types of the intestinal mucosa (Table 6). Such peptides exhibit comparable biologic properties and structural similarities to that of secretin and are classified together in the secretin family (see Figure 1).

Release of Secretin

An acid pH of 4 to 4.5 appears to be the upper end point below which secretin is released from the S cells into the circulation. The argument that the duodenum is only slightly acidified after a meal in normal subjects resulted in seriously questioning the originally proposed physiologic role of secretin. Inability to measure secretin below the detectability limits of the assay techniques available is largely responsible for the difficulties in accepting secretin as a hormone. It has recently been demonstrated that when acid enters the duodenum, secretin is synchronously released to achieve neutralization by stimulating pancreatic bicarbonate secretion. Acid is still the most effective releaser of secretin. Secretin is also released by alcohol and glucose, but not by fats or amino acids.

Metabolism

The half-life for secretin is 3 to 6 min. The kidney is the major site of secretin catabolism.

Biologic Actions

The full molecule of secretin is required for biologic activity. Loss of activity occurs when only the histidine residue at the amino terminal is removed. In addition to its own ability to stimulate and inhibit gastric secretory function, secretin is also synergistic to CCK in stimulating pancreatic exocrine secretion. The effects on pancreatic secretion are greater when CCK and secretin are given in combination than the sum of the two when each is given separately. Table 7 lists the actions known to secretin.

Table 7
BIOLOGIC ACTIONS OF SECRETIN

Water and electrolyte secretion
Pancreas
Liver
Small intestine
Inhibition of water and electrolyte secretion
Stomach
Enzyme secretion
Pancreas[a]
Stomach
Inhibition of smooth muscle
Lower esophageal sphincter
Stomach
Small intestine
Release of hormones
Gastrin
Insulin

[a] Primarily potentiate the effect of CCK.

Pathophysiology

No known secretin-secreting tumors have been identified. Patients with Zollinger-Ellison syndrome who have high basal acid secretion typically manifest hypersecretinemia. This supernormal secretin level in the blood reflects the continuous release of secretin from S cells in response to the highly acidic duodenum in these patients.

Despite many difficulties, a reliable radioimmunoassay has been developed to detect even subthreshold levels of plasma secretin as a stimulant for pancreatic secretion.

VASOACTIVE INTESTINAL PEPTIDE (VIP)[39-41]

VIP is a peptide of 28 amino acids (Figure 1) which is found in the entire gut, in varying concentrations from the salivary glands down to the rectum. The highest concentration occurs in the intestine. D_1 cells are the site of origin of this peptide. The peptide is structurally and functionally related to secretin and thus is a member of the secretin family.

Release of VIP

Ingestion of a meal or digested chemical products (except fat) fails to cause the release of VIP into the circulation. The present status of VIP as a hormone is uncertain.

Recent evidence strongly suggests that VIP possesses multiple neuronal functions and is a valid candidate for having a neurotransmitter function in the central and peripheral nervous system. VIP is elevated in the plasma in response to electrical vagal stimulation or administration of acetylcholine.

Metabolism

The circulating half-life is short, about 1 min in man. It is doubtful that the liver contributes to the inactivation of VIP and data about its metabolism are sparse.

Biologic Actions

The full molecule is not essential for biologic activity. Smaller fragments, though weaker, still carry VIP activity.

Despite the inability to demonstrate its release in response to a meal, infusion of VIP mimics the actions of secretin on pancreatic exocrine secretion and produces other biologic actions which are outlined herein (Table 8).

Table 8
BIOLOGIC ACTIONS OF VIP

Inhibition of gastric acid secretion
Stimulation of intestinal water and electrolyte secretion
Stimulation of pancreatic bicarbonate secretion
Stimulation of hepatic bile flow
Stimulation of hepatic glycogenolysis and lipolysis
Relaxation of smooth muscle

Pathophysiology

Some pancreatic endocrine tumors and neuroblastomas are known to contain a large quantity of VIP. Controversy still exists as to whether a VIP-secreting tumor is the underlying cause of all chronic watery diarrhea syndromes (watery diarrhea syndrome is used synonymously with pancreatic cholera, Verner-Morrison syndrome and WDHA syndrome). In the majority of cases reported of the Verner-Morrison syndrome, there is a positive correlation between the VIP level and the clinical features. Supportive evidence includes a decline in circulating VIP following removal of the tumor or chemotherapy. VIP may be a reliable indicator of this disease state, but a sensitive VIP radioimmunoassay coupled with a clearer definition of the syndrome, whether other hormonal peptides besides VIP are involved, would help settle these differences.

Due to the immense complexity of dual role it may play as a hormone in addition to that of a neurotransmitter, much is to be learned about VIP.

GASTRIC INHIBITORY PEPTIDE (GIP, GLUCOSE-DEPENDENT INSULINOTROPIC PEPTIDE)[42-43]

GIP is a distinct peptide that has structural and functional similarities to those of secretin. This peptide of 43 amino acid (Figure 3) has been localized in K cells throughout the entire small intestine, with the highest concentration in the jejunum.

Release of GIP

GIP is released into the circulation after a meal and a rise in its blood level has been demonstrated by intraduodenal perfusion of glucose, fat or amino acids.

Metabolism

Studies on GIP have been limited because of the unavailability of a synthetic compound. The structural requirements, if any, for its biologic activity and site of inactivation are not known.

Biologic Actions

Intravenous infusion of GIP augments an insulin release which has been previously stimulated by glucose. This insulinotropic property parallels that seen with glucose load, although a threshold level of glucose needs to be attained for GIP to become effective. With increasing glucose load, the insulinotropic efficacy of GIP also increases. For this reason, renaming GIP as a glucose-dependent insulinotropic peptide has been proposed. An outline of its biologic actions is found in Table 9.

Pathophysiology

No known GIP-secreting tumor has been identified. Despite its strong insulinotropic action, the role it may play in glucose metabolism is not well understood. Hypersecretion of GIP in maturity-onset diabetes has been observed. A significantly higher level of GIP is released in response to a meal in obese but not in normal subjects. Since the insulin level in both maturity-onset diabetes and obesity is higher than normal, it may be that GIP is partly responsible for the hyperinsulinemia that is observed.

Tyr-Ala-Glu-Gly-Thr-Phe-Ile-Ser-Asp-Tyr-Ser-Ile-Ala-Met-Asp-Lys-Ile-Arg-Gln-Gln-Asp-Phe-Val-Asn-

Trp-Leu-Leu-Ala-Gln-Gln-Lys-Gly-Lys-Lys-Ser-Asp-Trp-Lys-His-Asn-Ile-Thr-Gln (CARBOXYL TERMINAL)

FIGURE 3. Gastric inhibitory peptide.

SOMATOSTATIN (GROWTH HORMONE-RELEASING INHIBITORY HORMONE, GH-RIH, OR SOMATOTROPIN RELEASE-INHIBITING FACTOR, SRIF)[44-50]

The occurrence of somatostatin, a peptide of 14 amino acids, in the D cells of the stomach, pancreas and intestine has led to speculation about its functional role in the digestive system (Figure 4). Somatostatin-containing neurons are also present in the gut.

Recent morphologic evidence strongly supports the possibility that somatostatin may also have paracrine function in the gut. The basic concept of the paracrine system is that biologically active substances secreted from one cell can exert their influence on adjacent target cells by a local cytoplasmic diffusion pathway. This is different from the endocrine system in which the active substance is carried by the circulation to the target tissue. Long cytoplasmic process endings from somatostatin-containing cells are known to terminate on neighboring cell types including the parietal cells, gastrin-secreting cells, and chief cells. It is likely that this is one way in which gastric functions are regulated by somatostatin.

The view of a cell to cell communication by way of local chemical messengers released from cytoplasmic endings is now used to support the findings of a reciprocal relationship between the release of gastrin and somatostatin from the antrum. Similarly, in the pancreas, a close proximity of somatostatin cells to both α and β cells has been described. This could permit a paracrine modulation of glucagon and insulin release by somatostatin with great precision.

Release of Somatostatin

Considerable effort has been focused on factors involved in the release of somatostatin. Table 10 shows a list of releasers and inhibitors for its release.

Metabolism

The circulating half-life for somatostatin is about 4 min. It can undergo minor amino acid residue replacement without significant loss of biologic activity in the stomach and pancreas. Little is known of its degradation by organs in the body.

Biologic Actions

Despite a reported wide range of biologic effects, we have no hard evidence of specific physiologic roles for somatostatin. The kinetics of inhibitory effects of somatostatin on gastric and pancreatic secretions appear to be of a competitive type. There is a lack of structural analogy with some of the known stimulants of those organs. The ability to precisely measure local peptide level will facilitate our understanding of somatostatin.

A catalog of somatostatin-induced effects is available in Table 11.

Pathophysiology

Hypersomatostatinemia as the result of somatostatinoma of the pancreas has been described. The elevated somatostatin level is associated with a decrease in secretion of both insulin and glucagon.

Table 9
BIOLOGIC ACTIONS OF GIP

Inhibition of gastric acid and pepsin secretion
Inhibition of gastric motility
Stimulation of intestinal water and electrolyte secretion[a]
Stimulation of insulin release[b]

[a] Inhibition can also occur, depending on concentrations used.
[b] Insulin release is glucose-dependent.

Patients with duodenal ulcer have been found to have hyposomatostatinemia. This is presumably responsible for a diminished inhibition in the release of gastrin. The latter observation further substantiates the modulatory role that somatostatin may have as a paracrine peptide on the endocrine activity of other gut peptides.

MOTILIN (INTERDIGESTIVE HORMONE)[51-52]

Motilin, a peptide containing 22 amino acid residues (Figure 5), is present within specific enterochromaffin cells (EC_2) in the gut, with the highest concentration in the upper small intestine.

Release of Motilin

Alkalinization of the upper small intestine can trigger the release of motilin. It has been proposed that it be renamed the "interdigestive hormone" because of a decrease in its release during the feeding period. A positive correlation between its circulating level and the occurrence of an interdigestive motor complex has been observed. The interdigestive motor complex is a type of vigorous, sweeping motor activity of the gut initiated from the stomach in a caudad direction towards the ileum during nonfeeding period. The period of strong activity is interrupted with long periods of quiescence.

The metabolism and fate of motilin are obscure.

Biologic Actions

The circulating half-life for motilin is 5 min or less. The ability of motilin to stimulate gastric acid and pancreatic exocrine secretions is relatively weak in comparison with the actions of gastrin and secretin on their major target organ. For this reason, the functions of motilin are unclear.

An outline of the probable biologic actions of motilin is presented in Table 12.

Pathophysiology

No known excessive secretion or deficiency of motilin has been described or correlated with any disease state.

PANCREATIC POLYPEPTIDE (PP)[53-54]

As the name implies, pancreatic polypeptide is a 36 amino acid polypeptide from the pancreas, localized primarily within specific PP cells of the exocrine portion of the gland. Low concentrations are found in the islet tissues and also in the stomach and small intestine (Figure 6).

Release of PP

Claims of gastrin, CCK, and secretin as PP releasers have been made. These contentions are presently uncertain. A possible neural stimulation of PP release is also poorly

Ala-Gly-Cys-Lys-Asn-Phe-Phe-Trp-Lys-Thr-Phe-Thr-Ser-Cys

FIGURE 4. Somatostatin — molecular weight: 1638.

Phe-Val-Pro-Ile-Phe-Thr-Tyr-Gly-Glu-Leu-Gln-Arg-Met-Gln-Glu-Lys-Glu-Arg-Asn-Lys-Gly-Gln

FIGURE 5. Motilin — molecular weight: 2699.

understood. Both cephalic phase stimuli and a stretch-initiated reflex from gastric distention have been said to elevate PP in the circulation. Truncal vagotomy eliminates a response of PP to food, but the inhibition is slowly reversible with time. Eventually vagotomized patients may regain their ability to release PP after ingestion of a meal. Proteins, amino acids, VIP, bombesin, and GIP have been demonstrated to release PP.

Biologic Actions

A wide range of activities has been reported. They are listed in Table 13. The metabolism and fate are poorly understood.

Pathophysiology

No known clinical conditions related to any excessive or deficient secretion of PP have been proved. In severe chronic pancreatitis, the PP level remains unchanged in response to food. Because of its wide distribution in both endocrine and exocrine segments of the pancreas, attempts have been made to relate the circulating PP level to the overall pancreatic function. A rise in PP concentration has been said to occur in patients with a variety of pancreatic endocrine tumors, but the data are inconclusive. The use of PP variations as a diagnostic measure of pancreatic function may conceivably yield promising results in years ahead.

BOMBESIN[55-56]

Bombesin is a tetradecapeptide originally isolated from the skin of the amphibian *Bombina bombina.* It has subsequently been identified immunohistochemically in the P endocrine cells of the mammalian gastric antrum and upper intestinal mucosa (Figure 7).

Release of Bombesin

The intraduodenal instillation of crude liver extract can cause a rise in circulating gastrin. This is taken as indirect evidence for bombesin release because this effect is abolished by antrectomy. No known direct acting stimulant for bombesin has been reported.

Biologic Actions

Little is known about the release of pancreatic hormones by bombesin; reports are inconclusive. The most interesting effect of bombesin is its ability to stimulate release of gastrin in a magnitude greater than that induced by proteins being digested. It is not certain, however, whether other effects of bombesin are directly related to bombesin itself or to whether they are secondary to the gastrin released into the circulation. In isolated smooth muscle preparations, bombesin has a direct contractile effect. The biologic actions claimed in the literature are outlined in Table 14.

Table 10
FACTORS AFFECTING RELEASE OF SOMATOSTATIN

Increase	Decrease
Gastrin	Glucose
Secretin	Insulin
VIP	Glucagon
Hyperosmolarity	
Bombesin[a]	
Neurotensin[a]	

[a] Conflicting results

Table 11
BIOLOGIC ACTIONS OF SOMATOSTATIN

Inhibition of gastric acid and pepsin secretion
Inhibition of gastric emptying
Inhibition of pancreatic exocrine secretion
Inhibition of release of gastrin, cholecystokinin, motilin, insulin, glucagon, secretin, and VIP
Inhibition of gallbladder contraction
Inhibition of intestinal secretion
Inhibition of hepatic bile secretion
Stimulation of interdigestive myoelectric complex

Pathophysiology

Clinical conditions resulting from any abnormal bombesin secretion have not been reported. In view of the weak evidence that proposes its release into the circulation and the recent finding of immunoreactive bombesin neurons in the gut plexus, the role it may play as an endocrine peptide needs to be re-examined.

NEUROTENSIN[57-58]

Neurotensin is a tridecapeptide (Figure 8) present in the hypothalamus and the small bowel. Immunohistochemical studies have shown that the gut contains N cells reacting with antibodies to neurotensin. In the rat about 85% of the body's neurotensin is located in the distal part of the small intestine.

Release of Neurotensin

Circulating neurotensin becomes elevated in response to ingestion of food, but direct evidence is lacking concerning the true identity of this peptide.

Biologic Actions

No plausible physiologic function has been ascribed to the gut neurotensin, but its cellular location suggests a hormonal role. The target tissue for neurotensin in a hormonal role has not been identified.

A catalog of biologic actions of neurotensin include inhibition of antral motor activity, inhibition of gastric acid secretion, increase in gut blood flow, and at higher doses, an increase in blood glucose concentration by a release of glucagon. Depending on the concentrations used, its effect on gut smooth muscle may be one of stimulation or inhibition.

All neurotensin-like immunoreactivity has been found thus far exclusively in the gut endocrine cells. There is no evidence for its existence in the enteric plexus neurons.

Table 12
BIOLOGIC ACTIONS OF MOTILIN

Stimulation of gastric acid and pepsin secretion
Inhibition of gastric emptying
Stimulation of pancreatic exocrine secretion
Stimulation of smooth muscle
Stimulation of interdigestive myoelectric complex

Table 13
BIOLOGIC ACTIONS OF PANCREATIC POLYPEPTIDE

Stimulation of basal but inhibition of gastrin-induced gastric acid secretion
Inhibition of basal pancreatic exocrine secretion and CCK-induced enzyme secretion
Stimulation of secretin-induced pancreatic water and electrolyte secretion
Stimulation of gastric motility and emptying
Stimulation of intestinal motility
Inhibition of gallbladder contraction and stimulation of choledocalduodenal contraction

Table 14
BIOLOGIC ACTIONS OF BOMBESIN

Stimulation of gastric acid secretion
Stimulation of pancreatic exocrine secretion
Stimulation of release of gastrin, cholecystokinin, insulin, and glucagon
Stimulation of smooth muscle

Pathophysiology

Hyperneurotensinemia is noted in patients with celiac disease. The significance of this observation is obscure. No other clinical condition related to abnormal secretion of neurotensin is known.

SUBSTANCE P (SP)[59-60]

Substance P is an undecapeptide (Figure 9) found in particularly high concentrations in the brain and spinal afferent neurons. In the gut, SP content is low in the esophagus and stomach, high in the duodenum and jejunum, and there are moderate amounts in the ileum and large intestine. It is estimated that 45 to 70% of immunoreactive SP in plasma is derived from the intestinal tract. The SP endocrine cells are a population of enterochromaffin cells (EC_1), which presumably also store serotonin (5-HT).

Release of SP

Electrical stimulation of the vagus releases SP into an antral perfusate. Acetylcholine and epinephrine, administered intravenously, stimulate SP release. Its possible endocrine function is uncertain. The source of its release may be neuronal.

Biologic Actions

SP displays multiple extra-gastrointestinal activities. It has recently been implicated as a neurotransmitter, and within the digestive system stimulates salivation and induces retching, vomiting, and defecation. Its ability to stimulate pancreatic exocrine enzyme secretion has been documented. It is also a potent smooth muscle stimulant. Little is known of its biologic half-life in the circulation despite the fact that SP is inactivated by both liver and kidney.

Ala-Pro-Leu-Glu-Pro-Gln-Tyr-Pro-Gly-Asp-Asp-Ala-Thr-Pro-Glu-Gln-Met-Ala-Gln-Tyr-Ala-Ala-Glu-Leu-

Arg-Arg-Tyr-Ile-Asn-Met-Leu-Thr-Arg-Pro-Arg-Tyr-NH_2

FIGURE 6. Pancreatic polypeptide — Bovine pancreatic peptide — molecular weight: 4200.

Glp-Gln-Arg-Leu-Gly-Asn-Gln-Trp-Ala-Val-Gly-His-Leu-Met-NH_2

FIGURE 7. Bombesin — molecular weight: 1620.

Glp-Leu-Tyr-Glu-Asn-Lys-Pro-Arg-Arg-Pro-Tyr-Ile-Leu

FIGURE 8. Neurotensin — molecular weight: 1673.

Arg-Pro-Lys-Pro-Gln-Gln-Phe-Phe-Gly-Leu-Met-NH_2

FIGURE 9. Substance — molecular weight: 1347.

Pathophysiology

Both neural and endocrine disorders have been associated with SP. The SP content in the aganglionic portion of the rectosigmoid in Hirschsprung's disease is lower than in the adjacent neurohistologically normal segments. In carcinoid tumors, both 5-HT and SP are secreted. This is not surprising in view of the dual existence of these two substances within the same cell type. Enteroglucagon immunoreactivity has also been demonstrated within these carcinoid tissues, suggesting that the defect may be of multipeptide origin.

ENTEROGLUCAGON (GLYCETIN, GUT-GLUCAGON-LIKE-IMMUNOREACTIVITY, GUT-GLI)[61-62]

Enteroglucagon is a peptide found within the L endocrine cells throughout the intestine. High concentrations are found in the ileum and colon. The exact chemical structure is not known, but it has been estimated to be a peptide that consists of 22 to 27 amino acids.

It appears that glucagon exists in at least two forms in the gut. One has a molecular weight of 3,500 and resembles that of pancreatic glucagon. This component is given the name of gut-glucagon. The other form is at least twice as large and is called gut-glucagon-like-immunoreactivity or Gut-GLI. The larger of the two forms is more abundant in the gut and is considered to be the precursor form (progut-glucagon).

Release of Gut-GLI

Enteroglucagon is released into the blood upon food ingestion. The following stimulants, when administered intraduodenally or intravenously, can cause release of gut-GLI: fats, glucose, fructose, xylose, mannose, galactose, calcium, magnesium, and hypertonic sodium solutions.

Biologic Actions

A lack of synthetic enteroglucagon has made the assignment of biologic actions difficult. Its well known pancreatic counterpart displays a wide range of effects in the gut. Some of these effects resemble those of secretin, which is expected because of their structural similarities. A glycogenolytic property has been ascribed to enteroglucagon.

Pathophysiology

In patients with the dumping syndrome, the enteroglucagon level is raised in the blood. This is suggestive of a massive release of enteroglucagon when the small bowel is rapidly exposed to a large glucose load. A decrease in intestinal transit has been noted to occur during the period of hyperenteroglucagonemia. Glucagonoma is a known disease entity; however, it remains to be demonstrated whether there is secretion of enteroglucagon from such a tumor.

A full understanding of the role of enteroglucagon in the digestive system awaits the availability of synthetic enteroglucagon.

CONCLUDING REMARKS

Significant contributions to our understanding of modern gut endocrinology have come from many areas. Sophisticated biochemical techniques have made simple purification, isolation, and ultimate synthesis a reality. Sensitive radioimmunoassay methods have provided valuable information on circulating levels of gut hormones in health and disease. Immunohistochemical localization of peptide-secreting cells and peptide-containing neurons have now given special meanings to these biologically active substances. The digestive system, which can be appropriately called the cradle of endocrinology, has reached a degree of complexity far beyond any possible imaginings of the original discoverers.

The gut now boasts within its system no less than 16 different, histologically identifiable cells, capable of secreting up to as many as 27 possible hormone-like substances. Many of the biologic actions derived from studies of these peptides are not firmly established, but there is great impetus in moving ahead despite the many difficulties. Little is known of multihormonal interaction — a situation which closely resembles that of a normal response to a meal. Interactions, not just between peptides, but also between peptides and their respective target cells, are still poorly understood. However, some progress is being seen with radioligand-receptor binding studies. The classical model of hormonal interaction with the autonomic nervous system also needs to be re-examined in light of the strong evidence supporting the existence of peptidergic neural pathways throughout the gut. The paracrine control by way of a short diffusion pathway across intercellular space for some of the cells secreting these peptides has added a new dimension in understanding the control system for digestive activity.

ACKNOWLEDGMENT

The author wishes to thank Pat Lingle for her help in the preparation of this manuscript.

REFERENCES

1. **Rehfeld, J. F.,** Gastrointestinal Hormones, in *Gastrointestinal Physiology III,* Vol. 19, Crane, R. K., Ed., University Park, Baltimore, 291, 1979.
2. **Grossman, M. I.,** Neural and hormonal regulation of gastrointestinal function: an overview, *Ann. Rev. Physiol.,* 41, 27, 1979.
3. **Dockray, G. J.,** Comparative biochemistry and physiology of gut hormones, *Ann. Rev. Physiol.,* 41, 83, 1979.
4. **Walsh, J. H.,** Gastrointestinal hormones in clinical disease: recent developments, *Ann. Intern. Med.,* 90, 817, 1979.

5. **Walsh, J. H.**, Gastrointestinal peptide hormones and other biologically active peptides, in *Gastrointestinal Disease, Pathophysiology, Diagnosis and Management,* Vol. 1, 2nd ed., Sleisenger, M. H. and Fordtran, J. S., Eds., W. B. Saunders, Philadelphia, 1978, 107.
6. **McGuigan, J. E.**, Gastrointestinal hormones, *Ann. Rev. Med.*, 29, 307, 1978.
7. **Dockray, G. J. and Gregory, R. A.**, Relations between neuropeptides and gut hormones, *Proc. R. Soc. (London),* B210, 151, 1980.
8. **Bloom, S. R.**, Gastrointestinal Hormones, in *Gastrointestinal Physiology II,* Vol. 12, Crane, R. K., Ed., University Park, Baltimore, 72, 1977.
9. **Grossman, M. I., Speranza, V., Basso, N., and Lezoche, E.**, Gastrointestinal hormones and pathology of the digestive system, in *Advances in Experimental Medicine and Biology,* Vol. 106, Plenum Press, New York, 1978.
10. **Barrington, E. J. W. and Dockray, G. J.**, Gastrointestinal hormones, *J. Endocrinol.*, 69, 299, 1976.
11. **Rayford, P. L., Miller, T. A., and Thompson, J. C.**, Secretin, cholecystokinin and newer gastrointestinal hormones, *N. Engl. J. Med.*, 294, 1093, 1976.
12. **Rehfeld, J. F.**, Radioimmunoassay in diagnosis, localization and treatment of endocrine tumors in gut and pancreas, *Scand. J. Gastroent. 14,* Suppl., 53, 33, 1979.
13. **Thompson, J. C., Ed.**, Gastrointestinal hormones, A Symposium, University of Texas, Austin, 1975.
14. **Chey, W. Y. and Brooks, F. P.**, *Endocrinology of the Gut,* Charles B. Slack, Thorofare, New Jersey, 1974.
15. **Jorpes, J. E. and Mutt, V.**, *Handbook of Experimental Pharmacology,* Vol. 34, Springer-Verlag, Basel, 1973.
16. **Makhlouf, G. M.**, The neuroendocrine design of the gut, *Gastroenterology,* 67, 159, 1974.
17. **Grossman, M. I. et al.**, Candidate hormones of the gut, *Gastroenterology,* 67, 730, 1974.
18. **Gardner, J. D.**, Receptors for gastrointestinal hormones, *Gastroenterology,* 76, 202, 1979.
19. **Johnson, L. R.**, Trophic actions of gastrointestinal hormones, *Gastroenterology,* 70, 278, 1976.
20. **Larsson, L.-I. and Schwartz, T. W.**, Radioimmunocytochemistry — a novel immunocytochemical principle, *J. Histochem. Cytochem.*, 25, 1140, 1977.
21. **Walsh, J. H. and Grossman, M. I.**, Gastrin, *N. Engl. J., Med.*, 292, 1324, 1975.
22. **Walsh, J. H.**, Circulating gastrin, *Ann. Rev. Physiol.*, 37, 81, 1975.
23. **Rehfeld, J. F. and Uvnas-Wallensten, K.**, Gastrins in cat and dog: evidence for a biosynthetic relationship between the large molecular forms of gastrin, *J. Physiol.*, 283, 181, 1978.
24. **Rehfeld, J. F. and Larsson, L.-I.**, The predominating molecular form of gastrin and cholecystokinin in the gut is a small peptide resembling the COOH-terminal tetrapeptide amide, *Acta Physiol. Scand.*, 104, 37, 1979.
25. **Devaney, C. W., Devaney, K. S., Jaffe, B. M., Jones, R. S. and Way, L. W.**, The use of calcium and secretin in the diagnosis of gastrinoma, *Ann. Inter. Med.*, 87, 680, 1977.
26. **Rehfeld, J. F., Schwartz, T. W., and Stadil, F.**, Immunochemical studies on macromolecular gastrins: evidence that "big big gastrin" in blood and mucosa is artifactual — but truly present in some large gastrinomas, *Gastroenterology,* 72, 469, 1977.
27. **Polak, J. M., Pearse, A. G. E., Bloom, S. R., Buchan, A. M. J., Rayford, P. L., and Thompson, J. C.**, Identification of cholecystokinin-secreting cells, *Lancet,* 2, 1016, 1975.
28. **Schlegel, W., Raptis, W., Harvey, R. F., Oliver, J. M., and Pfeiffer, E. F.**, Inhibition of cholecystokinin-pancreozymin release by somatostatin, *Lancet,* 2, 166, 1977.
29. **Demol, P., Laugier, R., Dagorn, J. C., and Sarles, H.**, Inhibition of rat pancreatic secretion by neurotensin: mechanism of action, *Arch. Int. Pharmacodyn. Ther.*, 242, 139, 1979.
30. **Lin, T.M.**, Actions of gastrointestinal hormones and related peptides on the motor function of the biliary tract, *Gastroenterology,* 69, 1006, 1975.
31. **Thompson, J. C., Fender, H. R., Ramus, N. I., Villar, H. V., and Rayford, P. L.**, Cholecystokinin metabolism in man and dogs, *Ann. Surg.*, 182, 496, 1975.
32. **Meyer, J. H., Kelly, G. A., Spingola, L. J., and Jones, R. S.**, Canine gut receptors mediating pancreatic responses to luminal L-amino acids, *Am. J. Physiol.*, 231, 669, 1976.
33. **Grossman, M. I. and Konturek, S. J.**, Gastric acid does drive pancreatic bicarbonate secretion, *Scand. J. Gastroent.*, 9, 299, 1974.
34. **Cutis, P. J., Fender, H. R., Rayford, P. L., and Thompson, J. C.**, Catabolism of secretin by the liver and kidney, *Surgery,* 80, 259, 1976.
35. **Fahrenkrug, J., Schaffalitzky de Muckadell, O. B., and Rehfeld, J. F.**, Production and evaluation of antibodies for radioimmunoassay of secretin, *Scand. J. Clin. Lab. Invest.*, 36, 281, 1976.
36. **Straus, E. and Yalow, R. S.**, Hypersecretinemia associated with marked basal hyperchlorhydria in man and dog, *Gastroenterology,* 72, 992, 1977.
37. **Schafflitzky de Muckadell, O. B. and Fahrenkrug, J.**, Secretion pattern of secretin in man: regulation by gastric acid, *Gut,* 19, 812, 1988.
38. **Pelletier, M. J., Chayvialle, J. A. P., and Minaire, Y.**, Uneven and transient secretin release after a liquid test meal, *Gastroenterology,* 75, 1124, 1978.

39. **Fahrenkrug, J.**, Vasoactive intestinal polypeptide: measurement, distribution and putative neurotransmitter function, *Digestion*, 19, 149, 1979.
40. **Fahrenkrug, J. and Schafflitzky de Muckadell, O. B.**, Verner-Morrison syndrome and vasoactive intestinal polypeptide, *Scand. J. Gastroent.*, 14, Suppl., 53, 1979.
41. **Alumets, J., Schaffalitzky de Muckadell, O., Fahrenkrug, J., Sundler, F., Hakanson, R., and Uddman, R.**, A rich VIP nerve supply is characteristic of sphincters, *Nature*, 280, 155, 1979.
42. **Buffa, R., Polak, J. M., Pearse, A. G. E., Solcia, E., Grimelius, L., and Capella, C.**, Identification of the intestinal cell storing gastric inhibitory peptide, *Histochemistry*, 43, 249, 1975.
43. **Helman, C. A. and Barbezat, G. O.**, The effect of gastric inhibitory polypeptide on human jejunal water and electrolyte transport, *Gastroenterology*, 73, 376, 1977.
44. **Efendic, S., Enzumann, F., Nylen, A., Uvnas-Wallensten, K., and Luft, R.**, Effect of glucose-sulfonylurea interaction on release of insulin, glucagon, and somatostatin from isolated perfused rat pancreas, *Proc. Natl. Acad. Sci., U.S.A.*, 76, 5901, 1979.
45. **Alumets, J., Ekelund, M., El Munshid, H. A., Hakanson, R., Loren, I., and Sundler, F.**, Topography of somatostatin cells in the stomach of the rat: possible functional significance, *Cell Tissue Res.*, 202, 177, 1979.
46. **Hermansen, K. and Schwartz, T. W.**, Differential sensitivity to somatostatin of pancreatic polypeptide, glucagon, and insulin secretion from the isolated perfused canine pancreas, *Metabolism*, 28, 1229, 1979.
47. **Chiba, T., Taminato, T., Kadowaki, S., Inoue, Y., Mori, K., Seino, Y., Abe, H., Chihara, K., Matsukara, S., Fujita, T., and Goto, Y.**, Effects of various gastrointestinal peptides on gastric somatostatin release, *Endocrinology*, 106, 145, 1980.
48. **Furness, J. B. and Costa, M.**, Actions of somatostatin on excitatory and inhibitory nerves in the intestine, *Eur. J. Pharmacol.*, 56, 69, 1979.
49. **Meyer, W. C., Hanks, J. B., and Jones, R. S.**, Inhibition of basal and meal-stimulated choleresis by somatostatin, *Surgery*, 86, 301, 1979.
50. **Krejs, G. J., Orci, L., Conlon, J. M., Ravazzola, M., Davis, G. R., Raskin, P., Collins, S. M., McCarthy, D. M., Baetens, D., Rubenstein, A., Aldor, T. A., and Unger, R. H.**, Somatostatinoma syndrome: biochemical, morphologic and clinical features, *N. Engl. J. Med.*, 301, 385, 1979.
51. **Demling, L. and Domschke, W., Eds.**, Motilin, origin, chemistry, and actions, *Scand. J. Gastroent.*, *11*, Suppl., 39, 1976.
52. **Itoh, E., Takeuchi, S., Aizawa, I., Mori, K., Taminato, T., Seino, Y., Imura, H., and Yanaihara, N.**, Changes in plasma motilin concentration and gastrointestinal contractile activity in conscious dogs, *Am. J. Dig. Dis.*, 23, 929, 1978.
53. **Adrian, T. E., Bloom, S. R., Barnes, A. J., Besterman, H. S., Russell, C. R., Cooke, T. J., and Faber, G. R.**, Mechanism of pancreatic polypeptide release in man, *Lancet*, 1, 161, 1977.
54. **Modlin, I. M., Lamers, C. B. H., and Walsh, J. H.**, Stimulation of canine pancreatic polypeptide, gastrin, and gastric acid secretion by ranatensin, litorin, bombesin nonapeptide and substance P, *Reg. Pep.*, 1, 279, 1980.
55. **Polak, J. M., Bloo, S. R., Hobbs, S., Solcia, E., and Pearse, A. E. G.**, Distribution of a bombesin-like peptide in human gastrointestinal tract, *Lancet*, 1, 1109, 1976.
56. **Modlin, I. M., Lamers, C., and Walsh, J. H.**, Mechanisms of gastrin release by bombesin and food, *J. Surg. Res.*, 28, 539, 1980.
57. **Rosell, S. and Rokaeus, A.**, The effect of ingestion of amino acids, glucose and fat on circulating neurotensin-like immunoreactivity (NTLI) in man, *Acta Physiol. Scand.* , 107, 263, 1979.
58. **Hammer, R. A., Leeman, S. E., Carraway, R., and Williams, R. H.**, Isolation of human intestinal neurotensin, *J. Biol. Chem.*, 255, 2476, 1980.
59. **Franco, R., Costa, M., and Furness, J. B.** Evidence for the release of endogenous substance P from intestinal nerves, Naunyn Schmiedebergs, *Arch. Pharmacol.*, 306, 195, 1979.
60. **Hokfelt, T., Lundberg, J. M., Schultzberg, M., Johansson, O., Skirboll, L., Angard, A., Fredholm, B., Hamberger, B., Pernow, B., Rehfeld, J., and Goldstein, M.**, Cellular localization of peptides in neural structures, *Proc. R. Soc. London*, B210, 63, 1980.
61. **Ralphs, D. N. L., Bloom, S. R., Lawson-Smith, C., and Thompson, J. P. S.**, The relationship between gastric emptying rate and plasma enteroglucagon concentration, *Gut*, 16, 406, 1975.
62. **Modlin, I. M.**, Endocrine tumors of the pancreas, *Surg. Gynecol. Obstet.*, 149, 751, 1979.

PANCREAS

Jimmie L. Valentine

INTRODUCTION

The mammalian pancreas forms as an outgrowth of a duodenal and hepatic diverticula and begins its function as an endocrine organ early in utero.[1-5] In very early development the human pancreas can be differentiated as two buds, the ventral and dorsal pancreas. In later development the ventral and dorsal process fuses, and generally the duct systems fuse to form a common duct opening into the common bile duct. This development emphasizes the fact that the pancreas has an intimate relationship with the digestive tract and the pancreas also is involved with digestive processes in addition to its endocrine function.

The human adult pancreas functions as both an exocrine (external secreting) and endocrine (internal secreting) gland. The endocrine function will be emphasized herein, although exocrine secretions from this gland are affected in part by the endocrine secretions. Its exocrine secretions aid in digestion of nutrients within the gut and its endocrine secretions are concerned primarily with glucose homeostasis in the blood. Glucose is used by the central nervous system as its principal energy source and a constant supply must be available at all times. In man, glucose in blood must be maintained at about 100 mg/dℓ to prevent hypoglycemia or hyperglycemia, respectively, in spite of the variable dietary intake of glucose. To maintain this homeostasis, intestinal absorption of glucose, cellular uptake, and release from storage sites must be regulated by endocrine secretions of the pancreas as well as by hormones from other glands.

ANATOMIC FEATURES

Location and General Appearance

The pancreas is an acinous (grape bunches-like) appearing gland located in the retroperitoneum below the liver and stomach (Figure 1). The gland is subdivided arbitrarily into various anatomical portions: head, neck, body, and tail. The head of the gland, which is thicker, adheres to the duodenum. The gland then projects slightly upward and curves (neck) transversely across the peritoneum (body) gradually tapering to a narrower portion (tail) in close proximity to the spleen.

Beginning in the tail, a large duct (of Wirsung) runs throughout the length of the gland, receiving many tributary branches along its course. The duct enlarges as it passes through the gland. It travels toward the intestine from the pancreas head and becomes a branch of the common bile duct from the liver, terminating in the duodenum (ampulla of Vater). Secretions from the ducts are controlled by the sphincter of Oddi.

Due to embryonic developmental differences, a branch of the duct of Wirsung may have its own opening to the duodenum. This branch, termed the duct of Santorini, is independent of the duct of Wirsung.[6-8]

Histologic Considerations

Through the lobular appearing pancreas there pass blood vessels, nerves, lymph, and excretory ducts. Two broad categories of tissue can be distinguished (1) pancreatic acini; composed of cells which surround a collecting duct for exocrine secretion; and (2) islands (islets) of Langerhans which are groups of cells not in close proximity to collecting ducts, but which can secrete into extensive blood vessels (endocrine secretions) lying in contiguous areas. The islets are more numerous in the pancreas tail than in the body or head.

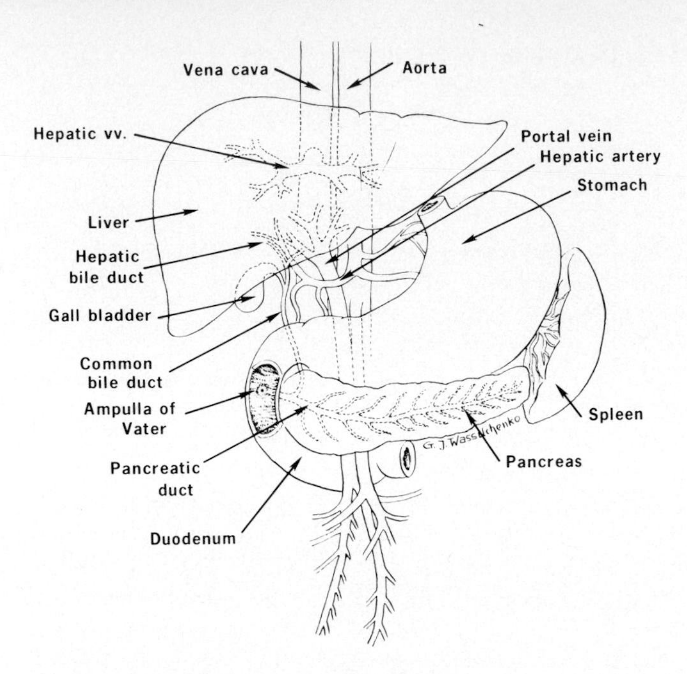

FIGURE 1. Relationship of the pancreas to adjacent organs. The pancreas lies behind the stomach but in this depiction is pulled forward to reveal its shape and the pancreatic ducts junction with the common bile duct.

Three distinct types of cells can be identified in the islets, A (or α), B (or β) and D (or δ). Other types of cells are present, such as PP (pancreatic polypeptide) cells,[9,10] endothelial cells, nerve cells, and fibroblasts. The function of the PP cells is at present uncertain, although the function of the other hormones contained within the endocrine islets has been elucidated.

Microanatomy of the Islets

Variations in the arrangement and amount of cell types exist in different species.[11] Most histologic characterization of the islets has been performed in the rat or man. Therefore, the subsequent discussion will focus upon information derived primarily from these two species.

B cells are located predominantly in a central position within the islets and comprise 65 to 85% of their volume.[12-14] The concentration of B cells can change with obesity, as demonstrated in normal mice (80% of the volume),[15] and in obese mice,[16] where the percentage of these cells appear to increase. Those B cells which are located toward the periphery of each islet are juxtaposed to A, D, and possibly PP cells, but the majority are in close contact with other B cells. In human islets, invagination of vascular connective tissue into the islet periphery produces septa along which the B cells are located. Thus, some B cells are located closer to a vascular supply than others. In man the invagination of vascular connective tissue tends to subdivide the islet into lobules.

A and D cells, and occasionally a PP cell, are found around the periphery of the islet, surrounding the clustered B cells. In general, the D and PP cells are found in a more intermediate position, between the B cells and the more peripherally situated A cells. These relationships of cell types have been demonstrated by various techniques and are amply illustrated by many workers.[17-22]

Localization of Hormone Function

The various cell types found within the islets, with the exception of PP cells, have been well characterized as to their hormone content. Various techniques have been used to verify the exact hormones present, but the immunocytochemical techniques have proved to be most useful. Both light microscopic and ultrastructural studies have amply demonstrated that glucagon is the primary hormone within the A cells,[23-27] insulin in the B cells,[25,26,28-29] and somatostatin in the D cells.[30-39]

Intracellular Communication Between Cell Types Within the Islets

Histologic examination of the junction between various cell types within the islets, particularly A and B cells, has demonstrated three types of intercellular junctions: desmosome, tight, and gap. In addition, various microtubules have been found within the cells. The desmosomes were the first junction recognized within the islets[40] and were later shown to be involved in cellular adhesion.[41-42]

Orci and co-workers have extensively investigated the juncture between A and B cells. Using islets which had been treated with uranyl acetate or lanthanum hydroxide, they clearly demonstrated that junctures were found between A and B cells.[43] These junctures are generally uniform in width, although at various points they do narrow. The narrowed points are referred to as gap junctions. The interruption of the juncture line by a traversing of leaflets of adjacent plasma membranes is termed a tight junction.[43] Freeze-fracture techniques have shown the gap junction to contain many aggregates of particles or globular subunits, whereas the tight junction consists of a network of linear ridges or fibrils.[43-47] Such junctures are probably involved in the transport of ions or of small molecules between the cells.

Microtubules have been demonstrated in the B cells,[48-51] as well as in other body tissues. The microtubules are scattered throughout the cytoplasm of B cells. They have a hollow-halo appearance and often are located near secretory granules. A role for the participation of the microtubules in insulin release has been proposed.[52]

Innervation

Evidence for neural control of pancreatic function has been obtained by finding chemical mediators of the autonomic nervous system in pancreatic homogenates as well as by using histochemical methods. Both the vagus nerves and the celiac ganglion complex are the main nerves which innervate the pancreas. Most likely, the nerves are concerned primarily with exocrine secretions.

Nerves appear close to arteries in all parts of the gland. With classical staining techniques the presence of nerve branches can be identified in both acinar cells and islets.[53] Nerve branches appear to extend from the acinar cells to the islets, thus demonstrating an autonomic relationship.[54] In juxtaposition to the islets there are autonomic nerve cells termed " complexe neuroinsulaives".[55]

Various authors have studied the distribution of adrenergic and cholinergic nerves in different cell types within the islets.[40,56] The interior cells of the islets, i.e., the B cells, appear to have very little innervation whereas the peripheral cells (A, D, and PP) are either innervated or are in close proximity to nerve endings.

Some workers speculate on a mode of pancreatic innervation in which the control is mediated by a released transmitter substance, termed a paracrine secretion. An example would be adrenergic stimulation of a D cell, causing it to release somatostatin[57] which would then inhibit release of insulin and glucagon from A and B secretory cells.[54] For a more detailed discussion of islet innervation, the reader is referred to two reviews.[54,58]

BIOSYNTHESIS OF THE HORMONES WITHIN VARIOUS CELL TYPES OF THE ISLETS

The secretory hormones which are ultimately released from islet cells are biosynthesized within each cell, then stored until a signal occurs for release. For the three major hormones, insulin, glucagon, and somatostatin, several stages of processing are required prior to the final formation of the hormone. In each case the ultimate end-product represents a degradation of a larger peptide.

Insulin Biosynthesis

Insulin, which is secreted from the B cells, is formed by successive degradation of larger peptides, some of which have been well characterized. The immediate precursor of insulin is termed proinsulin. Human proinsulin has an 86 amino acid sequence and is linked by disulfide bridges between amino acid residues 72, 19, and 85.[59] Residues 1-32 are referred to as the B-chain, 64-86 as the A-chain and 33-64 as the C-peptide. The A-chain has, in addition, an intra-disulfide bridge between residues 71—76.

Proinsulin is formed on ribosomes in the rough endoplasmic reticulum of the B cell.[60,61] Once formed it is transported in an energy requiring step to the Golgi apparatus[62] and then incorporated in a B cell granula.[63] The granula is maturated from the Golgi apparatus after a short period of time. Upon incorporation in the granula, proteolysis of proinsulin begins, to form insulin and C-peptide.[64]

Enzymes which cleave proinsulin have not been totally elucidated but the process can be explained by extrusion of four amino acids (3 agrinine and 1 lysine), using a trypsin-like and a carboxypeptidase B-like enzyme (see References 65 and 67 for diagrams of this process). C-peptide is retained in the granula following the proteolytic conversion in equimolar amounts.[66]

Species variations in proinsulin, insulin, and C-peptides have been reviewed.[62]

Evidence indicates that another precursor of proinsulin exists within the B cell. This is a peptide which has been designated preproinsulin. It appears to have a 24 amino acid residue extension on the NH_2 terminal end of proinsulin.[67] Information concerning gene expression to give preproinsulin and proinsulin has been reviewed.[67,68,85]

Glucagon Biosynthesis

The primary structure of porcine glucagon has been known for some time.[69] Its structure is the same in many other species, such as cow, rat, rabbit, and man. Structural differences in animals have been reviewed.[62]

At present, only fragmented information is available on the biosynthesis of glucagon, within the A cell. Trager et al.[67] summarized their work on isolating proglucagon. It appears that a sequence of proteolytic degradations similar to those for insulin in the B cell exists in the A cell. Recent studies indicate that the biosynthesis of glucagon has a pattern similar to that of insulin.[70-74]

Biosynthesis of glucagon has also been shown to take place in the intestine[67] and the salivary glands.[75]

Somatostatin Biosynthesis

Somatostatin is a 14 amino acid polypeptide, originally isolated from bovine hypothalamus.[76,77] Later this hormone was found in the D cells of pancreatic islets (see previous section) as well as in many other tissues.[39,78]

Like insulin and glucagon, biosynthesis of somatostatin takes place in islet cells through a degradation of larger peptides. Evidence supports the concept of a prosomatostatin, which is contained in the D cell of the islets and which acts as precursor of somatostatin.

FACTORS INVOLVED IN HORMONE RELEASE FROM VARIOUS CELL TYPES WITHIN THE ISLET

The biochemistry of the role which glucose plays in stimulating the release of insulin is well defined. More recently, the relationships which exist among insulin, glucagon and somatostatin, and the factors which control the release of these hormones, have been elucidated. Many factors, including extrapancreatic hormones, e.g., the catecholamines, various drugs, and also dietary substances, are known to inhibit or stimulate the release of the pancreatic hormones, with resulting effects upon glucose homeostasis.

Glucose and Somatostatin

Since glucose is a primary energy source, a constancy of this sugar must be maintained in the blood delivery system despite a variable dietary intake. Thus, a high level of glucose appearing in the blood will stimulate release of insulin from the B cells, eventuating in glucose burning or storage.

Insulin facilitates membrane permeability of various cells to glucose and permits each cell so penetrated to utilize the sugar for energy. If blood glucose levels fall below normal, release of glucagon from A cells is triggered, which then catabolizes glycogen stores to release more glucose. Thus, insulin can act as a delayed stimulator of glucagon and vice versa.[84]

Somatostatin inhibits the release of both insulin and glucagon, even in the presence of glucose stimulation.[79] Somatostatin has been shown to exhibit a 20 times greater inhibitor effect on glucagon than does insulin.[80]

The action of somatostatin on A and B cells is not fully understood. Adrenergic blockade does not prevent somatostatin-induced inhibition of insulin release.[81] This suggests that insulin release may not be mediated by the autonomic nervous system. A possible mechanism is proposed by Gerich and coworkers[80] to the effect that somatostatin modifies cAMP dependent systems rather than altering cAMP levels. This view is based on the fact that somatostatin inhibits glucagon response to isoproterenol (an activator of adenylate cyclase) and theophylline (an elevator of intracellulor cAMP).

Catecholamines

The islets have numerous nerve endings, which indicates that they are under the control of the autonomic nervous system. To demonstrate whether A, B, and D cells are under the control of the autonomic system, Samols et al.[82] used a gut-free perfused canine pancreas and determined the effect of various autonomic agonist and antagonist drugs on insulin, glucagon, and somatostatin release. Insulin and glucagon were stimulated in a manner analogous to a high or low glucose perfusate, respectively, when challenged with a β-agonist; somatostatin was moderately stimulated. Use of the β-blocker propanolol abolished the β-agonist stimulation. Experiments with epinephrine, an α-adrenergic agonist (in the presence of a β-blocker), produced a potent inhibition of insulin release, but a lesser degree of somatostatin release. This suggests that D cells have fewer α-receptors than do B cells. The effect on A cells is not clear in this work.[82,83] Acetylcholine in these experiments induced marked stimulation of insulin and mild inhibition of somatostatin. Thus, autonomic control of B cells is demonstrated, but a similar control of A and D cells needs clarification.

Drugs

Many drugs are potent stimulators of insulin. Common examples are tolbutamide (and other oral hypoglycemic agents), colchicine, and theophylline. Presumably, these drugs exert some effect on the B cells. At present very little is known about the effect which most drugs have on insulin, glucagon, and somatostatin release. With the present availability of radioimmunoassay techniques for insulin, glucagon, and somatostatin, fertile ground for research exists.

REFERENCES

1. **Pronina, T. S. and Sapronova, A. Y.,** Development of the function of endocrine pancreas in the human foetus, in *The Evolution of Pancreatic Islets,* Grillo, T. A., Leibson, L., and Epple, A., Eds., Pergamon Press, New York, 1976, 25.
2. **Fujimoto, W. Y. and Williams, L. H.,** Insulin release from cultured fetal human pancreas, *Endocrinology,* 91, 1133, 1972.
3. **Kaplan, S. L., Grumbach, M. M., and Shepard, T. H.,** The ontogenesis of human fetal hormone. Growth hormone and insulin, *J. Clin. Invest.,* 12, 3080, 1973.
4. **Milner, R. D., Ashoworth, M. A., and Barson, A. J.,** Insulin release from human foetal pancreas in response to glucose, leucine, and arginine, *J. Endocrinol.,* 52, 497, 1972.
5. **Wellman, K. F., Volk, B. W., and Brancato, P.,** Ultrastructure and insulin content of the endocrine pancreas in the human fetus, *Lab. Invest.,* 25, 97, 1971.
6. **Berman, L. G., Prior, J. T., Abramow, S. M., and Ziegler, D. D.,** A study of the pancreatic duct system in man by the use of vinyl acetate cast of postmortem preparations, *Surg. Gynecol. Obstet.,* 110, 391, 1960.
7. **Kleitsh, W. P.,** Anatomy of the pancreas: a study with special reference to the duct system, *Arch. Surg.,* 71, 795, 1955.
8. **Lytle, W. J.,** The common bile duct groove in the pancreas, *Br. J. Surg.,* 48, 209, 1959.
9. **Pelletier, G. and Leclerc, R.,** Immunohistochemical localization of human pancreatic polypeptide (HPP) in the human endocrine pancreas, *Gasteroenterology,* 72, 569, 1977.
10. **Larsson, K. I., Sundler, F., and Hakansson, R.,** Immunohistochemical localization of human pancreatic polypeptide (HPP) to a population of islet cells, *Cell Tiss. Res.,* 156, 167, 1975.
11. **Epple, A. and Lewis, T. L.,** Comparative histophysiology of the pancreatic islets, *Am. Zool.,* 13, 567, 1973.
12. **Carpenter, A. -M. and Lazarow, A.,** Effects of hyper- and hypoglycemia on beta cell degranulation and glycogen infiltration in normal, subdiabetic and diabetic rats, *Diabetes,* 16, 493, 1967.
13. **Dean, P. M.,** Ultrastructural morphometry of the pancreatic beta cell, *Diabetologia,* 9, 115, 1973.
14. **Hellman, B.,** The total volume of the pancreatic tissue at different ages in the rat, *Acta Pathol. Microbiol. Scand.,* 47, 35, 1959.
15. **Hedeskov, C. J.,** Mechanism of glucose-induced insulin secretion, *Physiol. Rev.,* 60, 442, 1980.
16. **Hellman, B.,** Studies in obese-hyperglycemic mice, *Ann. New York Acad. Sci.,* 131, 541, 1965.
17. **Erlandsen, S. L., Hegre, O. D., Parsons, J. A., McEvoy, R. C., and Elde, R. P.,** Pancreatic islet cell hormones: distribution of cell types in the islet and evidence for the presence of somatostatin and gastrin within the D cell, *J. Histochem. Cytochem.,* 24, 883, 1976.
18. **Hellman, B. and Taljedal, I-B.,** Histochemistry of the pancreatic islet cells, in *Handbook of Physiology, Section 7,* Endocrinology, Steiner, D. F. and Freinkel, N., Eds., American Physiological Society, Washington, D.C., 1972, 91.
19. **Lazarow, A.** Cell types of the islets of Langerhans and the hormones they produce, *Diabetes,* 6, 222, 1957.
20. **Kito, H. and Hosoda, S.,** Triple staining for simultaneous visualization of cell types in islet of Langerhans of pancreas, *J. Histochem. Cytochem.,* 25, 1019, 1977.
21. **Orci, L.,** The microanatomy of the islets of Langerhans, *Metabolism,* 25, 1303, 1976.
22. **Unger, R. H., Raskin, P., Srikant, C. B., and Orci, L.,** Glucagon and the A cells, *Rec. Prog. Horm. Res.,* 33, 477, 1977.
23. **Baum, J., Simons, B. E., Jr., Unger, R. H., and Madison, L. L.,** Localization of glucagon in the alpha cells in the pancreatic islets by immunofluorescent technics, *Diabetes,* 11, 371, 1962.
24. **Bussolati, G., Capella, C., Vassallo, G., and Solcia, E.,** Histochemical and ultrastructural studies on pancreatic A cells. Evidence for glucagon and non-glucagon components of the granule, *Diabetologia,* 7, 181, 1971.
25. **Erlandsen, S. L., Parsons, J. A., Burke, J. P., Redick, J. A., Van Orden, D. E., and Van Orden, L. S.,** A modification of the unlabeled antibody enzyme method using heterologous antisera for the light microscopic and ultrastructural localization of insulin, glucagon, and growth hormone, *J. Histochem. Cytochem.,* 23, 666, 1975.

26. **Lange, R. H., Ali, S. S., Klein, C., and Trandaburu, T.**, Immunohistological demonstration of insulin and glucagon in islet tissue of reptiles, amphibians, and teleosts using epoxy-embedded material and antiporcine hormone sera, *Acta Histochem.*, 52, 71, 1975.
27. **Okada, N., Takaki, R., and Kitagawa, M.**, Histologic and immunofluorescent studies on the site of origin of glucagon in mammalian pancreas, *J. Histochem. Cytochem.*, 16, 405, 1968.
28. **Lacy, P. E. and Davies, J.**, Demonstration of insulin in mammalian pancreas by the fluorescent antibody method, *Stain Technol.*, 34, 85, 1959.
29. **Misugi, K., Howell, S. L., Greider, M. H., Lacy, P. E., and Sorenson, G. D.**, The pancreatic beta cell. Demonstration with peroxidase-labeled antibody technique, *Arch. Pathol.*, 89, 97, 1970.
30. **Dubois, P. M., Paulin, C., Assan, R., and Dubois, M. P.**, Evidence for immunoreactive somatostatin in the endocrine cells of human foetal pancreas, *Nature*, 26, 731, 1975.
31. **Dubois, M. P.**, Immunoreactive somatostatin is present in discrete cells of the endocrine pancreas, *Proc. Natl. Acad. Sci. U.S.A.*, 72, 1340, 1975.
32. **Goldsmith, P. C., Rose, J. C., Arimura, A., and Ganong, W. F.**, Ultrastructural localization of somatostatin in pancreatic islets of the rat, *Endocrinology*, 97, 1061, 1975.
33. **Hokfelt, T., Efendic, S., Hellerstrom, C., Johansson, O., Luft, R., and Arimura, A.**, Cellular localization of somatostatin in endocrine-like cells and neurons of the rat with special references to the A_1 cells of the pancreatic islets and to the hypothalamus, *Acta Endocrinol. (Kbh).*, (Suppl.) 200, 1975.
34. **Luft, R., Efendic, S., Hokfelt, T., Johansson, O., and Arimura, A.**, Immunohistochemical evidence for the localization of somatostatin-like immunoreactivity in a cell population of the pancreatic islets, *Med. Biol.*, 52, 428, 1974.
35. **Orci, L., Beretens, D., Dubois, M. P., and Rufener, C.**, Evidence for the D-cell of the pancreas secreting somatostatin, *Horm. Metab. Res.*, 7, 400, 1975.
36. **Pelletier, G., Leclerc, R., Arimura, A., and Schally, A. V.**, Immunohistochemical localization of somatostatin in the rat pancreas, *J. Histochem. Cytochem.*, 23, 699, 1975.
37. **Polak, J. M., Grimelius, L., Pearse, A. G. E., Bloom, S. R., and Arimura, A.**, Growth-hormone release-inhibiting hormone in gastrointestinal and pancreatic D-cells, *Lancet*, 1, 1220, 1975.
38. **Refener, C., Amherdt, M., Dubois, M. P., and Orci, L.**, Ultrastructural immunocytochemical localization of somatostatin in rat pancreatic monolayer culture, *J. Histochem. Cytochem.*, 23, 866, 1975.
39. **Efendic, S., Hokfelt, T., and Luft, R.**, Somatostatin, *Adv., Metab. Disord.*, 9, 367, 1978.
40. **Lacy, P. E. and Greider, M. H.**, Ultrastructural organization of mammalian pancreatic islets, *Handbo. Physiol.*, 1, 77, 1972.
41. **McNutt, N. S. and Weinstein, R. S.**, Membrane ultrastructure at mammalian intercellular junctions, *Prog. Biophys. Mol. Biol.*, 26, 45, 1973.
42. **Staehelin, L. A.**, Structure and function of intercellular junctions, *Int. Rev. Cytol.*, 39, 191, 1974.
43. **Orci, L., Malaisse-Lagae, F., Ravazzola, M., Rouiller, D., Renold, A. E., Perrelet, A., and Unger, R.**, A morphological basis for intercellular communication between α- and β-cells in the endocrine pancreas, *J. Clin. Invest.*, 56, 1066, 1975.
44. **Orci, L., Malaisse-Lagae, F., Amherdt, M., Ravazzola, M., Weisswange, A., Dobbs, R., Perrelet, A., and Unger, R.**, Cell contacts in human islets of Langerhans, *J. Clin. Endocrinol. Metab.*, 41, 841, 1975.
45. **Orci, L., Unger, R. H., and Renold, A. E.**, Structural basis for intercellular communications between cells of the islets of Langerhans, *Experientia*, 29, 777, 1973.
46. **Orci, L., Unger, R. H., and Renold, A. E.**, Structural coupling between pancreatic islet cells, *Experientia*, 29, 1015, 1973.
47. **Orci, L.**, A portrait of the pancreatic B-cell, *Diabetologia*, 10, 163, 1974.
48. **Lacy, P. E., Howell, S. L., Young, D. A., and Fink, C. J.**, New hypothesis of insulin secretion, *Nature*, 219, 1177, 1968.
49. **Orci, L., Stauffacher, W., Beaven, D., Lambert, A. E., Renold, A. E., and Rouiller, C.**, Ultrastructural events associated with the action of tolbutamide and glybenclamide on pancreatic B-cells in vivo and in vitro, *Acta Diabet. Lat.*, 6, 271, 1968.
50. **Bencosme, S. A. and Martinez-Palomo, A.**, Formation of secretory granules in pancreatic islet B cells of cortisone-treated rabbits, *Lab. Invest.*, 18, 746, 1968.
51. **Malaisse-Lagae, F., Greider, M. H., Malaisse, W. J., and Lacy, P. E.**, The stimulus-secretion coupling of glucose-induced insulin release. IV. The effect of vincristine and deuterium oxide on the microtubular system of the pancreatic beta cell, *J. Cell. Biol.*, 49, 530, 1971.
52. **Malaisse, W. J., Malaisse-Lange, F., Van Obberghen, E., Somers, G., Devis, G., Ravazzola, M., and Orci, L.**, Role of microtubules in the phasic pattern of insulin release, *Ann. New York Acad. Sci.*, 253, 630, 1975.
53. **Richins, C. A.**, The innervation of the pancreas, *J. Comp. Neurol.*, 83, 223, 1945.
54. **Tiscornia, O. M.**, The neural control of exocrine and endocrine pancreas, *Am. J. Gastroenterol.*, 67, 541, 1977.

55. **Simard, L. C.,** Les complexes neuro-insulaires du pancreas humain; (Neurocrinie et fonction paraganglionnaire), *Arch. Anat. Microsc.,* 33, 4, 1937.
56. **Woods, S.W. and Porte, D.,** Neural control of the endocrine pancreas, *Physiol. Rev.,* 54, 596, 1974.
57. **Orci, L. and Unger, R. H.,** Functional subdivision of islets of Langerhans and possible role of D cells, *Lancet,* 1, 1243, 1975.
58. **Forssmann, W. G. and Greenberg, J.,** Innervation of the endocrine pancreas in primates, in *Peripheral Neuroendocrine Interaction,* Coupland, R. E. and Forssmann, W. G., Eds., Springer-Verlag, Basel, 1978, 124.
59. **Oyer, P. E., Cho, S., Peterson, J. D.,and Steiner, D. F.,** Studies on human proinsulin. Isolation and amino acid sequence of the human pancreatic C-peptide, *J. Biol. Chem.,* 246, 1375, 1971.
60. **Permutt, M. A. and Kipnis, D. M.,** Insulin biosynthesis: studies of islet polyribosomes, *Proc. Natl. Acad. Sci. U.S.A.,* 69, 505, 1972.
61. **Sorenson, R. L., Steffes, W., and Lindall, A. W.,** Subcellular localization of proinsulin to insulin conversion in isolated rat islets, *Endocrinology,* 86, 88, 1970.
62. **Trager, H. S. and Steiner, D. F.,** Peptide hormones, *Ann. Rev. Biochem.,* 43, 509, 1974.
63. **Howell, S. L., Kostianovsky, M., and Lacy, P. E.,** Beta granule formation in isolated islets of Langerhans. A study by electron microscopic radioautography, *J. Cell. Biol.,* 42, 695, 1969.
64. **Kemmler, W. and Steiner, D. F.,** Conversion of proinsulin to insulin in a subcellular fraction from rat islets, *Biochem. Biophys. Res. Commun.,* 41, 1223, 1970.
65. **Kemmler, W., Peterson, J. D., and Steiner, D. F.,** Studies on the conversion of proinsulin to insulin. I. Conversion in vitro with trypsin and carboxypeptidase B, *J. Biol. Chem.,* 246, 6786, 1971.
66. **Kemmler, W., Steiner, D. F., and Borg, J.,** Studies on the conversion of proinsulin to insulin. III. Studies in vitro with a crude secretion granule fraction isolated from rat islets of Langerhans, *J. Biol. Chem.,* 248, 4544, 1973.
67. **Tager, H. S., Patzelt, C., Assoian, R. K., Chan, S. J., Duguid, J. R., and Steiner, D. F.,** Biosynthesis of islet cell hormones, *Ann. New York Acad. Sci.,* 343, 133, 1980.
68. **Steiner, D. F.,** Insulin today, *Diabetes,* 26, 322, 1977.
69. **Bromer, W. W., Sinn, L. G., and Behrens, O. K.,** *J. Am. Chem. Soc.,* 79, 2807, 1957.
70. **Patzelt, C.,** Identification and processing of proglucagon in pancreatic islets, *Nature,* 282, 260, 1979.
71. **Fujii, S.,** Development of pancreatic endocrine cells in the rat fetus, *Arch. Histol. (Japan),* 42, 467, 1979.
72. **Tullis, R. H., Gutierrez, R., and Rubin, H.,** Specific detection of human and rabbit glucagon mRNA using a synthetic oligodeoxynucleotide, *Biochem. Biophy. Res. Commun.,* 93, 941, 1980.
73. **Lund, P. K.,** Glucagon precursors identified by immunoprecipitation of products of cell-free translation of messenger RNA, *Diabetes,* 29, 583, 1980.
74. **Ostenson, C. G.,** Glucagon biosynthesis in isolated pancreatic islets of mice and guinea pigs, *Diabet. Metab.,* 6, 141, 1980.
75. **Perez-Castillo, A.,** Synthesis and release of glucagon by human salivary glands, *Diabetologia,* 19, 123, 1980.
76. **Brazeau, P., Vale, W., Burgus, R., Ling, N., Butcher, M., Rivier, J. and Guillemin, R.,** Hypothalamic polypeptide that inhibits the secretion of immunoreactive pituitary growth hormone, *Science,* 179, 77, 1973.
77. **Burgus, R., Ling, N., Butcher, M., and Guillemin, R.,** Primary structure of somatostatin, a hypothalamic peptide that inhibits the secretion of pituitary growth hormone, *Proc. Natl. Acad. Sci. U.S.A.,* 70, 684, 1973.
78. **Track, N. S., Creutzfeldt, C., Litzenberger, J., Neuhoff, C., Arnold, R., and Creutzfeldt, W.,** Appearance of gastrin and somatostatin in the human fetal stomach, duodenum and pancreas, *Digestion,* 19, 292, 1979.
79. **Gerich, J. E., Lorenzi, M., Schneider, V., and Forsham, P. H.,** Effect of somatostatin on plasma glucose and insulin responses to glucagon and tolbutamide in man, *J. Clin. Endocrinol. Metab.,* 39, 1057, 1974.
80. **Gerich, J. E., Lovinger, R., and Grodsky, G. M.,** Inhibition by somatostatin of glucagon and insulin release from the perfused rat pancreas in response to arginine, isoproterenol and theophylline: evidence for a preferential effect on glucagon secretion, *Endocrinology,* 96, 749, 1975.
81. **Efendic, S. and Luft, R.,** Studies on the mechanism of somatostatin action on insulin release in man. I. Effect of blockade of α-adrenergic receptors, *Acta Endocrinol.,* 78, 516, 1975.
82. **Iversen, J.,** Adrenergic receptors and the secretion of glucagon and insulin from the isolated, perfused canine pancreas, *J. Clin. Invest.,* 52, 2102, 1973.
83. **Gerich, J. E., Langlois, M., Noacco, C., Schneider, V., and Forsham, P. H.,** Adrenergic modulation of pancreatic glucagon secretion in man, *J. Clin. Invest.,* 53, 1441, 1974.
84. **Unger, R. H. and Dobbs, R. E.,** Insulin, glucagon and somatostatin secretion in the regulation of metabolism, *Ann. Rev. Physiol.,* 40, 307, 1978.
85. **Hedeskov, C. J.,** Mechanism of glucose-induced insulin secretion, *Physiol. Rev.,* 60, 442, 1980.

INDEX

A

B

C

D

E

F

G

H

I

K

L

N

O

P

R

S

T

U

V

W

Y

Z

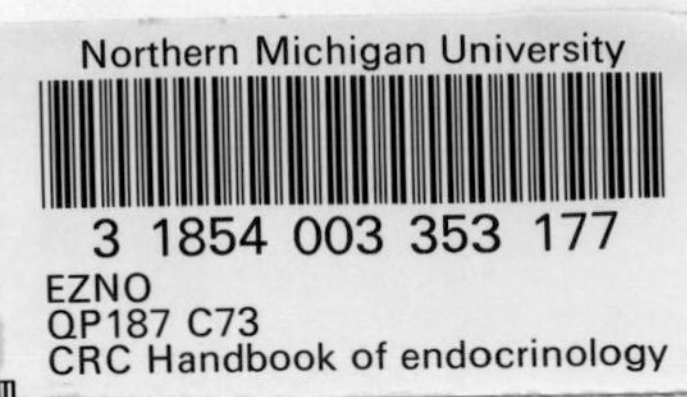